GRAY'S
Clinical
Neuroanatomy
The Anatomic Basis for Clinical Neuroscience

GRAY'S
Clinical
Neuroanatomy
The Anatomic Basis for Clinical Neuroscience

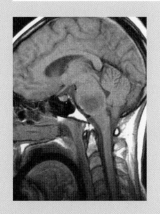

Editor

Elliott L. Mancall, MD
Emeritus Professor of Neurology
Department of Neurology
Thomas Jefferson University
Jefferson Medical College
Philadelphia, Pennsylvania

Associate Editor

David G. Brock, MD, CIP
Medical Director
Neuronetics, Inc.
Malvern, Pennsylvania

Excerpts from *Gray's Anatomy*
Susan Standring, Editor-in-Chief
Alan Crossman, Section Editor

ELSEVIER
SAUNDERS

1600 John F. Kennedy Blvd.
Ste 1800
Philadelphia, PA 19103-2899

GRAY'S CLINICAL NEUROANATOMY: THE ANATOMIC BASIS FOR CLINICAL
NEUROSCIENCE   ISBN: 978-1-4160-4705-6

Notices

Knowledge and best practice in this field are constantly changing. As new research and experience
broaden our understanding, changes in research methods, professional practices, or medical treatment
may become necessary.

Practitioners and researchers must always rely on their own experience and knowledge in evaluating
and using any information, methods, compounds, or experiments described herein. In using such
information or methods, they should be mindful of their own safety and the safety of others, including
parties for whom they have a professional responsibility.

With respect to any drug or pharmaceutical products identified, readers are advised to check the most
current information provided (i) on procedures featured or (ii) by the manufacturer of each product to be
administered to verify the recommended dose or formula, the method and duration of administration,
and contraindications. It is the responsibility of practitioners, relying on their own experience and
knowledge of their patients, to make diagnoses, to determine dosages and the best treatment for each
individual patient, and to take all appropriate safety precautions.

To the fullest extent of the law, neither the Publisher nor the authors, contributors, or editors assume
any liability for any injury and/or damage to persons or property as a matter of products liability,
negligence or otherwise, or from any use or operation of any methods, products, instructions, or ideas
contained in the material herein.

International Standard Book Number 978-1-4160-4705-6

Acquisitions Editor: Madelene Hyde
Developmental Editor: Christine Abshire
Publishing Services Manager: Anne Altepeter
Team Leader: Radhika Pallamparthy
Senior Project Manager: Cheryl A. Abbott
Project Manager: Vijay Vincent
Design Direction: Steven Stave

Printed in China

Last digit is the print number: 9 8 7 6 5 4 3 2 1

Dedication
To our wives, J.C.M. and C.A.S.—thank you for your support.
Elliott L. Mancall
David G. Brock

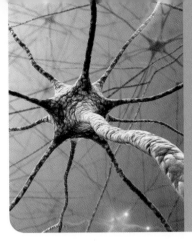

Contributors

Michael W. Devereaux, MD
Professor of Neurology
Department of Neurology
Case Western Reserve School of Medicine;
Staff Neurologist
Case Medical Center
Cleveland, Ohio

Karl Doghramji, MD
Professor of Psychiatry and Human Behavior, Neurology, and Medicine
Program Director, Fellowship in Sleep Medicine
Thomas Jefferson University;
Medical Director, Jefferson Sleep Disorders Center
Thomas Jefferson University Hospital
Philadelphia, Pennsylvania

Keith Dombrowski, MD
Fellow, Neurocritical Care
Department of Medicine, Division of Neurology
Duke University Medical Center
Durham, North Carolina

Laurie Gutmann, MD
Professor
Neurology and Exercise Physiology
West Virginia University School of Medicine;
Professor/CNP Fellowship Program Director
Neurology
Ruby Memorial Hospital
Morgantown, West Virginia

John Khoury, MD
Fellow in Sleep Medicine
Thomas Jefferson University Hospital
Philadelphia, Pennsylvania

Daniel Kremens, MD, JD
Assistant Professor of Neurology
Thomas Jefferson University Hospital
Philadelphia, Pennsylvania

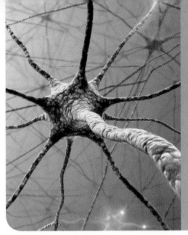

Preface

Gray's Anatomy has been a cornerstone of medical education since its original appearance in 1858. It has provided a remarkably authoritative description of both gross and microscopic anatomy of the human body for many generations of medical students and practicing medical scientists on a worldwide basis. It has been, and remains, cherished not only as a primary source of anatomical knowledge but also as a reliable resource to which the student or practitioner might return for many years, indeed, throughout the entire length of a medical career. Although the classical text is regularly updated, recent major developments in both basic and clinical medicine have prompted a major reconsideration of the utility of a single large volume devoted to all of human anatomy. Concerns are especially related to the increasing specialization, if not frank fragmentation, of the medical arts with which the contemporary physician must deal on a day-to-day basis. As a consequence of such a reappraisal, a decision has been made to extract focused portions of the major text devoted to specific conceptual domains. *Gray's Anatomy* itself will remain as authoritative as ever but will be expanded by the inclusion of clinical case material to illustrate in depth, whenever possible, the application of anatomical principles to the bedside. The field of neuroanatomy lends itself particularly well to such a departure from the more traditional approach to human anatomy, with the original *Gray's* material being utilized as the foundation for such an enhanced pedagogical approach. In *Gray's Clinical Neuroanatomy,* virtually all the original neuroanatomical text in the thirty-ninth edition is preserved, although it is transposed and rearranged to meet innovative structural guidelines and is complemented by a host of clinical case vignettes, which in turn are augmented by visual materials designed to strengthen the link between the clinic and the dissecting room. It must be emphasized that there has been no attempt to develop yet another comprehensive textbook of neurology as such; the neurological disorders cited here are entirely exemplary and directly relevant to the underlying anatomical principles of the traditional *Gray's.*

Organizationally, *Gray's Clinical Neuroanatomy* begins with a selection of general, non-systematized topics that lack a specific regional approach—for example, the general vasculature of the brain and spinal cord, the ventricular system and the meninges, as well as the general microstructure of the nervous system. A detailed review of neuroembryology and development is also provided; the extraordinary length here reflects the perceived need for in-depth coverage of these topics, which is not available elsewhere. Following these introductory topics, the remaining sections are devoted to the systematized gross and microscopic anatomy of the central and peripheral nervous systems, considered on a regional and clinically pertinent basis, with direct relevance to the bedside and the clinic and thus with direct applicability to the clinician treating a patient with a neurological disease.

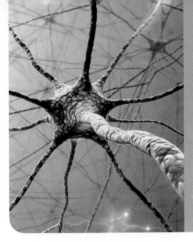

Acknowledgments

Dr. David Brock accepted the role of Associate Editor without hesitation and has played a major role not only in refining the clinical parameters of this new *Gray's* but also in resolving a number of technical issues inherent in a departure of this sort. This project would never have developed as it did without the input of the other major clinical contributors, Drs. Michael Devereaux and Laurie Gutmann, who took time away from their busy academic and clinical lives to provide the clinical and supplemental illustrative material so vital to this effort. Drs. Keith Dombrowski and Karl Doghramji contributed additional clinical material for inclusion, and Drs. Daniel Kremens and John Khoury reviewed manuscript and provided clinical images for which we are grateful. Finally, I would be remiss if I did not cite those who contributed so successfully to the parent *Gray's Anatomy*, the remarkable work from which *Gray's Clinical Neuroanatomy* is derived.

Special thanks go to the members of the Elsevier community: Susan Pioli, who in a very real sense was vital to the initiation of this project, and Madelene Hyde, Christine Abshire and Cheryl Abbott, who managed to keep us on track and guided us through the intricacies of the contemporary publishing world. Last, Valerie Cabrera handled the secretarial tasks so essential to a project of this sort.

Elliott L. Mancall, MD

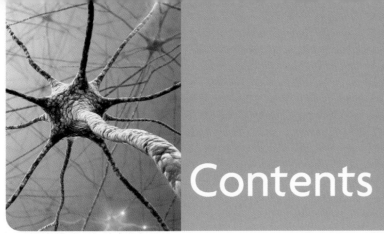

Contents

Section I

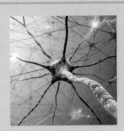

General

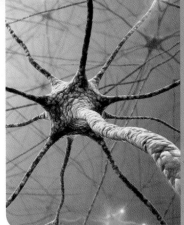

Overview of the Organization of the Nervous System

The human nervous system is the most complex product of biological evolution. The constantly changing patterns of activity of its billions of interactive units represent the fundamental physical basis of every aspect of human behaviour and experience. Many thousands of scientists and clinicians around the world, whether driven by intellectual curiosity or the quest for better methods of disease prevention and treatment, have studied the nervous system over many years. However, our understanding of complex neural organization and function is still quite rudimentary, as is our ability to deal with its many pathologies. Multidisciplinary research into the nervous system is one of the most active areas of contemporary biology and medicine, and rapid advances across a range of fronts bring the realistic prospect of better prevention and treatment of many neurological disorders in the future.

The functional capabilities of the nervous system are a product of its vast population of intercommunicating nerve cells, or neurones, estimated to number on the order of 10^{10}. Neurones encode information, conduct it, sometimes over considerable distances, and then transmit it to other neurones or to non-neural tissues (muscles or glandular cells). Most neurones consist of a central mass of cytoplasm within a limiting cell membrane (the cell body or soma) from which a number of branched processes, termed neurites, extend (Fig. 1.1). One of these, the axon, is usually much longer than the others and normally conducts information away from the cell body. The other processes are termed dendrites, and these typically conduct information toward the soma. The nerve cell membrane is polarized, the inside of the cell being around 70 mV negative with respect to the outside. Information is coded in the form of patterns of transient depolarizations and repolarizations of this membrane potential, known as nerve impulses or action potentials. These are conducted along the axon, which may have collateral branches that permit information to be distributed simultaneously to several targets (Fig. 1.2). Axons possess specialized endings, or axon terminals, that come into close apposition with the membrane of the target cell at synapses, where information passes from one cell to another. Axon terminals may form synaptic contacts with dendrites (axodendritic), cell bodies (axosomatic), other axons (axoaxonic) or non-neural tissue such as muscle cells (neuromuscular junction). Transmission of information to other cells is brought about when action potentials cause the release of specific neurotransmitter substances stored in synaptic vesicles within the presynaptic nerve terminal. Specialized receptors are located on the postsynaptic target cell membrane. The neurotransmitter binds to these and, depending on the nature of the chemical and the receptor, either elicits an excitatory (depolarizing) or inhibitory (hyperpolarizing) response or modulates intracellular second messenger systems.

The huge complexity of the nervous system reflects the fact that individual neurones may make synaptic contact with hundreds or even thousands of other neurones via profuse axonal and dendritic branching (arborization). This is exemplified by the extensive dendritic field of the cerebellar Purkinje cell, which is traversed by thousands of axons, each of which makes synaptic contact as it passes. At the level of the individual neurone, competing incoming excitatory and inhibitory synaptic potentials are summated in time (temporal summation) and between synapses (spatial summation). If the postsynaptic neurone is depolarized above a certain threshold, it fires action potentials that are conducted along the axon to the next target cells.

The nervous system contains far more supporting cells (neuroglia) than neurones. Glia are responsible for creating and maintaining an appropriate environment in which the neurones can operate efficiently; they are not electrically excitable in the same way as neurones.

The nervous system consists of three basic functional types of neurone: afferent (sensory), efferent (motor) and interneurones. At the simplest level of interpretation, they allow the nervous system to detect changes in the internal and external environments and to respond appropriately. The sensory elements are able to detect a wide range of stimuli and subserve the general senses (touch, pressure, temperature, etc.) and the special senses (vision, hearing, smell, taste, vestibular sensation). Motor neurones send axons from the central nervous system to effector organs, chiefly muscles and glands.

Neurones that are confined to the central nervous system and that possess neither sensory nor motor terminals are called interneurones. They greatly outnumber sensory and motor neurones and confer on the nervous system its prodigious capacity to analyse, integrate and store information.

The nervous system is customarily divided into two major parts: the central nervous system (CNS) and the peripheral nervous system (PNS). The CNS consists of the brain and spinal cord. The PNS is composed of cranial nerves and spinal nerves together with their ramifications and certain groupings of cell bodies that constitute the peripheral ganglia. Another convention divides the nervous system into somatic and autonomic components. Anatomically, both of these have elements in the CNS and PNS. The autonomic nervous system, which consists of sympathetic and parasympathetic divisions, is made up of neurones concerned primarily with control of the internal environment through innervation of secretory glands and cardiac and smooth muscle. It is considered in detail in Chapter 21. The wall of the gastrointestinal tract contains neurones capable of sustaining local reflex activity independent of the CNS, which are known as the enteric nervous system.

CENTRAL NERVOUS SYSTEM

The brain and spinal cord (Fig. 1.3) contain the great majority of neuronal cell bodies in the nervous system. In many parts of the CNS the cell bodies of neurones are grouped together and are more or less segregated from axons. The generic term for such collections of cell bodies is grey matter. Smaller aggregations of neuronal cell bodies, which usually share a common functional role, are termed nuclei. It follows that neuronal dendrites and synaptic interactions are mostly confined to grey matter. Axons tend to be grouped together to form white matter, so called because axons are often ensheathed in myelin, which confers a paler colouration. Axons that pass between similar sources or destinations within the CNS tend to run together in defined pathways or tracts. These often cross the midline (decussate), which means that half of the body is, in many respects, controlled by and sends information to the opposite side of the brain.

Some groups of neurones in the spinal cord and brain stem that subserve similar functions are organized into longitudinal columns. The neurones in these columns may be concentrated into discrete, discontinuous nuclei in some areas, such as the cranial nerve nuclei of the brain stem, or they may form more or less continuous longitudinal bands, as in much of the spinal cord (Fig. 1.4). Efferent neurones constitute three such columns. The somatic motor column contains motor neurones, the axons of which serve muscles derived from head somites. The two other columns are related to specialized features of head morphology. Of these, the branchial motor column innervates muscles derived from the wall of the embryonic pharynx (branchial muscles), and the visceral motor column supplies preganglionic parasympathetic fibres to glands and visceral smooth muscle. There are four longitudinal cell columns related to sensory functions. The general somatic sensory column essentially deals with information from the head. Special somatic sensory neurones are related to the special senses and receive vestibular and auditory input. General visceral sensory neurones deal with information from widespread and varied visceral sensory endings, and special visceral sensory neurones are related to the special sense of taste.

The brain and spinal cord receive information from, and send it to, the rest of the body through cranial and spinal nerves, respectively. These contain afferent fibres carrying information from sensory receptors and efferent fibres running to effector organs. Through inherent connections of varying complexity between afferent and efferent components of spinal and cranial nerves, the spinal cord and brain stem have the innate capacity to control many aspects of body function and respond to external and internal stimuli by reflex action. Such functions are under the modulatory influence of rich descending connections from the brain. In addition, afferent input to the spinal cord and brain stem is channelled into various ascending pathways, some of which eventually impinge on the cerebral cortex, conferring conscious awareness.

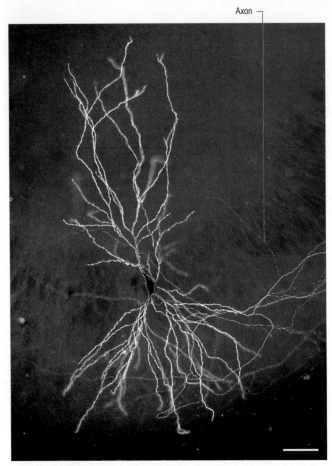

Fig. 1.1 *Dark-field illuminated micrograph of a CA3 pyramidal cell in a hippocampal slice culture, intracellularly injected with the dye biocytin. Scale bar 50 μm. (Courtesy of R. Anne McKinney, McGill University, and Mathias Abegg, Brain Research Institute, University of Zurich.)*

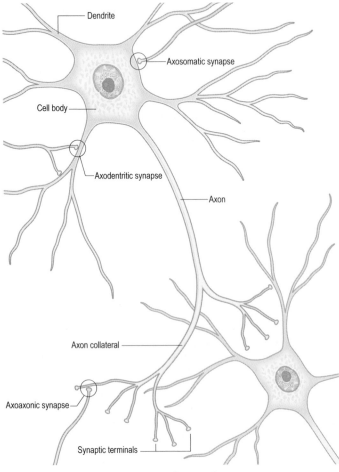

Fig. 1.2 *Structure of a typical neurone.*

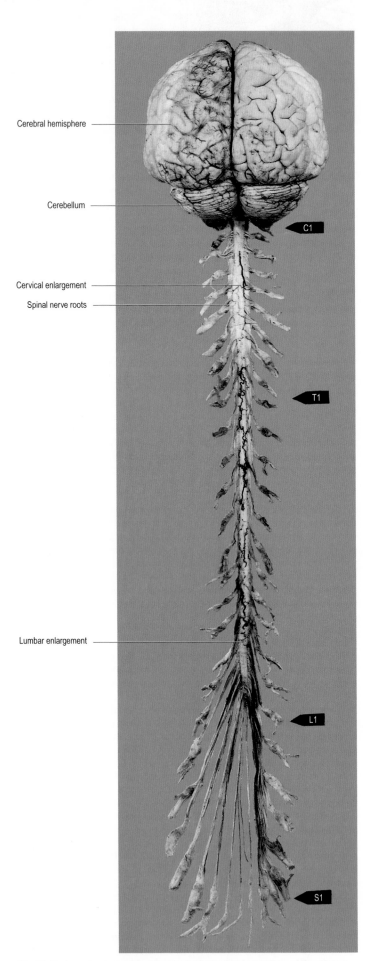

Fig. 1.3 *Brain and spinal cord with attached spinal nerve roots and dorsal root ganglia, photographed from the dorsal aspect. (Photograph by Kevin Fitzpatrick on behalf of GKT School of Medicine, London.)*

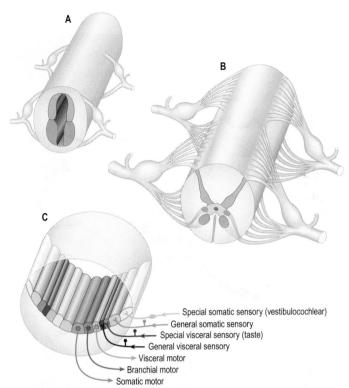

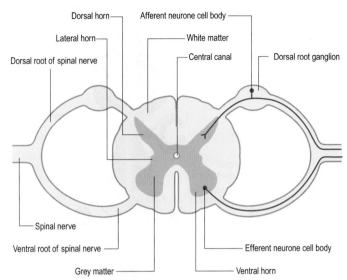

Fig. 1.5 *Transverse section through the spinal cord illustrating the disposition of grey and white matter and the attachment of dorsal and ventral spinal nerve roots.*

Fig. 1.4 *Arrangement of sensory and motor cell columns in the spinal cord and brain stem. A, Organization of the primitive spinal cord with a dorsal sensory column (blue), a ventral column (red) and segmentally arranged dorsal and ventral nerve roots. B, Arrangement of adult spinal cord serving the thorax, with sensory and somatic motor columns colour-coded in the same way as in A, with an additional intermediate (lateral) visceral motor column (orange). C, Arrangement of multiple longitudinal columns in the brain stem, where the motor column is now subdivided into three parts and the sensory column into four. For further information about the embryological aspects of the early nervous system, consult Chapter 3. See also Fig. 10.1.*

To sustain the energy required by constant neuronal activity, the CNS has a high metabolic rate and a rich blood supply. The blood–brain barrier controls the neuronal environment and imposes severe restrictions on the types of substances that can pass from the blood stream into nervous tissue.

Spinal Cord

The spinal cord is located within the vertebral column, lying in the upper two-thirds of the vertebral canal (Ch. 8). It is continuous rostrally with the medulla oblongata. For the most part, the spinal cord controls the functions of, and receives afferent input from, the trunk and limbs. Afferent and efferent connections travel in 31 pairs of segmentally arranged spinal nerves. These attach to the cord as dorsal and ventral rootlets that unite to form the spinal nerves proper (Fig. 1.5). The dorsal and ventral roots are functionally distinct. Dorsal roots carry primary afferent nerve fibres from cell bodies located in dorsal root ganglia. Ventral roots carry efferent fibres from cell bodies located in the spinal grey matter.

Internally, the spinal cord is differentiated into a central core of grey matter surrounded by white matter. The grey matter is configured in a characteristic H, or butterfly, shape that has projections known as dorsal and ventral horns (Fig. 1.6). In general, neurones situated in the dorsal horn are primarily concerned with sensory functions, and those in the ventral horn are mostly associated with motor activities. At certain levels of the spinal cord a small lateral horn is also present, marking the location of the cell bodies of preganglionic sympathetic neurones. The central canal, which is a vestigial component of the ventricular system, lies at the centre of the spinal grey matter and runs the length of the cord. The white matter of the spinal cord consists of ascending and descending axons that link spinal cord segments to one another and link the spinal cord to the brain.

Brain

The brain (encephalon) lies within the cranium. It receives information from, and controls the activities of, the trunk and limbs, mainly through rich connections with the spinal cord. It possesses 12 pairs of cranial nerves through which it communicates mostly with structures of the head and neck. The brain is divided into major regions on the basis of ontogenetic growth in individuals and phylogenetic principles (Figs. 1.7–1.9; see also

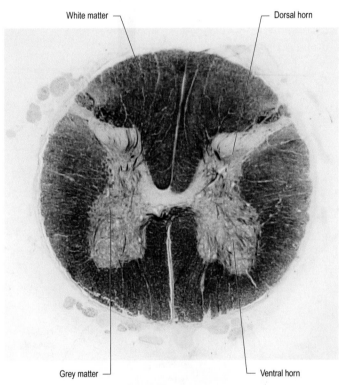

Fig. 1.6 *Transverse section through the human spinal cord at the lumbar level, stained to demonstrate myelinated nerve fibres in the white matter (blue-black). Grey matter remains relatively unstained. (Figure enhanced by B. Crossman.)*

Fig. 6.8). Ascending in sequence from the spinal cord, the principal divisions are the rhombencephalon or hindbrain, the mesencephalon or midbrain and the prosencephalon or forebrain.

The rhombencephalon is subdivided into the myelencephalon or medulla oblongata, the metencephalon or pons and the cerebellum. The medulla oblongata, pons and midbrain are collectively referred to as the brain stem, which lies on the basal portions of the occipital and sphenoid bones (clivus). The medulla oblongata is the most caudal part of the brain stem and is continuous with the spinal cord below the level of the foramen magnum. The pons lies rostral to the medulla and is distinguished by a mass of transverse nerve fibres that connect it to the cerebellum. The midbrain is a short segment of brain stem, rostral to the pons. The cerebellum consists of paired hemispheres united by a median vermis; it lies within the posterior cranial fossa, dorsal to the pons, medulla and caudal midbrain, areas with which it has rich fibre connections.

The prosencephalon may be subdivided into the diencephalon and the telencephalon. The diencephalon comprises mostly the thalamus and

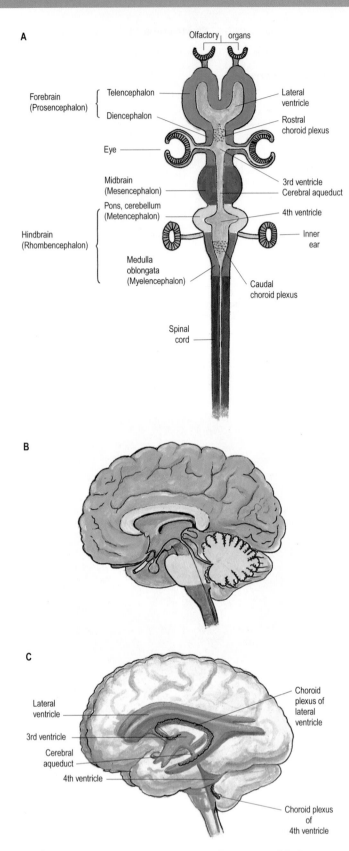

A

Olfactory organs

Forebrain (Prosencephalon)
- Telencephalon
- Diencephalon

Eye

Midbrain (Mesencephalon)

Pons, cerebellum (Metencephalon)

Hindbrain (Rhombencephalon)

Medulla oblongata (Myelencephalon)

Spinal cord

Lateral ventricle

Rostral choroid plexus

3rd ventricle
Cerebral aqueduct

4th ventricle

Inner ear

Caudal choroid plexus

B

C

Lateral ventricle

3rd ventricle

Cerebral aqueduct

4th ventricle

Choroid plexus of lateral ventricle

Choroid plexus of 4th ventricle

Fig. 1.7 *Nomenclature and arrangement of the different areas of the brain.* **A,** *Major features of the basic brain plan, including the relationship of its parts to the major special sensory organs of the head.* **B,** *Arrangement of the same regions in the adult brain, seen in sagittal section.* **C,** *Organization of the ventricular system in the brain.*

hypothalamus but also includes the smaller epithalamus and subthalamus. The telencephalon is composed mainly of the two cerebral hemispheres or cerebrum. The diencephalon is almost completely embedded in the cerebrum and is therefore largely hidden. The cerebrum constitutes the major portion of the volume of the human brain. It occupies the anterior and middle cranial fossae and is directly related to the cranial vault. It consists of two cerebral hemispheres. The surface of each hemisphere is convoluted in a complex

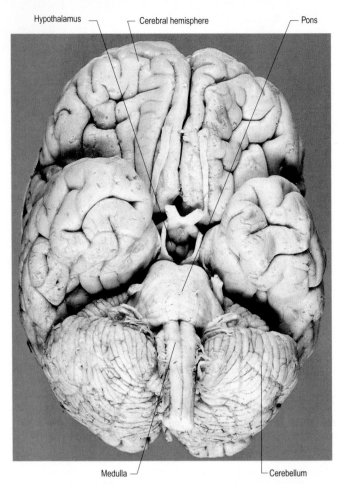

Hypothalamus — Cerebral hemisphere — Pons

Medulla — — Cerebellum

Fig. 1.8 *Base of the brain. The midbrain, lying between the pons and the hypothalamus, cannot be seen in this photograph. (Photograph by Kevin Fitzpatrick on behalf of GKT School of Medicine, London.)*

pattern of ridges (gyri) and furrows (sulci). Internally, each hemisphere has an external layer of grey matter, called the cerebral cortex, beneath which lies a dense mass of white matter (Fig. 1.10). One of the most important components of the cerebral white matter is the internal capsule, which contains nerve fibres that pass to and from the cerebral cortex. Several large nuclei of grey matter, usually referred to as the basal ganglia, are partly embedded in the subcortical white matter. Connections between corresponding areas of the two sides of the brain cross the midline within commissures. By far the largest commissure is the corpus callosum, which links the two cerebral hemispheres.

During prenatal development, the walls of the neural tube thicken greatly but never completely obliterate the central lumen. Although the latter remains in the spinal cord as the narrow central canal, it becomes greatly expanded in the brain to form a series of interconnected cavities called the ventricular system. In two regions, the forebrain and the hindbrain, parts of the neural tube roof do not generate nerve cells but become thin, folded sheets of highly vascular secretory tissue, the choroid plexuses. These secrete cerebrospinal fluid, which fills the ventricles. The cavity of the rhombencephalon becomes expanded to form the fourth ventricle, which lies dorsal to the pons and upper half of the medulla. Caudally, the fourth ventricle is continuous with a canal in the caudal medulla and, through this, with the spinal central canal. At its rostral extent, the fourth ventricle is continuous with a narrow channel, the cerebral aqueduct, which passes through the midbrain. The rostral end of the cerebral aqueduct opens out into the median third ventricle, a narrow slit-like cavity bounded laterally by the diencephalon. At the rostral end of the third ventricle, a small aperture (foramen of Monro) on each side leads into the large lateral ventricle located within each cerebral hemisphere.

Overview of Ascending Sensory Pathways

Sensory modalities are conventionally described as either special senses or general senses. The special senses are olfaction, vision, taste, hearing and vestibular function. Afferent information is encoded by highly specialized sense organs and transmitted to the brain in certain cranial nerves (I, II, VII, VIII and IX). The special senses are described in Chapter 12.

Thalamus — ⌐ Hypothalamus

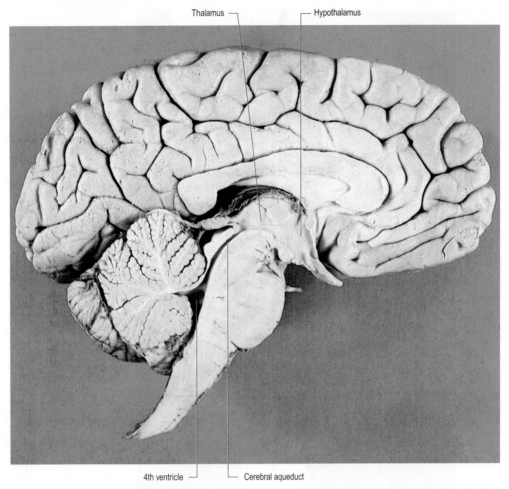

4th ventricle — └ Cerebral aqueduct

Fig. 1.9 *Sagittal section of the brain. (Photograph by Kevin Fitzpatrick on behalf of GKT School of Medicine, London.)*

The general senses include touch, pressure, vibration, pain, thermal sensation and proprioception (perception of posture and movement). Stimuli from the external and internal environments activate a diverse range of receptors in the skin, viscera, muscles, tendons and joints. Afferent impulses from the trunk and limbs are conveyed to the spinal cord in spinal nerves, and those from the head are carried to the brain in cranial nerves. The detailed anatomy of the complex pathways by which the various general senses impinge on conscious levels is better understood with reference to certain overall organizational principles. Although undoubtedly oversimplified and subject to many exceptions, this schema is helpful in emphasizing the essential similarities between the ascending sensory systems.

In essence, ascending sensory projections related to the general senses consist of a sequence of three neurones extending from the peripheral receptor to the contralateral cerebral cortex (Fig. 1.11). These are often referred to as primary, secondary and tertiary sensory (afferent) neurones or first-, second- and third-order neurones, respectively. Primary afferents have peripherally located sensory endings, and their cell bodies lie in dorsal root ganglia or the ganglia associated with certain cranial nerves. Their axons enter the CNS through ipsilateral spinal or trigeminal nerves. Within the CNS they terminate ipsilateral to their side of entry, on the cell bodies of second-order neurones. The precise location of this termination depends on the modality.

Primary afferent fibres carrying pain, temperature and coarse touch or pressure information from the trunk and limbs terminate in the dorsal horn of the spinal grey matter, near their point of entry into the spinal cord. Homologous fibres from the head terminate in the trigeminal sensory nucleus of the brain stem. The cell bodies of second-order neurones are located in the dorsal horn and trigeminal sensory nucleus. Their axons decussate and ascend to the thalamus. The ascending second-order axons from the spinal cord form the spinothalamic tract. Those from the trigeminal sensory nucleus constitute the trigeminothalamic tract.

Primary afferent fibres carrying proprioceptive information and fine (discriminative) touch from the trunk and limbs ascend ipsilaterally in the spinal cord without synapse. The ascending fibres constitute the dorsal columns (fasciculus gracilis and fasciculus cuneatus). They end in the dorsal column nuclei (nucleus gracilis and nucleus cuneatus) of the medulla. The

dorsal column nuclei contain the cell bodies of second-order neurones. Their axons decussate in the medulla and then ascend as the medial lemniscus. Similarly, a homologous projection exists for afferents derived from the head.

Within the thalamus, ascending second-order sensory neurones terminate in the ventral posterior nucleus, making synaptic contact with the cell bodies of third-order neurones. The axons of third-order neurones pass through the internal capsule to reach the cerebral cortex, where they terminate in the postcentral gyrus of the parietal lobe, also known as the primary somatosensory cortex.

Overview of Descending Motor Pathways

The concept of upper and lower motor neurones is fundamental to the clinical description of the effects of lesions of the motor system. The term 'lower motor neurones' refers to the alpha motor neurones that innervate the extrafusal muscle fibres of skeletal muscle. The term 'upper motor neurones' in theory refers collectively to all the descending pathways that impinge on the activity of lower motor neurones. In common parlance, however, the term is often equated with the corticospinal (pyramidal) tract (Fig. 1.12). This pathway originates from widespread regions of the cerebral cortex, including the primary motor cortex of the frontal lobe, where the opposite half of the body is represented in a detailed somatotopic fashion. Corticofugal fibres descend through the internal capsule and pass into the brain stem, where some of them (designated corticobulbar fibres) terminate. Corticobulbar fibres control the activity of brain stem neurones, including motor neurones within the cranial nerve nuclei. Corticospinal fibres descend through the brain stem. The majority of them cross to the contralateral side in the pyramidal decussation of the medulla and continue as the lateral corticospinal tract of the spinal cord. This terminates in association with interneurones and motor neurones of the spinal grey matter. The principal function of the corticospinal and corticobulbar tracts is the control of fine, fractionated movements, particularly of those parts of the body where delicate muscular control is required. These tracts are particularly important in speech (corticobulbar tract) and movement of the hand (corticospinal tract).

The terms 'upper motor neurone lesion' and 'lower motor neurone lesion' are used clinically to distinguish, for example, between the effects of a stroke in the internal capsule (a typical upper motor neurone lesion) and those of

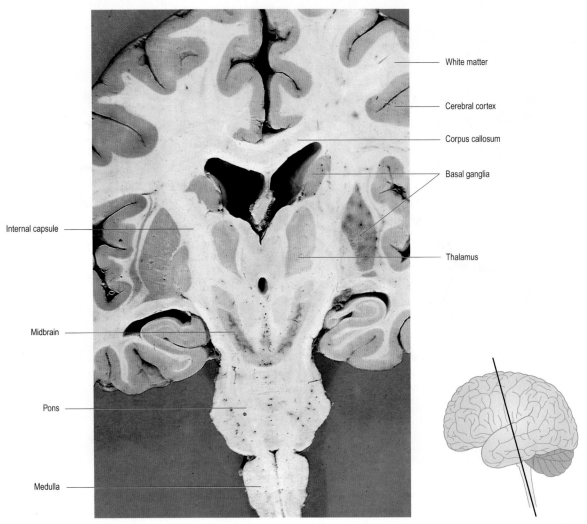

White matter

Cerebral cortex

Corpus callosum

Basal ganglia

Internal capsule

Thalamus

Midbrain

Pons

Medulla

Fig. 1.10 *Section through the cerebral hemisphere and brain stem showing the disposition of grey and white matter, the basal ganglia and the internal capsule. (Photograph by Kevin Fitzpatrick on behalf of GKT School of Medicine, London.)*

motor neurone disease (a typical lower motor neurone lesion). These produce very different signs and symptoms (summarized below), which are indicative of the anatomical site of the lesion.

Lower motor neurone lesions cause paralysis or paresis of specific muscles due to loss of innervation, loss or reduction of tendon reflex activity, reduced muscle tone, spontaneous muscular contraction (fasciculation) and atrophy of muscles over time. Upper motor neurone lesions cause paralysis or paresis of movements due to loss of higher control, increased tendon reflex activity, increased muscle tone and positive plantar reflex (Babinski's sign); there is no atrophy of muscles. The combination of paralysis, increased tendon reflex activity and hypertonia is referred to as spasticity.

The pathophysiology of upper motor neurone lesions is complex. This is because many descending pathways other than the corticospinal tract exist, and they also influence lower motor neurone activity. These pathways include rich corticofugal projections to the brain stem (e.g., corticoreticular, corticopontine) that traverse the internal capsule, and numerous pathways that originate within the brain stem itself (e.g., reticulospinal, vestibulospinal). Clearly, these pathways may be compromised to varying extents, determined by the site of a lesion. Their involvement is believed to be important in the pathophysiological mechanisms underlying the generation of spasticity. Pure corticospinal tract lesions, which are exceedingly rare in humans because corticospinal tract fibres lie in close proximity to other pathways throughout most of their course, are believed to cause deficits in delicate, fractionated movements and to induce the positive plantar reflex.

Two other major systems that contribute to the control of movement are the basal ganglia and the cerebellum. The basal ganglia are a group of large subcortical nuclei, the major components of which are the caudate nucleus, putamen and globus pallidus (see Fig. 1.10; Ch. 14). These structures have important connections with the cerebral cortex, certain diencephalic nuclei of the thalamus and subthalamus and the brain stem. They appear to be involved in the selection of appropriate movements and the suppression of inappropriate ones. Disorders of the basal ganglia cause either too little movement (akinesia) or abnormal involuntary movements (dyskinesia), as well

as tremor and abnormalities of muscle tone. The basal ganglia are sometimes described as being part of the so-called extrapyramidal (motor) system. This term is used to distinguish between the effects of basal ganglia disease and the effects of damage to the pyramidal (corticospinal) system. However, the progressive elucidation of basal ganglia anatomy and the pathophysiology of motor disorders has revealed the close functional interrelationship between the two 'systems' and has rendered the terms that distinguish them largely obsolete (Brodal 1981). The cerebellum has rich connections with the brain stem, particularly the reticular and vestibular nuclei, and with the thalamus. It is concerned with the coordination of movement. Among the clinical signs of cerebellar disorders are ataxia, hypotonia and the so-called intention tremor.

PERIPHERAL NERVOUS SYSTEM

The PNS is composed mainly of spinal nerves, cranial nerves, their ganglia and their ramifications, which carry afferent and efferent neurones between the CNS and the rest of the body. It also includes the peripheral parts of the autonomic nervous system, notably the sympathetic trunks and ganglia, and the enteric nervous system, which is composed of plexuses of nerve fibres and cell bodies in the wall of the alimentary tract.

Spinal Nerves

Spinal nerves are the means by which the CNS receives information from, and controls the activities of, the trunk and limbs. Spinal nerves are considered in detail elsewhere. In brief, there are 31 pairs of spinal nerves (8 cervical, 12 thoracic, 5 lumbar, 5 sacral, 1 coccygeal) that contain a mixture of sensory and motor fibres. They originate from the spinal cord as continuous lines of dorsal and ventral nerve rootlets. Adjacent groups of rootlets fuse to form dorsal and ventral roots, which then merge to form the spinal nerves proper. The dorsal roots of spinal nerves contain afferent nerve fibres from cell bodies located in dorsal root ganglia. These cells give off both centrally and peripherally directed processes and do not have synapses on their cell bodies. The ventral roots of spinal nerves contain efferent fibres from cell bodies

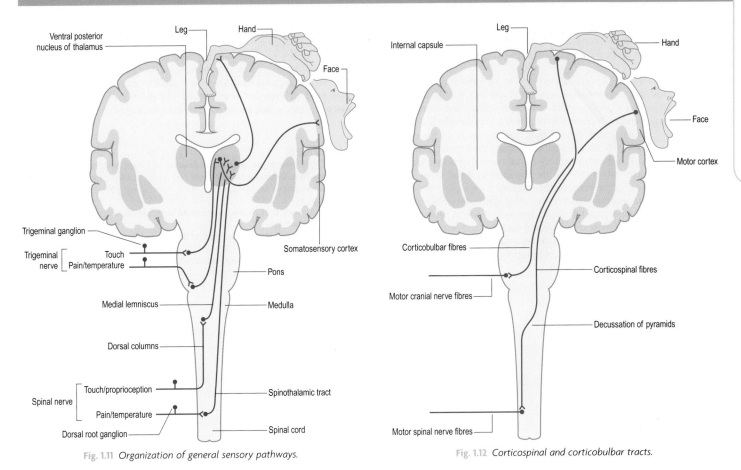

Fig. 1.11 *Organization of general sensory pathways.*

Fig. 1.12 *Corticospinal and corticobulbar tracts.*

Table 1.1 *Summary of cranial nerves*

Number	Name	Function
I	Olfactory	Olfaction
II	Optic	Vision
III	Oculomotor	Eye movement Parasympathetic innervation of eye
IV	Trochlear	Eye movement
V	Trigeminal	General sensation from head Motor innervation to muscles of mastication
VI	Abducens	Eye movement
VII	Facial	Taste Facial movement Parasympathetic innervation of salivary and lacrimal glands
VIII	Vestibulocochlear	Vestibular sense Hearing
IX	Glossopharyngeal	Taste General sensory and motor innervation of pharynx Visceral innervation from carotid body and sinus Parasympathetic innervation of salivary gland
X	Vagus	General sensory and motor innervation of pharynx, larynx and oesophagus Visceral innervation from thorax and abdomen, including aortic body and arch Parasympathetic innervation of thoracic and abdominal viscera
XI	Accessory	Movement of head and shoulders
XII	Hypoglossal	Movement of tongue

located in the spinal grey matter. They include motor neurones innervating skeletal muscle and preganglionic autonomic neurones.

Spinal nerves exit from the vertebral canal via their corresponding intervertebral foramina. They then divide to form a large ventral ramus and a much smaller dorsal ramus. In general terms, the ventral ramus innervates the limbs, together with the muscles and skin of the anterior part of the trunk. The posterior ramus innervates the postvertebral muscles and the skin of the back. The anterior rami serving the upper and lower limbs are redistributed within the brachial and lumbosacral plexuses, respectively.

Cranial Nerves

Cranial nerves are the means by which the brain receives information from, and controls the activities of, the head and neck and, to a lesser extent, the thoracic and abdominal viscera. The cranial nerves' component fibres, their route of exit from the cranial cavity, their subsequent peripheral course and their distribution and functions are considered in detail elsewhere. Their origins, destinations and connections within the CNS are considered in this section.

Briefly, there are 12 pairs of cranial nerves. They are individually named and numbered (I to XII) in a rostrocaudal sequence (Table 1.1). Unlike spinal nerves, only some are mixed in function and carry both sensory and motor fibres. Others are purely sensory or purely motor. The first cranial nerve (I; olfactory) has an ancient lineage and is derived from the forerunner of the cerebral hemisphere. It retains this unique position through the connections of the olfactory bulb, and it is the only sensory cranial nerve that projects directly to the cerebral cortex rather than via the thalamus, as do all other sensory modalities. The areas of cerebral cortex involved have a primitive cellular organization and are an integral part of the limbic system, which is concerned with the emotional aspects of behaviour. The second cranial nerve (II; optic) consists of the axons of second-order visual neurones and terminates in the thalamus. The other 10 pairs of cranial nerves attach to the brain stem. Most of the component fibres originate from or terminate in named cranial nerve nuclei.

The sensory fibres in individual spinal and cranial nerves have characteristic, but often overlapping, peripheral distributions. As far as the innervation of the body surface is concerned, the area supplied by a particular spinal or cranial nerve is referred to as a dermatome. Detailed dermatome maps are described on a regional basis. The motor axons of individual spinal and cranial nerves tend to innervate anatomically and functionally related groups of skeletal muscles, which are referred to as myotomes.

References

Brodal, A., 1981. Neurological Anatomy in Relation to Clinical Medicine, third ed. Oxford University Press, Oxford. *Unconventional but highly readable neuroanatomy text, with an emphasis on clinical relevance. Particularly good account of motor pathways.*

Crossman, A.R., Neary, D. 2000. Neuroanatomy: An Illustrated Colour Text, second ed. Churchill Livingstone, Edinburgh.

England, M.A., Wakely, J. 1991. A Colour Atlas of the Brain and Spinal Cord. Wolfe Publishing Ltd, London.

Haines, D.E. 2000. Neuroanatomy: An Atlas of Structures, Sections and Systems, fifth ed. Lippincott Williams & Wilkins, Philadelphia.

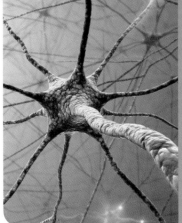

Overview of the Microstructure of the Nervous System

The nervous system has two major divisions, the central nervous system (CNS) and the peripheral nervous system (PNS). The CNS consists of the brain and spinal cord and contains the majority of neuronal cell bodies. The PNS includes all nervous tissue outside the CNS and is subdivided into the cranial and spinal nerves, autonomic nervous system (ANS) (including the enteric nervous system (ENS) of the gut wall) and special senses (taste, olfaction, vision, hearing and balance). It is composed mainly of the axons of sensory and motor neurones that pass between the CNS and the body. However, the ENS contains as many intrinsic neurones in its ganglia as the entire spinal cord, is not connected directly to the CNS, and may be considered separately as a third division of the nervous system.

The CNS is derived from the neural tube (Ch. 3). The cell bodies of neurones are often grouped together in areas termed nuclei, or they may form more extensive layers or masses of cells collectively called grey matter. Neuronal dendrites and synaptic activity are mostly confined to areas of grey matter, and they form part of its meshwork of neuronal and glial processes that is collectively termed the neuropil (Fig. 2.1). Their axons pass into bundles of nerve fibres that tend to be grouped separately to form tracts. In the spinal cord, cerebellum, cerebral cortices and some other areas, concentrations of tracts constitute the white matter, so called because the axons are often ensheathed in myelin, which is white when fresh (see Figs. 8.16, 8.19).

The PNS is composed of the axons of motor neurones situated inside the CNS and the cell bodies of sensory neurones (grouped together as ganglia) and their processes. Sensory cells in dorsal root ganglia give off both centrally and peripherally directed processes; there are no synapses on their cell bodies. Ganglionic neurones of the ANS receive synaptic contacts from various sources. Neuronal cell bodies in peripheral ganglia are all derived embryologically from cells that migrate from the neural crest (Ch. 3).

When the neural tube is formed during prenatal development, its walls thicken greatly but do not completely obliterate the cavity within. The latter remains in the spinal cord as the narrow central canal, and in the brain it becomes greatly expanded to form a series of interconnected cavities called the ventricular system. In the fore- and hindbrains, parts of the neural tube roof do not generate nerve cells but become thin, folded sheets of secretory tissue that are invaded by blood vessels and are called the choroid plexuses. The plexuses secrete cerebrospinal fluid (CSF), which fills the ventricles and subarachnoid spaces (Ch. 4). and penetrates the intercellular spaces of the brain and spinal cord to create their interstitial fluid. The CNS has a rich blood supply, which is essential to sustain its high metabolic rate. The blood–brain barrier places considerable restrictions on the substances that can diffuse from the blood stream into the nervous tissue.

Neurones encode information, conduct it over considerable distances and then transmit it to other neurones or to various non-neural cells. The movement of this information within the nervous system depends on the rapid conduction of transient electrical impulses along neuronal plasma membranes. Transmission to other cells is mediated by secretion of neurotransmitters at special junctions either with other neurones (synapses) or with cells outside the nervous system, such as muscle cells (neuromuscular junctions), gland cells and adipose tissue, and this causes changes in their behaviour.

The nervous system contains large populations of non-neuronal cells, neuroglia or glia that, although not electrically active in the same way, are responsible for creating and maintaining an appropriate environment in which neurones can operate efficiently. In the CNS, glia outnumber neurones by 10 to 50 times and consist of microglia and macroglia. Macroglia are further subdivided into three main types: oligodendrocytes, astrocytes and ependymal cells. The principal glial cell of the PNS is the Schwann cell. Satellite cells surround each neuronal soma in ganglia.

NEURONES

Most of the neurones in the CNS are either clustered into nuclei, columns or layers or dispersed within grey matter. Neurones of the PNS are confined to ganglia. Irrespective of location, neurones share many general features, which are discussed here in the context of central neurones. Special characteristics of ganglionic neurones and their adjacent tissues are discussed later in this chapter.

Neurones exhibit great variability in size (cell bodies range from 5 to 100 μm diameter) and shape. Their surface areas are extensive because most neurones display numerous narrow, branched cell processes. They usually have a rounded or polygonal cell body (perikaryon or soma). This is a central mass of cytoplasm that encloses a nucleus and gives off long, branched extensions, with which most intercellular contacts are made. Typically, one of these processes, the axon, is much longer than the others, the dendrites (Fig. 2.2). Dendrites conduct electrical impulses toward a soma, whereas axons conduct impulses away from it.

Neurones can be classified according to the number and arrangement of their processes. Multipolar neurones (Fig. 2.3; see also Fig. 16.9) are common; they have an extensive dendritic tree, which arises either from a single primary dendrite or directly from the soma, and a single axon. Bipolar neurones, which typify neurones of the special sensory systems (e.g., retina), have only a single dendrite that emerges from the soma opposite the axonal pole. Unipolar neurones that transmit general sensation (e.g., dorsal root ganglion neurones) have a single short process that bifurcates into peripheral and central processes, an arrangement that arises by the fusion of the proximal axonal and dendritic processes of a bipolar neurone during development.

Neurones are postmitotic cells and, with few exceptions, are not replaced when lost.

Soma

The plasma membrane of the soma is unmyelinated and contacted by inhibitory and excitatory axosomatic synapses; very occasionally, somasomatic and dendrosomatic contacts may be made. The non-synaptic surface is covered by either astrocytic or satellite oligodendrocyte processes.

The cytoplasm of a typical soma (see Fig. 2.2) is rich in rough and smooth endoplasmic reticulum and free polyribosomes, which reveals a high level of protein synthetic activity. Free polyribosomes often congregate in large groups associated with the rough endoplasmic reticulum. These aggregates of RNA-rich structures are visible by light microscopy as basophilic Nissl (chromatin) bodies or granules (Fig. 2.4). They are more obvious in large, highly active cells such as spinal motor neurones, which contain large stacks of rough endoplasmic reticulum and polyribosome aggregates. Maintenance and turnover of cytoplasmic and membranous components are necessary in all cells; the huge total volume of cytoplasm within the soma and processes of many neurones requires a considerable commitment of protein synthetic machinery. Neurones synthesize other proteins (e.g., enzyme systems) involved in the production of neurotransmitters and in the reception and transduction of incoming stimuli. Various transmembrane channel proteins and enzymes are located at the surfaces of neurones, where they are associated with ion transport. The apparatus for protein synthesis (including RNA and ribosomes) occupies the soma and dendrites but is usually absent from axons.

The nucleus is characteristically large, round and euchromatic, with one or more prominent nucleoli, as is typical of all cells engaged in substantial levels of protein synthesis. The cytoplasm contains many mitochondria and moderate numbers of lysosomes. Golgi complexes are typically seen close to the nucleus, near the bases of the main dendrites and opposite the axon hillock.

The neuronal cytoskeleton is a prominent feature of its cytoplasm, and it gives shape, strength and rigidity to the dendrites and axons. Neurofilaments (the intermediate filaments of neurones) and microtubules are abundant; they occur in the soma and extend along dendrites and axons, in proportions that vary with the type of neurone and cell process. Bundles of neurofilaments constitute neurofibrils, which can be seen by light microscopy in silver stained sections. Neurofilaments are heteropolymers of proteins assembled from three polypeptide subunits: NF-L (68 kDa), NF-M (160 kDa) and NF-H (200 kDa). NF-M and NF-H have long C-terminal domains that project as side arms from the assembled neurofilament and bind to neighbouring filaments. They can be

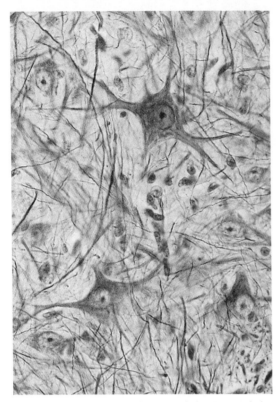

Fig. 2.1 *Neuronal somata, dendrites and axons in the CNS neuropil; their cytoskeleton has been stained using a gold method. The toluidine blue counterstaining reveals the nuclei of surrounding glial cells. (By permission from Young, B., Heath, J.W., 2000. Wheater's Functional Histology. Churchill Livingstone, Edinburgh.)*

heavily phosphorylated, particularly in the highly stable neurofilaments of mature axons, and are thought to give axons their tensile strength. Some axons are almost filled by neurofilaments. Dendrites usually have more microtubules than axons.

Microtubules are important in axonal transport. Centrioles persist in mature postmitotic neurones, where they are concerned with the generation of microtubules rather than cell division. Centrioles are associated with cilia on the surfaces of developing neuroblasts. Their significance, other than at some sensory endings (e.g., the olfactory mucosa), is not known.

Pigment granules appear in certain regions (e.g., neurones of the substantia nigra contain neuromelanin), probably a waste product of catecholamine synthesis. In the locus coeruleus a similar pigment, rich in copper, gives neurones a bluish colour. Some neurones are unusually rich in certain metals, which may form a component of enzyme systems, such as zinc in the hippocampus and iron in the oculomotor nucleus. Ageing neurones, especially in spinal ganglia, accumulate granules of lipofuscin (senility pigment). They represent residual bodies, which are lysosomes packed with partially degraded lipoprotein material (corpora amylacea).

Dendrites

Dendrites are highly branched, usually short processes that project from the soma (see Fig. 2.2). The branching patterns of many dendritic arrays are probably established by random adhesive interactions between dendritic growth cones and afferent axons that occur during development. There is an over-production of dendrites in early development, which is pruned in response to functional demand as the individual matures and information is processed through the dendritic tree. There is evidence that dendritic trees may be plastic structures throughout adult life, expanding and contracting as the traffic of synaptic activity varies through afferent axodendritic contacts. Groups of neurones with similar functions have a similar stereotypical tree structure (Fig. 2.5), suggesting that the branching patterns of dendrites are important determinants of the integration of afferent inputs that converge on the tree.

Dendrites differ from axons in many respects. They represent the afferent rather than the efferent system of the neurone, and they receive both excitatory and inhibitory axodendritic contacts. They may also make dendroden-dritic and dendrosomatic connections (see Fig. 2.8), some of which are reciprocal. Synapses occur either on small projections called dendritic spines or on the smooth dendritic surface. Dendrites contain ribosomes, smooth endoplasmic reticulum, microtubules, neurofilaments, actin filaments and

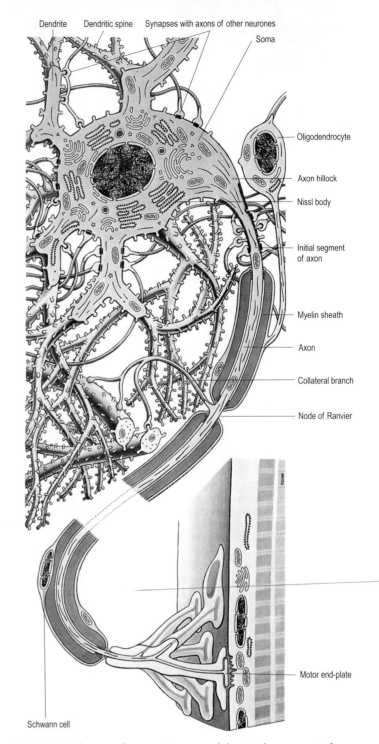

Fig. 2.2 *Typical neurone (here, a motor neurone) showing the soma; part of the dendritic tree, with dendritic spines and synaptic contacts; and an axon myelinated by oligodendrocytes and (in the PNS) Schwann cells and ending at a neuromuscular junction.*

Golgi complexes. The neurofilament proteins of dendrites are poorly phosphorylated. Dendrite microtubules express the microtubule-associated protein (MAP-2) almost exclusively, in comparison with axons.

Dendritic spine shapes range from simple protrusions to structures with a slender stalk and expanded distal end. Most spines are no more than 2 μm long and have one or more terminal expansions, but they can also be short and stubby, branched or bulbous. Free ribosomes and polyribosomes are concentrated at the base of the spine. Ribosomal accumulations near synaptic sites provide a mechanism for activity-dependent synaptic plasticity through the local regulation of protein synthesis.

Axons

The axon originates either from the soma or from the proximal segment of a dendrite, at a specialized region called the axon hillock (see Fig. 2.2), which is free of Nissl granules. Action potentials are initiated here. The axonal plasma

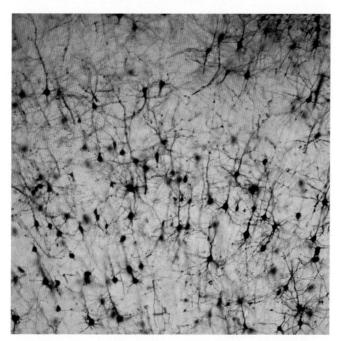

Fig. 2.3 *Section through the cerebral cortex (mouse) stained by the Golgi method, which demonstrates only a small proportion of the total neuronal population. (Specimen prepared by Martin Sadler, Division of Anatomy and Cell Biology, GKT School of Medicine, London.)*

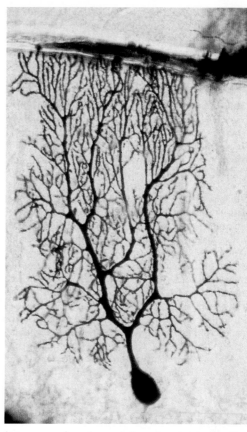

Fig. 2.5 *Purkinje neurone from the cerebellum of a rat stained by the Golgi–Cox method, showing the extensive two-dimensional array of dendrites. (Courtesy of Martin Sadler and M. Berry, Division of Anatomy and Cell Biology, GKT School of Medicine, London.)*

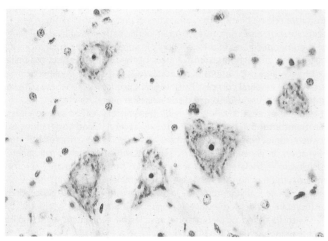

Fig. 2.4 *Large multipolar neuronal perikarya in the magnocellular part of the feline red nucleus, showing prominent Nissl granules, bases of dendrites and axon hillocks. The nuclei are euchromatic and vesicular, with prominent nucleoli. The small nuclei scattered in the surrounding neuropil are characteristic of the various categories of neuroglial cell. (Photograph by Kevin Fitzpatrick on behalf of GKT School of Medicine, London.)*

tissue. They may themselves be contacted by other axons, forming axo-axonal presynaptic inhibitory circuits. Further details of neuronal microcircuitry are given in Kandel and Schwartz (2000).

Axons contain microtubules, neurofilaments, mitochondria, membrane vesicles, cisternae and lysosomes; they do not usually contain ribosomes or Golgi complexes, except at the axon hillock. However, ribosomes are found in the neurosecretory fibres of hypothalamo-hypophysial neurones, which contain the mRNA of neuropeptides. Organelles are differentially distributed along axons; for instance, there is a greater density of mitochondria and membrane vesicles in the axon hillock, at nodes and in presynaptic endings. Axonal microtubules are interconnected by cross-linking microtubule-associated proteins (MAPs), of which tau is the most abundant. Microtubules have an intrinsic polarity: in axons, all microtubules are uniformly oriented with their rapidly growing ends directed away from the soma and toward the axon terminal. Neurofilament proteins ranging from high to low molecular weights are highly phosphorylated in mature axons, whereas growing and regenerating axons express a calmodulin-binding membrane-associated phosphoprotein and growth-associated protein-43 (GAP-43), as well as poorly phosphorylated neurofilaments.

Axons respond differently to injury, depending on whether the damage occurs in the CNS or PNS. The glial microenvironment of a damaged central axon does not facilitate regrowth, and reconnection with original synaptic targets does not normally occur. In the PNS the glial microenvironment is capable of facilitating axonal regrowth; however, the functional outcome of clinical repair of a large mixed peripheral nerve, especially if the injury occurs some distance from the target organ or produces a long defect in the damaged nerve, is frequently unsatisfactory.

Axoplasmic Flow

Neuronal organelles and cytoplasm are in continual motion. Bidirectional streaming of vesicles along axons results in a net transport of materials from the soma to the terminals, with more limited movement in the opposite direction. Two major types of transport occur—one slow, and one relatively fast. Slow axonal transport is a bulk flow of axoplasm only in the anterograde direction, carrying cytoskeletal proteins and soluble, non-membrane-bound proteins at a rate of 0.1 to 3 mm a day. In contrast, fast axonal transport carries vesicular material at approximately 200 mm a day in the retrograde direction and 40 mm a day anterogradely.

membrane (axolemma) is undercoated at the hillock by a concentration of cytoskeletal molecules, including spectrin and actin fibrils, which are thought to be important in anchoring numerous voltage-sensitive channels to the membrane. The axon hillock is unmyelinated and often participates in inhibitory axo-axonal synapses. This region of the axon is unique because it contains ribosomal aggregates immediately below the postsynaptic membrane.

When present, myelin begins at the distal end of the axon hillock. Myelin thickness and internodal segment lengths are positively correlated with axon diameter. In the PNS unmyelinated axons are embedded in Schwann cell cytoplasm; in the CNS they lie free in the neuropil. Nodes of Ranvier are specialized constricted regions of myelin-free axolemma where action potentials are generated and where an axon may branch. The density of sodium channels in the axolemma is highest at the nodes of Ranvier and very low along internodal membranes. In contrast, sodium channels are spread more evenly within the axolemma of unmyelinated axons. Fast potassium channels are also present in the paranodal regions of myelinated axons. Fine processes of glial cytoplasm (astrocyte in the CNS, Schwann cell in the PNS) surround the nodal axolemma. The terminals of an axon are unmyelinated. They expand into presynaptic boutons, which may form connections with axons, dendrites, neuronal somata or, in the periphery, muscle fibres, glands and lymphoid

Rapid flow depends on microtubules. Vesicles with side projections line up along microtubules and are transported along them by their side arms. Two microtubule-based motor proteins with ATPase activity are involved in fast transport. Kinesin family proteins are responsible for the fast component of anterograde transport, and cytoplasmic dynein is responsible for retrograde transport. Fast anterograde transport carries vesicles, including synaptic vesicles containing neurotransmitters, from the soma to the axon terminals. Retrograde axonal transport accounts for the flow of mitochondria, endosomes and lysosomal autophagic vacuoles from the axon terminals into the soma. Retrograde transport mediates the movement of neurotrophic viruses (e.g., herpes zoster, rabies, polio) from peripheral terminals and their subsequent concentration in the neuronal soma.

Synapses

Transmission of impulses across specialized junctions (synapses) between two neurones is largely chemical. It depends on the release of neurotransmitters from the presynaptic side; this causes a change in the electrical state of the postsynaptic neuronal membrane, resulting in either its depolarization or its hyperpolarization.

The patterns of axonal termination vary considerably. A single axon may synapse with one neurone, such as climbing fibres ending on cerebellar Purkinje neurones; more often, it synapses with many, such as cerebellar parallel fibres, which provide an extreme example of this phenomenon. In synaptic glomeruli (e.g., in the olfactory bulb) and synaptic cartridges, groups of synapses between two or more neurones form interactive units encapsulated by neuroglia (Fig. 2.6).

Electrical synapses (direct communication via gap junctions) are rare in the human CNS and are confined largely to groups of neurones with tightly coupled activity, such as the inspiratory centre in the medulla. They are not discussed further here.

Classification of Chemical Synapses

Chemical synapses have an asymmetric structural organization (Figs 2.7, 2.8), in keeping with the unidirectional nature of their transmission. Typical chemical synapses share a number of important features. They all display an area of presynaptic membrane apposed to a corresponding postsynaptic membrane; the two are separated by a narrow (20 to 30 nm) gap, the synaptic cleft. Synaptic vesicles containing neurotransmitters lie on the presynaptic side, clustered near an area of dense material on the cytoplasmic aspect of the presynaptic membrane. A corresponding region of submembrane density is present on the postsynaptic side. Together these define the active zone, the area of the synapse where neurotransmission takes place.

Chemical synapses can be classified according to a number of different parameters, including the neuronal regions forming the synapse, their ultrastructural characteristics, the chemical nature of their neurotransmitters and their effects on the electrical state of the postsynaptic neurone. The classification described here is limited to associations between neurones. Neuromuscular junctions share many (although not all) of these parameters

and are often referred to as peripheral synapses. They are described separately in Chapter 22.

Synapses can occur between almost any surface regions of the participating neurones. The most common type occurs between an axon and either a dendrite or a soma, when the axon is expanded as a small bulb or bouton (see Figs. 2.7, 2.8). This may be a terminal of an axonal branch (terminal bouton) or one of a row of bead-like endings, with the axon making contact at several points and often with more than one neurone (bouton de passage). Boutons may synapse with dendrites, including dendritic spines or the flat surface of a dendritic shaft; a soma, usually on its flat surface, but occasionally on spines; the axon hillock and the terminal boutons of other axons.

The connection is classified according to the direction of transmission, with the incoming terminal region named first. Most common are axodendritic synapses, although axosomatic connections are frequent. All other possible combinations are found, but they are less common: axoaxonic, dendroaxonic, dendrodendritic, somatodendritic and somatosomatic. Axodendritic and axosomatic synapses occur in all regions of the CNS and in autonomic ganglia, including those of the ENS. The other types appear to be restricted to regions of complex interaction between larger sensory neurones and microneurones, such as in the thalamus.

Ultrastructurally, synaptic vesicles may be internally clear or dense and of different sizes (loosely categorized as small or large) and shape (round, flat or pleomorphic, i.e., irregularly shaped). The submembranous densities may be thicker on the postsynaptic than on the presynaptic side (asymmetric synapses) or equivalent in thickness (symmetric synapses). Synaptic ribbons are found at sites of neurotransmission in the retina and inner ear. They have a distinctive morphology, in that the synaptic vesicles are grouped around a ribbon- or rod-like density oriented perpendicular to the cell membrane (see Fig. 2.8).

Synaptic boutons make obvious close contacts with postsynaptic structures, but many other terminals lack specialized contact zones. Areas of transmitter release occur in the varicosities of unmyelinated axons, where the effects are sometimes diffuse (e.g., the aminergic pathways of the basal ganglia and in autonomic fibres in the periphery). In some instances, such axons may ramify widely throughout extensive areas of the brain and affect the behaviour of very large populations of neurones (e.g., the diffuse cholinergic innervation of the cerebral cortices). Pathological degeneration of these pathways can therefore cause widespread disturbances in neural function.

Neurones express a variety of neurotransmitters, either as one class of neurotransmitter per cell or, more often, as several. Good correlations exist between some types of transmitters and specialized structural features of synapses. In general, asymmetric synapses with relatively small spherical vesicles are associated with acetylcholine (ACh), glutamate, serotonin (5-hydroxytryptamine, or 5-HT) and some amines; those with dense-core vesicles include many peptidergic synapses and other amines (e.g., noradrenaline (norepinephrine), adrenaline (epinephrine), dopamine). Symmetric synapses with flattened or pleomorphic vesicles have been shown to contain either γ-aminobutyric acid (GABA) or glycine.

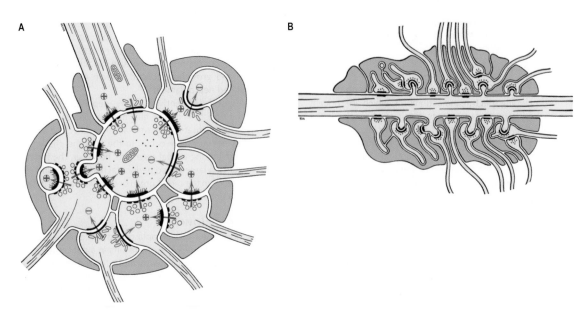

Fig. 2.6 *Arrangement of complex synaptic units.* **A**, *Synaptic glomerulus with excitatory (+) and inhibitory (−) synapses grouped around a central dendritic terminal expansion. The directions of transmission are shown by the arrows.* **B**, *Synaptic cartridge with a group of synapses surrounding a dendritic segment. Each complex unit is enclosed within a glial capsule* (green).

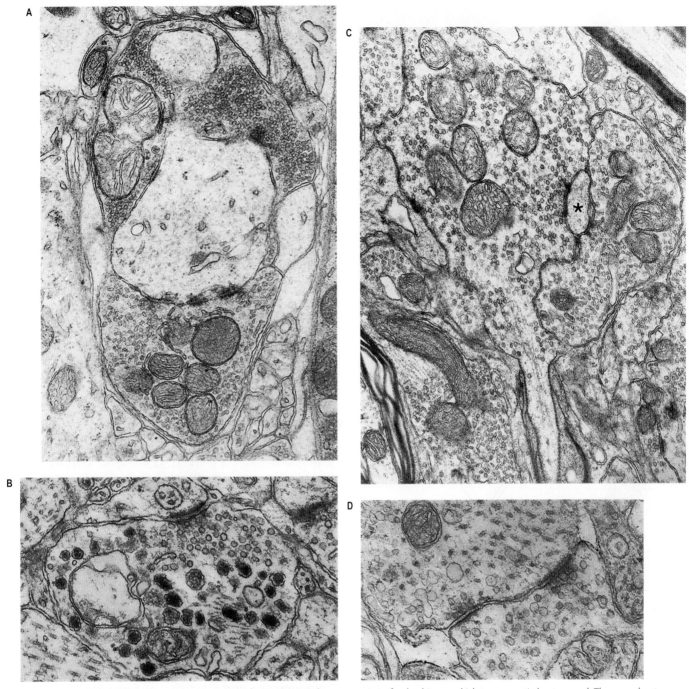

Fig. 2.7 *Electron micrographs demonstrating various types of synapses. A, Pale cross-section of a dendrite on which two synaptic boutons end. The upper bouton contains round vesicles, and the lower bouton contains flattened vesicles of the small type. A number of pre- and postsynaptic thickenings mark the specialized zones of contact. B, Type I synapse containing both small, round, clear vesicles and large, dense-core vesicles of the neurosecretory type. C, Large terminal bouton of an optic nerve afferent fibre, making contact with a number of postsynaptic processes, in the dorsal lateral geniculate nucleus of a rat. One of the postsynaptic processes (*) also receives a synaptic contact from a bouton containing flattened vesicles (right). D, Reciprocal synapses between two neuronal processes in the olfactory bulb. (A and C, Courtesy of A.R. Lieberman, Department of Anatomy, University College, London.)*

The neurosecretory endings found in various parts of the brain and in neuroendocrine glands have many features in common with presynaptic boutons. They all contain peptides or glycoproteins within dense-core vesicles of characteristic size and appearance. These are often ellipsoidal or irregular in shape and relatively large; for example, oxytocin and vasopressin vesicles in the neurohypophysis may be up to 200 nm across.

Synapses may cause depolarization or hyperpolarization of the postsynaptic membrane, depending on the neurotransmitter released and the classes of receptor molecule in the postsynaptic membrane. Depolarization of the postsynaptic membrane results in excitation of the postsynaptic neurone, whereas hyperpolarization has the effect of transiently inhibiting electrical activity. Subtle variations in these responses may also occur at synapses where mixtures of neuromediators are present and their effects are integrated.

Type I and II Synapses

There are two broad categories of synapse: type I synapses, in which the subsynaptic zone of dense cytoplasm is thicker than on the presynaptic side,

and type II synapses, in which the two zones are more symmetric but thinner. Other differences include the widths of the synaptic clefts, which are approximately 30 nm in type I and 20 nm in type II synapses, and their vesicle content. Type I boutons contain a predominance of small spherical vesicles approximately 50 nm in diameter, and type II boutons contain a variety of flat forms. The general principle that broadly applies throughout the CNS classifies type I synapses as excitatory and type II as inhibitory. In a few instances, type I and II synapses are found in close proximity, oriented in opposite directions across the synaptic cleft (a reciprocal synapse).

Mechanisms of Synaptic Activity

Synaptic activation begins with the arrival of one or more action potentials at the presynaptic bouton, which causes the opening of voltage-sensitive calcium channels in the presynaptic membrane. The response time in typical fast-acting synapses is then very rapid; classic neurotransmitter (e.g., ACh) is released in less than a millisecond, which is faster than the activation time of a classic second messenger system on the presynaptic side. The influx of

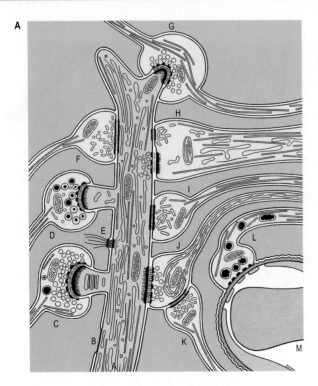

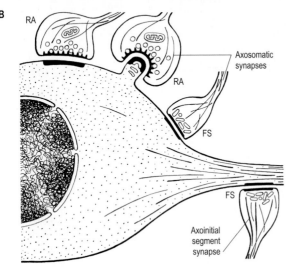

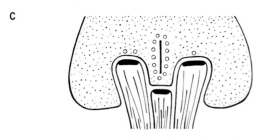

Fig. 2.8 *Structural arrangements of different types of synaptic contact.* **A,** *The gap junction (B) and the desmosome (E) have no synaptic significance. Excitatory synaptic boutons are shown (C and G), containing small, spherical, translucent vesicles. Also depicted are a bouton with dense-core, catecholamine-containing vesicles (D); an inhibitory synapse containing small flattened vesicles (F); a reciprocal synaptic structure between two dendritic profiles, inhibitory toward the dendrite (A) and excitatory in the opposite direction (H); an inhibitory synapse containing large flattened vesicles (I); two serial synapses—one (J) excitatory to the dendrite and one (K) inhibitory to J; and a neurosecretory ending (L) adjacent to a vascular channel (M), surrounded by a fenestrated endothelium. All the boutons in this diagram are of the terminal type except for G, which is a bouton de passage.* **B,** *Axosomatic and axoinitial segment synapses. FS, symmetric synapses with flattened vesicles; RA, asymmetric synapses with rounded vesicles.* **C,** *Ribbon synapse: triad at the base of a retinal rod.*

calcium activates Ca^{2+}-dependent protein kinases. This uncouples synaptic vesicles from a spectrin–actin meshwork within the presynaptic ending, to which they are bound via synapsins I and II. The vesicles dock with the presynaptic membrane, through processes not yet fully understood, and their membranes fuse to open a pore through which neurotransmitter diffuses into the synaptic cleft.

Once the vesicle has discharged its contents, its membrane is incorporated into the presynaptic plasma membrane and is then more slowly recycled back into the bouton by endocytosis around the edges of the active site. The time between endocytosis and re-release may be approximately 30 seconds; newly recycled vesicles compete randomly with previously stored vesicles for the next cycle of neurotransmitter release. The fusion of vesicles with the presynaptic membrane is responsible for the observed quantal behaviour of neurotransmitter release, both during neural activation and spontaneously, in the slightly leaky resting condition.

Postsynaptic events vary greatly, depending on the receptor molecules and their related molecular complexes. Receptors are generally classed as either ionotropic or metabotropic. Ionotropic receptors function as ion channels, so that conformational changes induced in the receptor protein when it binds the neurotransmitter cause the opening of an ion channel within the same protein assembly, thus causing a voltage change within the postsynaptic cell. Examples are the nicotinic ACh receptor and the *N*-methyl-D-aspartate (NMDA) glutamate receptor. Alternatively, the receptor and ion channel may be separate molecules coupled by G-proteins, some via a complex cascade of chemical interactions (a second messenger system), such as the adenylate cyclase pathway. Postsynaptic effects are generally rapid and short lived because the transmitter is quickly inactivated either by an extracellular enzyme (e.g., acetylcholinesterase, or AChE) or by uptake by neuroglial cells. Examples of such metabotropic receptors are the muscarinic ACh receptor and 5-HT receptor.

Neurohormones

Neurohormones are included in the range of transmitter activities. They are synthesized in neurones and released into the blood circulation by exocytosis at synaptic terminal–like structures. As with classic endocrine gland hormones, they may act at great distances from their site of secretion. Neurones secrete neurohormones into the CSF or local interstitial fluid to affect other cells, either diffusely or at a distance. To encompass this wide range of phenomena, the general term neuromediation has been used, and the chemicals involved are called neuromediators.

Neuromodulators — Some neuromediators do not appear to affect the postsynaptic membrane directly, but they can affect its responses to other neuromediators, either enhancing their activity (increasing the size of the immediate response or causing a prolongation) or perhaps limiting or inhibiting their action. These substances are called neuromodulators. A single synaptic terminal may contain one or more neuromodulators in addition to a neurotransmitter, usually (although not always) in separate vesicles. Neuropeptides (see later) are nearly all neuromodulators, at least in some of their actions. They are stored within dense granular synaptic vesicles of various sizes and appearances.

Development and Plasticity of Synapses

Embryonic synapses first appear as inconspicuous dense zones flanking synaptic clefts. Immature synapses often appear after birth, suggesting that they may be labile and are reinforced if transmission is functionally effective or withdrawn if redundant. This is implicit in some theories of memory, which postulate that synapses are modifiable by frequency of use to establish preferential conduction pathways. Evidence from hippocampal neurones suggests that even brief synaptic activity can increase the strength and sensitivity of the synapse for some hours or longer (long-term potentiation). During early postnatal life, the normal developmental increase in the number and size of synapses and dendritic spines depends on the degree of neural activity and is impaired in areas of damage or functional deprivation.

Neurotransmitters

Until recently the molecules known to be involved in chemical synapses were limited to a fairly small group of classic neurotransmitters—ACh, noradrenaline, adrenaline, dopamine and histamine—all of which had well-defined rapid effects on other neurones, muscle cells or glands. However, many synaptic interactions cannot be explained on the basis of classic neurotransmitters, and it now appears that other substances, particularly some amino acids such as glutamate, glycine, aspartate, GABA and the monoamine serotonin, also function as transmitters. Substances first identified as hypophysial hormones or as part of the dispersed neuroendocrine system of the alimentary tract can be detected widely throughout the CNS and PNS, often associated with functionally integrated systems. Many of these are peptides: more than 50 (together with other candidates) function mainly as neuromodulators and influence the activities of classic transmitters.

Acetylcholine — ACh is perhaps the most extensively studied neurotransmitter of the classic type. Its precursor, choline, is synthesized in the neuronal soma and transported to the axon terminals, where it is acetylated by the enzyme choline acetyltransferase (ChAT) and stored in clear spherical vesicles approximately 50 nm in diameter. ACh is synthesized by motor neurones and released at all their motor terminals on skeletal muscle and at synapses in parasympathetic and sympathetic ganglia. Many parasympathetic, and some sympathetic, ganglionic neurones are also cholinergic.

In some sites, such as at neuromuscular junctions, ACh is also associated with the degradative extracellular enzyme AChE. The effects of ACh on nicotinic receptors (i.e., those in which nicotine is an agonist) are rapid and excitatory. In the peripheral ANS, the slower, more sustained excitatory effects of cholinergic autonomic endings are mediated by muscarinic receptors via a second messenger system.

Monoamines — Monoamines include the catecholamines (noradrenaline, adrenaline and dopamine), the indoleamine serotonin (5-HT) and histamine. Neurones that synthesize the monoamines include sympathetic ganglia and their homologues, the chromaffin cells of the suprarenal medulla and paraganglia. Within the CNS, their somata lie chiefly in the brain stem, although their axons spread and ramify widely into all parts of the nervous system. Monoaminergic cells are also present in the retina.

Noradrenaline is the chief transmitter present in sympathetic ganglionic neurones with endings in various tissues, notably smooth muscle and glands, and in other sites, including adipose and haemopoietic tissues and the corneal epithelium. It is also found at widely distributed synaptic endings within the CNS, many of them terminals of neuronal somata situated in the locus coeruleus in the medullary floor. The actions of noradrenaline depend on its site of action and vary with the type of postsynaptic receptor. In some cases, such as the neurones of the submucosal plexus of the intestine and of the locus coeruleus, it is strongly inhibitory via actions on the α_2-adrenergic receptor, whereas the β-receptors of vascular smooth muscle mediate depolarization and therefore vasoconstriction. Adrenaline is present in central and peripheral nervous pathways and occurs with noradrenaline in the suprarenal medulla. Both these monoamines are found in dense-core synaptic vesicles measuring approximately 50 nm in diameter.

Dopamine is a neuromediator of considerable clinical importance. It is present mainly in the CNS, where it is found in neurones with cell bodies in the telencephalon, diencephalon and mesencephalon. A major dopaminergic neuronal population in the midbrain constitutes the substantia nigra, so called because its cells contain neuromelanin, a black granular by-product of dopamine synthesis. Dopaminergic endings are particularly numerous in the corpus striatum, limbic system and cerebral cortex. Pathological reduction in dopaminergic activity has widespread effects on motor control, affective behaviour and other neural activities, as seen in Parkinson's syndrome. Structurally, dopaminergic synapses contain numerous dense-core vesicles resembling those of noradrenaline.

Serotonin and histamine are found in neurones mainly in the CNS. Serotonin is synthesized chiefly in small median neuronal clusters of the brain stem, mainly in the raphe nuclei, whose axons spread and branch extensively throughout the entire brain and spinal cord. Synaptic terminals contain round, clear vesicles approximately 50 nm in diameter and are of the asymmetric type. Histaminergic neurones appear to be relatively sparse and are restricted largely to the hypothalamus.

Amino acids — The best understood amino acid is GABA, which is a major inhibitory transmitter released at the terminals of local circuit neurones within the brain stem and spinal cord (e.g., recurrent inhibitory Renshaw loop; Ch. 8), cerebellum (as the main transmitter of Purkinje neurones) and elsewhere. It is stored in flattened or pleomorphic vesicles within symmetric synapses; it may be inhibitory to the postsynaptic neurone, or it may mediate either presynaptic inhibition or facilitation, depending on the synaptic arrangement.

Glutamate and aspartate are major excitatory transmitters present widely in the CNS, including the major projection pathways from the cortex to the thalamus, tectum, substantia nigra and pontine nuclei. They are found in the central terminals of the auditory and trigeminal nerves, and glutamate is present in the terminals of parallel fibres ending on Purkinje cells in the cerebellum. Structurally, they are associated with asymmetric synapses containing small (approximately 30 nm), round, clear synaptic vesicles.

Glycine is a well-established inhibitory transmitter of the CNS, particularly the lower brain stem and spinal cord, where it is found mainly in local circuit neurones.

Nitric oxide — Nitric oxide (NO) is of considerable importance at autonomic and enteric synapses, where it mediates smooth muscle relaxation. NO has been implicated in the mechanism of long-term potentiation. The gas is able to diffuse freely through cell membranes, so it is not subject to the tight quantal control of vesicle-mediated neurotransmission.

Neuropeptides — Many neuropeptides coexist with other neuromediators in the same synaptic terminals. As many as three peptides often share a particular ending with a well-established neurotransmitter, in some cases within the same synaptic vesicles. Some peptides occur in both the CNS and PNS, particularly in the ganglion cells and peripheral terminals of the ANS, whereas others are entirely restricted to the CNS. Only a few examples are given here.

Most of the neuropeptides are classified according to the site where they were first discovered; for example, the gastrointestinal peptides were initially found in the gut wall, and a group first associated with the pituitary gland includes releasing hormones, adenohypophysial and neurohypophysial hormones. Some of these peptides are closely related to one another in terms of their chemistry because they are derived from the same gene products (e.g., the pro-opiomelanocortin group), which are cleaved to produce smaller peptides.

Substance P (SP) was the first peptide to be characterized as a gastrointestinal neuromediator. It consists of 11 amino acid residues and is a major neuromediator in the brain and spinal cord. It occurs in approximately 20% of dorsal root and trigeminal ganglion cells, particularly in small nociceptive neurones. It is also present in some fibres of the facial, glossopharyngeal and vagal nerves. Within the CNS, SP is present in several apparently unrelated major pathways. It is contained within large granular synaptic vesicles. Its known action is prolonged postsynaptic excitation.

Vasoactive intestinal polypeptide (VIP), another gastrointestinal peptide, is widely present in the CNS, where it is probably an excitatory neurotransmitter or neuromodulator. Its distribution includes distinctive bipolar neurones of the cerebral cortex; small dorsal root ganglion cells, particularly of the sacral region; the median eminence of the hypothalamus, where it may be involved in endocrine regulation; and intramural ganglion cells of the gut wall and sympathetic ganglia.

Somatostatin (ST, or somatotropin release inhibiting factor) has a broad distribution within the nervous system and may be a central neurotransmitter or neuromodulator. It occurs in small dorsal root ganglion cells.

β-Endorphin, leu- and met-enkephalins and the dynorphins belong to a group of peptides (naturally occurring opiates) that have aroused much interest because of their analgesic properties. They bind to opiate receptors in the brain, where their action seems to be inhibitory. The enkephalins have been localized in many areas of the brain, particularly the septal nuclei, amygdaloid complex, basal ganglia and hypothalamus. From this, it has been inferred that they are important mediators in the limbic system and in the control of endocrine function. They have been strongly implicated in the central control of pain pathways because they are found in the periaqueductal grey matter of the midbrain, a number of reticular raphe nuclei, the spinal nucleus of the trigeminal nerve and the substantia gelatinosa of the spinal cord. The enkephalinergic pathways exert an important presynaptic inhibitory action on nociceptive afferents in the spinal cord and brain stem. Like many other neuromediators, the enkephalins also occur widely in other parts of the brain in lower concentrations.

CENTRAL GLIA

Glial (neuroglial) cells vary considerably in type and number in different regions of the CNS. There are two major groups, classified according to origin. Macroglia arise within the neural plate, in parallel with neurones, and constitute the great majority of glial cells. Microglia are smaller cells, generally considered to be monocytic in origin, and are derived from haemopoietic tissue (Fig. 2.9).

Astrocytes

Astrocytes are star-shaped glia whose processes ramify through the entire central neuropil (see Fig. 2.9). Their processes are functionally coupled at gap junctions and form an interconnected network that ensheathes all neurones, except at synapses and along the myelinated segments of axons. Astrocyte processes terminate as end-feet at the basal lamina of blood vessels and where they form the glia limitans (glial-limiting membrane) at the pial surface (Fig. 2.10). Ultrastructurally, astrocytes typically have a pale nucleus with a narrow rim of heterochromatin, although this is variable. They have pale cytoplasm containing glycogen, lysosomes, Golgi complexes and bundles of glial intermediate filaments within their processes (the last are found particularly in fibrous astrocytes, which occur predominantly in white matter). Glial intermediate filaments are formed from glial fibrillary acidic protein (GFAP); its presence can be used clinically to identify tumour cells of glial origin. A second morphological type of astrocyte, the protoplasmic astrocyte, is found mainly in grey matter. The significance of these subtypes is unclear: there are

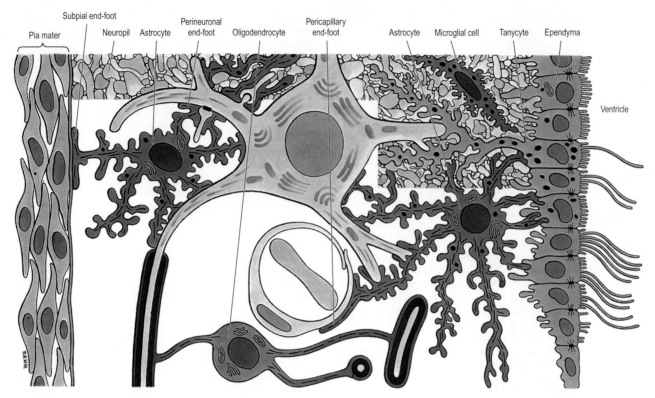

Fig. 2.9 *Different types of non-neuronal cells in the CNS and their structural organization and interrelationships with one another and with neurones.*

few known functional differences between fibrous and protoplasmic astrocytes.

Astrocytes are thought to provide a network of communication in the brain via interconnecting low-resistance gap junctional complexes. They signal to one another using intracellular calcium wave propagation, triggered by synaptically released glutamate. Functionally, this may coordinate astrocyte activities, including ion (particularly potassium) buffering, neurotransmitter uptake and metabolism (e.g., of excess glutamate, which is excitotoxic), membrane transport and the secretion of peptides, amino acids, trophic factors, etc, essential for efficient neuronal activity.

Injury to the CNS induces astrogliosis, which is seen as local increases in the number and size of cells expressing GFAP and in the extent of their meshwork of processes, forming a glial scar. It is thought that the local glial scar environment, which may include oligodendrocytes and myelin debris, inhibits the regeneration of CNS axons or fails to provide the necessary stimuli for axonal regrowth.

Pituicytes are glial cells found in the neural parts of the pituitary gland, the infundibulum and neurohypophysis. They resemble astrocytes, but their processes end mostly on endothelial cells in the neurohypophysis and tuber cinereum.

Blood–Brain Barrier

Proteins circulating in the blood enter most tissues of the body except those of the brain, spinal cord or peripheral nerves. This concept of a blood–brain barrier (and blood–nerve barrier) covers many substances, some of which are actively transported across the blood–brain barrier, whereas others are actively excluded. The blood–brain barrier is located at the capillary endothelium within the brain. It depends on the presence of tight junctions between endothelial cells and a relative lack of transcytotic vesicular transport. The tightness of the barrier depends on the close apposition of astrocytes to blood capillaries (Figs. 2.10C, 2.11).

The blood–brain barrier develops during embryonic life but may not be fully completed by birth. Moreover, there are certain areas of the adult brain in which the endothelial cells do not have tight junctions, and a free exchange of molecules occurs between blood and adjacent brain. Most of these areas are situated close to the ventricles and are known as circumventricular organs. Otherwise, unrestricted diffusion through the blood–brain barrier is possible only for substances that can cross biological membranes because of their lipophilic character. Lipophilic molecules may be actively re-exported by the brain endothelium.

Breakdown of the blood–brain barrier occurs following brain damage caused by ischaemia or infection, and this permits an influx of fluid, ions, protein and other substances into the brain. It is also associated with primary

and metastatic cerebral tumours. Computed tomography (CT) and magnetic resonance imaging (MRI) scans can demonstrate such breakdown of the blood–brain barrier clinically. A similar breakdown of the blood–brain barrier may be seen post mortem in patients who were jaundiced. Normally, the brain, spinal cord and peripheral nerves remain unstained by bile, except for the choroid plexus, which is often stained a deep yellow. However, areas of recent infarction (1 to 3 days) are stained by bile pigment as a result of localized breakdown of the blood–brain barrier.

Oligodendrocytes

Oligodendrocytes myelinate CNS axons and are most commonly seen as intrafascicular cells in myelinated tracts (Figs 2.12, 2.13). They usually have round nuclei, and their cytoplasm contains numerous mitochondria, microtubules and glycogen. They display a spectrum of morphological variation, from large euchromatic nuclei and pale cytoplasm to heterochromatic nuclei and dense cytoplasm. Oligodendrocytes may enclose up to 50 axons in separate myelin sheaths: the largest calibre axons are usually ensheathed on a 1:1 basis. Some oligodendrocytes are not associated with axons and are either precursor cells or perineuronal (satellite) oligodendrocytes whose processes ramify around neuronal somata.

Within tracts, interfascicular oligodendrocytes are arranged in long rows in which single astrocytes intervene at regular intervals. Groups of oligodendrocytes myelinate the surrounding axons: their processes are radially aligned to the axis of each row. Myelinated tracts therefore consist of cables of axons, which are predominantly myelinated by a row of oligodendrocytes running down the axis of each cable.

Oligodendrocytes originate from the ventricular neuroectoderm and the subependymal layer in the fetus and continue to be generated from the subependymal plate postnatally. Stem cells migrate and seed into white and grey matter to form a pool of adult progenitor cells that may later differentiate to replenish lost oligodendrocytes and possibly remyelinate pathologically demyelinated regions.

Nodes of Ranvier and Incisures of Schmidt–Lanterman

The territory ensheathed by an oligodendrocyte process defines an internode. The interval between internodes is called a node of Ranvier, and the territory immediately adjacent to the nodal gap is a paranode, where loops of oligodendrocyte cytoplasm abut the axolemma. Nodal axolemma is contacted by the end-feet of perinodal cells, which have been shown in animal studies to have a presumptive adult oligodendrocyte progenitor phenotype; their function is unknown (Butt and Berry 2000). Schmidt–Lanterman incisures are

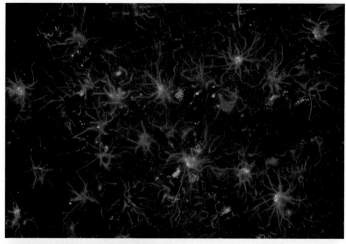

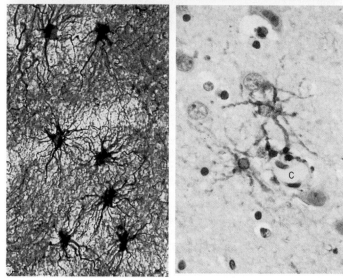

Fig. 2.10 *Astrocytes.* **A**, *Immunofluorescent technique showing astrocytes immunopositive for glial fibrillary acidic protein (GFAP) in the human cerebral cortex.* **B**, *Classic heavy-metal impregnation technique (Cajal method).* **C**, *Immunoperoxidase technique, GFAP. Note perivascular end-feet embracing the capillary (C). (**A**, Preparation by Jonathan Carlisle, Division of Anatomy and Cell Biology, GKT School of Medicine, London; **B** and **C**, by permission from Young, B., Heath, J.W., 2000. Wheater's Functional Histology. Churchill Livingstone, Edinburgh.)*

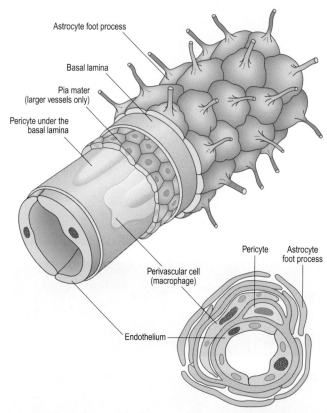

Fig. 2.11 *Relationship among the glia limitans, perivascular cells and blood vessels in the brain, in longitudinal and transverse section. A sheath of astrocytic end-feet wraps around the vessel and, in vessels larger than capillaries, its investment of pial meninges. Vascular endothelial cells are joined by tight junctions and supported by pericytes; perivascular macrophages lie outside the endothelial basal lamina.*

helical decompactions of internodal myelin where the major dense line of the myelin sheath splits to enclose a spiral of oligodendrocyte cytoplasm. Their function is unknown, but their structure suggests that they may play a role in the transport of molecules across the myelin sheath.

Myelin and Myelination

Myelin is secreted by oligodendrocytes (CNS) and Schwann cells (PNS). A single oligodendrocyte may ensheathe up to 50 separate axons, depending on their calibre, whereas myelinating Schwann cells ensheathe axons on a 1:1 basis.

In general, myelin is laid down around axons larger than 2 μm in diameter. However, the critical minimal axon diameter for myelination is smaller and more variable in the CNS than in the PNS and is approximately 0.2 μm (compared with 1 to 2 μm in the PNS). Because there is considerable overlap between the size of the smallest myelinated axons and the largest unmyelinated axons, axonal calibre is unlikely to be the only factor in determining myelination. Additionally, the first axons to become ensheathed ultimately reach larger diameters than do later ones. There is a reasonable linear relationship between axon diameter and internodal length and myelin sheath thickness. As the sheath thickens from a few lamellae to up to 200, the axon may also grow from 1 to 15 μm in diameter. Internodal lengths increase about 10-fold during the same time.

It is not known how myelin is formed in either the PNS or the CNS. The ultrastructural appearance of myelin (Fig. 2.14) is usually explained in terms of the spiral wrapping of a flat glial process around an axon and the subsequent extrusion of cytoplasm from the sheath at all points other than incisures and

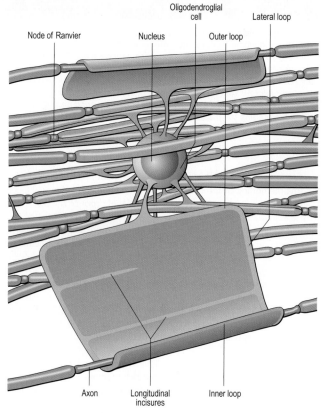

Fig. 2.12 *Ensheathment of a number of axons by the processes of an oligodendrocyte. The oligodendrocyte soma is shown in the centre, and its myelin sheaths are unfolded to varying degrees to show their extensive surface area. (Modified from Morell and Norton 1980 by Raine 1984, by permission.)*

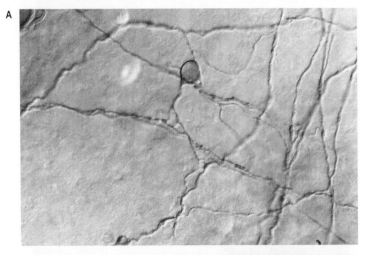

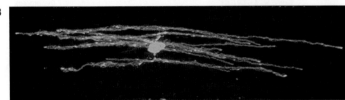

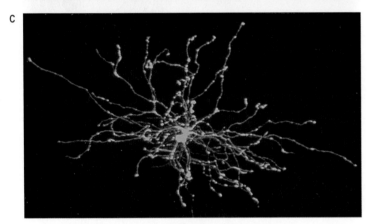

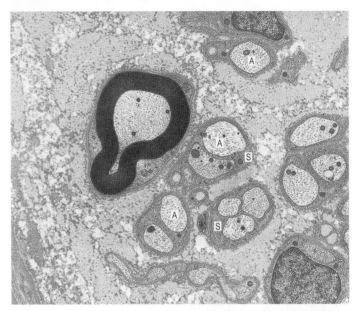

Fig. 2.14 Transverse section of sciatic nerve showing a myelinated axon and several non-myelinated axons (A), *ensheathed by Schwann cells* (S). *(Courtesy of Professor Susan Standring, GKT School of Medicine, London.)*

Fig. 2.13 *A, Oligodendrocyte enwrapping several axons with myelin, demonstrated in a whole-mounted rat anterior medullary velum, immunolabelled with antibody to an oligodendrocyte membrane antigen. B and C, Confocal micrographs of a mature myelin-forming oligodendrocyte (B) and astrocyte (C) iontophoretically filled in the adult rat optic nerve with an immunofluorescent dye by intracellular microinjection. (A, Courtesy of Fiona Ruge; B and C, prepared by Dr. A. Butt and Kate Colquhoun, Division of Physiology, and photographed by Sarah-Jane Smith using the pseudocolour technique, Division of Anatomy and Cell Biology, GKT School of Medicine, London.)*

paranodes. In this way, it is thought that the compacted external surfaces of the plasma membrane of the ensheathing glial cell produce the minor dense lines, and the compacted inner cytoplasmic surfaces produce the major dense lines, of the mature myelin sheath (Fig. 2.15). These correspond to the intraperiod and period lines, respectively, defined in X-ray studies of myelin. The inner and outer zones of occlusion of the spiral process are continuous with the minor dense line and are called the inner and outer mesaxons.

There are significant differences between central and peripheral myelin, reflecting the fact that oligodendrocytes and Schwann cells express different proteins during myelinogenesis. The basic dimensions of the myelin membrane are different. CNS myelin has a period repeat thickness of 15.7 nm, whereas PNS myelin has a period to period line thickness of 18.5 nm. The major dense line space is approximately 1.7 nm in CNS myelin, compared with 2.5 nm in PNS myelin.

Myelin membrane contains protein, lipid and water, which forms at least 20% of the wet weight. It is a relatively lipid-rich membrane and contains 70% to 80% lipid. All classes of lipid have been found, and the precise lipid composition of PNS and CNS myelin is different. The major lipid species are cholesterol (the most common single molecule), phospholipids and glycosphingolipids. Minor lipid species include galactosylglycerides, phosphoinositides and gangliosides. The major glycolipids are galactocerebroside and its sulphate ester sulphatide; these lipids are not unique to myelin but are present

in characteristically high concentrations. CNS and PNS myelin also contains low concentrations of acidic glycolipids, which constitute important antigens in some inflammatory demyelinating states. Gangliosides, which are glycosphingolipids characterized by the presence of sialic acid (*N*-acetylneuraminic acid), account for less than 1% of the lipid.

A relatively small number of protein species accounts for the majority of myelin protein. Some of these proteins are common to both PNS and CNS myelin, but others are different. Proteolipid protein and its splice variant DM20 are found only in CNS myelin, whereas myelin basic protein and myelin-associated glycoprotein (MAG) occur in both. MAG is a member of the immunoglobulin supergene family and is localized specifically in those regions of the myelin segment where compaction starts, namely, the mesaxons and inner periaxonal membranes, paranodal loops and incisures in both CNS and PNS sheaths. It is thought to have a functional role in membrane adhesion.

In the developing CNS, axonal outgrowth precedes the migration of oligodendrocyte precursors, and oligodendrocytes associate with and myelinate axons after their phase of elongation: oligodendrocyte myelin gene expression is not dependent on axon association. In marked contrast, Schwann cells in the developing PNS are associated with axons during the entire phase of outgrowth from CNS to target organ.

Myelination does not occur simultaneously in all parts of the body in late fetal and early postnatal development. White matter tracts and nerves in the periphery have their own specific temporal patterns, related to their degree of functional maturity.

Mutations of the major myelin structural proteins have now been recognized in a number of inherited human neurological diseases. As would be expected, these mutations produce defects in myelination and in the stability of nodal and paranodal architecture, consistent with the suggested functional roles of the relevant proteins in maintaining the integrity of the myelin sheath. The molecular organization of myelinated axons is described in Scherer and Arroyo (2002).

Ependyma

Ependymal cells line the ventricles and central canal of the spinal cord (Fig. 2.16). They form a single-layered epithelium that varies from squamous to columnar in form. At the ventricular surface, cells are joined by gap junctions and occasional desmosomes. Their apical surfaces have numerous microvilli and cilia, which contribute to the flow of CSF. There is considerable regional variation in the ependymal lining of the ventricles, but four major types have been described: the general ependyma that overlies grey matter, the general ependyma that overlies white matter, specialized areas of ependyma in the third and fourth ventricles and the choroidal epithelium.

The ependymal cells overlying areas of grey matter are cuboidal; each cell bears approximately 20 central apical cilia, surrounded by short microvilli. The cells are joined by gap junctions and desmosomes and do not have a basal lamina. Beneath them there may be a subependymal zone, two to three cells deep, consisting of cells that generally resemble ependymal cells.

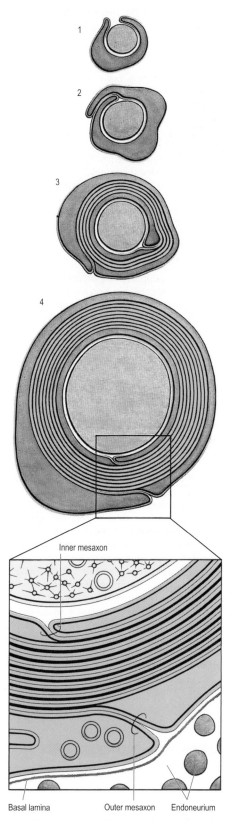

Fig. 2.15 *Stages in myelination of a peripheral axon.*

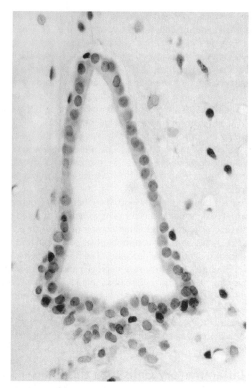

Fig. 2.16 *Ciliated cuboidal ependymal cells lining the central canal of the spinal cord. Similar cells line most of the ventricular system of the brain. (By permission from Kierszenbaum, A.L., 2002. Histology and Cell Biology. Mosby, St. Louis, and courtesy of Dr. Wan-hua Amy Yu.)*

cells are only rarely ciliated, and their ventricular surfaces bear many microvilli and apical blebs. They have numerous mitochondria, well-formed Golgi complexes and a rather flattened basal nucleus. They are joined laterally by tight junctions that form a barrier to the passage of materials across the ependyma and by desmosomes. Many of the cells are tanycytes (ependymal astrocytes) and have basal processes that project into the perivascular space surrounding the underlying capillaries. Significantly, these capillaries are fenestrated and therefore do not form a blood–brain barrier. It is believed that neuropeptides can pass from nervous tissue into the CSF by active transport through the ependymal cells in these specialized areas, giving them access to a wide population of neurones via the permeable ependymal lining of the rest of the ventricle.

The ependyma is highly modified where it lies adjacent to the vascular layer of the choroid plexus.

Choroid Plexus

The ependymal cells in the choroid plexus resemble those of the circumventricular organs, except that they do not have basal processes; instead, they form a cuboidal epithelium that rests on a basal lamina adjacent to the enclosed fold of pia mater and its capillaries (Figs. 2.17, 2.18). Capillaries of the choroid plexus are lined by a fenestrated endothelium. Cells have numerous long microvilli, with only a few cilia interspersed between them. They also have many mitochondria, large Golgi complexes and basal nuclei, consistent with their secretory activity: they produce most components of the CSF. They are linked by tight junctions that form a transepithelial barrier (a component of the blood–CSF barrier) and by desmosomes. Their lateral margins are highly folded.

The choroid plexus has a villous structure where the stroma is composed of pial meningeal cells, and it contains fine bundles of collagen and blood vessels. During fetal life, erythropoiesis occurs in the stroma, which is then occupied by bone marrow–like cells. In adult life, the stroma contains phagocytic cells, and these, together with the cells of the choroid plexus epithelium, phagocytose particles and proteins from the ventricular lumen.

Age-related changes occur in the choroid plexus that can be detected on imaging of the brain. Calcification of the choroid plexus can be detected by X-ray or CT scan in 0.5% of individuals in the first decade of life and in 86% in the eighth decade. There is a sharp rise in the incidence of calcification with age, from 35% of CT scans in the fifth decade to 75% in the sixth decade. The visible calcification is usually restricted to the glomus region of the choroid plexus, the vascular bulge in the choroid plexus as it curves to follow the anterior wall of the lateral ventricle into the temporal horn.

The capillaries beneath them have no fenestrations and few transcytotic vesicles, which is typical of the CNS. Where the ependyma overlies myelinated tracts of white matter, the cells are much flatter, and few are ciliated. There are gap junctions and desmosomes between cells, but their lateral margins interdigitate, unlike those overlying grey matter. No subependymal zone is present.

Specialized areas of ependymal cells are found in four areas around the margins of the third ventricle. These areas, called the circumventricular organs, consist of the lining of the median eminence of the hypothalamus, the subcommissural organ, the subfornical organ and the vascular organ of the lamina terminalis (Ch. 15). The area postrema, at the inferoposterior limit of the fourth ventricle, has a similar structure. In all these sites the ependymal

Microglia

Microglia are small dendritic cells found throughout the CNS (Fig. 2.19), including the retina. Evidence largely supports the view that they are derived from fetal monocytes or their precursors, which invade the developing nervous system. An alternative hypothesis holds that microglia share a lineage with ependymal cells and are thus neural tube derivatives. According to the monocyte theory, haematogenous cells pass through the walls of neural blood vessels and invade CNS tissue prenatally as amoeboid cells. Later they lose their motility and transform into typical microglia, bearing branched processes that ramify in non-overlapping territories within the brain. All microglial domains, defined by their dendritic fields, are equivalent in size and form a regular mosaic throughout the brain. The expression of microglia-specific antigens changes with age: many are downregulated as microglia attain the mature dendritic form.

Microglia have elongated nuclei with peripheral heterochromatin. The scant cytoplasm is pale staining and contains granules, scattered cisternae of rough endoplasmic reticulum and Golgi complexes at both poles. Two or three primary processes stem from opposite poles of the cell body and branch repeatedly to form short terminal processes. The function of microglia in the normal brain is obscure. Like astrocytes, microglia are activated by traumatic and ischaemic injury. In many diseases, including Parkinson's disease, Alzheimer's disease, multiple sclerosis, acquired immunodeficiency syndrome (AIDS), amyotrophic lateral sclerosis (motor neurone disease) and paraneoplastic encephalitis, they become phagocytic and are actively involved in synaptic stripping and clearance of neuronal debris. Some transform into amoeboid, motile cells.

Entry of Inflammatory Cells into the Brain

Although the CNS has long been considered an immunologically privileged site, lymphocyte surveillance of the brain may be a normal, low-grade activity that is enhanced in disease. Lymphocytes are able to enter the brain in response to viral infections and as part of the autoimmune response in multiple sclerosis. Activated, but not resting, lymphocytes pass through the endothelium of small venules, a process that requires the expression of recognition and adhesion molecules, which are induced following cytokine activation. They subsequently migrate into the brain parenchyma. Within the CNS, microglia and astrocytes can be induced by T-cell cytokines to act as efficient antigen-presenting cells. Lymphocytes probably drain along lymphatic pathways to regional cervical lymph nodes.

Polymorphonuclear leukocyte entry into the CNS is less common than lymphocyte entry, but it is seen in the early stages of infarction and autoimmune disease and, in particular, in pyogenic infections. These cells probably enter the nervous system following the expression of adhesion molecules on endothelium and pass through the endothelial layer. In the later stages of inflammation, monocytes may follow similar pathways.

Within the subarachnoid space, polymorphonuclear leukocytes and lymphocytes pass through the endothelium of large veins into the CSF during the inflammatory phase of meningitis.

PERIPHERAL NERVES

Afferent nerve fibres connect peripheral receptors to the CNS; their neuronal somata are located either in special sense organs (e.g. the olfactory epithelium) or in the sensory ganglia of craniospinal nerves. Efferent nerve fibres connect the CNS to the effector cells and tissues; they are the peripheral axons of neurones with somata in the central grey matter.

Widely variable numbers of peripheral nerve fibres are grouped into bundles (fasciculi). The size, number and pattern of fasciculi (Fig. 2.20) vary in different nerves and at different levels along their paths. Their number increases and their size decreases some distance proximal to a point of branching. Where nerves are subjected to pressure, such as deep to a retinaculum, fasciculi are increased in number but reduced in size, and the amount of associated connective tissue and degree of vascularity also increase. At these points, nerves may occasionally show a pink, fusiform dilatation, sometimes termed a pseudoganglion or gangliform enlargement.

Peripheral Nerve Fibres

The classification of peripheral nerve fibres is based on various parameters, such as conduction velocity, function and fibre diameter. Of the two classifications in common use, the first divides fibres into three major classes designated A, B and C, corresponding to peaks in the distribution of their conduction velocities. In humans, group A fibres are subdivided into α, β, δ and γ subgroups; group B fibres are preganglionic autonomic efferents, and group C fibres are unmyelinated. Fibre diameter and conduction velocity are proportional in most fibres. Group Aα fibres are the largest and conduct most rapidly, and group C fibres are the smallest and slowest.

The largest afferent axons (Aα fibres) innervate encapsulated cutaneous, joint and muscle receptors and some large alimentary enteroceptors. Aδ fibres innervate thermoreceptors and nociceptors, including those in dental pulp, skin and connective tissue. C fibres have thermoreceptive, nociceptive and interoceptive functions. The largest somatic efferent fibres (Aα) are up to

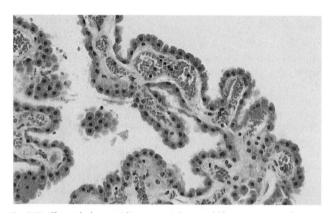

Fig. 2.17 *Choroid plexus within a ventricle. Frond-like projections of vascular stroma derived from the pial meninges are covered with a low columnar epithelium that secretes cerebrospinal fluid. (By permission from Stevens, A., Lowe, J.S., 1996. Human Histology, 2nd ed. Mosby, London.)*

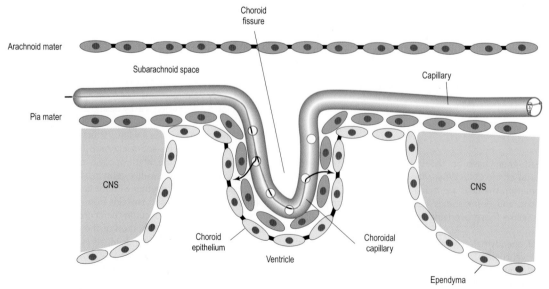

Fig. 2.18 *Schematic representation of the arrangement of tissues forming the choroid plexus. (By permission from Nolte, J., 2002. The Human Brain, 5th ed. Mosby, London.)*

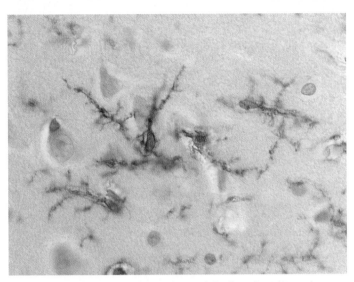

Fig. 2.19 *Micrograph showing activated microglial cells in the CNS, in a biopsy from a patient with Rasmussen's encephalitis, visualized using MHC class II antigen immunohistochemistry. (Courtesy of Dr. Norman Gregson, Division of Neurology, GKT School of Medicine, London.)*

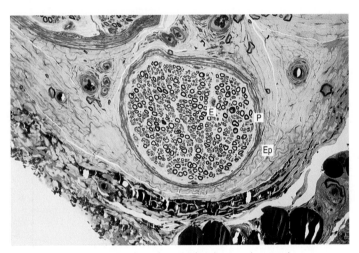

Fig. 2.20 *Transverse section through a peripheral nerve, showing the arrangement of its connective tissue sheaths. Individual axons, myelinated and unmyelinated, are arranged in a small fascicle bounded by a perineurium (P). E, endoneurium; Ep, epineurium. (Courtesy of Professor Susan Standring, GKT School of Medicine, London.)*

20 μm in diameter. They innervate extrafusal muscle fibres exclusively and conduct at a maximum of 120 m/s. Fibres to fast twitch muscles are larger than those to slow twitch muscles. Aβ fibres are restricted to collaterals of Aα fibres and form plaque endings on some intrafusal muscle fibres. Aγ fibres are exclusively fusimotor to plate and trail endings on intrafusal muscle fibres. C fibres are postganglionic sympathetic and parasympathetic axons. This scheme can be applied to all fibres of spinal and cranial nerves, except perhaps those of the olfactory nerve, whose fibres form a uniquely small and slow group.

A second classification, used for afferent fibres of somatic muscles, divides myelinated fibres into groups I, II and III. Group I fibres are large (12 to 22 μm) and include primary sensory fibres of muscle spindles (group Ia) and smaller fibres of Golgi tendon organs (group Ib). Group II fibres are the secondary sensory terminals of muscle spindles, with diameters of 6 to 12 μm. Group III fibres, 1 to 6 μm in diameter, have free sensory endings in the connective tissue sheaths around and within muscles and are believed to be nociceptive, relaying pressure pain in externally stimulated muscles. Paciniform (encapsulated) endings of muscle sheaths may also contribute fibres to this class. Group IV fibres are unmyelinated, with diameters of less than 1.5 μm; they include free endings in muscles and are primarily nociceptive.

Connective Tissue Sheaths

Nerve trunks, whether uni- or multifascicular, are surrounded by an epineurium. Individual fasciculi are enclosed by a multilayered perineurium, which in turn surrounds the endoneurium or intrafascicular connective tissue (see Fig. 2.20).

Epineurium

Epineurium is a condensation of loose (areolar) connective tissue and is derived from mesoderm. As a general rule, the more fasciculi present in a peripheral nerve, the thicker the epineurium. Epineurium contains fibroblasts, collagen (types I and III) and variable amounts of fat, and it cushions the nerve it surrounds. Loss of this protective layer may be associated with pressure palsies seen in wasted, bedridden patients. The epineurium also contains lymphatics (which probably pass to regional lymph nodes) and blood vessels—the vasa nervorum—which pass across the perineurium to communicate with a network of fine vessels within the endoneurium.

Perineurium

Perineurium extends from the CNS–PNS transition zone to the periphery, where it is continuous with the capsules of muscle spindles and encapsulated sensory endings. At unencapsulated endings and neuromuscular junctions, the perineurium ends openly. It consists of alternating layers of flattened polygonal cells, which are thought to be derived from fibroblasts, and collagen. It can often contain 15 to 20 layers of such cells, each layer enclosed by a basal lamina up to 0.5 μm thick. Cells within each layer interdigitate along extensive tight junctions, and their cytoplasm contains numerous pinocytotic vesicles and, often, bundles of microfilaments. These features indicate that the perineurium functions as a metabolically active diffusion barrier and, together with the blood–nerve barrier, probably plays an essential role in maintaining the osmotic milieu and fluid pressure within the endoneurium.

Endoneurium

Strictly speaking, the term endoneurium is restricted to interfascicular connective tissue, excluding the perineurial partitions within fascicles. Endoneurium consists of a fibrous matrix composed predominantly of type I collagen fibres, which are organized mainly in fine bundles lying parallel to the long axis of the nerve and condensed around individual Schwann cell–axon units and endoneurial vessels. The fibrous and cellular components of the endoneurium are bathed in endoneurial fluid at a slightly higher pressure than that outside in the surrounding epineurium. The major cellular constituents of the endoneurium are Schwann cells, associated with axons, and endothelial cells. Schwann cell–axon units and endothelial cells are enclosed within individual basal laminae. Other cells that are always present within the endoneurium are fibroblasts (constituting approximately 4% of the total endoneurial cell population), resident macrophages and mast cells.

Endoneurial arterioles have a poorly developed smooth muscle layer and do not autoregulate well. In sharp contrast, epineurial and perineurial vessels have a dense perivascular plexus of peptidergic, serotoninergic and adrenergic nerves.

Schwann Cells

Schwann cells are the major glial type in the PNS. *In vitro* they are fusiform in appearance. Both *in vitro* and *in vivo* they ensheathe peripheral axons and myelinate those greater than 2 μm in diameter. In a mature peripheral nerve fibre, they are distributed along the axons in longitudinal chains. The precise geometry of their association depends on whether the axon is myelinated or unmyelinated. In myelinated axons the territory of a Schwann cell defines an internode.

The molecular phenotype of mature myelin-forming Schwann cells is different from that of mature non-myelinating Schwann cells. Adult myelin-forming Schwann cells are characterized by the presence of several myelin proteins, some but not all of which are shared with oligodendrocytes and central myelin. In contrast, expression of the low-affinity neurotrophin receptor (p75[NTR]) and GFAP intermediate filament protein (which differs from the CNS form in its post-translational modification) characterizes adult non-myelin-forming Schwann cells.

Schwann cells arise during development from multipotent cells of the very early migrating neural crest, which also give rise to peripheral neurones. Axon-associated signals are critical in controlling the proliferation of developing Schwann cells and their precursors. Neurones may also regulate the developmentally programmed death of Schwann cell precursors, as a mechanism for matching numbers of axons and glia within each peripheral nerve bundle. Neuronal signals appear to control the production of basal laminae by Schwann cells, the induction and maintenance of myelination and, in the mature nerve, Schwann cell survival (few Schwann cells persist in chronically denervated nerves). Schwann cell signals may influence axonal calibre, and they are crucial in the repair of damaged peripheral nerves. The acute Schwann cell response to axonal injury and degeneration involves mitotic division and the elaboration of signals that promote the regrowth of axons.

Unmyelinated Axons

Unmyelinated axons are commonly 1 μm in diameter, although some may be 1.5 or even 2 μm in diameter. Groups of up to 10 small axons (0.15 to 2 μm in diameter) are enclosed within a chain of overlapping Schwann cells and surrounded by a basal lamina. Within each Schwann cell, individual axons are usually sequestered from their neighbours by delicate processes of cytoplasm (see Fig. 2.14). Axons move between Schwann cell chains as they pass proximodistally along a nerve fasciculus. It seems likely, on the basis of quantitative studies in subhuman primates, that axons from adjacent cord segments may share Schwann cell columns; this phenomenon may play a role in the evolution of neuropathic pain after nerve injury. In the absence of a myelin sheath and nodes of Ranvier, conduction along unmyelinated axons is not saltatory but electrotonic; the passage of impulses is therefore relatively slow (0.5 to 4 m/s).

Myelinated Axons

Myelinated axons (see Fig. 2.14) have a 1:1 relationship with their ensheathing Schwann cells. The territory of an individual Schwann cell defines an internode (Fig. 2.21): internodal length varies directly with the diameter of the fibre, from 150 to 1500 μm. The interval between two internodes is a node of Ranvier. In the PNS the myelin sheaths on either side of a node terminate in asymmetrically swollen paranodal bulbs. Schwann cell cytoplasm forms a continuous layer only in the perinuclear (mid-internodal) and paranodal regions. Between these sites, internodal Schwann cytoplasm forms a delicate network over the inner (abaxonal) surface of the myelin sheath. The outer (adaxonal) layer of Schwann cell cytoplasm is frequently discontinuous, and axons are surrounded by a narrow periaxonal space (15 to 20 nm), which, although nominally part of the extracellular space, is functionally isolated from it at the paranodes. For further details, see Scherer and Arroyo (2002).

Nodes of Ranvier (see Fig. 2.21) — PNS nodes of Ranvier are typically 0.8 to 1.1 μm long. The calibre of the nodal axon is characteristically reduced relative to that of the internodal axon; this is most marked in the largest calibre axons. Nodes are filled with an amorphous gap substance and processes of Schwann cell cytoplasm and are surrounded by a continuous basal lamina elaborated by the ensheathing Schwann cells. In large-calibre axons

the surfaces of the paranodal bulbs and of the underlying axon are fluted as they approach the nodes. The grooves in the external surface of the myelin sheath produced by this fluting are filled by Schwann cell cytoplasm, characterized by large numbers of mitochondria. In smaller fibres this arrangement is less obvious, although the paranodal cytoplasm usually contains mitochondria. Fine processes arise from the paranodal collar of Schwann cell cytoplasm and extend into the nodal gap substance, where they interdigitate with their counterparts from the adjacent Schwann cell. In small-calibre axons the processes contact the nodal axolemma. In large-calibre axons, where the processes are more numerous, they form regular hexagonal arrays that fill the nodal gap. Expanded terminal loops of paranodal Schwann cell cytoplasm either abut the paranodal axolemma directly or, in the case of the largest calibre myelinated axons, abut each other to form stacks with a typical 'ear of wheat' configuration.

Schmidt–Lanterman incisures — Schmidt–Lanterman incisures are helical decompactions of internodal myelin. The major dense line of the myelin sheath is split to enclose a continuous spiral band of granular cytoplasm that passes between the abaxonal and adaxonal layers of Schwann cell cytoplasm. The minor dense line of the incisural myelin sheath separates to create a long channel that connects the periaxonal space with the extracellular fluid in the endoneurium. The function of incisures is not known, but their structure suggests that they may participate in the transport of molecules across the myelin sheath.

Satellite Cells

Many non-neuronal cells of the nervous system have been called satellite cells. The list includes small, round extracapsular cells in peripheral ganglia, ganglionic capsular cells and Schwann cells. The term is sometimes used to describe all non-neuronal cells, both central and peripheral, that are closely associated with neuronal somata. The name is also given to precursor cells associated with striated muscle fibres. Within the nervous system, the term is most commonly reserved for the flat, epithelioid satellite cells (ganglionic glial cells, capsular cells) that surround the neuronal somata of peripheral ganglia (Fig. 2.22). The cytoplasm of capsular cells resembles that of Schwann cells, and their deep surfaces interdigitate with reciprocal infoldings in the membranes of the enclosed neurones. The capsular layer is continuous with

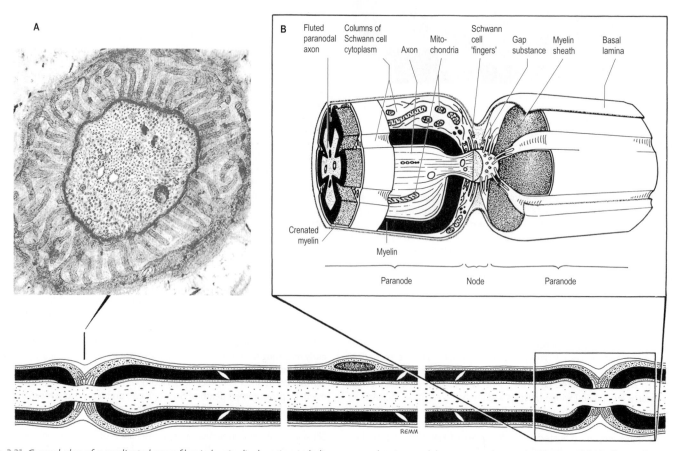

Fig. 2.21 *General plan of a myelinated nerve fibre in longitudinal section, including one complete internodal segment and two adjacent paranodal bulbs, used as a key for the more detailed microarchitecture of specific subregions.* ***A,*** *Transverse section through the centre of a node of Ranvier, with numerous finger-like processes of adjacent Schwann cells converging toward the nodal axolemma. Many microtubules and neurofilaments are visible within the axoplasm.* ***B,*** *Arrangement of the axon, myelin sheath and Schwann cell cytoplasm at the node of Ranvier and in the paranodal bulbs. (**A,** Courtesy of Professor Susan Standring, GKT School of Medicine, London; **B,** courtesy of P.L. Williams and D.N. Landon.)*

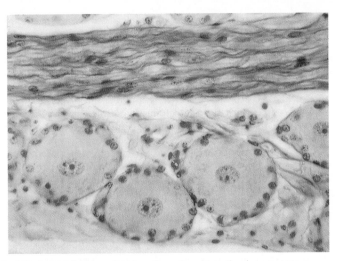

Fig. 2.22 Typical field in a dorsal root ganglion. Note the characteristic juxtaposition of large ovoid neuronal somata and the fascicles of myelinated and non-myelinated axons (top). Note also the nuclei of the capsular (satellite) cells that surround each neuronal soma (Grübler stain). (By permission from Dr. J.B. Kerr, Monash University, from Kerr, J.B., 1999. Atlas of Functional Histology. Mosby, London.)

similar cells that enclose the initial part of the dendroaxonal process in unipolar sensory neurones of the dorsal spinal roots and, subsequently, with the Schwann cells surrounding their peripheral and central processes.

Enteric Glia
Autonomic nerves of the ENS (Ch. 21) have more in common with central tracts than with other peripheral nerves. Enteric nerves do not have the collagenous coats of other peripheral nerves, and they lack an endoneurium. The enteric ganglionic neurones are supported by glia that closely resemble astrocytes and contain more GFAP than non-myelinating Schwann cells. The enteric glia also differ from Schwann cells, in that they do not produce a surrounding basal lamina.

Olfactory Ensheathing Glia
Olfactory ensheathing glia resemble Schwann cells in many respects but share a common origin with olfactory receptor neurones in the olfactory placode. They ensheathe olfactory sensory axons in a manner reminiscent of developing peripheral nerves because they surround, but do not segregate, bundles of up to 50 fine unmyelinated fibres to form approximately 20 fila olfactoria. Olfactory ensheathing glia accompany olfactory axons from the lamina propria of the olfactory epithelium to their synaptic contacts in the glomeruli of the olfactory bulbs. This unusual arrangement is quite unlike that seen at the CNS–PNS transition zone elsewhere in the nervous system, where there is an obvious boundary between the territories of peripheral and central glia.

Both ensheathing glia and the end-feet of astrocytes that lie between olfactory axon bundles contribute to the glia limitans at the pial surface of the olfactory bulbs. Ensheathing glia have a malleable phenotype; indeed, there may be more than one subtype. Some express GFAP as fine cytoplasmic filaments, and some express the low-affinity neurotrophin receptor.

Blood Supply of Peripheral Nerves
The blood vessels supply a nerve end in a capillary plexus that pierces the perineurium. Its branches run parallel with the fibres, connected by short transverse vessels, forming narrow, oblong meshes similar to those found in muscle. The blood supply of peripheral nerves is unusual. Endoneurial capillaries have atypically large diameters, and intercapillary distances are greater than in many other tissues. Peripheral nerves have two separate, functionally independent vascular systems: an extrinsic system (regional nutritive vessels and epineural vessels) and an intrinsic system (longitudinally running microvessels in the endoneurium). Anastomoses between the two systems produce considerable overlap in the territories of the segmental arteries. This unique pattern of vessels, together with a high basal nerve bloodflow relative to metabolic requirements, gives peripheral nerves a high degree of resistance to ischaemia.

Blood–Nerve Barrier
Just as the neuropil within the CNS is protected by a blood–brain barrier, the endoneurial contents of peripheral nerve fibres are protected by a blood–nerve barrier and by the cells of the perineurium. The blood–nerve barrier operates at the level of the endoneurial capillary walls. The endothelial cells are joined by tight junctions, are non-fenestrated and are surrounded by continuous basal laminae. The barrier is much less efficient in dorsal root and autonomic ganglia and in the distal parts of peripheral nerves.

GANGLIA
Ganglia are aggregations of neuronal somata. They occur in the dorsal roots of spinal nerves; in the sensory roots of the trigeminal, facial, glossopharyngeal, vagal and vestibulocochlear cranial nerves; in autonomic nerves and in the ENS. They vary in form and size. Each ganglion is enclosed within a capsule of fibrous connective tissue and contains neuronal somata and neuronal processes. Some ganglia, particularly in the ANS, contain fibres whose cell bodies lie elsewhere in the nervous system and pass through or terminate within them.

Sensory Ganglia
The sensory ganglia of dorsal spinal roots (see Fig. 2.22) and the ganglia of the trigeminal, facial, glossopharyngeal and vagal cranial nerves are enclosed in periganglionic connective tissue, which resembles the perineurium. Ganglionic neurones are unipolar. They have spherical or oval somata of varying sizes, which are aggregated in groups between fasciculi of myelinated and unmyelinated nerve fibres. For each neurone, the single axodendritic process bifurcates into central and peripheral processes; in myelinated fibres the junction occurs at a node of Ranvier. The peripheral process reaches a sensory ending, and because it conducts impulses toward the soma, strictly speaking, it functions as an elongated dendrite. However, because it has the typical structural and other functional properties of a peripheral axon, it is conventionally described as an axon.

Each soma has a capsule of satellite glial cells. Outside this lie the axodendritic process and its peripheral and central divisions, which are ensheathed by Schwann cells. The cells lie within a delicate vascular connective tissue that is continuous with the endoneurium of the nerve root.

Sensory ganglionic neurones are not entirely confined to discrete craniospinal ganglia. They often occupy heterotopic positions, either singly or in small groups, distal or proximal to their ganglia.

Herpes zoster — Primary infection with the varicella-zoster virus causes chickenpox. Following recovery, the virus remains dormant within dorsal root ganglia. Reactivation of the virus leads to shingles, which involves the dermatome supplied by the sensory nerve affected. Severe pain and a rash similar to chickenpox, often confined to one of the divisions of the trigeminal nerve or to a spinal nerve dermatome, are diagnostic. Herpes zoster involving the geniculate ganglion results in a lower motor neurone facial paralysis known as Ramsay Hunt syndrome. Occasionally, if the vestibulocochlear nerve is involved, there is vertigo, tinnitus and some deafness.

Autonomic Ganglia
Neurones in autonomic ganglia are multipolar and have dendritic trees on which preganglionic autonomic motor fibres synapse. They are surrounded by a mixed neuropil of afferent and efferent fibres, dendrites, synapses and non-neural cells. Autonomic ganglia are largely relay stations. A small fraction of their fibres traverses one or more ganglia without synapsing: some are efferent fibres en route to another ganglion, and some are afferents from the viscera and glands. There is considerable variation in the ratio between pre- and postganglionic fibres. Preganglionic sympathetic axons may synapse with many postganglionic neurones for the wide dissemination and perhaps amplification of sympathetic activity, a feature not found to the same degree in parasympathetic ganglia. Dissemination may also be achieved by connections with ganglionic interneurones or by the diffusion within the ganglion of transmitter substances produced locally (paracrine effect) or elsewhere (endocrine effect).

Most neurones of autonomic ganglia have somata ranging from 25 to 50 μm; a less common type is smaller, 15 to 20 μm, and often clustered in groups. Dendritic fields of these multipolar neurones are complex, and dendritic glomeruli have been observed in many ganglia. Clusters of small granular adrenergic vesicles occupy the soma and dendrites, probably representing the storage of catecholamines. Ganglionic neurones receive many axodendritic synapses from preganglionic nerve fibres; axosomatic synapses are less numerous. Postganglionic fibres commonly arise from the initial stem of a large dendrite and produce few or no collateral processes.

Enteric Ganglia
The ENS is composed of ganglionic neurones and associated nerves (Fig. 2.23) serving different functions, including regulation of gut motility and mucosal transport. Extrinsic autonomic fibres supply the gut wall, and together with intrinsic enteric ganglionic neurones and the endocrine and cardiovascular systems, they integrate the activities of the digestive system as a result of

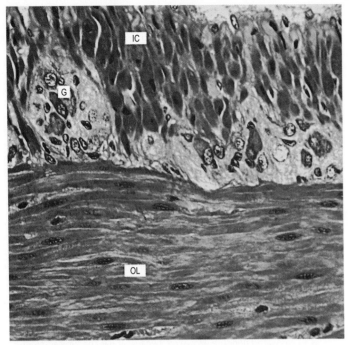

Fig. 2.23 *Myenteric plexus of ganglia (G) and fibres that lies between the inner circular (IC) and outer longitudinal (OL) smooth muscle layers of the gut wall.*

either interaction with enteric neurones (e.g. via vagal fibres) or direct regulation of the local bloodflow (via postganglionic sympathetic fibres).

Enteric ganglionic neurones are predominantly peptidergic or monoaminergic and can be classified accordingly. Other neurones express nitric oxide synthase and release NO. There are regional differences in the numbers of ganglia and the classes of neurone they contain. For example, myenteric plexus ganglia are less frequent in oesophageal smooth muscle (1.5 per centimeter) than in the small and large intestines (approximately 10 per centimeter of bowel length). Oesophageal enteric neurones all coexpress VIP and neuropeptide Y (NPY), whereas gastrin- and somatostatin-containing fibres are rare. In contrast, gastrin- and somatostatin-containing neurones are abundant in the small and large intestines, and although both types are present, very few VIP neurones coexpress NPY.

Correlations can be made between some phenotypical classes of enteric neurones and their functional properties, although much remains undetermined. Cholinergic neurones are excitatory, cause muscular contraction and mainly project orally. NO-releasing neurones are generally larger and project for longer distances, mainly anally. They are inhibitory neurones, some of which also express VIP, and they promote muscular relaxation.

SENSORY ENDINGS (Fig. 2.24)
General Features of Sensory Receptors
There are three major forms of sensory receptor: neuroepithelial, epithelial and neuronal.

A neuroepithelial receptor is a neurone with a soma situated near a sensory surface and an axon that conveys sensory signals into the CNS to synapse on second-order neurones. This is an evolutionarily primitive arrangement, and the only example in humans is the sensory neurone of the olfactory epithelium.

An epithelial receptor is a cell that is modified from non-nervous sensory epithelium and innervated by a primary sensory neurone, whose soma lies near the CNS. Examples are epidermal Merkel cells, auditory receptors and taste buds. Activity in this type of receptor elicits the passage of excitation from the receptor by neurotransmission across a synaptic gap. In taste receptors, individual cells are constantly being renewed from the surrounding epithelium. In many ways, visual receptors in the retina are similar in their form and relations. These cells are derived from the ventricular lining of the fetal brain and are not replaced.

A neuronal receptor is a primary sensory neurone with a soma in a craniospinal ganglion and a peripheral axon, the end of which is a sensory terminal. All cutaneous sensors (with the exception of Merkel cells) and proprioceptors are of this type; their sensory terminals may be encapsulated or linked to special mesodermal or ectodermal structures to form part of the sensory apparatus. The extraneural cells are not necessarily excitable, but they create the environment for excitation of the neuronal process.

The receptor stimulus is transduced into a graded change of electrical potential at the receptor surface (receptor potential), which initiates an all-or-none action potential transmitted to the CNS. This may occur in the receptor, where this is a neurone, or partly in the receptor and partly in the neurone innervating it, in the case of epithelial receptors.

Transduction varies with the modality of stimulus, usually causing depolarization of the receptor membrane (or, in the retina, hyperpolarization). In mechanoreceptors it may involve deformation of the membrane structure, which results in strain- or voltage-sensitive transducing protein molecules opening ion channels. In chemoreceptors, receptor action may resemble that for ACh at neuromuscular junctions. Visual receptors share similarities with chemoreceptors: light causes changes in receptor proteins, which activate G-proteins, resulting in the release of second messengers, and this affects membrane permeability.

The quantitative responses of sensory endings to stimuli vary greatly and increase the flexibility of sensory systems' functional design. Although increased excitation with an increasing stimulus level is a common pattern ('on' response), some receptors respond to decreased stimulation ('off' response). Even unstimulated receptors show varying degrees of spontaneous background activity against which an increase or decrease in activity occurs with changing levels of stimulus. In all receptors studied, when stimulation is maintained at a steady level, there is an initial burst (the dynamic phase), followed by gradual adaptation to a steady level (the static phase). Although all receptors show these two phases, one may predominate, providing a distinction between rapidly adapting endings, which accurately record the rate of stimulus onset, and slowly adapting endings, which signal the constant amplitude of a stimulus (e.g. position sense). Dynamic and static phases are reflected in the amplitude and duration of the receptor potential and also in the frequency of action potentials in the sensory fibres. The stimulus strength necessary to elicit a response in a receptor (i.e., its threshold level) varies greatly between receptors and provides an extra level of information about stimulus strength.

Functional Classification of Receptors
Receptors may be classified in several ways. They may be classified by the modalities to which they are sensitive, such as mechanoreceptors (which are responsive to deformation, e.g. touch, pressure, sound waves), chemoreceptors, photoreceptors and thermoreceptors. Some receptors respond selectively to more than one modality (polymodal receptors): they usually have high thresholds and respond to damaging stimuli associated with irritation or pain (nociceptors).

Another widely used classification divides receptors on the basis of their distribution in the body into exteroceptors, proprioceptors and interoceptors. Exteroceptors and proprioceptors are receptors of somatic afferent components of the nervous system, whereas interoceptors are receptors of the visceral afferent pathways.

Exteroceptors respond to external stimuli and are found at, or close to, body surfaces. They can be subdivided into the general or cutaneous sense organs and the special sensory organs. General sensory receptors include free and encapsulated terminals in skin and near hairs. Special sensory organs are the olfactory, visual, acoustic, vestibular and taste receptors.

Proprioceptors respond to stimuli to deeper tissues, especially of the locomotor system, and are concerned with detecting movement, mechanical stresses and position. They include Golgi tendon organs, neuromuscular spindles, Pacinian corpuscles, other endings in joints and vestibular receptors. Proprioceptors are stimulated by the contraction of muscles, the movement of joints and changes in the position of the body. They are essential for the coordination of muscles, the grading of muscular contraction and the maintenance of equilibrium.

Interoceptors are found in the walls of the viscera, glands and vessels, where their terminations include free nerve endings, encapsulated terminals and endings associated with specialized epithelial cells. Nerve terminals are found in the layers of visceral walls and the adventitia of blood vessels, but the detailed structure and function of many of these endings are not well established. Encapsulated (lamellated) endings occur in the heart, adventitia and mesenteries. Free terminal arborizations occur in the endocardium, loose connective tissue, the endomysium of all muscles and connective tissue generally.

Visceral nerve terminals are not usually responsive to stimuli that act on exteroceptors, and they do not respond to localized mechanical and thermal stimuli. Tension produced by excessive muscular contraction or by visceral distension often causes pain, particularly in pathological states; this pain is frequently poorly localized and of a deep-seated nature. Visceral pain is often referred to the corresponding dermatome.

Interoceptors include vascular chemoreceptors, such as the carotid body, and baroceptors, which are concerned with the regulation of bloodflow and

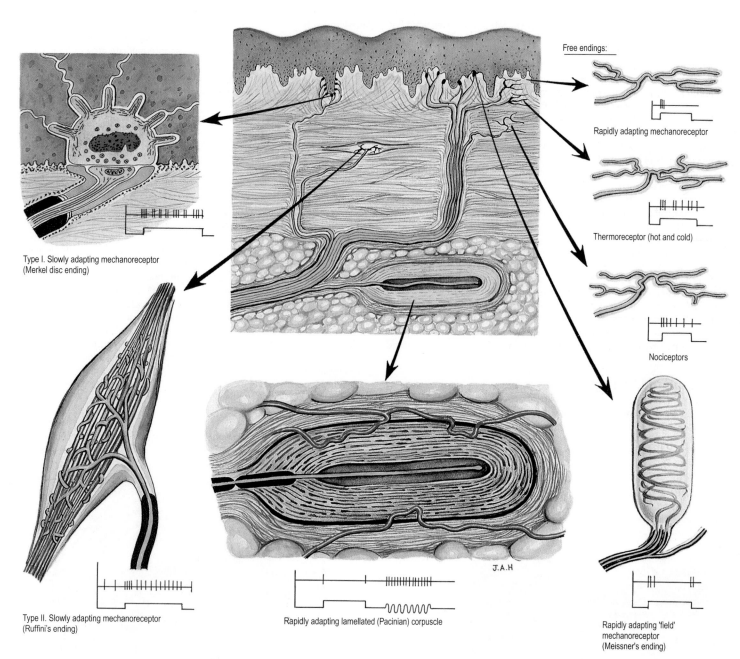

Free endings:

Rapidly adapting mechanoreceptor

Thermoreceptor (hot and cold)

Nociceptors

Type I. Slowly adapting mechanoreceptor
(Merkel disc ending)

Type II. Slowly adapting mechanoreceptor
(Ruffini's ending)

Rapidly adapting lamellated (Pacinian) corpuscle

Rapidly adapting 'field'
mechanoreceptor
(Meissner's ending)

J.A.H

Fig. 2.24 *Some major types of sensory endings of general afferent fibres (omitting neuromuscular, neurotendinous and hair-related types).*

pressure and with the control of respiration. Irritant receptors respond polymodally to noxious chemicals or damaging mechanical stimuli and are widely distributed in the epithelia of the alimentary and respiratory tracts; they may initiate protective reflexes.

Free Nerve Endings

Sensory endings that branch to form plexuses occur in many sites (see Fig. 2.24). They occur in all connective tissues, including those of the dermis, fasciae, capsules of organs, ligaments, tendons, adventitia of blood vessels, meninges, articular capsules, periosteum, perichondrium, Haversian systems in bone, parietal peritoneum, walls of viscera and endomysium of all types of muscle. They also innervate the epithelium of the skin, corneas, buccal cavity and alimentary and respiratory tracts and their glands. Within epithelia they lack Schwann cell ensheathment and are enveloped instead by epithelial cells. Afferent fibres from free terminals may be myelinated or unmyelinated but are always of small diameter and low conduction velocity. When afferent axons are myelinated, their terminal arborizations are not. These terminals serve several sensory modalities. In the dermis, they may be responsive to moderate cold or heat (thermoreceptors); light mechanical touch (mechanoreceptors); damaging heat, cold or deformation (unimodal nociceptors) and damaging stimuli of several kinds (polymodal nociceptors). Similar fibres in deeper tissues may also signal extreme conditions, and these are experienced, as with all nociceptors, as pain. Free endings in the corneas, dentine and periosteum may be exclusively nociceptive.

Special types of free endings are associated with epidermal structures in the skin. They include terminals associated with hair follicles (peritrichial receptors), which branch from myelinated fibres in the deep dermal cutaneous plexus; the number, size and form of the endings are related to the size and type of hair follicle innervated. These endings respond mainly to movement when hair is deformed and belong to the rapidly adapting mechanoreceptor group.

Merkel tactile endings lie at the base of the epidermis or around the apical ends of some hair follicles and are innervated by large myelinated axons. The axon expands into a disc, which is applied closely to the base of the Merkel cell in the basal layer of the epidermis. Merkel cells, which are believed to be derived from the neural crest, contain many large (50 to 100 nm) dense-core vesicles, presumably containing transmitters, which are concentrated near the junction with the axon. Merkel endings are slow-adapting mechanoreceptors and are responsive to sustained pressure and sensitive to the edges of applied objects.

Encapsulated Endings

Encapsulated endings are a major group of special endings, although they exhibit considerable variety in their size, shape and distribution. They all share a common feature, which is that the axon terminal is encapsulated by non-excitable cells. This category of ending includes lamellated corpuscles of various kinds (e.g. Meissner's, Pacinian), Golgi tendon organs, neuromuscular spindles and Ruffini endings (see Fig. 2.24).

Meissner's Corpuscles

Meissner's corpuscles are found in the dermal papillae of all parts of the hands and feet, the fronts of the forearms, lips, palpebral conjunctiva and

mucous membrane of the apical part of the tongue. They are most concentrated in thick, hairless skin, especially of the finger pads, where there may be up to 24 corpuscles/cm^2 in young adults. Mature corpuscles are cylindrical in shape, approximately 80 μm long and 30 μm across, with their long axes perpendicular to the skin surface. Each corpuscle has a connective tissue capsule and a central core (Fig. 2.25). Meissner's corpuscles are rapidly adapting mechanoreceptors, sensitive to shape and textural changes in exploratory and discriminatory touch; their acute sensitivity provides the neural basis for reading Braille text.

Pacinian Corpuscles

Pacinian corpuscles are situated subcutaneously in the palmar and plantar aspects of the hands and feet and their digits; in the external genitalia, arms, neck, nipple, periosteum, and interosseous membranes; near joints and in the mesentries. They are oval, spherical or irregularly coiled and are up to 2 mm long and 100 to 500 μm or more across; the larger ones are visible to the naked eye. Each corpuscle has a capsule, an intermediate growth zone and a central core that contains an axon terminal. The capsule is formed by approximately 30 concentrically arranged lamellae of flat cells approximately 0.2 μm thick (Fig. 2.26). Adjacent cells overlap, and successive lamellae are separated by an amorphous proteoglycan matrix that contains circularly oriented collagen fibres, closely applied to the surfaces of the lamellar cells. The amount of collagen increases with age. The intermediate zone is cellular, and its cells become incorporated into the capsule or core, so that it is not clearly defined in mature corpuscles. The core consists of approximately 60 bilateral, compacted lamellae that lie on both sides of a central nerve terminal.

Each corpuscle is supplied by a myelinated axon, which loses its myelin sheath and, at the junction with the core, its ensheathing Schwann cell. The naked axon runs through the central axis of the core and ends in a slightly expanded bulb. It is in contact with the innermost core lamellae, is transversely oval and sends short projections of unknown function into clefts in the lamellae. It contains numerous large mitochondria and minute vesicles approximately 5 nm in diameter, which aggregate opposite the clefts. The cells of the capsule and core lamellae are thought to be specialized fibroblasts, but some may be Schwann cells. Elastic fibrous tissue forms an overall external capsule to the corpuscle. Pacinian corpuscles are supplied by capillaries that accompany the axon as it enters the capsule.

Pacinian corpuscles act as very rapidly adapting mechanoreceptors. They respond only to sudden disturbances and are especially sensitive to vibration. The rapidity may be partly due to the lamellated capsule acting as a high pass frequency filter, damping slow distortions by fluid movement between lamellar cells. Groups of corpuscles respond to pressure changes, such as the grasping or releasing of an object.

Ruffini Endings

Ruffini endings are slowly adapting mechanoreceptors. They are found in the dermis of thin, hairy skin, where they function as dermal stretch receptors and

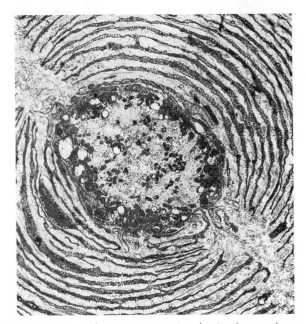

Fig. 2.26 *Pacinian corpuscle in transverse section, showing the central core region and lamellar cells surrounding the axon. Note the presence of large intercellular spaces between the lamellar cells and the numerous mitochondria in the axon (Rhesus monkey finger). (Material provided by W. Hamann, Department of Anaesthetics, Guy's Hospital Medical School, London.)*

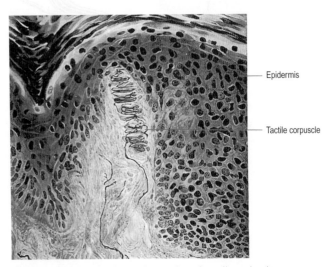

Epidermis

Tactile corpuscle

Fig. 2.25 *Tactile Meissner's corpuscle in a dermal papilla in the skin, demonstrated using the Gros–Bielschowsky technique. (Courtesy of N. Cauna, University of Pittsburgh.)*

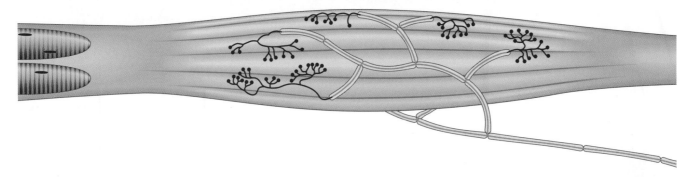

Fig. 2.27 Structure and innervation of a Golgi tendon organ. For clarity, the perineurium and endoneurium have been omitted to show the distribution of nerve fibres ramifying between the collagen fibre bundles of the tendon.

are responsive to maintained stresses in dermal collagen. They consist of highly branched, unmyelinated endings of myelinated afferents. They ramify between bundles of collagen fibres within a spindle-shaped structure that is enclosed partly by a fibrocellular sheath derived from the perineurium of the nerve. They appear electrophysiologically similar to Golgi tendon organs, which they resemble, although they are less organized structurally. Similar structures appear in joint capsules.

Golgi Tendon Organs

Golgi tendon organs are found mainly near musculotendinous junctions (Fig. 2.27), where more than 50 may occur at one site. Each terminal is closely related to a group of muscle fibres (up to 20) as they insert into the tendon. Golgi tendon endings are approximately 500 μm long and 100 μm in diameter and consist of small bundles of tendon fibres enclosed in a delicate capsule. The collagen bundles (intrafusal fasciculi) are less compact than elsewhere in the tendon; the collagen fibres are smaller, and the fibroblasts are larger and more numerous. One or more thickly myelinated axons enter the capsule and divide. Their branches, which lose their Schwann cell sheaths, terminate in leaf-like enlargements containing vesicles and mitochondria, which wrap around the tendon. A basal lamina or process of Schwann cell cytoplasm separates the nerve terminals from the collagen bundles that make up the tendon. The endings are activated by passive stretch of the tendon but are much more sensitive to active contraction of the muscle. They are important in providing proprioceptive information, complementing that from neuromuscular spindles. Their responses are slowly adapting, and they signal maintained tension.

Neuromuscular Spindles

Neuromuscular spindles are essential for the control of muscle contraction. Each spindle contains a few small, specialized intrafusal muscle fibres innervated by both sensory and motor nerve fibres (Figs. 2.28, 2.29). The whole is surrounded equatorially by a fusiform spindle capsule of connective tissue, consisting of an outer perineurial-like sheath of flattened fibroblasts and collagen and an inner sheath that forms delicate tubes around individual intrafusal fibres. A gelatinous fluid rich in glycosaminoglycans fills the space between the two sheaths.

There are usually 5 to 14 intrafusal fibres (the number varies between muscles) and two major types of fibre—nuclear bag and nuclear chain fibres—which are distinguished by the arrangement of nuclei in their sarcoplasm. In the former, the equatorial cluster of nuclei makes the fibre bulge slightly, whereas in the latter, the nuclei form a single axial row. Nuclear bag fibres are greater in diameter than chain fibres and extend beyond the surrounding capsule to the endomysium of nearby extrafusal muscle fibres. Nuclear chain fibres are attached at their poles to the capsule or to the sheaths of nuclear bag fibres.

The intrafusal fibres resemble typical skeletal muscle fibres, except that the zone of myofibrils is thin around the nuclei. One subtype of nuclear bag fibre (dynamic bag 1) generally lacks M lines, possesses little sarcoplasmic reticulum and has an abundance of mitochondria and oxidative enzymes but little glycogen. A second subtype of bag fibre (static bag 2) has distinct M lines and abundant glycogen. Nuclear chain fibres have marked M lines, sarcoplasmic reticulum and T-tubules, abundant glycogen, but few mitochondria. These variations reflect, as they do in muscle generally, the contractile properties of different intrafusal fibres (Boyd 1985).

The sensory innervation of muscle spindles is of two types, both of which involve the unmyelinated terminations of large myelinated axons. Primary (anulospiral) endings are equatorially placed and form spirals around the nucleated parts of intrafusal fibres. They are the endings of large sensory fibres (group Ia afferents), each of which sends branches to a number of intrafusal muscle fibres. Each terminal lies in a deep sarcolemmal groove in the spindle plasma membrane beneath its basal lamina. Secondary ('flower spray') endings, which may be spray shaped or anular, are largely confined to nuclear chain fibres and are the branched terminals of somewhat thinner myelinated (group II) afferents. They are varicose and spread in a narrow band on both sides of the primary endings. They lie close to the sarcolemma, although not in grooves. In essence, primary endings are rapidly adapting, whereas secondary endings have a regular, slowly adapting response to static stretch.

There are three types of motor endings in muscle spindles. Two are from fine, myelinated, fusimotor (γ) efferents, and one is from myelinated (β) efferent collaterals of extrafusal slow twitch muscle fibres. The fusimotor efferents terminate nearer the equatorial region, where their terminals either resemble the motor end-plates of extrafusal fibres (plate endings) or are more diffuse (trail endings). Stimulation of the fusimotor and β-efferents causes contraction of the intrafusal fibres and activation of their sensory endings.

Muscle spindles signal the length of extrafusal muscle both at rest and throughout contraction and relaxation, the velocity of their contraction and changes in velocity. These modalities may be related to the different behaviours of the three major types of intrafusal fibres and their sensory terminals. The sensory endings of one type of nuclear bag fibre (dynamic bag 1) are particularly concerned with signalling rapid changes in length that occur during movement, whereas those of the second type of bag fibre (static bag 2) are less responsive to movement. The afferents from chain fibres have relatively slowly adapting responses at all times. These elements can therefore detect complex changes in the state of the extrafusal muscle surrounding spindles and can signal fluctuations in length, tension, velocity of length change and acceleration. Moreover, they are under complex central control: efferent (fusimotor) nerve fibres, by regulating the strength of contraction, can adjust the length of the intrafusal fibres and thereby the responsiveness of spindle sensory endings. In summary, the organization of spindles allows them to actively monitor muscle conditions and compare intended and actual movements and thus provide detailed input to spinal, cerebellar, extrapyramidal and cortical centres about the state of the locomotor apparatus.

Joint Receptors

The arrays of receptors situated in and near articular capsules provide information on the position and movement of joints and the stresses acting on them. Structural and functional studies have demonstrated at least four types of joint receptors; their proportions and distribution vary by site. Three are encapsulated endings, and the fourth is a free terminal arborization.

Type I endings are capsulated corpuscles of the slowly adapting mechanoreceptor (Ruffini) type, situated in the superficial layers of fibrous joint capsules in small clusters and supplied by myelinated afferent axons. Being slowly adapting, they provide awareness of joint position and movement and respond to patterns of stress in articular capsules. They are particularly common in joints where static positional sense is necessary for the control of posture (e.g. hip, knee).

Type II endings are lamellated receptors and resemble small versions of the large Pacinian corpuscles found in general connective tissue. They occur in small groups throughout joint capsules, particularly in the deeper layers and other articular structures (e.g. fat pad of the temporomandibular joint). They are rapidly adapting, low-threshold mechanoreceptors, sensitive to movement and pressure changes, and they respond to joint movement and transient stresses in the joint capsule. They are supplied by myelinated afferent axons but are probably not involved in the conscious awareness of joint sensation.

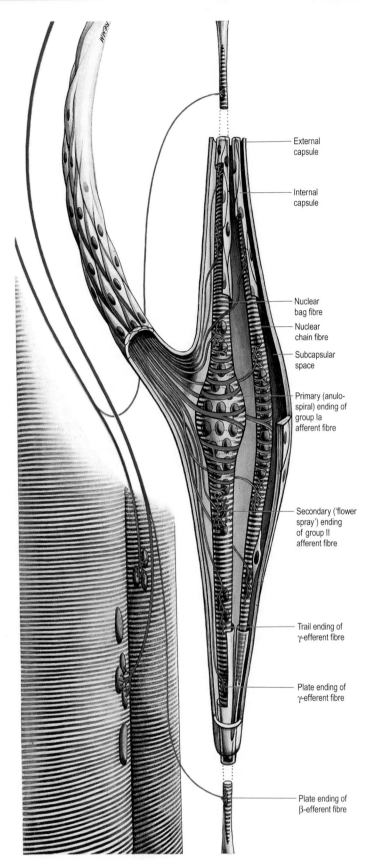

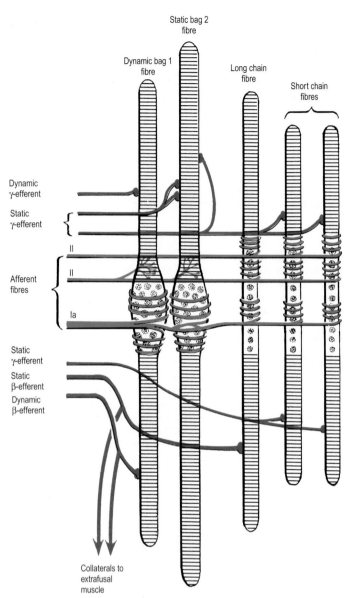

External
capsule

Internal
capsule

Nuclear
bag fibre

Nuclear
chain fibre

Subcapsular
space

Primary (anulo-
spiral) ending of
group Ia
afferent fibre

Secondary ('flower
spray') ending
of group II
afferent fibre

Trail ending of
γ-efferent fibre

Plate ending of
γ-efferent fibre

Plate ending of
β-efferent fibre

Fig. 2.28 *Schematic three-dimensional representation of a neuromuscular spindle, showing nuclear bag and nuclear chain fibres; these are innervated by the sensory anulospiral and 'flower spray' terminals (blue) and by the γ- and β-fusimotor terminals (red). See also Fig. 2.29.*

Dynamic bag 1
fibre

Static bag 2
fibre

Long chain
fibre

Short chain
fibres

Dynamic
γ-efferent

Static
γ-efferent

II

Afferent
fibres

II

Ia

Static
γ-efferent

Static
β-efferent

Dynamic
β-efferent

Collaterals to
extrafusal
muscle

Fig. 2.29 *Schematic three-dimensional representation of nuclear bag and nuclear chain fibres in a neuromuscular spindle. Dynamic β- and γ-efferents innervate dynamic bag 1 intrafusal fibres; whereas static β- and γ-efferents innervate static bag 2 and nuclear chain intrafusal fibres.*

blood vessels of the synovial layer. They are high-threshold, slowly adapting receptors and are thought to respond to excessive movements, providing a basis for articular pain.

NEUROMUSCULAR JUNCTIONS
See Chapter 22.

CNS–PNS TRANSITION ZONE
The transition between CNS and PNS usually occurs some distance from the point at which nerve roots emerge from the brain or the spinal cord. The segment of root that contains components of both CNS and PNS tissue is called the CNS–PNS transition zone. All axons in the PNS, other than post-ganglionic autonomic neurones, cross such a transition zone. Macroscopically, as a nerve root is traced toward the spinal cord or the brain, it splits into several thinner rootlets that may, in turn, subdivide into minirootlets. The transition zone is located within either a rootlet or a minirootlet (Fig. 2.30). The arrangement of roots and rootlets varies according to whether the root trunk is ventral, dorsal or cranial. Thus, in dorsal roots, the main root trunk separates into a fan of rootlets and minirootlets that enter the spinal cord in sequence along the dorsolateral sulcus. In certain cranial nerves, the miniroot-lets come together central to the transition zone and enter the brain as a stump of white matter.

Microscopically, the transition zone is characterized by an axial CNS compartment surrounded by a PNS compartment. The zone lies more periph-erally in sensory than in motor nerves, but in both, the apex of the transition

Type III endings are identical to Golgi tendon organs in structure and func-tion; they occur in articular ligaments but not in joint capsules. They are high-threshold, slowly adapting receptors that apparently serve, at least in part, to prevent excessive stresses at joints by reflex inhibition of the adjacent muscles. They are innervated by large myelinated afferent axons.

Type IV endings are free terminals of myelinated and unmyelinated axons. They ramify in articular capsules and the adjacent fat pads and around the

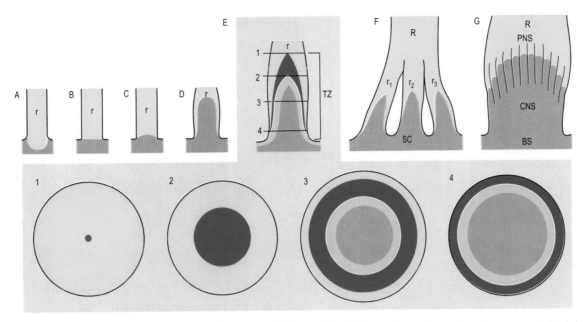

Fig. 2.30 *Schematic representation of the nerve root–spinal cord junction. **A–E**, Different CNS–PNS borderline arrangements. **A**, Concave borderline (white line) and inverted transitional zone (TZ). **B**, Flat borderline situated at the level of the rootlet (r)–spinal cord junction. **C** and **D**, Convex, dome-shaped borderline; the CNS expansion into the rootlet is moderate in **C** and extensive in **D**. Brown denotes CNS tissue. The glial fringe is not shown. **E**, Pointed borderline. The extent of the TZ is indicated. The cross-sectional appearance at four different TZ levels and the distribution of the different TZs are shown in the lower part of the illustration. Yellow, endoneurial zone; dark green, glial fringe; light green, mantle zone; brown, core zone. **F**, Root–spinal cord junction. The root (R) splits into rootlets (r), each with its own TZ and separate attachment to the spinal cord (SC). **G**, Arrangement noted in several cranial nerve roots (e.g., vestibulocochlear nerve). The PNS component of the root separates into a bundle of closely packed minirootlets, each equipped with a TZ. The minirootlets reunite centrally. BS, brain stem. (By permission from Dyck, P.J., et al, 1993. Peripheral Neuropathy, 3rd ed. WB Saunders, Philadelphia.)*

zone is described as a glial dome whose convex surface is directed distally. The centre of the dome consists of fibres with a typical CNS organization, surrounded by an outer mantle of astrocytes (corresponding to the glia limitans). From this mantle, numerous glial processes project into the endoneurial compartment of the peripheral nerve, where they interdigitate with its Schwann cells. The astrocytes form a loose reticulum through which axons pass. Peripheral myelinated axons usually cross the zone at a node of Ranvier, which is here termed a PNS–CNS compound node.

A cell type, the boundary cap cell, has recently been described in avian and mammalian species. Such cells transiently occupy the presumptive dorsal root transition zone of the embryonic spinal cord. Boundary cap cells are derived from the neural crest and are thought to prevent cell mixing at this interface and to help dorsal root ganglion afferents navigate their path to targets in the spinal cord. Further details are given in Golding and Cohen (1997).

References

Boyd, I.A., 1985. Muscle spindles and stretch reflexes. In: Swash, M., Kennard, C. (Eds.), Scientific Basis of Clinical Neurology. Churchill Livingstone, Edinburgh, pp. 74–97. *A detailed account of the functional aspects of neuromuscular spindles.*

Butt, A.M., Berry, M., 2000. Oligodendrocytes and the control of myelination in vivo: new insights from the rat anterior medullary velum. J. Neurosci. Res. 59, 477–488. *Describes the characteristics of a glial cell that contacts nodes of Ranvier in the CNS.*

Golding, J., Cohen, J., 1997. Border controls at the mammalian spinal cord: late-surviving neural crest boundary cap cells at dorsal root entry sites may regulate sensory afferent ingrowth and entry zone morphogenesis. Mol. Cell Neurosci. 9, 381–396. *Describes the characteristics of a novel type of cell concerned with establishing the boundary between the CNS and PNS during embryogenesis.*

Kandel, E.R., Schwartz, J.H., 2000. Principles of Neural Science, fourth ed. McGraw-Hill, New York.

Scherer, S.S., Arroyo, E.J., 2002. Recent progress on the molecular organization of myelinated axons. J. Periph. Nerv. Syst. 7, 1–12. *Review of the molecular architecture of myelinated peripheral axons and their myelin sheaths.*

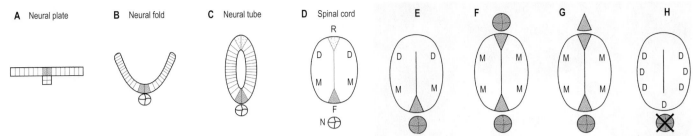

Fig. 3.7 *A–D, Successive stages in the development of the neural tube and spinal cord. **A**, The neural plate consists of epithelial cells. Cells in the midline of the neural plate are contacted directly by the notochord. More lateral regions of the neural plate overlie the paraxial mesenchyme (not shown). **B**, During neurulation, the neural plate bends at its midline, which elevates the lateral edges of the plate as the neural folds. Contact between the midline of the neural plate and the notochord is maintained at this stage. **C**, The neural tube is formed when the dorsal tips of the neural folds fuse. Cells in the region of fusion form the roof plate, which is a specialized group of dorsal midline cells. **D**, Cells at the ventral midline of the neural tube retain proximity to the notochord and differentiate into the floor plate. After neural tube closure, neuroepithelial cells continue to proliferate and eventually differentiate into defined classes of neurones at different dorsoventral positions within the spinal cord. For example, sensory relay, commissural and other classes of dorsal neurones (D) differentiate near the roof plate (R), and motor neurones (M) differentiate ventrally near the floor plate (F), which by this time is no longer in contact with the notochord (N). **E–H**, Summary of the results of experiments in chick embryos in which the notochord or floor plate is grafted to the dorsal midline of the neural tube or the notochord is removed before neural tube closure. **E**, The normal condition, showing the ventral location of motor neurones (M) and the dorsal location of sensory relay neurones (D). **F**, Dorsal grafts of a notochord result in induction of a floor plate in the dorsal midline and ectopic dorsal motor neurones (M). **G**, Dorsal grafts of a floor plate induce a new floor plate in the dorsal midline and ectopic dorsal motor neurones (M). **H**, Removal of the notochord results in the elimination of the floor plate and motor neurones and the expression of dorsal cells types (D) in the ventral region of the spinal cord. (After Jessell, Dodd. 1992. WB Saunders.)*

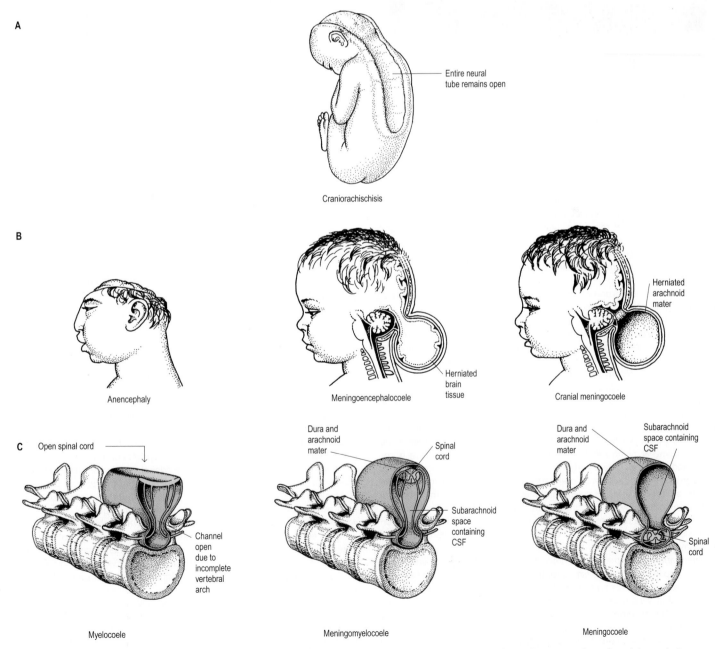

Fig. 3.8 *Defects caused by failure of neural tube formation. **A**, Total failure of neurulation. **B**, Failure of rostral neurulation. **C**, Failure of caudal neurulation.*

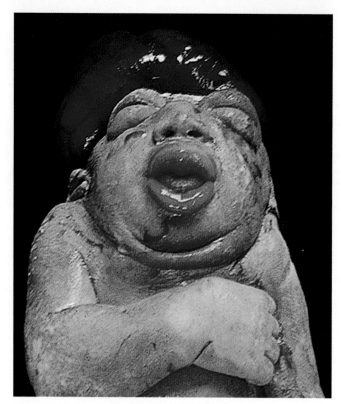

Fig. 3.9 *Anencephaly.*

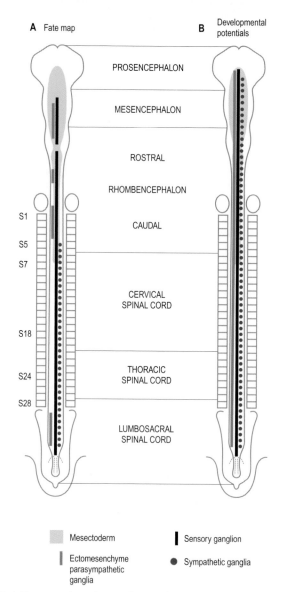

Fig. 3.10 *A, Fate map along the neural crest of the presumptive territories that yield the ectomesenchyme; the sensory, parasympathetic and sympathetic ganglia; and neural crest–derived mesenchyme in normal development. B, Developmental potentials for the same cell types. If neural crest cells from any level of the neural axis are implanted in the appropriate sites of a host embryo, they can give rise to almost all the cell types forming the various kinds of peripheral nervous system ganglia. This is not true for the neural crest–derived mesenchyme, whose precursors are confined to the cephalic area of the crest down to the level of somite (S) 5.*

Intermediate between the epibranchial and dorsolateral placodes are the profundal and trigeminal placodes, which fuse in humans to form a single entity. Prospective neuroblasts migrate from foci dispersed throughout the surface ectoderm lateral and ventrolateral to the caudal mesencephalon and metencephalon to contribute to the distal portions of the trigeminal ganglia.

PITUITARY GLAND (HYPOPHYSIS CEREBRI)

The hypophysis cerebri consists of the adenohypophysis and the neurohypophysis. Prior to neurulation the cell populations that give rise to these two portions of the pituitary gland are found next to each other within the rostral portion of the floor of the neural plate and the contiguous midline neural fold. As neurulation proceeds the future neurohypophysis remains within the floor of the prosencephalon, and the cells of the future adenohypophysis are displaced into the surface ectoderm, where they form the hypophysial placode.

The most rostral portion of the neural plate, which will form the hypothalamus, is in contact rostrally with the future adenohypophysis, in the rostral neural ridge, and caudally with the neurohypophysis, in the floor of the neural plate (see Fig. 3.11). After neurulation the cells of the anterior neural ridge remain in the surface ectoderm and form the hypophysial placode, which is in close apposition and adherent to the overlying prosencephalon.

Neural crest mesenchyme later moves between the prosencephalon and surface ectoderm, except at the region of the placode. Before rupture of the buccopharyngeal membrane, proliferation of the periplacodal mesenchyme results in the placode forming the roof and walls of a saccular depression. This hypophysial recess (Rathke's pouch; Figs. 3.14, 3.15) is the rudiment of the adenohypophysis. It lies immediately ventral to the dorsal border of the buccopharyngeal membrane, extending in front of the rostral tip of the notochord and retaining contact with the ventral surface of the prosencephalon. It is constricted by continued proliferation of the surrounding mesenchyme to form a closed vesicle, but it remains connected for a time to the ectoderm of the stomodeum by a solid cord of cells that can be traced down the posterior edge of the nasal septum. Masses of epithelial cells form mainly on each side and in the ventral wall of the vesicle, and development of the adenohypophysis progresses by the ingrowth of a mesenchymal stroma. Differentiation of epithelial cells into stem cells and three differentiating types is apparent during the early months of fetal development. It has been suggested that different types of cells arise in succession and that they may be derived in varying proportions from different parts of the hypophysial recess. A craniopharyngeal canal, which sometimes runs from the anterior part of the hypophysial fossa of the sphenoid to the exterior of the skull, often marks the original position of the hypophysial recess. Traces of the stomodeal end of the recess are usually present at the junction of the septum of the

nose and the palate. Some claim that the craniopharyngeal canal itself is a secondary formation caused by the growth of blood vessels and that it is unconnected to the stalk of the anterior lobe.

A small endodermal diverticulum, called Sessel's pouch, projects toward the brain from the cranial end of the foregut, immediately caudal to the buccopharyngeal membrane. In some marsupials this pouch forms a part of the hypophysis, but in humans it apparently disappears entirely.

Just caudal to, but in contact with, the adenohypophysial recess, a hollow diverticulum elongates toward the stomodeum from the floor of the neural plate just caudal to the hypothalamus (see Fig. 3.15B); this region of neural outgrowth is the neurohypophysis. It forms an infundibular sac, the walls of which increase in thickness until the contained cavity is obliterated except at its upper end, where it persists as the infundibular recess of the third ventricle. The neurohypophysis becomes invested by the adenohypophysis, which extends dorsally on each side of it. The adenohypophysis gives off two processes from its ventral wall that grow along the infundibulum and fuse to surround it, coming into contact with the tuber cinereum and forming the tuberal portion of the hypophysis. The original cavity of Rathke's pouch remains first as a cleft and later as scattered vesicles; it can be identified readily in sagittal sections through the mature gland. The dorsal wall of Rathke's pouch, which remains thin, fuses with the adjoining part of the neurohypophysis as the pars intermedia.

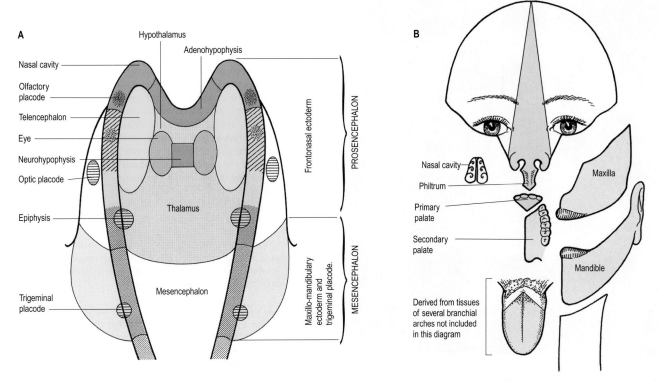

Fig. 3.11 *Fate map of the rostral region of the neural primordium as established by the quail–chick chimera system. **A,** The various territories yielding a rostral head are indicated on the neural plate and neural fold of a one- to three-somite embryo. **B,** Results obtained in the avian embryo have been extrapolated to the human head. Thus, the neural fold area* coloured green *yields the epithelium of the rostral roof of the mouth, the nasal cavities and part of the frontal area.*

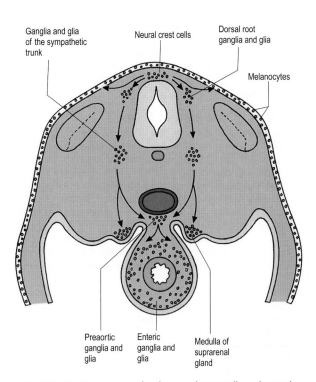

Fig. 3.12 *Migration routes taken by neural crest cells in the trunk.*

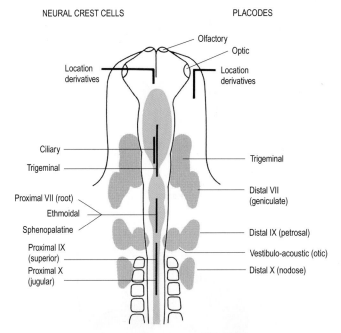

Fig. 3.13 *Positions of the neural crest and placodal cells in a stage 9.5 chick embryo. Neural crest cells are shown in the midline in green. Placodes are more laterally placed in grey. The otic placode is dorsolateral to the rhombencephalon, the trigeminal placode is placed intermediately and the epibranchial placodes (for facial, glossopharyngeal and vagus cranial nerves) are placed ventrolaterally and dorsal to the future pharyngeal grooves. (From D'Amico-Martel, A., Noden, D.M. 1983. Am. J. Anat. 166, 445–468. Reprinted by permission of Wiley-Liss Inc.)*

At birth the hypophysis is about one-sixth the weight of the adult gland; it increases to become about one-half the weight of the adult gland at 7 years and attains adult weight at puberty. Throughout postnatal life the gland is both larger and heavier in females.

NEUROGLIA

Glial cells that support neurones in the CNS and PNS are derived from three lineages: the neuroectoderm of the neural tube, the neural crest and the angioblastic mesenchyme. In the CNS, cells of the proliferating ventricular zone give rise to astrocyte and oligodendrocyte cell lines. After the proliferative phase, the cells remaining at the ventricular surface differentiate into ependymal cells, which are specialized in many regions of the ventricular

system as circumventricular organs. In the PNS, neural crest cells produce Schwann cells and astrocyte-like support cells in the enteric nervous system. Angioblastic mesenchyme gives rise to a variety of blood cell types, including circulating monocytes that infiltrate the brain as microglial cells later in development.

The ventricular zone lining the early central canal of the spinal cord and the cavities of the brain gives rise to neurones and glial cells (see Figs. 3.4, 3.5). One specialized form of glial cell is the radial glial cell, whose radial processes extend both outward, to form the outer limiting membrane deep to the pia

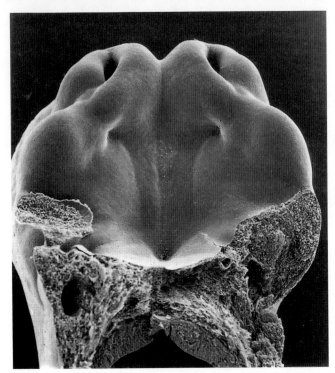

Fig. 3.14 *Scanning electron micrograph of the roof of the pharynx showing the invagination of placodal ectoderm to form the adenohypophysis (Rathke's pouch). (Photograph by P. Collins; printed by S. Cox, Electron Microscopy Unit, Southampton General Hospital.)*

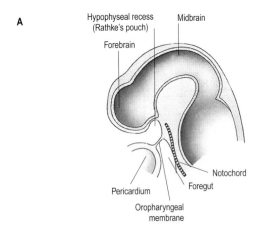

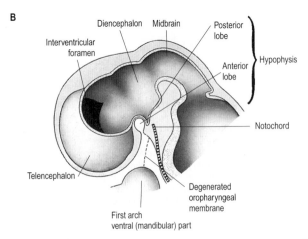

Fig. 3.15 *A and B, Sagittal sections of heads of early embryos showing the first stages in the development of the hypophysis.*

mater, and inward, to form the inner limiting membrane around the central cavity. The geometry of these cells may provide contact guidance paths for cell migrations, both neuroblastic and glioblastic. A secondary radial glial scaffold is formed in the late-developing cerebellum and dentate gyrus and serves to translocate neuroblasts, formed in secondary germinal centres, to

their definitive adult locations. Radial glia eventually lose their connections with both inner and outer limiting membranes, except for those that persist in the retina as Müller cells, in the cerebellum as Bergmann glia and in the hypothalamus as tanycytes. They can differentiate into neurones as well as astrocytes. They may partially clothe the somata of neighbouring developing neurones (between presumptive synaptic contacts) or similarly enwrap the intersynaptic surfaces of their neurites. Glial processes may expand around intraneural capillaries as perivascular end-feet. Other glioblasts retain an attachment (or form new expansions) to the pia mater, the innermost stratum of the meninges, as pial end-feet. Glioblasts also line the central canal and cavities of the brain as generalized or specialized ependymal cells, but they lose their peripheral attachments. In some situations, such as in the anterior median fissure of the spinal cord, ependymal cells retain their attachments to both the inner and outer limiting membranes. Thus, glia function as perineuronal satellites and provide cellular channels interconnecting extracerebral and intraventricular cerebrospinal fluid, the cerebral vascular bed, the intercellular crevices of the neuropil and the cytoplasm of all neural cell varieties.

Microglia appear in the CNS after it has been penetrated by blood vessels and invade it in large numbers from certain restricted regions. From there they spread in what have picturesquely been called 'fountains of microglia' to extend deeply among the nervous elements.

MECHANISMS OF NEURAL DEVELOPMENT

For more than a century the mechanisms that operate during development of the nervous system have been studied experimentally. Although much has been established, answers to many fundamental questions still remain obscure. In recent years, significant advances in our understanding of the development of vertebrates have come from work on amphibian, chicken, mouse and fish embryos and from the production of embryonic chimera (Le Douarin, Teillet and Catala, 1998). A combination of genetic, embryological, biochemical and molecular techniques has been used to elucidate the mechanisms operating in early neural populations.

The CNS has a fundamental structure of layers and cells that are all derived from a pluripotential neuroepithelium. Developing neuroblasts produce axons that traverse great distances to reach their target organs. Within the CNS they form myriad connections with other neuroblasts in response to locally secreted neurotrophins. The brain and spinal cord reveal an intrinsic metamerism, induced rostrally by genes and caudally by inductive influences from adjacent structures.

Histogenesis of the Neural Tube

The wall of the early neural tube consists of an internal ventricular zone (sometimes termed the germinal matrix) abutting the central lumen. It contains the nucleated parts of the pseudostratified columnar neuroepithelial cells and rounded cells undergoing mitosis. The early ventricular zone also contains a population of radial glial cells whose processes pass from the ventricular surface to the pial surface, thus forming the internal and external glia limitans (glial limiting membrane). As development proceeds, the early pseudostratified epithelium proliferates, and an outer layer (the marginal zone), devoid of nuclei but containing the external cytoplasmic processes of cells, is delineated. Subsequently, a middle mantle layer (the intermediate zone) forms as the progeny from the ventricular zone migrate ventriculofugally (see Fig. 3.5).

Most CNS cells are produced in the proliferative zone adjacent to the future ventricular system, and in some regions this area is the only actively mitotic zone. According to the monophyletic theory of neurogenesis, it is assumed to produce all cell types. The early neural epithelium, including the deeply placed ventricular mitotic zone, consists of a homogeneous population of pluripotent cells whose varying appearances reflect different phases in a proliferative cycle. The ventricular zone is considered to be populated by a single basic type of progenitor cell and to exhibit three phases. The cells show an 'elevator movement' as they pass through a complete mitotic cycle, progressively approaching and then receding from the internal limiting membrane (Fig. 3.16). DNA replication occurs while the cells are extended and their nuclei approach the pial surface; they then enter a premitotic resting period as the cells shorten and their nuclei pass back toward the ventricular surface. The cells now become rounded close to the internal limiting membrane and undergo mitosis. They then elongate, and their nuclei move toward the outer edge during the postmitotic resting period, after which DNA synthesis commences once more, and the cycle is repeated. The cells so formed may either start another proliferative cycle or migrate outward (i.e. radially) and differentiate into neurones as they approach and enter the adjacent stratum. This differentiation may be initiated as they pass outward during the postmitotic resting period. The proliferative cycle continues with the production of clones of neuroblasts and glioblasts. This sequence of events has been called

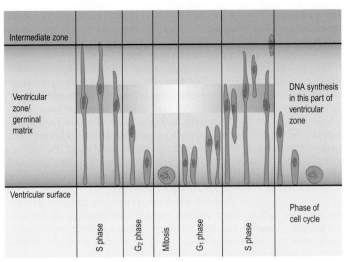

Fig. 3.16 *Cell cycle in the ventricular zone of the developing neural tube. The nuclei of the proliferating stem cells show interkinetic migration. (From Fujita, S. 1963. J. Comp. Neurol. 120, 37–42. Reprinted by permission from Wiley-Liss Inc.)*

interkinetic nuclear migration, and it eventually declines. At the last division, two postmitotic daughter cells are produced, and they differentiate at the ventricular surface into ependyma.

The progeny of some of these divisions move away from the ventricular zone to form an intermediate zone of neurones. The early spinal cord and much of the brain stem shows only these three main layers: ventricular, intermediate and marginal zones. However, in the telencephalon, the region of cellular proliferation extends deeper than the ventricular zone, where the escalator movement of interkinetic migration is seen, and a subventricular zone appears between the ventricular and intermediate layers (see Fig. 3.5). Here cells continue to multiply to provide further generations of neurones and glia, which subsequently migrate into the intermediate and marginal zones. In some regions of the nervous system (e.g. the cerebellar cortex) some mitotic subventricular stem cells migrate across the entire neural wall to form a subpial population and establish a new zone of cell division and differentiation. Many cells formed in this site remain subpial in position, but others migrate back toward the ventricle through the developing nervous tissue and finish their migration in various definitive sites where they differentiate into neurones or macroglial cells. In the cerebral hemispheres, a zone termed the cortical plate is formed outside the intermediate zone by radially migrating cells from the ventricular zone. The most recently formed cells migrate to the outermost layers of the cortical plate, so that earlier formed and migrating cells become subjacent to those migrating later. In the forebrain there is an additional transient stratum deep to the early cortical plate, the subplate zone.

Lineage and Growth in the Nervous System

Neurones come from two major embryonic sources: CNS neurones originate from the pluripotential neural plate and tube, whereas ganglionic neurones originate from the neural crest and ectodermal placodes. The neural plate also provides ependymal and macroglial cells. Peripheral Schwann cells and chromaffin cells arise from the neural crest. The origins and lineages of cells in the nervous system have been determined experimentally by the use of autoradiography, by microinjection or retroviral labelling of progenitor cells and in cell culture.

During development, neurones are formed before glial cells. The timing of events differs in various parts of the CNS and between species. Most neurones are formed prenatally in mammals, but some postnatal neurogenesis does occur (e.g. the small granular cells of the cerebellum, olfactory bulb and hippocampus, and neurones of the cerebral cortex). Gliogenesis continues after birth in periventricular and other sites. Autoradiographic studies have shown that different classes of neurones develop at specific times. Large neurones, such as principal projection neurones, tend to differentiate before small ones, such as local circuit neurones. However, their subsequent migration appears to be independent of the time of their initial formation. Neurones can migrate extensively through populations of maturing, relatively static cells to reach their destination; for example, cerebellar granule cells pass through a layer of Purkinje cells en route from the external pial layer to their final central position. Later, the final form of their projections, their cell volume and even their continuing survival depend on the establishment of patterns of functional connection.

Initially, immature neurones, termed neuroblasts, are rotund or fusiform. Their cytoplasm contains a prominent Golgi apparatus, many lysosomes, glycogen and numerous unattached ribosomes. As maturation proceeds, cells send out fine cytoplasmic processes that contain neurofilaments, microtubules and other structures, often including centrioles at their bases where microtubules form. Internally, endoplasmic reticulum cisternae appear, and attached ribosomes and mitochondria proliferate, whereas the glycogen content progressively diminishes. One process becomes the axon, and other processes establish a dendritic tree. Axonal growth, studied in tissue culture, may be as much as 1 mm per day.

Growth Cones

Ramón y Cajal (1890) was the first to recognize that the expanded end of an axon, the growth cone, is the principal sensory organ of the neurone. The growing tips of neuroblasts have been studied extensively in tissue culture. Classically, the growth cone is described as an expanded region that is constantly active, changing shape, extending and withdrawing small filopodia and lamellipodia that apparently 'explore' the local environment for a suitable surface along which extension can occur. These processes are stabilized in one direction, determining the direction of future growth, and after consolidation of the growth cone, the exploratory behaviour recommences. This continuous cycle resembles the behaviour at the leading edge of migratory cells such as fibroblasts and neutrophils. The molecular basis of this behaviour is the transmission of signals external to the growth cone via cell surface receptors to the scaffolding of microtubules and neurofilaments within the axon. Growing neuroblasts have a cortex rich in actin associated with the plasma membrane, along with a core of centrally located microtubules and sometimes neurofilaments. The assembly of these components, as well as the synthesis of new membrane, occurs in segments distal to the cell body and behind the growth cone, although some assembly of microtubules may take place near the cell body.

The driving force of growth cone extension is uncertain. One possible mechanism is that tension applied to objects by the leading edge of the growth cone is mediated by actin, and local accumulations of F-actin redirect the extension of microtubules. Under some culture conditions, growth cones can develop mechanical tension, pulling against other axons or the substratum to which they are attached. It is possible that tension in the growth cone acts as a messenger to mediate the assembly of cytoskeletal components. Adhesion to the substratum appears to be important for consolidation of the growth cone and elaboration of the cytoskeleton in that direction.

During development, the growing axons of neuroblasts navigate with precision over considerable distances, often pursuing complex courses to reach their targets. Eventually they make functional contact with their appropriate end-organs (neuromuscular endings, secretomotor terminals, sensory corpuscles or synapses with other neurones). During the outgrowth of axonal processes, the earliest nerve fibres are known to traverse appreciable distances over an apparently virgin landscape, often occupied by loose mesenchyme. A central problem for neurobiologists, therefore, has been understanding the mechanisms of axon guidance (Gordon-Weeks 2000). Axon guidance is thought to involve short-range local guidance cues and long-range diffusible cues, any of which can be either attractive and permissive for growth or repellent and inhibitory. Short-range cues require factors that are displayed on cell surfaces or in the extracellular matrix; for example, axon extension requires a permissive, physical substrate, the molecules of which are actively recognized by the growth cone. They also require negative cues that inhibit the progress of the growth cone. Long-range cues come from gradients of specific factors diffusing from distant targets, which cause neurones to turn their axons toward the source of the attractive signal. The evidence for this has come from *in vitro* co-culture studies. The floor plate of the developing spinal cord exerts a chemotropic effect on commissural axons that later cross it, whereas there is chemorepulsion of developing motor axons from the floor plate. These forces are thought to act *in vivo* in concert in a dynamic process to ensure the correct passage of axons to their final destinations and to mediate their correct bundling together en route.

Dendritic Tree

Once growth cones have arrived in their general target area, they have to form terminals and synapses. In recent years, much emphasis has been placed on the idea that patterns of connectivity depend on the death of inappropriate cells. Programmed cell death, or apoptosis, occurs during the period of synaptogenesis if neurones fail to acquire sufficient amounts of specific neurotrophic factors. Coincident firing of neighbouring neurones that have found the appropriate target region might be involved in eliciting the release of these factors, thus reinforcing correct connections. Such mechanisms may explain the numerical correspondence between neurones in a motor pool and the muscle fibres innervated. On a subtler level, pruning of collaterals may give rise to mature neuronal architecture. The projections of pyramidal neurones from the motor and visual cortices, for example, start out with a similar architecture; the mature repertoire of targets is produced by the pruning of collaterals, leading to loss of projections to some targets.

The final growth of dendritic trees is also influenced by patterns of afferent connections and their activity. If deprived of afferents experimentally, dendrites fail to develop fully and, after a critical period, may become permanently affected even if functional inputs are restored (e.g. in the visual systems of young animals that have been visually deprived). This is analogous to the results of untreated amblyopia in infants. Metabolic factors also affect the final branching patterns of dendrites; for instance, thyroid deficiency in perinatal rats results in a small size and restricted branching of cortical neurones. This may be analogous to the mental retardation of cretinism.

Once established, dendritic trees appear to be remarkably stable, and partial deafferentation affects only dendritic spines or similar small details. As development proceeds, plasticity is lost, and soon after birth a neurone is a stable structure with a reduced rate of growth.

Neurotrophins

If neurones lose all afferent connections or are totally deprived of sensory input, there is atrophy of much of the dendritic tree or even the whole soma. Different regions of the nervous system vary quantitatively in their responses to such anterograde transneuronal degeneration. Similar effects occur in retrograde transneuronal degeneration. Thus, neurones are dependent on peripheral structures for their survival. Loss of muscles or sensory nerve endings, such as in the developing limb, results in reduced numbers of motor and sensory neurones. The specific factor produced by these target organs is termed nerve growth factor (NGF). NGF is taken into nerve endings and transported back to the neuronal somata. It is necessary for the survival of many types of neurones during early development and for the growth of their axons and dendrites, and it promotes the synthesis of neurotransmitters and enzymes. Antibodies to NGF cause the death of neuronal subsets when they reach their targets, and added NGF rescues neurones that would otherwise die. Since the discovery of NGF, several other trophic factors have been identified, including brain-derived neurotrophic factor (BDNF), neurotrophin-3 (NT-3) and NT-4/5.

Neurotrophins exert their survival effects selectively on particular subsets of neurones. NGF is specific to sensory ganglion cells from the neural crest, sympathetic postganglionic neurones and basal forebrain cholinergic neurones. BDNF promotes the survival of retinal ganglion cells, motor neurones, sensory proprioceptive and placode-derived neurones, such as those of the nodose ganglion, which are unresponsive to NGF. NT-3 has effects on motor neurones and both placode- and neural crest–derived sensory neurones. Other growth factors that influence the growth and survival of neural cells include the fibroblast growth factors (FGFs) and ciliary neurotrophic factor (CNTF), all of which are unrelated in sequence to the NGF family. Members of the FGF family support the survival of embryonic neurones from many regions of the CNS. CNTF may control the proliferation and differentiation of sympathetic ganglion cells and astrocytes.

Each of the neurotrophins binds specifically to certain receptors on the cell surface. The receptor termed $p75^{NTR}$ binds all the neurotrophins with similar affinity. By contrast, members of the family of tyrosine kinase receptors bind with higher affinity and display binding preferences for particular neurotrophins. However, the presence of a tyrosine kinase receptor seems to be required for $p75^{NTR}$ function.

Nervous tissue influences the metabolism of its target tissues. If, during development, a nerve fails to connect with its muscle, both degenerate. If the innervation of slow (red) or fast (white) skeletal muscle is exchanged, the muscles change structure and properties to reflect the new innervation, indicating that the nerve determines muscle type, not vice versa.

Induction and Patterning of the Brain and Spinal Cord

The generation of neural tissue involves an inductive signal from the underlying chordamesoderm (notochord), termed the organizer. The observation by Spemann in 1925 that, in intact amphibian embryos, the presence of an organizer causes ectodermal cells to form nervous tissue, whereas in its absence they form epidermis, led to the discovery of neural induction. However, experiments performed much later in the century revealed that when ectodermal cells are dissociated, they also give rise to neural tissue. The paradox was resolved by the finding that intact ectodermal tissue is prevented from becoming neural by an inhibitory signal that is diluted when cells are dissociated. Many lines of evidence now indicate that this inhibitory signal is mediated by members of a family of secreted proteins, the bone morphogenetic proteins (BMPs). These molecules are found throughout ectodermal tissue during early development, and their inhibitory effect is antagonized by several neural inducers that are present within the organizer: noggin, chordin and follistatin. Each of these factors is capable of blocking BMP signalling, in some cases by preventing it from binding to its receptor.

The regional pattern of the nervous system is induced before and during neural tube closure. Early concepts about regional patterning envisaged that regionalization within mesenchymal populations that transmit inductive signals to the ectoderm imposes a similar mosaic of positional values on the overlying neural plate. For example, transplantation of caudal mesenchyme beneath the neural plate in Amphibia induced spinal cord, whereas rostral mesenchyme induced brain, as assessed by the morphology of the neuroepithelial vesicles. However, later work indicated a more complex scenario in which organizer grafts from early embryos induced mainly head structures, whereas later grafts induced mainly trunk structures. Subsequent molecular data tend to support a model in which neural-inducing factors released by the organizer, such as noggin, chordin and follistatin, neuralize the ectoderm and promote a mainly rostral neural identity. Later secreted signals then act to caudalize this rostral neural tissue, setting up an entire array of axial values along the neural tube. Candidates for these later caudalizing signals include retinoic acid, FGFs, and the WNT secreted proteins, which are present in the paraxial mesenchyme and later in its derivatives, the somites. This combination of signals does not seem to be sufficient to produce the most rostral forebrain structures. Other secreted proteins resident in the rostralmost part of the earliest ingressing axial populations of endoderm and mesenchyme are also capable of inducing markers of forebrain identity from ectodermal cells (Withington, Beddington and Cooke 2001).

As the neural tube grows and its shape is modified, a number of mechanisms refine the crude rostrocaudal pattern imposed during neurulation. Molecules that diffuse from tissues adjacent to the neural tube, such as the somites, have patterning influences. The neural tube possesses a number of intrinsic signalling centres, such as the midbrain–hindbrain boundary, which produce diffusible molecules capable of influencing tissue development at a distance. In this way extrinsic and intrinsic factors serve to subdivide the neural tube into a number of fairly large domains, on which local influences can then act. Domains are distinguished by their expression of particular transcription factors, which in many cases have been causally related to the development of particular regions. Examples of such genes are the *Hox* family, which are expressed in the spinal cord and hindbrain, and the *Dlx, Emx* and *Otx* families of genes, which are expressed in various regions of the forebrain. These are all developmental control genes that lie high up in the hierarchy and are capable of initiating cascades of expression of other genes to create a more fine-grained pattern of cellular differentiation. In contrast to the aforementioned secreted molecules, these genes encode proteins that are retained in the cell nucleus and thus can act on DNA to induce or repress further gene expression.

Segmentation in the Neural Tube

One mechanism involved in the process of regional differentiation of cell populations within the neural tube is segmentation, which is conspicuous in humans and other vertebrates in the serial arrangement of the vertebrae and axial muscles and in the periodicity of the spinal nerves. In the last century, the possibility that the neural tube might be divided into segments or neuromeres was entertained, but some contended that the bulges observed in the lateral walls of the neural tube were artifacts or were caused by mechanical deformation of the tube by adjacent structures. Recent years have seen a resurgence of interest in this subject and a detailed evaluation of the significance of neuromeres. A series of eight prominent bulges that appear bilaterally in the rhombencephalic wall early in development have been termed rhombomeres (see Fig. 3.3). (Whereas the term neuromere applies generally to putative 'segments' of the neural tube, the term rhombomere applies specifically to the rhombencephalon.) Many aspects of the patterning of neuronal populations and the elaboration of their axon tracts conform to a segmental plan, and rhombomeres have now been shown to constitute crucial units of pattern formation. Domains of expression of developmental control genes abut rhombomere boundaries, and perhaps most importantly, single-cell labelling experiments have revealed that cells within rhombomeres form segregated non-mixing populations (Fig. 3.17). The neural crest also shows intrinsic segmentation in the hindbrain and is segregated into streams at its point of origin in the dorsal neural tube. This may represent a mechanism whereby morphogenetic specification of the premigratory neural crest cells is conveyed to the pharyngeal arches. Although these segmental units lose their morphological prominence with subsequent development, they represent the fundamental ground plan of this part of the neuraxis, creating a series of semiautonomous units within which local variations in patterning can develop. The consequences of early segmentation for later developmental events, such as the formation of

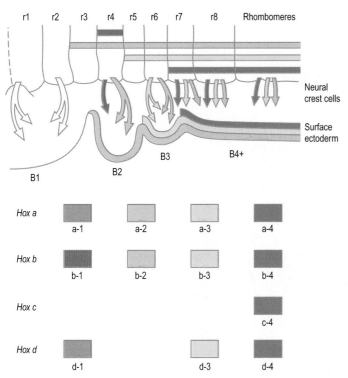

r1 r2 r3 r4 r5 r6 r7 r8 Rhombomeres

Neural crest cells

Surface ectoderm

B1 B2 B3 B4+

Hox a   a-1   a-2   a-3   a-4

Hox b   b-1   b-2   b-3   b-4

Hox c   c-4

Hox d   d-1   d-3   d-4

Fig. 3.17 Hox *gene expression domains in the branchiorhombomeric area in the mouse embryo at stage 9.5. The arrows* indicate neural crest cells migrating from the rhombencephalon and midbrain. At the former level, they are shaded to indicate the Hox *genes they express. The same combination of* Hox *genes is expressed in the rhombomeres and in the superficial ectoderm of the pharyngeal arches at the corresponding rostrocaudal levels. The four* Hox *clusters are represented below. (Modified by permission from Annual Review of Cell and Developmental Biology, Vol. 8. 1992. www.annualreviews.org.)*

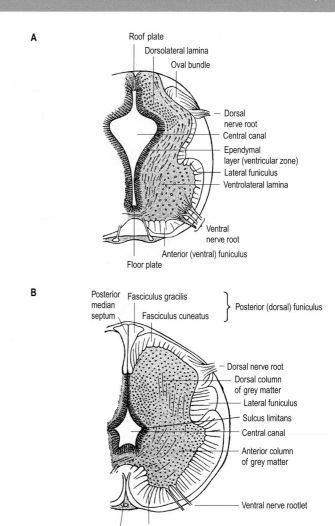

A

Roof plate
Dorsolateral lamina
Oval bundle
Dorsal nerve root
Central canal
Ependymal layer (ventricular zone)
Lateral funiculus
Ventrolateral lamina
Ventral nerve root
Anterior (ventral) funiculus
Floor plate

B

Posterior median septum
Fasciculus gracilis
Fasciculus cuneatus
Posterior (dorsal) funiculus
Dorsal nerve root
Dorsal column of grey matter
Lateral funiculus
Sulcus limitans
Central canal
Anterior column of grey matter
Ventral nerve rootlet
Anterior funiculus
Anterior median fissure

Fig. 3.18 *Transverse sections through the developing spinal cord of human embryos.* **A**, *Approximately 6 weeks old.* **B**, *Approximately 3 months old.*

definitive neuronal nuclei within the brain stem, and of peripheral axonal projections remain to be explored.

Other brain regions are not segmented in quite the same way as the hindbrain. However, morphological boundaries, domains of cell lineage restriction and of cell mixing and regions of gene expression that abut sharp boundaries are found in the diencephalon and telencephalon. It is thus likely that compartmentation of cell groups with some, if not all, of the features of rhombomeres plays an important role in the formation of various brain regions.

The significance of intrinsic segmentation in the hindbrain is underlined by the absence of overt segmentation of the adjacent paraxial mesenchyme. There is no firm evidence for intrinsic segmentation in the spinal cord. Instead, segmentation of the neural crest, the motor axons and eventually the spinal nerves is dependent on segmentation of the neighbouring somites. Both neural crest cell migration and motor axon outgrowth occur through only the rostral, not the caudal, sclerotome of each somite, so dorsal root ganglia form only at intervals. The caudal sclerotome possesses inhibitory properties that deter neural crest cells and motor axons from entering. This illustrates the general principle that the nervous system is closely interlocked, in terms of morphogenesis, with the periphery—that is, surrounding non-nervous structures—and each is dependent on the other for its effective structural and functional maturation.

Genes such as the *Hox* and *Pax* gene families, which encode transcription factor proteins, show intriguing expression patterns within the nervous system. Genes of the *Hox-b* cluster, for example, are expressed throughout the caudal neural tube and up to discrete limits in the hindbrain that coincide with rhombomere boundaries. The ordering of these genes within a cluster on the chromosome (5′–3′) is the same as the caudal-to-rostral limits of expression of consecutive genes. This characteristic pattern is surprisingly similar in fish, frogs, birds and mammals. *Hox* genes play a role in patterning of not only the neural tube but also much of the head region, consistent with their expression in neural crest cells and within the pharyngeal arches. Disruption of the *Hox a-3* gene in mice mimics DiGeorge syndrome, a congenital human disorder characterized by the absence (or near absence) of the thymus, parathyroid and thyroid glands; hypotrophy of the walls of the arteries derived from the aortic arches and subsequent conotruncal cardiac malformations. Some *Pax* genes are expressed in different dorsoventral domains within the neural tube. *Pax-3* is expressed in the alar lamina, including the neural crest, whereas *Pax-6* is expressed in the intermediate plate. The *Pax-3*

gene has the same chromosomal localization as the mouse mutation Splotch and the affected locus in the human Waardenburg's syndrome, both of which are characterized by neural crest disturbances with pigmentation disorders and occasional neural tube defects. Both *Hox* and *Pax* genes have restricted expression patterns with respect to the rostrocaudal and dorsoventral axes of the neural tube, consistent with roles in positional specification. (For reviews of the expression patterns of these genes, see Krumlauf et al 1993.)

Whereas craniocaudal positional values are probably conferred on the neuroepithelium at the neural plate or early neural tube stage, dorsoventral positional values may become fixed later. The development of the dorsoventral axis is heavily influenced by the presence of the underlying notochord. The notochord induces the ventral midline of the neural tube, the floor plate. This specialized region consists of a strip of non-neural cells with distinctive adhesive and functional properties. Notochord and floor plate together participate in inducing the differentiation of the motor columns. Motor neurone differentiation occurs early, giving some support to the idea of a ventral-to-dorsal wave of differentiation. The notochord–floor plate complex may also be responsible for allotting the values of more dorsal cell types within the tube (see Fig. 3.7). For example, the dorsal domain of *Pax-3* expression extends more ventrally in embryos experimentally deprived of notochord and floor plate, whereas grafting an extra notochord adjacent to the dorsal neural tube leads to the repression of *Pax-3* expression.

PERIPHERAL NERVOUS SYSTEM

Somatic Nerves

Spinal Nerves

Each spinal nerve is connected to the spinal cord by a ventral root and a dorsal root (Fig. 3.18). The fibres of the ventral roots grow out from cell bodies in the anterior and lateral parts of the intermediate zone. These pass through the overlying marginal zone and external limiting membrane. Some enter the

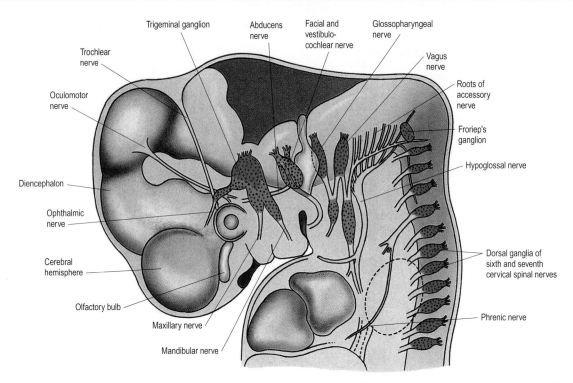

Trigeminal ganglion   Abducens nerve   Facial and vestibulo-cochlear nerve   Glossopharyngeal nerve

Trochlear nerve

Oculomotor nerve

Vagus nerve

Roots of accessory nerve

Froriep's ganglion

Hypoglossal nerve

Diencephalon

Ophthalmic nerve

Cerebral hemisphere

Dorsal ganglia of sixth and seventh cervical spinal nerves

Olfactory bulb

Maxillary nerve

Phrenic nerve

Mandibular nerve

Fig. 3.19 *Brain and cranial nerves of a human embryo, 10.2 mm long. Note the ganglia (stippled) associated with the trigeminal, facial, vestibulocochlear, glossopharyngeal, vagus and spinal accessory nerves. Froriep's ganglion, an occipital dorsal root ganglion, is inconstant and soon disappears.*

myotomes of the somites, and some penetrate the somites, reaching the adjacent somatopleure; in both sites they ultimately form the α-, β- and γ-efferents. At appropriate levels these are accompanied by the outgrowing axons of preganglionic sympathetic neuroblasts (segments T1–L2) or preganglionic parasympathetic neuroblasts (S2–4).

The fibres of the dorsal roots extend from cell somata in dorsal root ganglia into the spinal cord and also into the periphery. Neural crest cells are produced continuously along the length of the spinal cord, but gangliogenic cells migrate only into the rostral part of each somitic sclerotome, where they condense and proliferate to form a bilateral series of oval-shaped primordial spinal ganglia (dorsal root ganglia; see Fig. 3.12). Negative factors in the caudal sclerotome deter neural crest from entering. The rostral sclerotome has a mitogenic effect on the crest cells that settle within it. From the ventral region of each ganglion, a small part separates to form sympathochromaffin cells, whereas the remainder becomes a definitive spinal ganglion (dorsal root ganglion). The spinal ganglia are arranged symmetrically at the sides of the neural tube and, except in the caudal region, are equal in number to the somites. The cells of the ganglia, like the cells of the intermediate zone of the early neural tube, are glial and neuronal precursors. The glial precursors develop into satellite cells (which become closely applied to the ganglionic nerve cell somata), Schwann cells and possibly other cells. The neuroblasts, which are initially round or oval, soon become fusiform, and their extremities gradually elongate into central and peripheral processes. The central processes grow into the neural tube as the fibres of dorsal nerve roots, and the peripheral processes grow ventrolaterally to mingle with the fibres of the ventral root, thus forming a mixed spinal nerve. As development proceeds, the original bipolar form of the cells in the spinal ganglia changes, and the two processes become approximated until they ultimately arise from a single stem to form a unipolar cell. The bipolar form is retained in the ganglion of the vestibulocochlear nerve.

Cranial Nerves

Cranial nerves may contain motor, sensory or both types of fibres. With the exception of the olfactory and optic nerves, the cranial nerves develop in a manner similar in some respects to components of the spinal nerves. The somata of motor neuroblasts originate within the neuroepithelium; those of sensory neuroblasts are derived from the neural crest, with additional contributions in the head from ectodermal placodes (Fig. 3.19).

The motor fibres of the cranial nerves that project to striated muscle are the axons of cells originating in the basal plate of the midbrain and hindbrain. The functional and morphological distinction between the neurones within these various nerves is based on the types of muscle innervated. In the trunk, the motor roots of the spinal nerves all emerge from the spinal cord close to the ventral midline, to supply the muscles derived from the somites. In the head, the motor outflow is traditionally divided into two pathways (see

Figs. 3.2B, 3.19). General somatic efferent neurones exit ventrally in a similar manner to those of the spinal cord. Thus the oculomotor, trochlear, abducens and hypoglossal nerves parallel the organization of the somatic motor neurones in the spinal cord. The second motor component, the special branchial efferent, consists of the motor parts of the trigeminal, facial, glossopharyngeal and vagus nerves, which supply the pharyngeal (branchial) arches and the accessory nerve. All these nerves have nerve exit points more dorsally placed than in the somatic motor system.

The cranial nerves also contain general visceral efferent neurones (parasympathetic preganglionic neurones) that travel in the oculomotor, facial, glossopharyngeal and vagus nerves and leave the hindbrain via the same exit points as the special branchial efferent fibres. All three categories of motor neurones probably originate from the same region of the basal plate, adjacent to the floor plate. The definitive arrangement of nuclei reflects the differential migration of neuronal somata. It is not known whether all these cell types share a common precursor within the rhombencephalon; however, in the spinal cord, somatic motor and preganglionic autonomic neurones are linearly related.

These motor neurone types have been designated according to the types of muscles or structures they innervate. General somatic efferent nerves supply striated muscle derived from the cranial (occipital) somites and prechordal mesenchyme. Myogenic cells from the ventrolateral edge of the epithelial plate of occipital somites give rise to the intrinsic muscles of the tongue, and the prechordal mesenchyme gives rise to the extrinsic ocular muscles. Special branchial efferent nerves supply the striated muscles developing within the pharyngeal (branchial) arches, which are derived from parachordal mesenchyme between the occipital somites and the prechordal mesenchyme. All the voluntary muscles of the head originate from axial (prechordal) or paraxial mesenchyme, which renders the distinction between somatic efferent supply and branchial efferent supply somewhat artificial. However, because of the obviously special nature of the arch musculature, its patterning by the neural crest cells, its particularly rich innervation for both voluntary and reflex activity and the different origins from the basal plate of the branchial efferent nerves compared with the somatic efferent nerves, the distinction between the two is of some value.

General visceral efferent neurones (parasympathetic preganglionic neurones) innervate the glands of the head, the sphincter pupillae and ciliary muscles and the thoracic and abdominal viscera.

The cranial sensory ganglia are derived in part from the neural crest and in part from cells of the ectodermal placodes (see Figs. 3.13, 3.19). Generally, neurones distal to the brain are derived from placodes, and proximal ones are derived from the neural crest (see Fig. 3.19). Supporting cells of all sensory ganglia arise from the neural crest. The most rostral sensory ganglion, the trigeminal, contains both neural crest– and placode-derived neurones that mediate general somatic afferent functions. The same applies to the more caudal cranial nerves (facial, glossopharyngeal, vagus), but the two cell populations form separate ganglia in the case of each nerve. The proximal series of ganglia is derived from neural crest (forming the proximal ganglion of the facial nerve, the superior ganglion of the glossopharyngeal nerve and the jugular ganglion of the vagus nerve); the distal series is derived from placodal cells (forming the geniculate ganglion of the facial nerve, the petrosal ganglion of the glossopharyngeal nerve and the nodose ganglion of the vagus nerve). These ganglia contain neurones that mediate special, general visceral and somatic afferent functions. The vestibulocochlear nerve has a vestibular ganglion that contains both crest and placodal cells and an acoustic ganglion from placodal neurones only; it conveys special somatic afferents.

The neurones and supporting cells of the cranial autonomic ganglia in the head and trunk originate from neural crest cells. Caudal to the ganglion of the vagus nerve, the occipital region of the neural crest is concerned with the 'ganglia' of the accessory and hypoglossal nerves. Rudimentary ganglion cells may occur along the hypoglossal nerve in the human embryo; they subsequently regress. Ganglion cells are found on the developing spinal root of the accessory nerve, and these are believed to persist in the adult. The central processes of the cells of these various ganglia, where they persist, form some sensory roots of the cranial nerves and enter the alar lamina of the hindbrain. Their peripheral processes join the efferent components of the nerve to be distributed to the various tissues innervated. Some incoming fibres from the facial, glossopharyngeal and vagus nerves collect to form an oval bundle, the tractus solitarius, on the lateral aspect of the myelencephalon. This bundle is the homologue of the oval bundle of the spinal cord, but in the hindbrain it becomes more deeply placed by the overgrowth, folding and subsequent fusion of tissue derived from the rhombic lip on the external aspect of the bundle.

Autonomic Nervous System

Autonomic nerves, apart from the preganglionic motor axons arising from the CNS, are formed by the neural crest. The autonomic nervous system includes the sympathetic and parasympathetic neurones in the peripheral ganglia and their accompanying glia, the enteric nervous system and glia and the suprarenal medulla.

In the trunk at neurulation, neural crest cells migrate from the neural epithelium to lie transitorily on the fused neural tube. Thereafter, crest cells migrate laterally and then ventrally to their respective destinations (see Fig. 3.12). In the head, the neural crest cells migrate prior to neural fusion, producing a vast mesenchymal population as well as autonomic neurones.

The four major regions of neural crest cell distribution to the autonomic nervous system are cranial, vagal, trunk and lumbosacral. The cranial neural crest gives rise to the cranial parasympathetic ganglia, whereas the vagal neural crest gives rise to the thoracic parasympathetic ganglia. The trunk neural crest gives rise to the sympathetic ganglia, mainly the paravertebral ganglia, and suprarenomedullary cells. This category is often referred to as the sympathoadrenal lineage.

Neurones of the enteric nervous system are described as arising from the vagal crest—that is, the neural crest derived from somite levels 1 to 7, and the sacral crest caudal to the twenty-eighth somite. At all these levels the crest cells also differentiate into glial-like support cells alongside the neurones (Fig. 3.20).

Parasympathetic Ganglia

Neural crest cells migrate from the region of the mesencephalon and rhombencephalon prior to neural tube closure. From rostral to caudal, three populations of neural crest are described: cranial neural crest, cardiac neural crest and vagal neural crest. Migration of the sacral neural crest and formation of the caudal parasympathetic ganglia have attracted little research interest.

Neural crest cells from the caudal third of the mesencephalon and the rostral metencephalon migrate along or close to the ophthalmic branch of the trigeminal nerve and give rise to the ciliary ganglion. Cells migrating from the nucleus of the oculomotor nerve may also contribute to the ganglion; a few scattered cells are always demonstrable in postnatal life along the course of this nerve. Preotic myelencephalic neural crest cells give rise to the pterygopalatine ganglion, which may also receive contributions from the ganglia of the trigeminal and facial nerves. The otic and submandibular ganglia are also derived from myelencephalic neural crest and may receive contributions from the glossopharyngeal and facial cranial nerves, respectively.

Neural crest from the region located between the otic placode and the caudal limit of somite 3 has been termed cardiac neural crest. Cells derived from these levels migrate through pharyngeal arches 3, 4 and 6, where they provide, among other things, support for the embryonic aortic arch arteries, cells of the aorticopulmonary septum and truncus arteriosus. Some of these neural crest cells also differentiate into the neural anlage of the

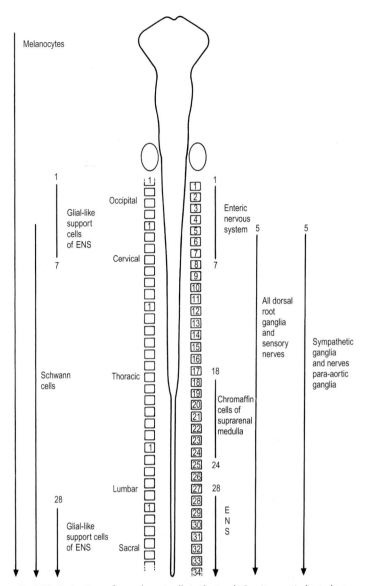

Fig. 3.20 *Derivatives of neural crest cells in the trunk. Somites are indicated on the right, and vertebral levels are indicated on the left. The fate of crest cells arising at particular somite levels is shown.*

parasympathetic ganglia of the heart. Sensory innervation of the heart is from the inferior ganglion of the vagus, which is derived from the nodose placodes. Neural crest cells migrating from the level of somites 1 to 7 are collectively termed vagal neural crest; they migrate to the gut along with the sacral neural crest.

Sympathetic Ganglia

Neural crest cells migrate ventrally within the body segments to penetrate the underlying somites and continue to the region of the future paravertebral and prevertebral plexuses, notably forming the sympathetic chain of ganglia as well as the major ganglia around the ventral visceral branches of the abdominal aorta (see Figs. 3.12, 3.20).

There is cell-specific recognition of postganglionic neurones and the growth cones of sympathetic preganglionic neurones. They meet during growth, and this may be important in terms of guidance to their appropriate target. The position of postganglionic neurones, and the exit point from the spinal cord of preganglionic neurones, may influence the types of synaptic connections made and the affinity for particular postganglionic neurones. When a postganglionic neuroblast is in place, it extends axons (and dendrites), and synaptogenesis occurs. The earliest axonal outgrowths from the superior cervical ganglion occur at about stage 14; although the axon is the first cell process to appear, the position of the neurones apparently does not influence the appearance of the cell processes.

The local environment is the major factor that controls the appropriate differentiation of the presumptive autonomic ganglion neurones. The factors responsible for subsequent adrenergic, cholinergic or peptidergic phenotype have yet to be identified, although it has been proposed that fibronectin and basal lamina components initiate adrenergic phenotypical expression at the expense of melanocyte numbers. Cholinergic characteristics are acquired relatively early, and the appropriate phenotypical expression may be promoted by cholinergic differentiation factor and CNTF.

Neuropeptides are expressed by autonomic neurones *in vitro* and may be stimulated by various target tissue factors in sympathetic and parasympathetic neurones. Some neuropeptides are expressed more intensely during early stages of ganglion formation.

Enteric Nervous System

The enteric nervous system is different from the other components of the autonomic nervous system because it can mediate reflex activity independently of control by the brain and spinal cord. The number of enteric neurones that develop is believed to be of the same magnitude as the number of neurones in the spinal cord. Preganglionic fibres that supply the intestine, and therefore modulate the enteric neurones, are much fewer.

The enteric nervous system is derived from the neural crest. The axial levels of crest origin are shown in Figure 3.20. Premigratory neural crest cells are not prepatterned for specific axial levels; rather, they attain their axial value as they leave the neuraxis. Once within the gut wall, there is a regionally specific pattern of enteric ganglia formation that may be controlled by the local splanchnopleuric mesenchyme. Cranial neural crest from somite levels 1 to 7 contributes to the enteric nervous system, forming both neuroblasts and glial support cells.

The most caudal derivatives of neural crest cells from the lumbosacral region, or somite 28 onward, form components of the pelvic plexus after migrating through the somites toward the level of the colon, rectum and cloaca. Initially the cells lie within the developing mesentery, then transiently between the layers of the differentiating muscularis externa, before finally forming a more substantial intramural plexus characteristic of the adult enteric nervous system.

Of the neural crest cells that colonize the bowel, some in the foregut may acquire the ability to migrate outward and colonize the developing pancreas.

Hirschsprung's disease appears to result from a failure of neural crest cells to colonize the gut wall appropriately. The condition is characterized by a dilated segment of colon proximally and lack of peristalsis in the segment distal to the dilatation. Infants with Hirschsprung's disease show delay in the passage of meconium, constipation, vomiting and abdominal distension. In humans, Hirschsprung's disease is often associated with other defects of neural crest development, including Waardenburg's syndrome type II, which includes deafness and facial clefts with megacolon.

Chromaffin Cells

Chromaffin cells are derived from the neural crest and found at numerous sites throughout the body. They are the classic chromaffin cells of the suprarenal medulla, bronchial neuroepithelial cells, dispersed epithelial endocrine cells of the gut (formerly known as argentaffin cells), carotid body cells and paraganglia.

The sympathetic ganglia, suprarenal medulla and chromaffin cells are all derived from the cells of the sympathoadrenal lineage. In the suprarenal medulla these cells differentiate into a number of types consisting of small and intermediate-sized neuroblasts or sympathoblasts and larger, initially rounded phaeochromocytoblasts.

Large cells with pale nuclei, thought to be the progenitors of chromaffin cells, can be detected from 9 weeks in human fetuses, and clusters of small neuroblasts are evident from 14 weeks.

Intermediate-sized neuroblasts differentiate into the typical multipolar postganglionic sympathetic neurones (which secrete noradrenaline at their terminals) of classic autonomic neuroanatomy. The smaller neuroblasts have been equated with types I and II small intensely fluorescent (SIF) cells, which store and secrete dopamine type I and are thought to function as true interneurones, synapsing with the principal postganglionic neurones. Type II cells probably operate as local neuroendocrine cells, secreting dopamine into the ganglionic microcirculation. Both types of SIF cells can modulate preganglionic–postganglionic synaptic transmission in the ganglionic neurones. The large cells differentiate into masses of columnar or polyhedral phaeochromocytes (classic chromaffin cells), which secrete either adrenaline (epinephrine) or noradrenaline (norepinephrine). These cell masses are termed paraganglia and may be situated near, on the surface of or embedded in the capsules of the ganglia of the sympathetic chain or in some of the large autonomic plexuses. The largest members of the latter are the para-aortic bodies, which lie along the sides of the abdominal aorta in relation to the inferior mesenteric artery. During childhood the para-aortic bodies and the paraganglia of the sympathetic chain partly degenerate and can no longer be isolated by gross dissection, but even in the adult, chromaffin tissue can still be recognized microscopically in these various sites. Both phaeochromocytes and SIF cells

belong to the amine precursor uptake and decarboxylation (APUD) series of cells and are paraneuronal in nature.

CENTRAL NERVOUS SYSTEM

Spinal Cord

In the future spinal cord the median roof plate (dorsal lamina) and floor plate (ventral lamina) of the neural tube do not participate in the cellular proliferation that occurs in the lateral walls, so they remain thin. Their cells contribute largely to the formation of the ependyma.

The neuroblasts of the lateral walls of the tube are large and initially round or oval (apolar). Soon they develop processes at opposite poles and become bipolar neuroblasts. However, one process is withdrawn, and the neuroblast becomes unipolar, although this is not invariably so in the case of the spinal cord. Further differentiation leads to the development of dendritic processes, and the cells become typical multipolar neurones. In the developing cord they occur in small clusters, representing clones of neurones. Development of a longitudinal sulcus limitans on each side of the central canal of the cord divides the ventricular and intermediate zones in each lateral wall into a basal (ventrolateral) plate or lamina and an alar (dorsolateral) plate or lamina (see Fig. 3.18). This separation indicates a fundamental functional difference. Neural precursors in the basal plate include the motor cells of the anterior (ventral) and lateral grey columns, whereas those of the alar plate exclusively form 'interneurones' (which possess both short and long axons), some of which receive the terminals of primary sensory neurones. Caudally the central canal of the cord ends as a fusiform dilatation, the terminal ventricle.

Anterior (Ventral) Grey Column

The cells of the ventricular zone are closely packed at this stage and arranged in radial columns (see Fig. 3.6). Their disposition may be determined in part by contact guidance along the earliest radial array of glial fibres that cross the full thickness of the early neuroepithelium. The cells of the intermediate zone are more loosely packed. They increase in number initially in the region of the basal plate. This enlargement outlines the anterior (ventral) column of the grey matter and causes a ventral projection on each side of the median plane; the floor plate remains at the bottom of the shallow groove produced. As growth proceeds, these enlargements, which are further increased by development of the anterior funiculi (tracts of axons passing to and from the brain), encroach on the groove until it becomes converted into the slit-like anterior median fissure of the adult spinal cord (see Fig. 3.18). The axons of some of the neuroblasts in the anterior grey column cross the marginal zone and emerge as bundles of ventral spinal nerve rootlets on the anterolateral aspect of the spinal cord. These constitute, eventually, both the α-efferents, which establish motor end-plates on extrafusal striated muscle fibres, and the γ-efferents, which innervate the contractile polar regions of the intrafusal muscle fibres of the muscle spindles.

Lateral Grey Column

In the thoracic and upper lumbar regions, some intermediate zone neuroblasts in the dorsal part of the basal plate outline a lateral column. Their axons join the emerging ventral nerve roots and pass as preganglionic fibres to the ganglia of the sympathetic trunk or related ganglia, the majority eventually myelinating to form white rami communicantes. The axons within the rami synapse on the autonomic ganglionic neurones, and axons of some of the latter pass as postganglionic fibres to innervate smooth muscle cells, adipose tissue or glandular cells. Other preganglionic sympathetic efferent axons pass to the cells of the suprarenal medulla. An autonomic lateral column is also laid down in the midsacral region. It gives origin to the preganglionic parasympathetic fibres that run in the pelvic splanchnic nerves.

The anterior region of each basal plate initially forms a continuous column of cells throughout the length of the developing cord. This soon develops into two columns (on each side): one is medially placed and concerned with innervation of axial musculature, and the other is laterally placed and innervates the limbs. At limb levels the lateral column enlarges enormously, but it regresses at other levels.

Axons arising from ventral horn neurones—that is, α-, β- and γ-efferent fibres—are accompanied at thoracic, upper lumbar and midsacral levels by preganglionic autonomic efferents from neuroblasts of the developing lateral horn. Numerous interneurones develop in these sites (including Renshaw cells); it is uncertain how many of these differentiate directly from ventrolateral lamina (basal plate) neuroblasts and how many migrate to their final positions from the dorsolateral lamina (alar plate).

In the human embryo, the definitive grouping of ventral column cells, which characterizes the mature cord, occurs early; by the fourteenth week (80 mm), all the major groups can be recognized. As the anterior and lateral grey columns assume their final form, the germinal cells in the ventral part of the ventricular zone gradually stop dividing. The layer becomes less thick until it ultimately forms the single-layered ependyma that lines the ventral part of the central canal of the spinal cord.

Posterior (Dorsal) Grey Column

The posterior (dorsal) column develops later; consequently, for a time, the ventricular zone is much thicker in the dorsolateral lamina (alar plate) than it is in the ventrolateral lamina (basal plate) (see Fig. 3.6).

While the columns of grey matter are being defined, the dorsal region of the central canal becomes narrow and slit-like, and its walls come into apposition and fuse with each other (see Fig. 3.18). In this way, the central canal becomes relatively reduced in size and somewhat triangular in outline.

About the end of the fourth week, advancing axonal sprouts invade the marginal zone. The first to develop are those destined to become short intersegmental fibres, derived from neuroblasts in the intermediate zone, and fibres of dorsal roots of spinal nerves that pass into the spinal cord, derived from neuroblasts of the early spinal ganglia. The earlier dorsal root fibres that invade the dorsal marginal zone arise from small dorsal root ganglionic neuroblasts. By the sixth week they form a well-defined oval bundle near the peripheral part of the dorsolateral lamina (see Figs. 3.6, 3.18). This bundle increases in size and, spreading toward the median plane, forms the primitive, fine-calibre posterior funiculus. Later, fibres derived from new populations of large dorsal root ganglionic neuroblasts join the dorsal root; they are destined to become fibres of much larger calibre. As the posterior funiculi increase in thickness, their medial surfaces come into contact, separated only by the posterior medial septum, which is ependymal in origin and neuroglial in nature. It is thought that the displaced primitive posterior funiculus may form the basis of the dorsolateral tract or fasciculus (of Lissauer).

Maturation of the Spinal Cord

Long intersegmental fibres begin to appear at about the third month, and corticospinal fibres are seen at about the fifth month. All nerve fibres at first lack myelin sheaths. Myelination starts in different groups at different times—the ventral and dorsal nerve roots about the fifth month, and the corticospinal fibres after the ninth month. In peripheral nerves the myelin is formed by Schwann cells (derived from neural crest cells), and in the CNS it is formed by oligodendrocytes (which develop from the ventricular zone of the neural tube). Myelination persists until overall growth of the CNS and PNS has ceased. In many sites, slow growth continues for long periods, even into the postpubertal years.

The cervical and lumbar enlargements appear at the time their respective limb buds develop.

In early embryonic life, the spinal cord occupies the entire length of the vertebral canal, and the spinal nerves pass at right angles to the cord. After the embryo has attained a length of 30 mm, the vertebral column begins to grow more rapidly than the spinal cord, and the caudal end of the cord gradually becomes more cranial in the vertebral canal (Fig. 3.21). Most of this relative rostral migration occurs during the first half of intrauterine life. By the twenty-fifth week the terminal ventricle of the spinal cord has altered in level from the second coccygeal vertebra to the third lumbar vertebra, a distance of nine segments. Because the change in level begins rostrally, the caudal end of the terminal ventricle, which is adherent to the overlying ectoderm, remains *in situ*, and the walls of the intermediate part of the ventricle and its covering pia mater become drawn out to form a delicate filament, the filum terminale. The separated portion of the terminal ventricle persists for a time, but it

usually disappears before birth. It occasionally gives rise to congenital cysts in the neighbourhood of the coccyx. In the definitive state, the upper cervical spinal nerves retain their position at roughly right angles to the cord. Proceeding caudally, the nerve roots lengthen and become progressively more oblique.

During gestation the relationship between the conus medullaris and the vertebral column changes, such that the conus medullaris gradually ascends to lie at higher vertebral levels. By 19 weeks of gestation the conus is adjacent to the fourth lumbar vertebra, and by full term (40 weeks) it is at the level of the second lumbar vertebra. By 2 months postnatally the conus medullaris has usually reached its permanent position at the level of the body of the first lumbar vertebra.

When performing a lumbar puncture, it is important to enter the spinal canal below the level of the tip of the conus medullaris. Although this is usually at or above the level of the second lumbar vertebra, in some individuals the cord may rarely extend as low as the third lumbar vertebra. It is therefore advisable for the needle to enter the canal below this level.

Brain

A summary of the derivatives of the cerebral vesicles from caudal to rostral is given in Table 3.1.

Rhombencephalon

By the time the midbrain flexure appears, the length of the hindbrain is greater than that of the combined extent of the other two brain vesicles. Rostrally it exhibits a constriction, the isthmus rhombencephali (see Fig. 3.2B), which is best viewed from the dorsal aspect. Ventrally the hindbrain is separated from the dorsal wall of the primitive pharynx only by the notochord, the two dorsal aortae and a small amount of mesenchyme; on each side it is closely related to the dorsal ends of the pharyngeal arches.

The pontine flexure appears to 'stretch' the thin epithelial roof plate, which becomes widened. The greatest increase in width corresponds to the region of maximal convexity, so the outline of the roof plate becomes rhomboidal. Due to the same change, the lateral walls become separated, particularly dorsally, and the cavity of the hindbrain, subsequently the fourth ventricle, becomes flattened and somewhat triangular in cross-section. The pontine flexure becomes increasingly acute until, at the end of the second month, the laminae of its cranial (metencephalic) and caudal (myelencephalic) slopes are opposed to each other (see Fig. 3.23); at the same time, the lateral angles of the cavity extend to form the lateral recesses of the fourth ventricle.

At about the end of the fourth week, when the pontine flexure is first discernible, a series of seven transverse rhombic grooves appears in the ventrolateral laminae (basal plate) of the hindbrain. Between the grooves, the intervening masses of neural tissue are termed rhombomeres. These are closely associated with the pattern of the underlying motor nuclei of certain cranial nerves. The general pattern of distribution of motor nuclei seems to be as follows: rhombomere 1 contains the trochlear nucleus, rhombomeres 2 and 3 the trigeminal nucleus, rhombomeres 4 and 5 the facial nucleus, rhombomere 5 the abducens nucleus, rhombomeres 6 and 7 the glossopharyngeal nucleus and rhombomeres 7 and 8 the vagal, accessory and hypoglossal nuclei. Rhombomeric segmentation represents the ground plan of development in this region of the brain stem and is pivotal for the development of regional identity. With further morphogenesis, however, the obvious constrictions of the rhombomere boundaries disappear, and the medulla once again assumes a smooth contour. Differentiation of the lateral walls of the hindbrain into basal (ventrolateral) and alar (dorsolateral) plates has a similar significance to the corresponding differentiation in the lateral wall of the spinal cord; ventricular, intermediate and marginal zones are formed in the same way.

Cells of the basal plate (ventrolateral lamina) — Cells of the basal plate form three elongated but interrupted columns positioned ventrally and dorsally, with an intermediate column between (Fig. 3.22). The most ventral column is continuous with the anterior grey column of the spinal cord and will supply muscles considered 'myotomic' in origin. It is represented in the caudal part of the hindbrain by the hypoglossal nucleus, and it reappears at a higher level as the nuclei of the abducens, trochlear and oculomotor nerves, which are somatic efferent nuclei. The intermediate column is represented in the upper part of the spinal cord and caudal brain stem (medulla oblongata and pons) and is for the supply of branchial (pharyngeal) and postbranchial musculature. It is interrupted and forms the elongated nucleus ambiguus in the caudal brain stem, which gives fibres to the ninth, tenth and eleventh cranial nerves. The latter continues into the cervical spinal cord as the origin of the spinal accessory nerve. At higher levels, parts of this column give origin to the motor nuclei of the facial and trigeminal nerves. These three nuclei are termed branchial (special visceral) efferent nuclei. The most dorsal column of the basal plate (represented in the spinal cord by the lateral grey column) innervates viscera. It too is interrupted, with its large caudal part forming some

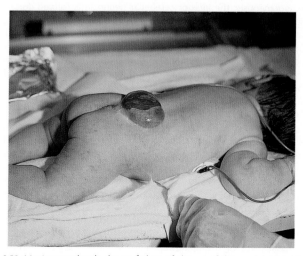

Fig. 3.21 *Meningomyelocele due to failure of closure of the caudal neural tube.*

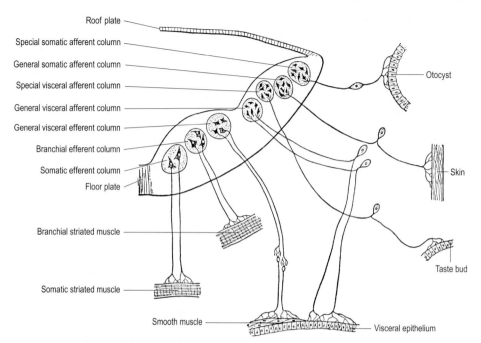

Roof plate

Special somatic afferent column

General somatic afferent column

Special visceral afferent column

General visceral afferent column

General visceral efferent column

Branchial efferent column

Somatic efferent column

Floor plate

Branchial striated muscle

Somatic striated muscle

Smooth muscle

Otocyst

Skin

Taste bud

Visceral epithelium

Fig. 3.22 *Transverse section through the developing hindbrain of a human embryo, 10.5 mm long, showing the relative positions of the columns of grey matter from which the nuclei associated with the different nerve components are derived. Postganglionic neurones are associated with the general visceral efferent column, bipolar neurones are associated with the otocyst and unipolar afferent neurones are associated with the other alar lamina columns.*

of the dorsal nucleus of the vagus and its cranial part the salivatory nucleus. These are termed general visceral (general splanchnic) efferent nuclei, and their neurones give rise to preganglionic, parasympathetic nerve fibres.

It should be noted here that the neurones of the basal plate and their three columnar derivatives are motor neurones only in the sense that some of them form either motor neurones or preganglionic parasympathetic neurones. The remainder, which greatly outnumber the former, differentiate into functionally related interneurones and, in some loci, neuroendocrine cells.

Cell columns of the alar plate (dorsolateral lamina) — Cell columns of the alar plate are interrupted and give rise to general visceral (general splanchnic) afferent, special visceral (special splanchnic) afferent, general somatic afferent and special somatic afferent nuclei (their relative positions, in simplified transverse section, are shown in Fig. 3.22). The general visceral afferent column is represented by part of the dorsal nucleus of the vagus nerve, the special visceral afferent column by the nucleus of the tractus solitarius, the general somatic afferent column by the afferent nuclei of the trigeminal nerve and the special somatic afferent column by the nuclei of the vestibulocochlear nerve. (The relatively simple functional independence of these afferent columns implied by the foregoing classification is mainly an aid to elementary learning. The emergent neurobiological mechanisms are in fact much more complex and less well understood.) Although they tend to retain their primitive positions, some of these nuclei are later displaced by differential growth patterns, by the appearance and growth of neighbouring fibre tracts and possibly by active migration.

It has been suggested that a neurone tends to remain as close as possible to its predominant source of stimulation and that when the possibility of separation arises as a result of the development of neighbouring structures, it migrates in the direction from which the greatest density of stimuli comes—a phenomenon termed neurobiotaxis. The curious courses of the fibres arising from the facial nucleus and the nucleus ambiguus have been held to illustrate this phenomenon. In the 10-mm embryo, the facial nucleus lies in the floor of the fourth ventricle, occupying the position of the special visceral efferent column, and it is placed at a higher level than the abducens nucleus. As growth proceeds, the facial nucleus migrates at first caudally and dorsally, relative to the abducens nucleus, and then ventrally to reach its adult position. As it migrates, the axons to which its somata give rise elongate, and their subsequent course is assumed to map out the pathway along which the facial nucleus has travelled. Similarly, the nucleus ambiguus initially arises immediately deep to the ventricular floor; in the adult it is more deeply placed, and its efferent fibres pass first dorsally and medially before curving laterally to emerge at the surface of the medulla oblongata.

Myelencephalon

The caudal slope of the embryonic hindbrain constitutes the myelencephalon, which develops into the medulla oblongata (see Fig. 3.2). The nuclei of the ninth, tenth, eleventh and twelfth cranial nerves develop in the positions

already indicated, and afferent fibres from the ganglia of the ninth and tenth nerves form an oval marginal bundle in the region overlying the alar (dorsolateral) lamina. Throughout the rhombencephalon, the dorsal edge of this lamina is attached to the thin expanded roof plate and is termed the rhombic lip. (The inferior rhombic lip is confined to the myelencephalon; the superior rhombic lip to the metencephalon.) As the walls of the rhombencephalon spread outward, the rhombic lip protrudes as a lateral edge that becomes folded over the adjoining area. The rhombic lip may later become adherent to this area, and its cells migrate actively into the marginal zone of the basal plate. In this way the oval bundle that forms the tractus solitarius becomes buried. Alar plate cells that migrate from the rhombic lip are believed to give rise to the olivary and arcuate nuclei and the scattered grey matter of the nuclei pontis. While this migration is in progress, the floor plate is invaded by fibres that cross the median plane (accompanied by neurones that cluster in and near this plane), and it becomes thickened to form the median raphe. Some of the migrating cells from the rhombic lip in this region do not reach the basal plate and form an oblique ridge: the corpus pontobulbare (nucleus of the circumolivary bundle) across the dorsolateral aspect of the inferior cerebellar peduncle.

The lower (caudal half) part of the myelencephalon has no role in the formation of the fourth ventricle, and in its development it closely resembles the spinal cord. The gracile and cuneate nuclei, and some reticular nuclei, are derived from the alar plate, and their efferent arcuate fibres and interspersed neurones play a large part in the formation of the median raphe.

At about the fourth month the descending corticospinal fibres invade the ventral part of the medulla oblongata to initiate formation of the pyramids. Contemporaneously, the inferior cerebellar peduncle is formed dorsally by ascending fibres from the spinal cord and by olivocerebellar and parolivocerebellar fibres, external arcuate fibres and two-way reticulocerebellar and vestibulocerebellar interconnections. (The reticular nuclei of the lower medulla probably have a dual origin from both basal and alar plates.) In the neonate the brain stem is more oblique and has a distinct bend as it passes through the foramen magnum to become the spinal cord.

Metencephalon

The rostral slope of the embryonic hindbrain is the metencephalon, from which both the cerebellum and the pons develop. Before formation of the pontine flexure, the dorsolateral laminae of the metencephalon are parallel with one another. After its formation, the roof plate of the hindbrain becomes rhomboidal, and the dorsal laminae of the metencephalon lie obliquely. They are close at the cranial end of the fourth ventricle but widely separated at the level of its lateral angles (Fig. 3.23). Accentuation of the flexure approximates the cranial angle of the ventricle to the caudal angle, and the alar plates of the metencephalon now lie almost horizontally.

The basal plate of the metencephalon becomes the pons. Ventricular, intermediate and marginal zones are formed in the usual way, and the nuclei

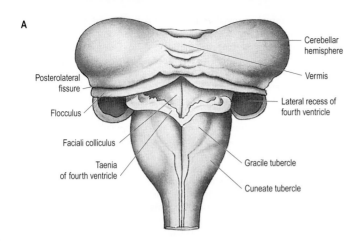

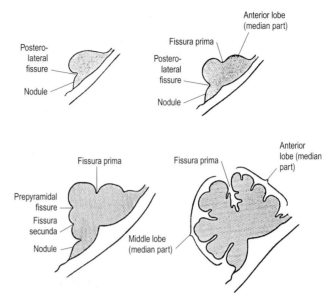

Fig. 3.24 *Median sagittal sections through the developing cerebellum, showing four different stages.*

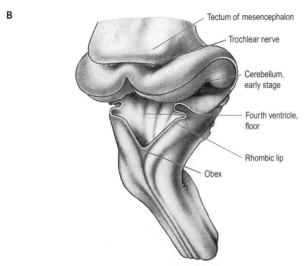

Fig. 3.23 *A, Cerebellum of a fetus in the fifth month. B, Dorsal aspect of the hindbrain of a human fetus approximately 3 months old, viewed partly from the right side.*

of the trigeminal, abducens and facial nerves develop in the intermediate layer. It is possible that the grey matter of the formatio reticularis is derived from the basal plate and that of the nuclei pontis from the alar plate by the active migration of cells from the rhombic lip. However, at about the fourth month the pons is invaded by corticopontine, corticobulbar and corticospinal fibres; it becomes proportionately thicker and takes on its adult appearance. It is relatively smaller in a full-term neonate.

The region of the isthmus rhombencephali undergoes a series of changes that are notoriously difficult to interpret but result in the incorporation of the greater part of the region into the caudal end of the midbrain. Only the roof plate, in which the superior medullary velum is formed, and the dorsal part of the alar plate, which is invaded by converging fibres of the superior cerebellar peduncles, remain as recognizable derivatives in the adult. Early in development, the decussation of the trochlear nerves is caudal to the isthmus, but as growth changes occur, it is displaced rostrally until it reaches its adult position.

Fourth ventricle and choroid plexus — Caudal to the developing cerebellum the roof of the fourth ventricle remains epithelial and covers an approximately triangular zone from the lateral angles of the rhomboid fossa to the median obex (see Fig. 3.23). Nervous tissue fails to develop over this region, and vascular pia mater is closely applied to the subjacent ependyma. At each lateral angle and in the midline caudally, the membranes break through, forming the lateral (Luschka) and median (Magendie) apertures of the roof of the fourth ventricle. These become the principal routes by which cerebrospinal fluid, produced in the ventricles, escapes into the subarachnoid space. The vascular pia mater (tela choroidea), in an inverted V formation cranial to the apertures, invaginates the ependyma to form vascular fringes, which become the vertical and horizontal parts of the choroid plexuses of the fourth ventricle.

Cerebellum

The cerebellum develops from the rhombic lip—the dorsal part of the alar plate of the metencephalon, which constitutes the rostral margin of the diamond-shaped fourth ventricle. Two rounded swellings develop that project partly into the ventricle at first (see Fig. 3.23), forming the rudimentary cerebellar hemispheres. The most rostral part of the roof of the metencephalon originally separates the two swellings, but it becomes invaded by cells derived from the alar plate, which form the rudiments of the vermis. At a later stage, extroversion of the cerebellum occurs, its intraventricular projection is reduced and the dorsal extraventricular prominence increases. The cerebellum now consists of a bilobar (dumbbell shaped) swelling stretched across the rostral part of the fourth ventricle (see Fig. 3.23). It is continuous rostrally with the superior medullary velum, formed from the isthmus rhombencephali, and caudally with the epithelial roof of the myelencephalon. With growth, a number of transverse grooves appear on the dorsal aspects of the cerebellar rudiment; these are the precursors of the numerous fissures that characterize the surface of the mature cerebellum (Fig. 3.24).

The first fissure to appear on the cerebellar surface (see Fig. 3.24) is the lateral part of the posterolateral fissure, which forms the border of a caudal region corresponding to the flocculi of the adult. The right and left parts of this fissure subsequently meet in the midline, where they form the boundary between the most caudal vermian lobule, the nodule and the rest of the vermis. The flocculonodular lobe can now be recognized as the most caudal cerebellar subdivision at this stage, and it serves as the attachment of the epithelial roof of the fourth ventricle. Because of the expansion of the other divisions of the cerebellum, the flocculonodular lobe comes to occupy an anteroinferior position in adults. At the end of the third month a transverse sulcus appears on the rostral slope of the cerebellar rudiment and deepens to form the fissura prima. This cuts into the vermis and both hemispheres and forms the border between the anterior and posterior lobes. Contemporaneously, two short transverse grooves appear in the caudal vermis. The first is the fissura secunda (postpyramidal fissure), which forms the rostral border of the uvula; the second, the prepyramidal fissure, demarcates the pyramid (see Fig. 3.24). The cerebellum now grows dorsally, rostrally, caudally and laterally, and the hemispheres expand much more than does the inferior vermis, which becomes buried at the bottom of a deep hollow, the vallecula. Numerous other transverse grooves develop, the most extensive being the horizontal fissure.

Cellular development of the cerebellum — The cerebellum consists of a cortex beneath which are buried a series of deep nuclei. The organization of the cerebellar cortex is similar to that of the cerebral cortex, except that the latter has six layers and the former has only three. However, whereas in the cerebral cortex neuroblasts originate from the ventricular zone and migrate ventriculofugally toward the pial surface (in an 'inside-out' fashion), early in cerebellar development a layer of cells derived exclusively from the metencephalic rhombic lip initially migrates ventriculofugally to form a layer beneath the glia limitans over the surface of the developing cerebellum. These cells form the external germinative layer, and later in development their progeny will migrate ventriculopetally (in an 'outside-in' manner) into the cerebellum. Thus, the cerebellum has an intraventricular portion (cells proliferating from the ventricular zone) and an extraventricular portion (cells proliferating from the external germinative layer) during development. The extraventricular portion becomes larger at the expense of the intraventricular part, the so-called extroversion of the cerebellum. Before the end of the third month the main mass of the cerebellum is extraventricular.

The developed cerebellar cortex contains three layers: the molecular layer, the Purkinje layer and the granular layer. The early bilateral expansion of the ventricular surface reflects the production, by the metencephalic alar plate ventricular epithelium, of neuroblasts that will give rise to the radial glia, cerebellar nuclei and efferent neurones of the cerebellar cortex (Purkinje cells) (Fig. 3.25). The radial glia play a role in guiding the Purkinje cells to the meningeal surface of the cerebellar anlage. During this early stage of cerebellar development, which is dominated by the production and migration of efferent cerebellar neurones, the surface of the cerebellar anlage remains smooth. Extroversion of the cerebellum begins later, when cells of the external granular layer, also termed the superficial matrix, begin proliferating and migrating. These cells produce the granule cells, which migrate inward along the radial glia and through the layers of Purkinje cells, settling deep to them in the granular layer. This stage coincides with the emergence of the transverse folial pattern. Proliferation and migration of granule cells lead to a great rostrocaudal expansion of the meningeal surface of the cerebellum, forming the transverse fissures and transforming the multicellular layer of Purkinje cells into a monolayer. Purkinje cells and nuclear cells are formed prior to the granule cells, and granule cells serve as the recipient of the main afferent (mossy fibre) system of the cerebellum. Thus, the development of efferent neurones of the cerebellar cortex and nuclei precedes the development of its afferent organization.

The early bilateral cerebellar anlage is changed into a unitary structure by fusion of the bilateral intraventricular bulges and the disappearance of the ependyma at this site, the merging of the left and right primitive cerebellar cortex over the midline and the development of the cerebellar commissure by ingrowth of afferent fibres and outgrowth of efferent axons of the medial cerebellar nucleus.

When the external germinative layer is initially formed, the multicellular Purkinje cell layer beneath is not uniform but is subdivided into clusters that form columns extending rostrocaudally (Fig. 3.26). The medial Purkinje cell clusters develop into the future vermis. These Purkinje cells will grow axons that connect to neurones in the vestibular nuclei and the fastigial nucleus. The lateral clusters belong to the future hemispheres and will grow axons terminating in the interposed and dentate nuclei. The sharp border in the efferent projections from the vermis and hemispheres is thus established at an early age. These clusters will give rise to Purkinje cell zones in the adult cerebellum that project to a single vestibular or cerebellar nucleus.

Mesencephalon

The mesencephalon or midbrain is derived from the intermediate primary cerebral vesicle. It persists for a time as a thin-walled tube enclosing a cavity of some size, separated from that of the prosencephalon by a slight constriction and from the rhombencephalon by the isthmus rhombencephali (Figs. 3.2, 3.27). Later, its cavity becomes relatively reduced in diameter, and in the adult brain it forms the cerebral aqueduct. The basal (ventrolateral) plate of the midbrain increases in thickness to form the cerebral peduncles, which are small at first but enlarge rapidly after the fourth month, when their numerous fibre tracts begin to appear in the marginal zone. The neuroblasts of the basal plate give rise to the nuclei of the oculomotor nerve and some grey masses of the tegmentum, while the nucleus of the trochlear nerve remains in the region of the isthmus rhombencephali. The cells giving rise to the trigeminal mesencephalic nucleus arise on either side of the dorsal midline, from the isthmus rhombencephali rostrally across the roof of the mesencephalon. Recent studies have shown that the progenitors of these cells do not express neural crest cell markers.

The cells of the dorsal part of the alar (dorsolateral) plates proliferate and invade the roof plate, which thickens and is later divided into corpora

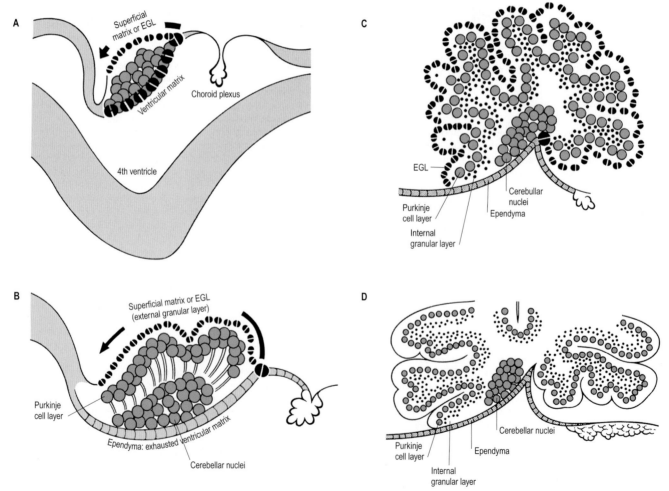

Fig. 3.25 *Four stages in the histogenesis of the cerebellar cortex and cerebellar nuclei.* **A**, *Purkinje cells and cells of the cerebellar nuclei are produced by the ventricular epithelium and are in the process of migrating to their future positions. The cells of the superficial matrix (external granular layer) originate from the ventricular epithelium at the caudal pole of the cerebellar anlage and migrate rostrally over its surface.* **B**, *After migration, the Purkinje cells constitute a multicellular layer beneath the external granular layer. Cell production in the ventricular epithelium has stopped. The remaining cells transform into ependymal cells.* **C**, *Granule cells are produced by the external granular layer and migrate inward through the Purkinje cell layer to their position in the granular layer. Purkinje cells spread into a monolayer.* **D**, *Adult position of cortical and nuclear neurones.*

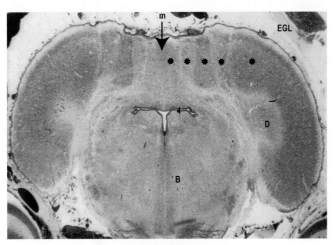

Fig. 3.26 Coronal section through the cerebellum and brain stem of a 65-mm human fetus. The Purkinje cells are located in five multicellular clusters (stars) *on both sides of the midline. The anlage of the dentate nucleus occupies the centre of the most lateral Purkinje cell cluster.* B, brain stem; D, dentate nucleus; EGL, external granular layer; m, midline; 4, fourth ventricle. *(Courtesy of the Schenk Collection, Dr. Johan M. Kros, Division of Neuropathology, Department of Pathology, Erasmus Medical Centre, Rotterdam, the Netherlands.)*

bigemina by a median groove. Caudally this groove becomes a median ridge, which persists in the adult as the frenulum veli. The corpora bigemina are later subdivided into the superior and inferior colliculi by a transverse furrow. The red nucleus, substantia nigra and reticular nuclei of the midbrain tegmentum may first be defined at the end of the third month. Their origins are probably mixed from neuroblasts of both basal and alar plates.

The detailed histogenesis of the tectum and its main derivatives, the colliculi, are not followed here, but in general, the principles outlined for the cerebellar cortex, the palaeopallium and neopallium also apply to this region. A high degree of geometric order exists in the developing retinotectal projection (the equivalent of the retinogeniculate projection) and in the tectospinal projection.

Prosencephalon

At an early stage, a transverse section through the forebrain shows the same parts displayed in similar sections of the spinal cord and medulla oblongata: thick lateral walls connected by thin floor and roof plates. Moreover, each lateral wall is divided into a dorsal area and a ventral area separated internally by the hypothalamic sulcus (see Fig. 3.27). This sulcus ends anteriorly at the medial end of the optic stalk. In the fully developed brain it persists as a slight groove extending from the interventricular foramen to the cerebral aqueduct. It is analogous to, if not the homologue of, the sulcus limitans. The thin roof plate remains epithelial but is invaginated by vascular mesenchyme, the tela choroidea of the choroid plexuses of the third ventricle. Later the lateral margins of the tela undergo a similar invagination into the medial walls of the cerebral hemispheres. The floor plate thickens as the nuclear masses of the hypothalamus and subthalamus develop.

At a very early period, before closure of the rostral neuropore, two lateral diverticula—the optic vesicles—appear, one on each side, at about the level of the prosencephalon. For a time they communicate with the cavity of the prosencephalon by relatively wide openings. The distal parts of the optic vesicles expand, and the proximal parts become the tubular optic stalks. The optic vesicles (which are described in the section on the development of the eye) are derived from the lateral walls of the prosencephalon before the telencephalon can be identified. They are usually regarded as derivatives of the diencephalon, and the optic chiasma is often regarded as the boundary between the diencephalon and telencephalon.

As the most rostral portion of the prosencephalon enlarges, it curves ventrally, and two additional diverticula rapidly expand from it, one on each side. These diverticula are rostrolateral to the optic stalks and subsequently form the cerebral hemispheres. Their cavities are the rudiments of the lateral ventricles, and they communicate with the median part of the forebrain cavity by relatively wide openings that ultimately become the interventricular foramina. The anterior limit of the median part of the forebrain consists of a thin sheet, the lamina terminalis (see Fig. 3.27), which stretches from the interventricular foramina to the recess at the base of the optic stalks. The anterior part of the forebrain, including the rudiments of the cerebral hemispheres, is the telencephalon (endbrain) and the posterior part of the diencephalon (between brain). Both contribute to the formation of the third

ventricle, although the latter predominates. The fate of the lamina terminalis is described later.

Diencephalon

The diencephalon is broadly divided by the hypothalamic sulcus into dorsal (pars dorsalis diencephali) and ventral (pars ventralis diencephali) parts; these, however, are composite, and each contributes to diverse neural structures. The dorsal part develops into the (dorsal) thalamus and metathalamus along the immediate suprasulcal area of its lateral wall, while the highest dorsocaudal lateral wall and roof form the epithalamus. The thalamus (see Fig. 3.27) is first visible as a thickening that involves the anterior part of the dorsal area. Caudal to the thalamus, the lateral and medial geniculate bodies, or metathalamus, are first recognizable as surface depressions on the internal aspect and as elevations on the external aspect of the lateral wall. As the thalami enlarge to become smooth ovoid masses, the wide interval between them gradually narrows into a vertically compressed cavity that forms the greater part of the third ventricle. After a time these medial surfaces may come into contact and become adherent over a variable area, the connection (single or multiple) constituting the interthalamic adhesion or massa intermedia. The caudal growth of the thalamus excludes the geniculate bodies from the lateral wall of the third ventricle.

At first the lateral aspect of the developing thalamus is separated from the medial aspect of the cerebral hemisphere by a cleft, but with growth, the cleft becomes obliterated (Fig. 3.28) as the thalamus fuses with the part of the hemisphere in which the corpus striatum is developing. Later, with the development of the projection fibres (corticofugal and corticopetal) of the neocortex, the thalamus becomes related to the internal capsule, which intervenes between it and the lateral part of the corpus striatum (lentiform nucleus). Ventral to the hypothalamic sulcus, the lateral wall of the diencephalon, in addition to median derivatives of its floor plate, forms a large part of the hypothalamus and subthalamus.

The epithalamus, which includes the pineal gland, the posterior and habenular commissures and the trigonum habenulae, develops in association with the caudal part of the roof plate and the adjoining regions of the lateral walls of the diencephalon. At an early period (12 to 20 mm crown–rump length), the epithalamus in the lateral wall projects into the third ventricle as a smooth ellipsoid mass, larger than the adjacent mass of the (dorsal) thalamus and separated from it by a well-defined epithalamic sulcus. In subsequent months, growth of the thalamus rapidly overtakes that of the epithalamus, and the intervening sulcus is obliterated. Thus, ultimately, structures of epithalamic origin are topographically relatively diminutive.

The pineal gland arises as a hollow outgrowth from the roof plate, immediately adjoining the mesencephalon. Its distal part becomes solid by cellular proliferation, but its proximal stalk remains hollow, containing the pineal recess of the third ventricle. In many reptiles the pineal outgrowth is two-fold. The anterior outgrowth (parapineal organ) develops into the pineal or parietal eye, whereas the posterior outgrowth is glandular in character. The posterior outgrowth is homologous with the pineal gland in humans. The anterior outgrowth also develops in the human embryo but soon disappears entirely.

The nucleus habenulae, which is the most important constituent of the trigonum habenulae, develops in the lateral wall of the diencephalon and is at first in close relationship with the geniculate bodies, from which it becomes separated by the dorsal growth of the thalamus. The habenular commissure develops in the cranial wall of the pineal recess. The posterior commissure is formed by fibres that invade the caudal wall of the pineal recess from both sides.

The ventral part of the diencephalon forms the subsulcal lateral walls of the third ventricle and takes part in the formation of the hypothalamus, including the mammillary bodies, the tuber cinereum and the infundibulum of the hypophysis. The mammillary bodies arise as a single thickening, which becomes divided by a median furrow during the third month. Anterior to them, the tuber cinereum develops as a cellular proliferation that extends forward as far as the infundibulum. In front of the tuber cinereum, a wide-mouthed diverticulum forms in the floor of the diencephalon. It grows toward the stomodeal roof and comes into contact with the posterior aspect of a dorsally directed ingrowth from the stomodeum (Rathke's pouch). These two diverticula together form the hypophysis cerebri (see Fig. 3.15). An extension of the third ventricle persists in the base of the neural outgrowth as the infundibular recess. The remaining caudolateral walls and floor of the ventral diencephalon are an extension of the midbrain tegmentum, the subthalamus. This forms the rostral limits of the red nucleus, substantia nigra, numerous reticular nuclei and a wealth of interweaving, ascending, descending and oblique nerve fibre bundles, which have many origins and destinations.

Third ventricle and choroid plexus — The roof plate of the diencephalon, rostral to the pineal gland (and continuing over the median telencephalon), remains thin and epithelial in character and is subsequently invaginated by

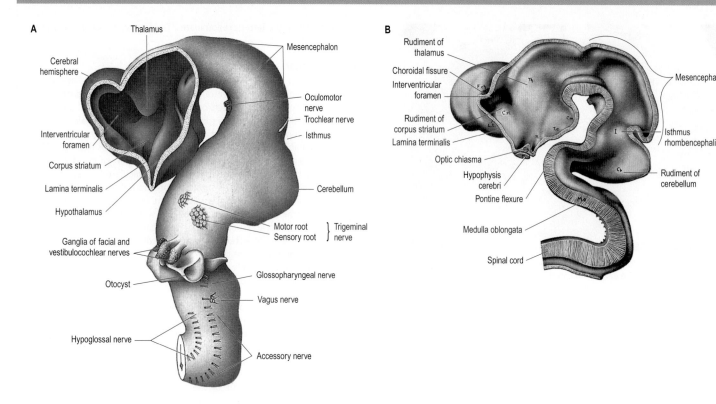

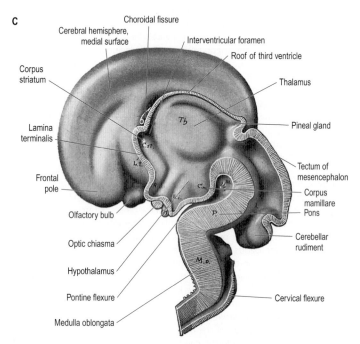

Fig. 3.27 *A, Brain of a human embryo, approximately 10.2 mm long. B, Medial surface of the right half of the brain of a human embryo, 13.6 mm long. The roof of the hindbrain has been removed. C, Medial surface of the right half of the brain of a human fetus, approximately 3 months old.*

the choroid plexuses of the third ventricle (Fig. 3.29). Before the development of the corpus callosum and the fornix, it lies at the bottom of the longitudinal fissure, between and reaching the two cerebral hemispheres. It extends as far rostrally as the interventricular foramina and lamina terminalis. Here and elsewhere, choroid plexuses develop by the close apposition of vascular pia mater and ependyma without intervening nervous tissue. With development, the vascular layer is infolded into the ventricular cavity and develops a series of small villous projections, each covered by a cuboidal epithelium derived from the ependyma. The cuboidal cells carry numerous microvilli on their ventricular surfaces; basally, the plasma membrane becomes complexly folded into the cell. The early choroid plexuses secrete a protein-rich cerebrospinal fluid into the ventricular system, which may provide a nutritive medium for the developing epithelial neural tissues. As the latter becomes increasingly vascularized, the histochemical reactions of the cuboidal cells and the character of the fluid change to the adult type. The remaining lining of the third ventricle does not simply form generalized ependymal cells. Many regions become highly specialized, developing concentrations of tanycytes or

other modified cells (e.g. those of the subfornical organ), the organum vasculosum (intercolumnar tubercle) of the lamina terminalis, the subcommissural organ and those lining the pineal, suprapineal and infundibular recesses, which are collectively termed the circumventricular organs.

Telencephalon

The telencephalon (endbrain) consists of two lateral diverticula connected by a median region (the telencephalon impar). The anterior part of the third ventricle develops from the impar and is closed below and in front by the lamina terminalis. The lateral diverticula are outpouchings of the lateral walls of the telencephalon; these may correspond to the alar lamina, although this is uncertain. Their cavities are the future lateral ventricles, and their walls are formed by the presumptive nervous tissue of the cerebral hemispheres. The roof plate of the median part of the telencephalon remains thin and is continuous behind with the roof plate of the diencephalon (see Fig. 3.27). The anterior parts of the hypothalamus, which include the optic chiasma, optic recess and related nuclei, develop in the floor plate and lateral walls of the

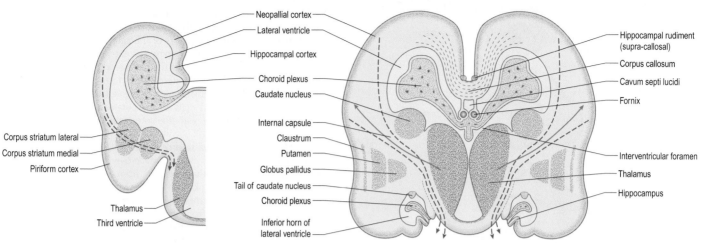

Fig. 3.28 Development of the basal nuclei and internal capsule. (Redrawn by permission from Hamilton, W.J., Boyd, J.D., Mossman, H.W. 1972. Human Embryology: Prenatal Development of Form and Function. Williams and Wilkins, Baltimore.)

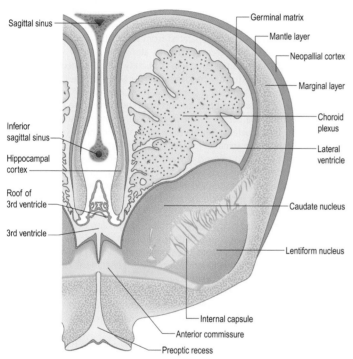

Fig. 3.29 Coronal section of the left cerebral hemisphere in a 73-mm fetus. (Redrawn by permission from Hamilton, W.J., Boyd, J.D., Mossman, H.W. 1972. Human Embryology: Prenatal Development of Form and Function. Williams and Wilkins, Baltimore.)

prosencephalon, ventral to the primitive interventricular foramina. The chiasma is formed by the meeting and partial decussation of the optic nerves in the ventral part of the lamina terminalis. The optic tracts subsequently grow backward from the chiasma to end in the diencephalon and midbrain.

Cerebral hemispheres — The cerebral hemispheres arise as diverticula of the lateral walls of the telencephalon, with which they remain in continuity around the margins of the initially relatively large interventricular foramina, except caudally, where they are continuous with the anterior part of the lateral wall of the diencephalon (see Figs. 3.2, 3.27). As growth proceeds, the hemisphere enlarges forward, upward and backward and acquires an oval outline, medial and superolateral walls and a floor. As a result, the medial surfaces approach, but are separated by, a vascularized mesenchyme and pia mater that fill the median longitudinal fissure (see Fig. 3.29). At this stage the floor of the fissure is the epithelial roof plate of the telencephalon, which is directly continuous caudally with the epithelial roof plate of the diencephalons.

At the early oval stage of hemispheric development, regions are named according to their future principal derivatives. The rostromedial and ventral floor becomes linked with the forming olfactory apparatus and is termed the primitive olfactory lobe. The floor (ventral wall, or base) of the larger remainder of the hemisphere forms the anlage of the primitive corpus striatum and

amygdaloid complex, including its associated rim of lateral and medial walls; this is the striate part of the hemisphere. The rest of the hemisphere—the medial, lateral, dorsal and caudal regions—is the suprastriate part of the hemisphere. Although largest in terms of surface area, it initially possesses comparatively thin walls. The rostral end of the oval hemisphere becomes the definitive frontal pole. As the hemisphere expands, its original posterior pole moves relatively in a caudoventral and lateral direction, following a curve like a ram's horn; it curves toward the orbit in association with the growth of the caudate nucleus (and other structures) to form the definitive temporal pole. A new posterior part persists as the definitive occipital pole of the mature brain (Fig. 3.30). The great expansion of the cerebral hemispheres is characteristic of mammals and especially of humans. In their subsequent growth they overlap, successively, the diencephalon and the mesencephalon and then meet the rostral surface of the cerebellum. The temporal lobes embrace the flanks of the brain stem.

Olfactory bulb — A longitudinal groove appears in the anteromedial part of the floor of each developing lateral ventricle at about the fifth week of embryonic development. This groove deepens and forms a hollow diverticulum that is continuous with the hemisphere by means of a short stalk. The diverticulum becomes connected on its ventral or inferior surface to the olfactory placode. Placodal cells give rise to afferent axons that terminate in the walls of the diverticulum. As the head increases in size, the diverticulum grows forward and, losing its cavity, is converted into the solid olfactory bulb. The forward growth of the bulb is accompanied by elongation of its stalk, which forms the olfactory tract. The part of the floor of the hemisphere to which the tract is attached constitutes the piriform area.

Lateral ventricles and choroid plexus — The early diverticulum or anlage of the cerebral hemisphere initially contains a simple spheroidal lateral ventricle that is continuous with the third ventricle via the interventricular foramen. The rim of the foramen is the site of the original evagination. The expanding ventricle develops the ram's horn shape of the surrounding hemisphere, becoming first roughly ellipsoid and then a curved cylinder that is convex dorsally (see Fig. 3.30). The ends of the cylinder expand toward, but do not reach, the frontal and (temporary) occipital poles; differentiating and thickening neural tissues separate the ventricular cavities and pial surfaces at all points, except along the line of the choroidal fissure. Pronounced changes in ventricular form accompany the emergence of a temporal pole. The original caudal end of the curved cylinder expands within its substance, and the temporal extensions in each hemisphere pass ventrolaterally to encircle both sides of the upper brain stem. Another extension may develop from the root of the temporal extension in the substance of the definitive occipital pole and pass caudomedially; it is quite variable in size, often asymmetric on the two sides and one or both may be absent. Although the lateral ventricle is a continuous system of cavities, specific parts are now given regional names. The central part (body) extends from the interventricular foramen to the level of the posterior edge (splenium) of the corpus callosum. Three cornua (horns) diverge from the body: anterior toward the frontal pole, posterior toward the occipital pole and inferior toward the temporal pole.

At these early stages of hemispheric development, the term pole is preferred, in most instances, to lobe. Lobes are defined by specific surface topographic features that will appear over several months, and differential growth patterns persist for a considerable period.

The pia mater covering the epithelial roof of the third ventricle at this stage is itself covered with loosely arranged mesenchyme and developing blood

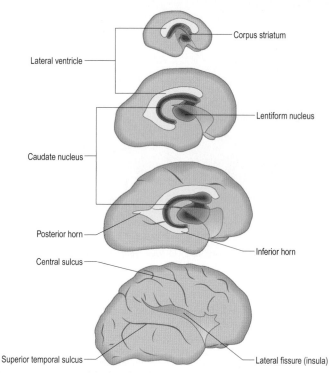

Lateral ventricle — Corpus striatum

Lentiform nucleus

Caudate nucleus

Posterior horn — Inferior horn

Central sulcus

Superior temporal sulcus — Lateral fissure (insula)

Fig. 3.30 *Formation of the basal nuclei and lateral ventricles as the telencephalon develops. (Redrawn by permission from Hamilton, W.J., Boyd, J.D., Mossman, H.W. 1972. Human Embryology: Prenatal Development of Form and Function. Williams and Wilkins, Baltimore.)*

vessels. These vessels subsequently invaginate the roof of the third ventricle on each side of the median plane to form its choroid plexuses. The lower part of the medial wall of the cerebral hemisphere, which immediately adjoins the epithelial roof of the interventricular foramen and the anterior extremity of the diencephalon, also remains epithelial. It consists of ependyma and pia mater; elsewhere the walls of the hemispheres are thickening to form the pallium. The thin part of the medial wall of the hemisphere is invaginated by vascular tissue that is continuous in front with the choroid plexus of the third ventricle and constitutes the choroid plexus of the lateral ventricle. This invagination occurs along a line that arches upward and backward, parallel with and initially limited to the anterior and upper boundaries of the interventricular foramen. This curved indentation of the ventricular wall, where no nervous tissue develops between ependyma and pia mater, is termed the choroidal fissure (see Figs. 3.27C, 3.28). Subsequent assumption of the definitive form of the choroidal fissure depends on related growth patterns in neighbouring structures. Of particular importance are the relatively slow growth of the interventricular foramen, the secondary 'fusion' between the lateral diencephalon and medial hemisphere walls, the encompassing of the upper brain stem by the forward growth of the temporal lobe and its pole toward the apex of the orbit and the massive expansion of two great cerebral commissures (the fornix and corpus callosum). The choroidal fissure is now clearly a caudal extension of the much reduced interventricular foramen, which arches above the thalamus and here is only a few millimetres from the median plane. Near the caudal end of the thalamus it diverges ventrolaterally, its curve reaching and continuing in the medial wall of the temporal lobe over much of its length (i.e. to the tip of the inferior horn of the lateral ventricle). The upper part of the arch will be overhung by the corpus callosum, and throughout its convexity it is bordered by the fornix and its derivatives.

Basal nuclei — At first, growth proceeds more actively in the floor and the adjoining part of the lateral wall of the developing hemisphere, and elevations formed by the rudimentary corpus striatum encroach on the cavity of the lateral ventricle (see Figs. 3.27, 3.28). The head of the caudate nucleus appears as three successive parts—medial, lateral and intermediate—which produce elevations in the floor of the lateral ventricle. Caudally these merge to form the tail of the caudate nucleus and the amygdaloid complex, both of which remain close to the temporal pole of the hemisphere. When the occipital pole grows backward and the general enlargement of the hemisphere carries the temporal pole downward and forward, the tail of the caudate is continued from the floor of the central part (body) of the ventricle into the roof of its temporal extension, the future inferior horn. The amygdaloid complex encapsulates its tip. Anteriorly the head of the caudate nucleus extends forward to the floor of the interventricular foramen, where it is separated from the developing anterior end of the thalamus by a groove; later the head expands

in the floor of the anterior horn of the lateral ventricle. The lentiform nucleus develops from two laminae of cells, medial and lateral, which are continuous with both the medial and lateral parts of the caudate nucleus. The internal capsule appears first in the medial lamina and extends laterally through the outer lamina to the cortex. It divides the laminae in two; the internal parts join the caudate nucleus, and the external parts form the lentiform nucleus. In the latter, the remaining medial lamina cells give rise mainly to the globus pallidus and the lateral lamina cells to the putamen. The putamen subsequently expands concurrently with the intermediate part of the caudate nucleus.

Fusion of diencephalic and telencephalic walls — As the hemisphere enlarges, the caudal part of its medial surface overlaps and hides the lateral surface of the diencephalon (thalamic part), from which it is separated by a narrow cleft occupied by vascular connective tissue. At this stage (about the end of the second month) a transverse section made caudal to the interventricular foramen would pass from the third ventricular cavity successively through the developing thalamus, the narrow cleft just mentioned, the thin medial wall of the hemisphere and the cavity of the lateral ventricle, with the corpus striatum in its floor and lateral wall (see Fig. 3.28).

As the thalamus increases in extent it acquires a superior surface in addition to medial and lateral surfaces. The lateral part of its superior surface fuses with the thin medial wall of the hemisphere so that this part of the thalamus is finally covered with the ependyma of the lateral ventricle immediately ventral to the choroidal fissure. As a result, the corpus striatum is approximated to the thalamus and is separated from it only by a deep groove that becomes obliterated by increased growth along the line of contact. The lateral aspect of the thalamus is now in continuity with the medial aspect of the corpus striatum, so that a secondary union between the diencephalon and telencephalon is effected over a wide area, providing a route for the subsequent passage of projection fibres to and from the cortex (see Fig. 3.28).

Development of the cortex — The migration and differentiation of neural progenitors to form nuclei are either minimal or limited throughout the brain stem, as they are in the spinal cord. Their progeny remain immediately extraependymal or partially displaced toward the pial exterior and are arrested deeply embedded in the myelinated fibre 'white matter' of the region. In marked contrast, proliferation and migration of neuroblasts in the cerebral hemisphere produce a superficial layer of grey matter. This occurs in both the striate and suprastriate regions, but not in the central areas of the original medial wall, where secondary fusion of the diencephalon occurs. The superficial layer of grey matter consists of neuronal somata, dendrites, the terminations of incoming (afferent) axons, the stems (or the whole) of efferent axons and glial cells and endothelial cells. Successive generations of neuroblasts migrate through the layers of earlier generations to attain subpial positions, so that the surface of the cerebral hemispheres expands at a rate greater than that of the hemispheres as a whole. Subsequent differentiation results in a highly organized subpial surface coat of grey matter termed the cortex or pallium.

The terminology used to describe regions of the cortex is based on evolutionary concepts. The oldest portions of cortex receive information concerned with olfaction; they are termed the archicortex (archipallium) and palaeocortex (palaeopallium), and both are subdivisions of an overall allocortex. The archicortex is the forerunner of the hippocampal lobe, and the palaeocortex gives rise to the piriform area. The remaining cortical surface expands greatly in mammals to form the neocortex (young cortex), which displaces the earlier cortices so that they come to lie partially internally in each hemisphere.

Formation of the insula — At the end of the third month, while the corpus striatum is developing, there is a relative restriction of growth between the frontal and temporal lobes. The region lateral to the striatum becomes depressed to form a lateral cerebral fossa, with a portion of cortex, the insula, at its base (see Fig. 3.30). As the temporal lobe continues to protrude toward the orbit, and with more rapid growth of the temporal and frontal cortices, the surface of the hemisphere expands at a rate greater than that of the hemisphere as a whole, and the cortical areas become folded, forming gyri and sulci. The insula is gradually overgrown by these adjacent cortical regions, and they overlap it to form the opercula, the free margins of which form the anterior part of the lateral fissure. This process is not completed until after birth. The lentiform nucleus remains deep to and coextensive with the insula.

Olfactory nerve, limbic lobe and hippocampus — The growth changes in the temporal lobe that help submerge the insula produce important changes in the olfactory and neighbouring limbic areas. As it approaches the hemispheric floor, the olfactory tract diverges into lateral, medial and (variable) intermediate striae. The medial stria is clothed with a thin archaeocortical medial olfactory gyrus. This curves up into other archaeocortical areas anterior to the lamina terminalis (paraterminal gyrus, prehippocampal rudiment, parolfactory gyrus, septal nuclei), and these continue into the indusium griseum. The lateral stria, clothed by the lateral olfactory gyrus, and, when present, the intermediate stria terminate in the rostral parts of the piriform area. This includes the olfactory trigone and tubercle, anterior perforated substance and uncus (hook) and entorhinal area of the anterior part of the future parahippocampal gyrus. Its lateral limit is indicated by the rhinal sulcus. The forward growth of the temporal pole and the general expansion of the neocortex cause the lateral olfactory gyrus to bend laterally, with the summit of the convexity lying at the anteroinferior corner of the developing insula (Fig. 3.31). During the fourth and fifth months, much of the piriform area

becomes submerged by the adjoining neocortex, and in the adult, only part of it remains visible on the inferior aspect of the cerebrum.

The limbic (bordering) lobe is the first part of the cortex to differentiate. At first it forms a continuous, almost circular strip on the medial and inferior aspects of the hemisphere. Below and in front, where the stalk of the olfactory tract is attached, it constitutes part of the piriform area. The portion outside the curve of the choroid fissure (Fig. 3.32) constitutes the hippocampal formation. In this region the neural progenitors of the developing cortex proliferate and migrate, and the wall of the hemisphere thickens and produces

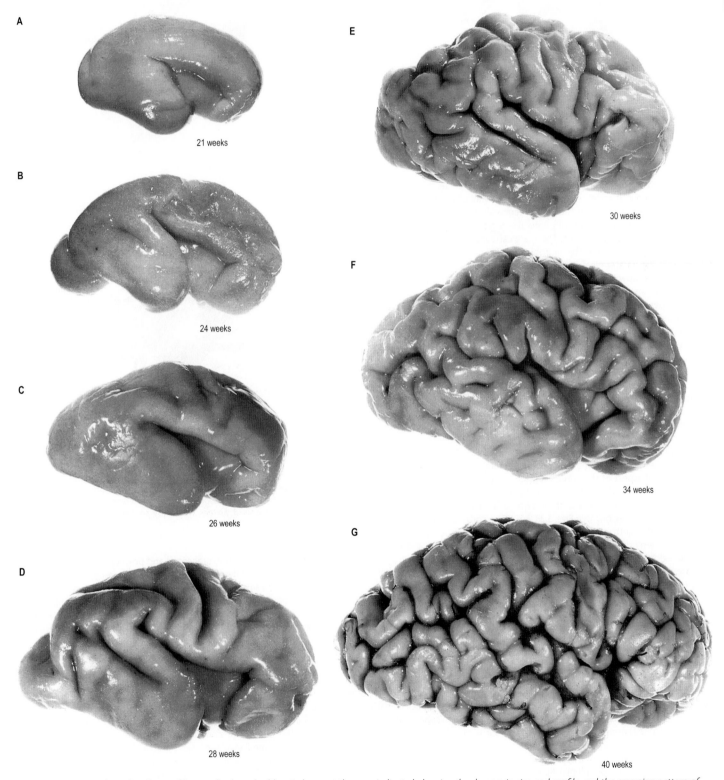

A
21 weeks

B
24 weeks

C
26 weeks

D
28 weeks

E
30 weeks

F
34 weeks

G
40 weeks

Fig. 3.31 A–G, Superolateral surfaces of human fetal cerebral hemispheres at the ages indicated, showing the changes in size and profile and the emerging pattern of cerebral sulci with increasing maturation. Note the changing prominence and relative positions of the frontal, occipital and particularly temporal poles of the hemisphere. At the earliest stage (A), the lateral cerebral fossa is already obvious; its floor covers the developing corpus striatum in the depths of the hemisphere and progressively matures into the cortex of the insula. The fossa is bounded by overgrowing cortical regions—the frontal, temporal and parietal opercula—which gradually converge to bury the insula; their approximation forms the lateral cerebral sulcus. By the sixth month, the central, pre- and postcentral, superior temporal, intraparietal and parieto-occipital sulci are all clearly visible. In the subsequent stages shown, all the remaining principal and subsidiary sulci rapidly appear, and by 40 weeks (G), all the features that characterize the adult hemisphere in terms of surface topography are present in miniature. (Photographs provided by Dr. Sabina Strick, The Maudsley Hospital, London.)

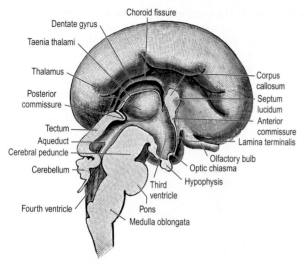

Fig. 3.32 *Medial aspect of the left half of the brain of a human fetus, 16 weeks old.*

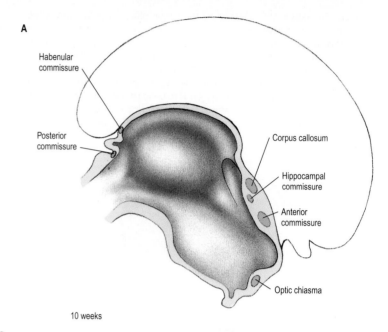

10 weeks

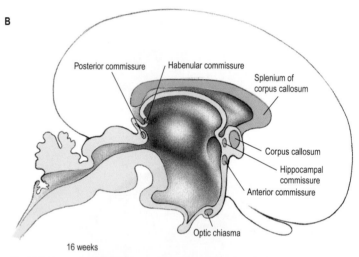

16 weeks

Fig. 3.33 *Formation of the commissures. The telencephalon gives rise to commissural tracts that integrate the activities of the left and right cerebral hemispheres. These include the anterior and hippocampal commissures and the corpus callosum. The small posterior and habenular commissures arise from the epithalamus. A, Ten weeks. B, Sixteen weeks. (By permission from Larsen.)*

an elevation that projects into the medial side of the ventricle: this elevation is the hippocampus. It appears first on the medial wall of the hemisphere in the area above and in front of the lamina terminalis (paraterminal area) and gradually extends backward, curving into the region of the temporal pole, where it adjoins the piriform area. The marginal zone in the neighbourhood of the hippocampus is invaded by neuroblasts to form the dentate gyrus. Both extend from the paraterminal area backward, above the choroid fissure, and follow its curve downward and forward toward the temporal pole, where they continue into the piriform area. A shallow groove (the hippocampal sulcus) crosses the medial surface of the hemisphere throughout the hippocampal formation.

The efferent fibres from the cells of the hippocampus collect along its medial edge and run forward immediately above the choroid fissure. Anteriorly they turn ventrally and enter the lateral part of the lamina terminalis to gain the hypothalamus, where they end in and around the mammillary body and neighbouring nuclei. These efferent hippocampal fibres form the fimbria hippocampi and the fornix.

Projection fibres and internal capsule — The growth of the neocortex and its enormous expansion during the latter part of the third month are associated with the initial appearance of corticofugal and corticopetal projection fibres and the pathway they follow, the internal capsule. These fibres follow the route provided by the apposition of the lateral aspect of the thalamus with the medial aspect of the corpus striatum, and as they do so, they divide the latter almost completely into a lateral part, the lentiform nucleus, and a medial part, the caudate nucleus; these two nuclei remain confluent only in their anteroinferior regions (see Figs. 3.28, 3.30). The corticospinal tracts begin to develop in the ninth week of fetal life and have reached their caudal limits by the twenty-ninth week. The fibres destined for the cervical and upper thoracic regions and involved in innervation of the upper limbs are in advance of those concerned with the lower limbs, which in turn are in advance of those concerned with the face. The appearance of reflexes in these three parts of the body follows a comparable sequence.

The majority of subcortical nuclear masses receive terminals from descending fibres of cortical origin. These are joined by thalamocortical, hypothalamocortical and other afferent ascending bundles. The internal capsular fibres pass lateral to the head and body of the caudate nucleus, anterior cornu and central part of the lateral ventricle, rostroventral extensions and body of the fornix and dorsal thalamus and dorsal choroidal fissure; they pass medial to the lentiform nucleus (see Fig. 3.28).

Formation of gyri and sulci — Apart from the shallow hippocampal sulcus and the lateral cerebral fossa, the surfaces of the hemisphere remain smooth and uninterrupted until early in the fourth month (see Fig. 3.31). The parieto-occipital sulcus appears at about that time on the medial aspect of the hemisphere. Its appearance seems to be associated with an increase in the number of splenial fibres in the corpus callosum. Over the same period, the posterior part of the calcarine sulcus appears as a shallow groove extending forward from a region near the occipital pole. It is a true infolding of the cortex in the long axis of the striate area and produces an elevation, the calcar avis, on the medial wall of the posterior horn of the ventricle.

During the fifth month the cingulate sulcus appears on the medial aspect of the hemisphere, and sulci appear on the inferior and superolateral aspects

in the sixth month. The central, precentral and postcentral sulci appear, each in upper and lower parts; these two parts usually coalesce shortly afterward, although they may remain discontinuous. The superior and inferior frontal, intraparietal, occipital, superior and inferior temporal, occipitotemporal, collateral and rhinal sulci all make their appearance during the same period. By the end of the eighth month all the important sulci can be recognized (see Fig. 3.31).

Development of commissures — The development of the commissures causes a profound alteration in the medial wall of the hemisphere. At the time of their appearance, the two hemispheres are connected to each other by the median part of the telencephalon. The roof plate of this area remains epithelial, while its floor becomes invaded by the decussating fibres of the optic nerves and developing hypothalamic nuclei. These two routes are thus not available for the passage of commissural fibres from hemisphere to hemisphere across the median plane; these fibres therefore pass through the anterior wall of the interventricular foramen, the lamina terminalis. The first commissures to develop are those associated with the palaeocortex and archicortex. Fibres of the olfactory tracts cross in the ventral or lower part of the lamina terminalis and, together with fibres from the piriform and prepiriform areas and the amygdaloid bodies, form the anterior part of the anterior commissure (Figs. 3.32, 3.33). In addition, the two hippocampi become interconnected by transverse fibres that cross from fornix to fornix in the upper part of the lamina terminalis as the commissure of the fornix. Various other decussating fibre bundles (known as the supraoptic commissures, although they are not true commissures) develop in the lamina terminalis immediately dorsal to the optic chiasma, between it and the anterior commissure.

The commissures of the neocortex develop later and follow the pathways already established by the commissures of the limbic system. Fibres from the tentorial surface of the hemisphere join the anterior commissure and constitute its larger posterior part. All the other commissural fibres of the neocortex associate themselves closely with the commissure of the fornix and lie on its dorsal surface. These fibres increase enormously in number, and the bundle rapidly outgrows its neighbours to form the corpus callosum (see Figs. 3.32, 3.33).

The corpus callosum originates as a thick mass connecting the two cerebral hemispheres around and above the anterior commissure. (This site has been called the precommissural area, but this term has been rejected here because of increasing use of the adjective 'precommissural' to denote the position of parts of the limbic lobe—prehippocampal rudiment, septal areas and nuclei and strands of the fornix—in relation to the anterior commissure of the mature brain.) The upper end of this neocortical commissural area extends backward to form the trunk of the corpus callosum. The rostrum of the corpus callosum develops later and separates part of the rostral end of the limbic area from the remainder of the cerebral hemisphere. Further backward growth of the trunk of the corpus callosum then results in the entrapped part of the limbic area becoming stretched out to form the bilateral septum pellucidum. As the corpus callosum grows backward, it extends above the choroidal fissure, carrying the commissure of the fornix on its undersurface. In this way a new floor is formed for the longitudinal fissure, and additional structures come to lie above the epithelial roof of the third ventricle. In its backward growth, the corpus callosum invades the area hitherto occupied by the upper part of the archaeocortical hippocampal formation, and the corresponding parts of the dentate gyrus and hippocampus are reduced to vestiges, the indusium griseum and the longitudinal striae (see Figs. 3.32, 3.33). However, the posteroinferior (temporal) archaeocortical regions of both the dentate gyrus and the hippocampus persist and enlarge.

Cellular Development of the Cerebrum

The wall of the earliest cerebral hemisphere consists of a pseudostratified epithelium whose cells exhibit interkinetic nuclear migration as they proliferate to form clones of germinal cells. The columnar cells elongate, and their non-nucleated peripheral processes now constitute a marginal zone, while their nucleated, paraluminal and mitosing regions constitute the ventricular zone. Some of their progeny leave the ventricular zone and migrate to occupy an intermediate zone. The proliferative phase continues for a considerable period of fetal life. Ultimately, groups of progenitor cells form: at first, generations of definitive neurones, and later, glial cells that migrate to and mature in their final positions. These phases of proliferation, migration, differentiation and maturation overlap one another in space and time and are not precisely sequential.

The earliest migration of neuronal precursors from the ventricular and intermediate zones occurs radially until they approach, but do not reach, the pial surface. Their somata become arranged as a transient cortical plate. Subsequently, proliferation wanes in the ventricular zone but persists for considerable periods in the immediately subjacent subventricular zone. From the pial surface inward, the following zones may be defined: marginal, cortical plate, subplate, intermediate, subventricular and ventricular (see Fig. 3.5). The marginal zone gives rise to the outermost layer of the cerebral cortex, and the neuroblasts of the cortical plate and subplate form the neurones of the remaining cortical laminae (the complexity varies in different locations and with further additions of neurones from the deeper zones). The intermediate zone gradually transforms into the white matter of the hemisphere. Meanwhile, other deep progenitor cells produce generations of glioblasts that also migrate into the more superficial layers. As proliferation wanes and finally ceases in the ventricular and subventricular zones, their remaining cells differentiate into general or specialized ependymal cells, tanycytes or subependymal glial cells.

The phases of proliferation vary spatiotemporally with location and cell type. The first groups of cells to migrate are destined for the deep cortical laminae, and later groups pass through them to more superficial regions. The subplate zone, a transient feature that is most prominent during mid-gestation, contains neurones surrounded by a dense neuropil; it is the site of the most intense synaptogenesis in the cortex. The cumulative effect of this radial and tangential growth is evident in a marked increase in cortical thickness and surface area.

In the pallial walls of the mammalian cerebral hemisphere, the phylogenetically oldest regions, which are the first to differentiate during ontogeny, are those that border the interventricular foramen and its extension the choroidal fissure, the lamina terminalis and the piriform lobe. An increasingly complex level of organization, from three to six tangential laminae, is encountered in

passing from the dentate gyrus and cornu ammonis through the subiculum to the general neocortex. (Many investigators find the simple progression from three to six major laminae a gross oversimplification, and numerous subdivisions have been proposed.)

Mechanisms of cortical development — Rakic (2003) initially demonstrated the migration of neuroblasts along radial glial processes, and this has subsequently been seen to occur in three phases. First, the neuroblasts become apposed to the radial glial cells and establish an axis of polarity away from the ventricular surface. Next, they are propelled along the glial surface until they 'recognize' their final destination, whereupon they cease locomotion and detach from the glial processes. They then continue to differentiate according to their final position, and later-born neuroblasts migrate past them toward the pial surface (see Fig. 3.5, Figs. 3.34, 3.35). Cortical neurones or cerebellar granule cells appear equally capable of migrating on hippocampal or cerebellar Bergmann glia, indicating conservation of migration mechanisms in different brain regions.

Various lines of evidence support the proposal that the laminar fate of neurones is determined prior to migration. In the mutant reeler mouse, laminar formation is inverted so that layers form in an outside-in rather than inside-out array, yet axonal connections and neuronal properties appear normal, suggesting that the cells differentiate according to their time of origin rather than their location. Likewise, the prevention of neuronal migration by irradiation leads to the production of cells that remain apposed to the ventricular surface but develop an appropriate phenotype and efferent projections. Transplantation of labelled cells suggests that commitment to a particular cortical lamina occurs shortly after S phase. Neurones of preexisting laminae that have begun axonogenesis may provide feedback on the forming cortical layers, providing a sort of developmental clock for histogenesis.

In a plane perpendicular to its laminae (i.e. tangentially-circumferentially), the cortex is divided into a number of areas, displaying a hierarchy of organization. These include primary areas such as the motor cortex, unimodal association areas concerned with the integration of information from one of the primary areas and multimodal association areas that integrate information from more than one modality. There are also areas concerned with functions that are even less well understood, such as the frontal lobes, concerned with goal-orientation responsibility and long-term planning. The primary areas are further divided into somatotopic maps. At the finest level, the cortex is known to consist of a series of 'columns' 50 to 500 μm wide, within which cells on a vertical traverse display common features of modality and electrophysiological responses to stimuli (e.g. the ocular dominance columns of the visual cortex). Despite the precise stacking of neurones in these columns, only 80% to 85% of cells migrate radially along the glial cells; a subpopulation is thought to move tangentially in the intermediate zone (O'Rourke et al 1995). Moreover, some neurones may migrate tangentially on the radial glial cells, as a result of glial cell branching in the cortical plate. The ventricular zone is not the only source of cortical neurones, because striatal and GABAergic neurones are known to migrate from the lateral ganglionic eminence into the developing cortex.

Two models have been proposed to explain the development of this complex cortical organization. The 'protocortex' model assumes that the proliferative ventricular epithelium is a 'tabula rasa' that generates homogeneous layers of neurones that are patterned solely by the ingrowth of processes from the thalamus. The 'protomap' hypothesis proposes that the intrinsic differences between the various areas are specified prior to cell migration (Rakic 1988, 2003). The radial glial cells translate this map from the ventricular zone to the cortical plate, where the pattern is refined by innervating axons. In this 'radial unit' model, the tangential coordinates of the different areas are determined by the position of their ventricular ancestors, whereas their radial position is determined by their time of birth and rate of migration.

But what would constitute such a protomap? The investigation of gene expression patterns shows that the early cortex is not homogeneous and that it expresses some markers that are transient and some that persist into adulthood. For example, the mouse gene *Id2* marks the transition between the motor and somatosensory cortices in the embryo, whereas limbic-associated membrane protein (LAMP) delineates the limbic cortex throughout life. LAMP expression is regulated by transforming growth factor-α, which is expressed by the lateral ganglionic eminence at the lateral edge of the cortex; the medial edge or cortical hem expresses signalling molecules of the WNT and BMP families. Any or all of these may be the components of short-range signalling centres along the edges of the cortex. Coupled with the gradients of transcription factors such as Emx2 and Lhx2, there is evidence to support the protomap hypothesis (Donoghue and Rakic 1999).

However, studies of cell migration are consistent with the idea that cortical areas might not be rigidly determined. Manipulations of the developing cortex by deafferentation or manipulation of inputs give some indication of the state of commitment of cortical areas. In two independent sets of experiments,

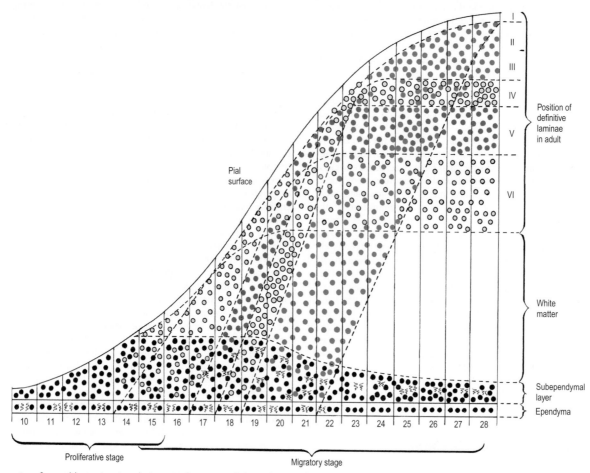

Fig. 3.34 *Dynamics of neuroblast migration during transformation of the early cranial neural tube to form the cerebral neocortex of the rat through days 10 to 28. Note the successive waves of migration. Symbolic metaphase chromosomes, mitotic cells; full black discs, ventricular and subventricular zone neuroblasts; full yellow discs, infragranular neuroblasts destined for lamina VI; full magenta discs, infragranular neuroblasts destined for lamina V; open black circles, granular neuroblasts destined for lamina IV; full blue discs, supragranular neuroblasts destined for laminae III and II. (Redrawn and colour-coded from data provided by Professor M. Berry [1974], Anatomy Department, Guy's Hospital Medical School, London.)*

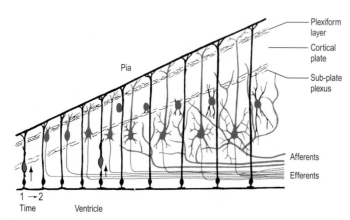

Fig. 3.35 *Initial stages of the formation of apical and basal dendrites of pyramidal neurones and of stellate neurone dendrites in the cortical plate. Note radial glial cells (black) extending from the internal to external limiting membrane; these provide contact guidance paths for neuroblasts. 1, Migration of a presumptive pyramidal neurone (magenta); 2, migration of a presumptive stellate neurone (purple). Time increments are from left to right. (After Berry, M. 1982. Cellular differentiation. Neurosci. Res. Prog. Bull. 20, 451–461.)*

somatosensory or auditory cortex was induced to process visual information by misrouting retinal axons to somatosensory thalamus or auditory thalamus (von Melchner, Pallas and Sur, 2000). When the lateral geniculate nucleus and the visual cortex were ablated and space was created in the medial geniculate by ablating the inferior colliculus, cells in the somatosensory or auditory cortex were visually driven, and receptive field and response properties resembled those seen in the visual cortex. These results suggest that the modality of a sensory thalamic nucleus or cortical area can be specified by inputs during development.

The development of cortical projections has been investigated in terms of both laminar and area-specific connectivity. Recently, attention has focused on the idea that connections might be influenced by the existence of a transient population of subplate neurones that later dies. The cortex develops within a preplate, consisting of corticopetal nerve fibres and the earliest generated neurones. This zone is then split into two zones—the subplate underneath the cortical plate, and the marginal zone at the pial surface—by the arrival of cortical neurones. Subplate neurones extend axons via the internal capsule to the thalamus and superior colliculus before other cortical neurones have been born.

How are region-specific projections generated? Layer 5 neurones in various cortical areas extend axons to different repertoires of targets. For instance, layer 5 neurones of the visual cortex project to the tectum, pons and mesencephalic nuclei, whereas those in the motor cortex project to mesencephalic and pontine targets, the inferior olive and dorsal column nuclei and the spinal cord. An interesting feature of these cortical projections is that they arise by collateral formation rather than by projection of the primary axon or by growth cone bifurcation. In the case of the corticopontine projection, collaterals are elicited by a diffusible, chemotrophic agent. Retrograde labelling of neurones at various times in development has shown that rather than being generated *de novo*, these patterns seem to arise by the pruning of collaterals from a more widespread projection. Visual cortical neurones possess a projection to the spinal cord early in development, which is later eliminated. This late emergence of the specificity of projections could be driven by intrinsic programming of the neurones to be pruned or by a response to position-dependent factors. There is evidence that the latter is the case. When pieces of visual cortex were transplanted into motor areas and the resulting layer 5 projections were labeled later in development, projections to the spinal cord persisted rather than being eliminated, as in normal development. Thus, position plays an important role in the modelling of cortical projections, implying that the same classes of neurones exist in different tangential regions of the cortex. Regressive events such as axon and synapse elimination and neuronal death thus play an important part in modelling the cortex. For example, in rodents, approximately 30% of cortical neurones die, and the number of cells in layer 4 is governed by thalamic input.

Human cortical malformations are thought to arise as neuronal migration disorders. Lissencephaly constitutes a broad class of neuronal migration disorders in which the cortex has a normal thickness but a decreased number of neurones and a smooth surface with a decreased number of gyri. The mutated protein in some forms of the disorder, LIS-1, is expressed in the ventricular neuroepithelium and is responsible for regulating levels of the lipid messenger platelet-activating factor. How this translates into a cell migration defect remains obscure. Conversely, polymicrogyria manifests as a highly convoluted cerebrum with a nearly normal surface area but a thinner cortex. It is thought that the normal number of proliferative units and thus ontogenetic columns is established, but each column contains fewer neurones, implying either a reduced rate of proliferation and cell migration or an enhanced level of cell death.

Neonatal Brain and Reflexes

The brain of the full-term neonate ranges from 300 to 400 g, with an average of 350 g; the brains of male neonates are slightly heavier than those of females. Because the head is large at birth, measuring one-quarter of the total body length, the brain is also proportionally larger and constitutes 10% of body weight, compared with 2% in the adult. At birth the volume of the brain is 25% of its adult volume. The greatest increase occurs during the first year, at the end of which the volume of the brain has increased to 75% of its adult volume. This growth can be accounted for partly by the increased size of nerve cell somata, by the profusion and dimensions of their dendritic trees, axons and collaterals and by the growth of neuroglial cells and cerebral blood vessels; however, it mainly reflects the acquisition of myelin sheaths by the axons. The sensory pathways—visual, auditory and somatic—myelinate first; the motor fibres myelinate later. During the second and subsequent years, growth proceeds much more slowly. The brain reaches 90% of its adult size by age 5 years and 95% by 10 years. The brain attains adult size by the seventeenth or eighteenth year. This is largely due to continued myelination of various groups of nerve fibres.

The sulci of the cerebral hemispheres appear from the fourth month of gestation (see Fig. 3.31), and at full term the general arrangement of sulci and gyri is present, but the insula is not completely covered. The central sulcus is situated farther rostrally and the lateral sulcus is more oblique than in the adult. Most of the developmental stages of sulci and gyri have been identified in the brains of premature infants. Of the cranial nerves, the olfactory and the optic at the chiasma are much larger than in the adult, whereas the roots of the other nerves are relatively smaller.

The brain occupies 97.5% of the cranial cavity from birth to 6 years of age, after which the space between the brain and the skull increases in volume until the adult brain occupies only 92.5% of the cranial cavity. Although the cerebral ventricles are larger in the neonate than in the adult, the newborn has a total of 10 to 15 ml of cerebrospinal fluid when delivered vaginally and 30 ml when delivered by caesarean section.

Myelination — Myelination in the PNS occurs over a protracted period, beginning during the second trimester. Motor roots myelinate before sensory roots in the PNS, whereas sensory nerves myelinate before the motor systems. The cranial nerves of the midbrain, pons and medulla oblongata begin myelination at about 6 months' gestation. Myelination is not complete at birth; its most rapid phase occurs during the first 6 months of postnatal life, after which it continues at a slower rate up to puberty and beyond. The sequence of myelination of the motor pathways may explain, at least in part, the order of development of muscle tone and posture in the premature infant and neonate. Myelination of the various subcorticospinal pathways—vestibulospinal, reticulospinal, olivospinal and tectospinal (often grouped as bulbospinal tracts)—occurs from 24 to 30 weeks' gestation for the medial groups and extends to 28 to 34 weeks' gestation for the lateral groups. Myelination of the corticospinal tracts occurs some 10 to 14 days after birth in the internal capsule and cerebral peduncles and then proceeds simultaneously in both tracts. Longer axons appear to myelinate first. Thus, in the preterm infant, axial extension precedes flexion, whereas finger flexion precedes extension. By term, the neonate at rest has a strong flexor tone accompanied by adduction of all limbs. Neonates also display a distinct preference for a head position facing to the right, which appears to be independent of handling practices and may reflect the normal asymmetry of cerebral function at this age.

Reflexes present at birth — A number of reflexes are present at birth, and their demonstration is used to indicate normal development of the nervous system and responding muscles. Five tests of neurological development are most useful in determining gestational age. The pupillary reflex is consistently absent before 29 weeks' gestation and present after 31 weeks; the glabellar tap, a blink in response to a tap on the glabella, is absent before 32 weeks

and present after 34 weeks; the neck righting reflex appears between 34 and 37 weeks; the traction response, in which flexion of the neck or arms occurs when the baby is pulled up by the wrists from the supine position, appears after 33 weeks; head turning in response to light appears between 32 and 36 weeks. The spinal reflex arc is fully developed by the eighth week of gestation, and lower limb flexor tone is detectable from about 29 weeks. The extensor plantar (Babinski's) response, which involves extension of the great toe with spreading of the remaining toes in response to stimulation of the lateral aspect of the sole of the foot, is elicited frequently in neonates; it reflects poor cortical control of motor function by the immature brain. Generally, reflexes develop as muscles gain tone. They appear in a sequential manner from caudal to cephalic, in the lower limb before the upper, and centripetally, with distal reflexes appearing before proximal ones (Allen and Capute 1990).

The usual reflexes that can be elicited in the neonate include Moro, asymmetric tonic neck response, rooting–sucking, grasp, placing (contacting the dorsum of the foot with the edge of a table produces a 'stepping over the edge' response), stepping and trunk incurvation (elicited by stroking down the paravertebral area with the infant in the prone position). Examination of the motor system and evaluation of these reflexes allow an assessment of the nervous system in relation to gestational age. The neonate also exhibits complex reflexes such as nasal reflexes and sucking and swallowing.

Nasal reflexes produce apnoea via the diving reflex, sneezing, sniffing and both somatic and autonomic reflexes. Stimulation of the face or nasal cavity with water or local irritants produces apnoea in neonates. Breathing stops in expiration, with laryngeal closure, and infants exhibit bradycardia and a lowering of cardiac output. Bloodflow to the skin, splanchnic areas, muscles and kidneys decreases, whereas flow to the heart and brain is protected. Different fluids produce different effects when introduced into the pharynx of preterm infants. A comparison of the effects of water and saline in the pharynx showed that apnoea, airway obstruction and swallowing occur far more frequently with water than with saline, suggesting the presence of an upper airway chemoreflex. Reflex responses to the temperature of the face and nasopharynx are necessary to start pulmonary ventilation. Midwives have for many years blown on the faces of neonates to induce the first breath.

Sucking and swallowing involve a particularly complex set of reflexes, partly conscious and partly unconscious. As a combined reflex, sucking and swallowing require the coordination of several of the 12 cranial nerves. The neonate can, within the first couple of feeds, suck at the rate of once per second, swallow after five or six sucks, and breathe during every second or third suck. Air moves in and out of the lungs via the nasopharynx, and milk crosses the pharynx en route to the oesophagus without apparent interruption of breathing and swallowing or significant misdirection of air into the stomach or fluids in the trachea.

Swallowing movements are first noted at about 11 weeks' gestation; *in utero* fetuses swallow 450 ml of amniotic fluid per day. Sucking and swallowing in premature infants (1700 g) are not associated with primary peristaltic waves in the intestine; however, in older babies and full-term neonates, at least 90% of swallows initiate primary peristaltic waves.

Sucking develops, generally, slightly later than swallowing, although mouthing movements have been detected in premature babies as early as 18 to 24 weeks' gestation, and infants delivered at 29 to 30 weeks' gestation make sucking movements a few days after birth. Coordinated activities are not noted before 33 to 34 weeks. The concept of non-nutritive and nutritive sucking has been introduced to account for the different rates of sucking seen in neonates. Non-nutritive sucking, when rhythmic negative intraoral pressures are initiated that do not result in the delivery of milk, can be spontaneous or stimulated by an object in the mouth. This type of sucking tends to be twice as fast as nutritive sucking: the sucking frequency for non-nutritive sucking is 1.7 sucks/second in 37- to 38-week premature babies, 2 sucks/second in term neonates and 2.7 sucks/second at 7 to 9 months postnatally. Corresponding times for nutritive sucking are about 1 suck/second in term neonates, increasing to 1.5 sucks/second by 7 months postnatally.

The taste of the fluid as well as its nutrient content affects the efficiency of nutritive sucking in the early neonatal period. There is more sucking with milk than with 5% dextrose; however, sucking activities increase with solutions that are determined to be sweet by adult appraisal.

In full-term neonates the placing of a spoon or food onto the anterior part of the tongue elicits an extrusion reflex: the lips are pursed, and the tongue pushes vigorously against the object. By 4 to 6 months the reflex changes: food deposited on the anterior part of the tongue is moved to the back of the tongue, into the pharynx, and swallowed. Rhythmic biting movements occur by 7 to 9 months postnatally, even in the absence of teeth.

Difficulties in sucking and swallowing in infancy may be an early indication of disturbed nervous system function. There is an interesting correlation between the feeding styles of neonates and later eating habits. Children who were obese at 1 and 2 years of age, as measured by triceps skinfold thickness, had a feeding pattern in the first month of life that was characterized by sucking more rapidly, producing higher pressures during prolonged bursts of sucking and having shorter periods between bursts of sucking. Fewer feeds and higher sucking pressure seem to be associated with greater adiposity.

Meninges

The meningeal layers originate from paraxial mesenchyme in the trunk and caudal regions of the head and from the neural crest in regions rostral to the mesencephalon (the prechordal plate may also make a contribution). Those skull bones formed from neural crest, such as the base of the skull rostral to the sella turcica and the frontal, parietal and squamous temporal bones, overlie meninges that are also formed from crest cells.

During development the meninges can be divided into the pachymeninx (dura mater) and the leptomeninges (arachnoid mater, subarachnoid space with arachnoid cells and fibres and pia mater). All meningeal layers are derived from loose mesenchyme that surrounds the developing neural tube, termed the meninx primitiva or primary meninx. (For a detailed account of development of the meninges in the human, consult O'Rahilly and Muller 1986.)

The first indication of pia mater, consisting of a plexus of blood vessels that forms on the neural surface, is seen at stage 11 (24 days) around the caudalmost part of the medulla; this extends to the mesencephalic level by stage 12. Mesenchymal cells projecting from the rostral end of the notochord, and those in the region of the prechordal plate, extend rostrally into the mesencephalic flexure and form the earliest cells of the tentorium cerebelli; at the beginning of its development, the medial part of the tentorium is predominantly leptomeningeal. By stage 17 (41 days), dura mater can be seen in the basal areas where the future chondrocranium is also developing. Precursors of the venous sinuses lie within the pachymeninx at stage 19 (48 days), and by stage 20, cell populations in the region of the future falx cerebri are proliferating, although the dorsal regions of the brain are not yet covered with putative meninges.

By stage 23 (57 days), the dura is almost complete over the rhombencephalon and mesencephalon but is present only laterally around the prosencephalon. Subarachnoid spaces and most of the cisternae are present from this time, after the arachnoid mater becomes separated from the primitive dura mater by the accumulation of cerebrospinal fluid (which now has a net movement out of the ventricular system). The medial part of the tentorium is becoming thinner. A dural component of the tentorium is seen from stage 19. The earlier medial portion disappears, leaving an incomplete partition that separates a subarachnoid area containing the telencephalon and diencephalon from one containing the cerebellum and rhombencephalon.

There is a very close relationship, during development, between the mesenchyme from which the cranial dura mater is formed and that which is chondrified and ossified, or ossified directly, to form the skull. These layers are clearly differentiated only as the venous sinuses develop. The relationship between the developing skull and the underlying dura mater continues during postnatal life while the bones of the calvaria are still growing.

Growth of the cranial vault is initiated from ossification centres within the desmocranial mesenchyme. A wave of osteodifferentiation moves radially outward from these centres, stopping when adjacent bones meet at regions where sutures are induced to form. Once sutures are formed, a second phase of development occurs in which growth of the cranial bones occurs at the sutural margins. This growth forms most of the skull. A number of hypotheses have been generated to explain the process of suture morphogenesis. It has been suggested that the dura mater contains fibre tracts that extend from fixed positions in the cranial base to sites of dural reflection underlying each of the cranial sutures, and the tensional forces so generated dictate the position of the sutures and locally inhibit precocious ossification. Other hypotheses support the concept of local factors in the calvaria that regulate suture morphogenesis. Following removal of the entire calvaria, the skull regenerates and sutures and bones develop in anatomically correct positions, suggesting that the dura can dictate suture position at least in regeneration of the neonatal calvaria. In transplants of sutures in which the fetal dura mater was left intact, a continuous fibrous suture remained between developing vault bones, whereas in transplants in which the fetal dura mater was removed, bony fusion occurred (Opperman et al 1993).

The presence of fetal dura is not required for initial suture morphogenesis, which appears to be controlled by mesenchymal cell proliferation and fibrous extracellular matrix synthesis induced by overlapping of the advancing osteo-inductive fronts of the calvarial bones. It is thought that following overlap of the bone fronts, a signal is transferred to the underlying dura that induces changes in localized regions beneath the sutures. Once a suture has formed, it serves as a primary site for cranial bone growth, but constant interaction with the dura is required to avoid ossiferous obliteration.

Cranial Arteries (Fig 3.36)

The internal carotid artery is formed progressively from the third arch artery, the dorsal aorta cranial to this and a further forward continuation that differentiates, at the time of regression of the first and second aortic arches, from the capillary plexus extending to the walls of the forebrain and midbrain. At its anterior extremity this primitive internal carotid artery divides into cranial and caudal divisions. The former terminates as the primitive olfactory artery and supplies the developing regions implied. The latter sweeps caudally to reach the ventral aspect of the midbrain; its terminal branches are the primitive mesencephalic arteries. Simultaneously, bilateral longitudinal channels differentiate along the ventral surface of the hindbrain from a plexus fed by intersegmental and transitory presegmental branches of the dorsal aorta and its forward continuation. The most important of the presegmental branches is closely related to the fifth nerve, the primitive trigeminal artery. Otic and hypoglossal presegmental arteries occur and may persist. The longitudinal channels later connect cranially with the caudal divisions of the internal carotid arteries (each of which gives rise to an anterior choroidal artery supplying branches to the diencephalon, including the telae choroideae and midbrain) and caudally with the vertebral arteries through the first cervical intersegmental arteries. Fusion of the longitudinal channels results in formation of the basilar artery, and the caudal division of the internal carotid artery becomes the posterior communicating artery and the stem of the posterior cerebral artery. The remainder of the posterior cerebral artery develops comparatively late, probably from the stem of the posterior choroidal artery, which is annexed by the caudally expanding cerebral hemisphere; its distal portion becomes a choroidal branch of the posterior cerebral artery. The posterior choroidal artery supplies the tela choroidea at the future temporal end of the choroidal fissure; its rami advance through the tela to become confluent with branches of the anterior choroidal artery. The cranial division of the internal carotid artery gives rise to anterior choroidal, middle cerebral and anterior cerebral arteries. The stem of the primitive olfactory artery remains as a small medial striate branch of the anterior cerebral artery. The cerebellar arteries, of which the superior is the first to differentiate, emerge from the capillary plexus on the wall of the rhombencephalon.

The source of the blood supply to the territory of the trigeminal nerve varies at different stages of development. When the first and second aortic arch arteries begin to regress, the supply to the corresponding arches is derived from a transient ventral pharyngeal artery that grows from the aortic sac. It terminates by dividing into mandibular and maxillary branches.

Meningeal Arteries

At stages 20 to 23 (7 to 8 weeks' gestation), further expansion of the cerebral hemispheres completes the circle of Willis, with development of the anterior communicating arteries by 8 weeks' gestation. An anular network of meningeal arteries originates, mainly from each middle cerebral artery, and passes over each developing cerebral hemisphere. Caudally, similar meningeal branches

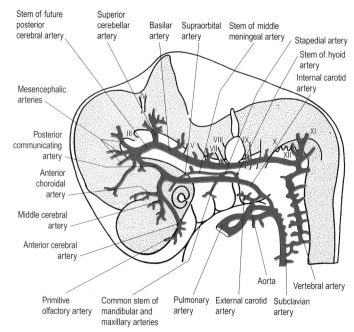

Fig. 3.36 *Origins of the main cranial arteries. (After Padget, D.H. 1948. The development of cranial arteries in the human embryo. Contrib. Embryol. Carnegie Inst. Washington 32, 205–261, by permission.)*

arise from the vertebral and basilar arteries and embrace the cerebellum and brain stem. The further development of the telencephalon somewhat obscures this early pattern over the cerebrum.

The meningeal arteries so formed have been classified into three groups: paramedian, short circumferential and long circumferential arteries. They can be described both supratentorially and infratentorially: all give off fine side branches and end as penetrating arteries. Of the supratentorial vessels, the paramedian arteries have a short course prior to penetrating the cerebral neuropil (e.g. branches of the anterior cerebral artery); the short circumferential arteries have a slightly longer course before becoming penetrating arteries (e.g. the striate artery); the long circumferential arteries reach the dorsal surface of the hemispheres. Infratentorial meningeal arteries are very variable. The paramedian arteries, after arising from the basilar or vertebral arteries, penetrate the brain stem directly. The short circumferential arteries end at the lateral surface of the brain before penetration, and the long circumferential arteries later form the range of cerebellar arteries. These vessels, arranged as a series of loops over the brain, arise from the circle of Willis and brain stem vessels on the base of the brain.

At 16 weeks' gestation the anterior, middle and posterior cerebral arteries contributing to the formation of the circle of Willis are well established. The meningeal arteries arising from them display a simple pattern, with little tortuosity and very few branches. With increasing age of the fetus and acquisition of the gyral pattern on the surface of the brain, their tortuosity, diameter and number of branches all increase. The branching pattern is complete by 28 weeks' gestation, and the number of branches does not increase further. Numerous anastomoses (varying in size from 200 to 760 μm) occur between the meningeal arteries in the depths of the developing sulci, nearly always in the cortical boundary zones of the three main cerebral arteries supplying each hemisphere. The number, diameter and location of these anastomoses change as fetal growth progresses, reflecting the regression and simplification of the complex embryonic cerebral vascular system. The boundary zones between the cerebral arteries may be the sites of inadequate perfusion in the premature infant.

Vascularization of the Brain

The brain becomes vascularized by angiogenesis (angiotrophic vasculogenesis) rather than by direct invasion by angioblasts. Blood vessels form by sprouting from vessels in the pial plexus that surrounds the neural tube from an early stage. These sprouts form branches that elongate at the junction between the ventricular and marginal zones; the branches project laterally within the inter-rhombomeric boundaries and longitudinally adjacent to the median floor plate. Subsequently, additional sprouts penetrate the inter-rhombomeric regions on the walls and floor of the hindbrain. Branches from the latter elongate toward and join the branches in the inter-rhombomeric junctions, forming primary vascular channels between rhombomeres and longitudinally on each side of the median floor plate. Later, additional sprouts invade the hindbrain within the rhombomeres, anastomosing in all directions.

The meningeal perforating branches pass into the brain parenchyma as cortical, medullary and striate branches (Fig. 3.37). The cortical vessels supply the cortex via short branches that may form precapillary anastomoses, whereas the medullary branches supply the white matter. The latter converge toward the ventricle but rarely reach it; they often follow a tortuous course as they pass around bundles of nerves. The striate branches, which penetrate the brain through the anterior perforated substance, supply the basal nuclei and internal capsule via a sinuous course; they are larger than the medullary branches, and the longest ones reach close to the ventricle. The periventricular region and basal nuclei are also supplied by branches from the tela choroidea, which develops from the early pial plexus but becomes medially and deeply placed as the telencephalon enlarges.

The cortical and medullary branches irrigate a series of corticosubcortical cone-shaped areas, centred around a sulcus containing an artery. They supply a peripheral portion of the cerebrum and are grouped as ventriculopetal arteries. Striate branches, in contrast, arborize close to the ventricle and supply a more central portion of the cerebrum; together with branches from the tela choroidea, they give rise to ventriculofugal arteries. The latter supply the ventricular zone (germinal matrix of the brain) and send branches toward the cortex. The ventriculopetal and ventriculofugal arteries run toward each other but do not make any connections or anastomoses (see Fig. 3.37); however, the ventriculopetal arteries form networks of small arterioles. The ventriculopetal vessels supply relatively more mature regions of the brain compared with the ventriculofugal vessels, which are subject to constant remodelling and do not develop tunicae mediae until ventricular zone proliferation is complete. The boundary zone between these two systems (outer centripetal and inner centrifugal) has practical implications related to the location of ischaemic lesions (periventricular leukomalacia [PVL]) in the white matter of premature infants' brains. Although it was

thought that the distribution of ischaemic lesions in PVL coincided with the demarcation zone between the centrifugal and centripetal vascular arterial systems, this is no longer thought to provide the complete answer. Three major interacting factors contribute to the pathology seen in PVL: the incomplete state of development of the vasculature in the ventricular zone, the maturation-dependent impairment of cerebral bloodflow regulation in premature infants and the vulnerability of oligodendroblasts in the periventricular region, which are particularly affected by swings in cerebral ischaemia and reperfusion (Volpe 2001).

The same pattern of centripetal and centrifugal arteries develops around the fourth ventricle. The ventriculofugal circulation is more extensive in the cerebellum than in the telencephalon. The arteries arise from the various cerebellar arteries and course, with the cerebellar peduncles, directly to the centre of the cerebellum, bypassing the cortex. The ventriculopetal arteries are derived from the meningeal vessels over the cerebellar surface, and most terminate in the white matter.

At 24 weeks' gestation there is a relatively well-developed blood supply to the basal nuclei and internal capsule through a prominent Heubner's artery (arteria recurrens anterior), a branch of the anterior cerebral artery. The cortex and the white matter regions are rather poorly vascularized at this stage. The distribution of arteries and veins on the lateral aspects of the cerebral hemispheres is affected by formation of the lateral fissure and development of the cerebral sulci and gyri. Between 12 and 20 weeks' gestation the middle cerebral artery and its branches are relatively straight, branching in an open-fan pattern. At the end of 20 weeks, the arteries become more curved as the opercula begin to appear and submerge the insular cortex. The area supplied by the middle cerebral artery becomes dominant when compared with the territories supplied by the anterior and posterior cerebral arteries. Early arterial anastomoses appear around 16 weeks' gestation and increase in size with age. The sites of anastomoses between the middle and anterior cerebral arteries move from the convexity of the brain toward the superior sagittal sinus. Anastomotic connections between the middle and posterior cerebral arteries shift toward the basal aspect of the brain.

By 32 to 34 weeks, marked involution of the ventricular zone (germinal matrix) has occurred, and the cortex acquires its complex gyral pattern and an increased vascular supply. Ventricular zone capillaries are gradually remodelled to blend with the capillaries of the caudate nucleus. Heubner's artery eventually supplies only a small area at the medial aspect of the head of the caudate nucleus. In the cortex there is progressive elaboration of cortical blood vessels (see Fig. 3.37), and toward the end of the third trimester, the balance of cerebral circulation shifts from one that is central and basal nuclei oriented to one that predominantly serves the cortex and white matter. These changes in the pattern of cerebral circulation are of major significance in the pathogenesis and distribution of hypoxic-ischaemic lesions in the developing human brain. In a premature brain the majority of ischaemic lesions occur in the boundary zone between the centripetal and centrifugal arteries, that is, in the periventricular white matter. In the full-term infant the cortical boundary zones and watershed areas between different arterial blood supplies are similar to those in adults.

Vessels of the ventricular zone (germinal matrix) — The germinal matrix (ventricular zone) is the end zone or border zone between the cerebral arteries and the collection zone of the deep cerebral veins. The germinal matrix is probably particularly prone to ischaemic injury in immature infants because of its unusual vascular architecture. The subependymal veins (septal, choroidal, thalamostriate and posterior terminal) flow toward the interventricular foramen, with a sudden change of flow at the level of the foramen, where the veins recurve at an acute angle to form the paired internal cerebral veins. The capillary channels in the germinal matrix open at right angles directly into the veins, and it has been postulated that these small vessels may be points of vascular rupture and the site of subependymal haemorrhage.

The capillary bed in the ventricular zone is supplied mainly by Heubner's artery and terminal branches of the lateral striate arteries from the middle cerebral artery. The highly cellular structure of the ventricular zone is a temporary feature, and the vascular supply to this area displays some primitive features. It has the capacity to remodel when the ventricular zone cells migrate, and the remaining cells differentiate as ependyma toward the end of gestation.

Vessel density is relatively low in the ventricular zone, suggesting that this area may normally have a relatively low bloodflow. Immature vessels, without a complex basal lamina or glial sheet, have been described up to 26 weeks' gestation in the zone; the endothelium of these vessels is apparently thinner than in the cortical vessels. In infants of less than 30 weeks' gestation, the vessels in the ventricular zone contain no smooth muscle, collagen or elastic fibres. Collagen and smooth muscle are seen in other regions after 30 weeks' gestation but are not detected in the remains of the germinal matrix. The lack of these components could make the vessels in this zone vulnerable to

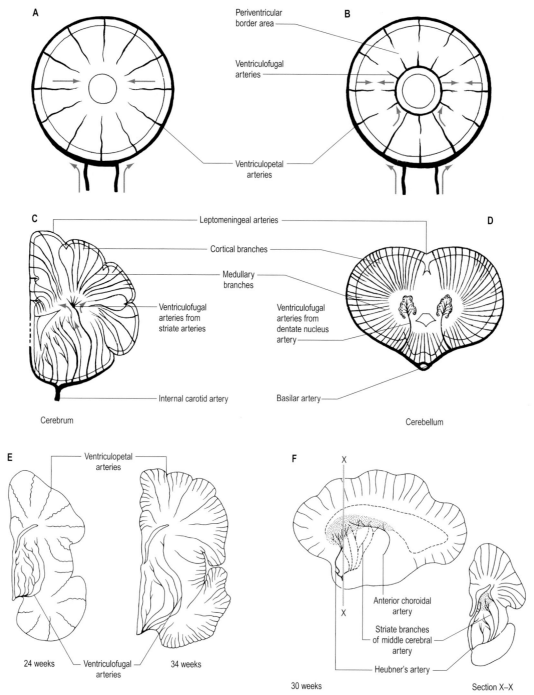

Fig. 3.37 *Development of cerebral blood vessels. **A**, The brain is surrounded by a system of leptomeningeal arteries from afferent trunks at the base of the brain. Intracerebral arteries arise from this system and converge (ventriculopetally) toward the ventricle (the inner circle in this diagram). **B**, A few deep penetrating vessels supply the brain close to the ventricle and send ventriculofugal arteries toward the ventriculopetal vessels without making anastomoses. **C**, Arrangement of ventriculopetal and ventriculofugal vessels around a cerebral hemisphere. **D**, Similar arrangement of vessels around the cerebellum. **E**, Changes in the arterial pattern of the human cerebrum between 24 and 34 weeks' gestation. **F**, Arterial supply to the basal nuclei at 30 weeks' gestation. (**A**–**D**, by permission from Van den Bergh, R., Van der Eecken, H. 1968. Anatomy and embryology of cerebral circulation. Prog. Brain Res. 30, 1–25; **E** and **F**, from Hambleton, G., Wigglesworth, J.S. 1976. Origin of intraventricular haemorrhage in the preterm infant. Arch. Dis. Child. 51, 651–659, by permission from the BMJ Publishing Group.)*

changes in intraluminal pressure, and the lack of smooth muscle would preclude them from participating in autoregulatory processes. Cerebral vessels in premature infants lack elastic fibres and have a disproportionately small number of reticulin fibres. Comparison of the cortical and germinal plate blood vessels shows that in infants between 25 and 32 weeks' gestation, the germinal matrix vessels commonly consist of one or two endothelial cells with an occasional pericyte, and the capillary lumina are larger than those of the vessels in the cortex. In more mature infants, the basal lamina is thicker and more irregular when compared with cortical vessels.

Glial fibrillary acidic protein–positive cells have been detected around blood vessels in the germinal matrix from 23 weeks' gestation. Glial cells may contribute to changes in the nature of endothelial intercellular junctions in brain capillaries.

Cerebral veins — From 16 weeks onward, cerebral veins can be identified. The superior, middle, inferior, anterior and posterior cerebral veins appear more tortuous than meningeal arteries. Veins draining the cortex, white matter and deeper structures are recognized in the mid-trimester. Subcortical veins drain the deep white matter, deep cortical tissue and subcortical superficial tissue; they terminate, together with cortical veins that drain the cortex, in the meningeal veins. The deep white matter and central nuclei are drained by longer veins that meet and join subependymal veins from the ventricular zone. Anastomoses between various groups of cortical veins can be recognized by 16 weeks' gestation. The inferior anastomotic vein (of Labbé), an anastomosis between the middle and inferior cerebral veins, becomes recognizable at 20 weeks' gestation, but the superior anastomotic vein (of Trolard), connecting the superior and middle cerebral veins, does not appear before the end of 30 weeks' gestation.

Rapid cortical development is correlated with the regression of the middle cerebral vein and its tributaries and the development of ascending and descending cortical veins and intraparenchymal (medullary) arteries and veins.

Cerebral venous drainage in a full-term infant is essentially composed of two principal venous arrays: the superficial veins and the deep Galenic venous system. Anastomoses between these two systems persist into adult life.

Veins of the Head

The earliest vessels form a transitory primordial hindbrain channel that drains into the precardinal vein (Fig. 3.38). This is soon replaced by the primary head vein, which runs caudally from the medial side of the trigeminal ganglion, lateral to the facial and vestibulocochlear nerves and otocyst, then medial to the vagus nerve, to become continuous with the precardinal vein. A lateral anastomosis subsequently brings it lateral to the vagus nerve. The cranial part of the precardinal vein forms the internal jugular vein.

The primary capillary plexus of the head becomes separated into three fairly distinct strata by the differentiation of the skull and meninges. The superficial vessels, draining the skin and underlying soft parts, eventually discharge in large part into the external jugular system. They retain some connections with the deeper veins through so-called emissary veins. Deep to this is the venous plexus of the dura mater, from which the dural venous sinuses differentiate. This plexus converges on each side into anterior, middle and posterior dural stems (see Fig. 3.37). The anterior stem drains the prosencephalon and mesencephalon and enters the primary head vein rostral to the trigeminal ganglion. The middle stem drains the metencephalon and empties into the primary head vein caudal to the trigeminal ganglion, while the posterior stem drains the myelencephalon into the start of the precardinal vein. The deepest capillary stratum is the pial plexus, from which the veins of the brain differentiate. It drains at the dorsolateral aspect of the neural tube into the adjacent dural venous plexus. The primary head vein also receives, at its cranial end, the primitive maxillary vein, which drains the maxillary prominence and region of the optic vesicle.

The vessels of the dural plexus undergo profound changes, largely to accommodate the growth of the cartilaginous otic capsule of the

membranous labyrinth and expansion of the cerebral hemispheres. With growth of the otic capsule, the primary head vein is gradually reduced, and a new channel joining the anterior, middle and posterior dural stems appears dorsal to the cranial nerve ganglia and the capsule. Where this new vessel joins the middle and posterior stems, together with the posterior dural stem itself (see Fig. 3.37B), the adult sigmoid sinus is formed.

A curtain of capillary veins—the sagittal plexus—forms between the growing cerebral hemispheres and along the dorsal margins of the anterior and middle plexuses, in the position of the future falx cerebri. Rostrodorsally, this plexus forms the superior sagittal sinus. It is continuous behind with the anastomosis between the anterior and middle dural stems, which forms most of the transverse sinus. Ventrally, the sagittal plexus differentiates into the inferior sagittal and straight sinuses and the great cerebral vein, and it drains, most commonly, into the left transverse sinus.

The vessels along the ventrolateral edge of the developing cerebral hemisphere form the transitory tentorial sinus, which drains the convex surface of the cerebral hemisphere and basal ganglia, and the ventral aspect of the diencephalon to the transverse sinus. With expansion of the cerebral hemispheres and, in particular, the emergence of the temporal lobe, the tentorial sinus becomes elongated, attenuated and eventually disappears, and its territory is drained by enlarging anastomoses of pial vessels. The latter become the basal veins, which are radicles of the great cerebral vein.

The anterior dural stem disappears, and the caudal part of the primary head vein dwindles; it is represented in the adult by the inferior petrosal sinus. The cranial part of the primary head vein, medial to the trigeminal ganglion, persists and still receives the stem of the primitive maxillary vein. The latter has now lost most of its tributaries to the anterior facial vein, and its stem becomes the main trunk of the primitive supraorbital vein, which will form the superior ophthalmic vein in the adult. The main venous drainage of the orbit and its contents is now carried via the augmented middle dural stem, the pro-otic sinus, into the transverse sinus and, at a later stage, into the cavernous sinus. The cavernous sinus is formed from a secondary plexus derived from the primary head vein and lying between the otic and basioccipital cartilages. The plexus forms the inferior petrosal sinus, which drains through the primordial hindbrain channel into the internal jugular vein. The superior petrosal sinus arises later from a ventral metencephalic tributary of the pro-otic sinus, and it communicates secondarily with the cavernous sinus. Meanwhile, the pro-otic sinus has developed a new and more caudally situated stem draining into the sigmoid sinus; this new stem is the petrosquamosal sinus. With progressive ossification of the skull, the pro-otic sinus becomes diploic in position. Development of the venous drainage and portal system of the hypophysis cerebri is closely associated with that of the venous sinuses.

DEVELOPMENT OF THE EYE

Development of the eye involves a series of interactions between neighbouring tissues in the head. These are the neuroectoderm of the forebrain, which forms the sensory retina and accessory pigmented structures; the surface ectoderm, which forms the lens and cornea; and the intervening neural crest mesenchyme, which contributes to the fibrous coats of the eye. These interactions lead to the potential to form optic vesicles throughout a broad anterior domain of neuroectoderm. Subsequent interactions between mesenchyme and neuroectoderm subdivide this region into bilateral domains at the future sites of the eyes. The parallel process of lens determination appears to depend on a brief period of inductive influence that spreads through the surface ectoderm from the rostral neural plate and elicits a lens-forming area of the head. Reciprocal interactions necessary for the complete development of both tissues take place as the optic vesicle forms and contacts the potential lens ectoderm (Saha et al 1992). Vascular tissue of the developing eye may form by local angiogenesis or vasculogenesis of angiogenetic mesenchyme. (Accounts of eye development are given in O'Rahilly 1966 and 1983.)

Embryonic Components of the Eye

The first morphological sign of eye development is a thickening of the diencephalic neural folds at 22 days' postovulation, when the embryo has seven or eight somites. This optic primordium extends on both sides of the neural plate and crosses the midline at the primordium chiasmatis. A slight transverse indentation, the optic sulcus, appears in the inner surface of the optic primordium on each side of the brain. During the period when the rostral neuropore closes, at about 24 days, the walls of the forebrain at the optic sulcus begin to evaginate, projecting laterally toward the surface ectoderm so that, by 25 days, the optic vesicles are formed. The lumen of each vesicle is continuous with that of the forebrain. Cells delaminate from the walls of the optic vesicle and, probably joined by head mesenchyme and cells derived from the mesencephalic neural crest, invest the vesicle in a sheath of mesenchyme. By 28 days, regional differentiation is apparent in each of the source tissues of the eye. The optic vesicle is visibly differentiated into its three primary parts.

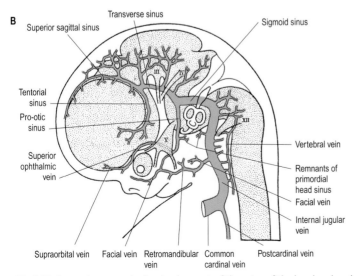

A Anterior dural stem   Middle dural stem   Otocyst   Primary head sinus

Primitive maxillary vein

Posterior dural stem

Intersegmental veins

Precardinal vein

Postcardinal vein

Ventral pharyngeal vein   Common cardinal vein

B Transverse sinus   Sigmoid sinus

Superior sagittal sinus

Tentorial sinus

Pro-otic sinus

Superior ophthalmic vein

Vertebral vein

Remnants of primordial head sinus

Facial vein

Internal jugular vein

Supraorbital vein   Facial vein   Retromandibular vein   Common cardinal vein   Postcardinal vein

Fig. 3.38 *Successive stages in the development of the veins of the head and neck. **A**, At approximately 8 mm crown–rump length. **B**, At approximately 24 mm crown–rump length.*

Thus, a thick-walled region marks the future optic stalk at the junction with the diencephalon; laterally, the tissue that will become the sensory retina forms a flat disc of thickened epithelium in close contact with the surface ectoderm; and the thin-walled part of the vesicle that lies between these regions will later form the pigmented layer of the retina. The area of surface ectoderm that is closely apposed to the optic vesicle also thickens to form the lens placode. The mesenchymal sheath of the vesicle begins to show signs of angiogenesis. Between 32 and 33 days' postovulation, the lens placode and optic vesicle undergo coordinated morphogenesis. The lens placode invaginates, forming a pit that pinches off from the surface ectoderm to form the lens vesicle. The surface ectoderm re-forms a continuous layer that will become the corneal epithelium. The lateral part of the optic vesicle also invaginates to form a cup, the inner layer of which—facing the lens vesicle—will become the sensory retina, and the outer layer of which will become the pigmented retinal epithelium. As a result of these folding movements, what were the apical (luminal) surfaces of the two layers of the cup now face each other across a much reduced lumen, the intraretinal space. The pigmented layer becomes attached to the mesenchymal sheath, but the junction between the pigmented and sensory layers is less firm and is the site of pathological detachment of the retina. The two layers are continuous at the lip of the cup, which, at the end of the third month, grows around the front of the lens and forms the pigmented iris. Between the base of the cup and the brain, the narrow part of the optic vesicle forms the optic stalk. The anteroventral surface of the vesicle and distal part of the stalk are also infolded, forming a wide groove—the choroid fissure—through which mesenchyme extends with the associated hyaloid artery. As growth proceeds, the fissure closes, and the artery is included in the distal part of the stalk. Failure of the optic fissure to close is a rare anomaly that is always accompanied by a corresponding deficiency in the choroid and iris (congenital coloboma).

Differentiation of the Functional Components of the Eye

The developments just described bring the embryonic components of the eye into the spatial relationships necessary for the passage, focusing and sensing of light. The next phase of development involves further patterning and cell type differentiation to develop the specialized structures of the adult organ.

The optic cup becomes patterned, from the base to the rim, into regions with distinct functions (Fig. 3.39). The external stratum remains as a rather thin layer of cells that begin to acquire pigmented melanosomes and form the pigmented epithelium of the retina at around 36 days. In a parallel process that began before invagination, the cells of the inner layer of the cup proliferate to form a thick epithelium. The inner layer forms neural tissue over the base and sides of the cup and non-neural tissue around the lip. The non-neural epithelium is further differentiated into the components of the prospective iris at the rim and the ciliary body a little farther back adjacent to the neural area. The development of this pattern is reflected in regional differences in the expression of various genes that encode transcriptional regulators and are therefore likely to play key roles in controlling and coordinating development. Each of these genes is expressed prior to overt cell type differentiation. For example, PAX6 is expressed in the prospective ciliary and iris regions of the optic cup. Individuals heterozygous for mutations in PAX6 lack an iris, which suggests a causal role for this gene in the development of the iris. The genes expressed in the eye are also active at a variety of other specific sites in the embryo, and this may account, in part, for the co-involvement of the eye and other organs in syndromes that result from single genetic lesions.

Neural Retina

The neural retina comprises an outer nuclear zone and an inner marginal zone that is devoid of nuclei. At around 36 days, the cells of the nuclear zone invade the marginal zone, and by 44 days, the nervous stratum of the retina consists of inner and outer neuroblastic layers. The inner neuroblastic layer gives rise to the ganglion cells, the amacrine cells and the somata of the 'fibrous' sustentacular cells (of Müller); the outer neuroblastic layer is the source of the horizontal and rod-and-cone bipolar neurones and probably the rod-and-cone cells, which first appear in the central part of the retina. By the eighth month, all the named layers of the retina can be identified. However, the retinal photoreceptor cells continue to form after birth, generating an array of increasing resolution and sensitivity.

The divergent differentiation of the pigmented and sensory layers of the retina depends on interactions mediated by diffusible molecules. For example, soluble factors from the retina elicit the polarized distribution of plasma membrane proteins and the formation of tight junctions in the pigmented epithelium. Neural retinal differentiation appears to be mediated by FGFs. However, the pigmented epithelium retains the potential to become neural retina and will do so if the embryonic retina is wounded.

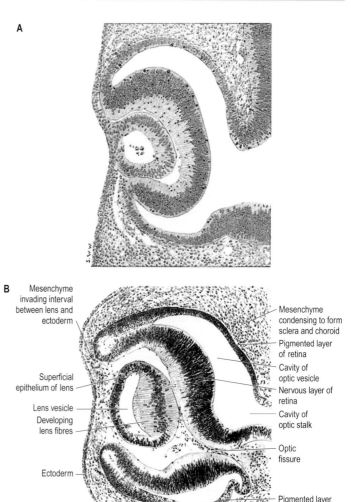

A

B
Mesenchyme invading interval between lens and ectoderm

Mesenchyme condensing to form sclera and choroid

Pigmented layer of retina

Cavity of optic vesicle

Superficial epithelium of lens

Nervous layer of retina

Lens vesicle
Developing lens fibres

Cavity of optic stalk

Optic fissure

Ectoderm

Pigmented layer of retina

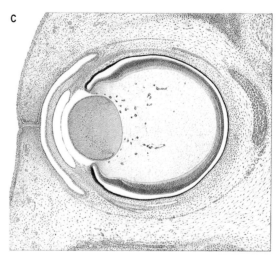

C

Fig. 3.39 *Sections through the developing eyes of human embryos. **A**, At 8 mm crown–rump length, the thick nervous layer and the thinner pigmented layers of the retina and the developing lens are shown (haematoxylin-eosin stain). **B**, At 13.2 mm crown–rump length. **C**, At 40 mm crown–rump length, note the layers of the retina, developing lens, pupillary membrane, cornea, conjunctival sac, anterior and posterior aqueous chambers, developing vitreous body, condensing circumoptic mesenchyme and fused eyelids (haematoxylin-eosin stain). (**A**, from material loaned by Professor R. J. Harrison; **B**, by permission from Streeter, G.L. 1948. Developmental horizons in human embryos. Contrib. Embryol. Carnegie Inst. Washington 32, 133–203.)*

Optic Nerve

The optic nerve develops from the optic stalk. The centre of the optic cup, where the optic fissure is deepest, later forms the optic disc. Here the neural retina is continuous with the corresponding invaginated cell layer of the optic stalk; consequently, the developing nerve fibres of the ganglion cells pass directly into the wall of the stalk and convert it into the optic nerve. The fibres of the optic nerve begin to acquire their myelin sheaths shortly before birth, but the process is not completed until sometime later. The optic chiasma is formed by the meeting and partial decussation of the fibres of the two optic nerves in the ventral part of the lamina terminalis at the junction of the telencephalon and the diencephalon in the floor of the third ventricle. Beyond the chiasma, the fibres are continued backward as the optic tracts and pass principally to the lateral geniculate bodies and to the superior tectum.

Ciliary Body

The ciliary body is a compound structure. Its epithelial components are the region of the inner layer of the retina between the iris and the neural retina and the adjacent outer layer of pigmented epithelium. The cells here differentiate in close association with the surrounding mesenchyme to form highly vascularized folds that secrete fluid into the globe of the eye. The inner surface of the ciliary body also forms the site of attachment of the lens, whereas the outer layer is associated with smooth muscle derived from mesenchymal cells in the choroid lying between the anterior scleral condensation and the pigmented ciliary epithelium.

Iris

The iris develops from the tip of the optic cup, where the two layers remain thin and are associated with vascularized, muscular connective tissue. The muscles of the sphincter and dilator pupillae are unusual, being of neuroectodermal origin, and develop from the cells of the pupillary part of the optic cup. The mature colour of the iris develops after birth and is dependent on the relative contributions of the pigmented epithelium on the posterior surface of the iris and the chromatophore cells in the mesenchymal stroma of the iris. If only epithelial pigment is present, the eye appears blue; if there is an additional contribution from the chromatophores, the eye appears brown.

Lens

The lens develops from the lens vesicle (see Fig. 3.39A). Initially, this is a ball of actively proliferating epithelium that encloses a clump of disintegrating cells; by 37 days, there is a discernible difference between the thin anterior (outward-facing) epithelium and the thickened posterior epithelium. Cells of the posterior wall lengthen and fill the vesicle (see Fig. 3.39B, C) and reduce the original cavity to a slit by about 44 days. The posterior cells become filled with a very high concentration of proteins (crystallins), which renders them transparent. They also become densely packed within the lens as primary lens fibres. Cells at the equatorial region of the lens elongate and contribute secondary lens fibres to the body of the lens in a process that continues into adult life, sustained by continued proliferation of cells in the anterior epithelium. The polarity and growth of the lens appear to depend on the differential distribution of soluble factors that promote either cell division or lens fibre differentiation and are present in the anterior chamber and vitreous humour, respectively.

The developing lens is surrounded by a vascular mesenchymal condensation, the vascular capsule; the anterior part is called the pupillary membrane. The posterior part of the capsule is supplied by branches from the hyaloid artery, and the anterior part is supplied by branches from the anterior ciliary arteries. During the fourth month, the hyaloid artery gives off retinal branches. By the sixth month, all the vessels have atrophied except the hyaloid artery. The latter becomes occluded during the eighth month of intrauterine life, although its proximal part persists in the adult as the central artery of the retina. Atrophy of the hyaloid vasculature and of the pupillary membrane appears to be an active process of programmed tissue remodelling that is macrophage dependent. The hyaloid canal, which carries the vessels through the vitreous, persists after the vessels have become occluded. In the newborn it extends more or less horizontally from the optic disc to the posterior aspect of the lens, but when the adult eye is examined with a slit lamp, it can be seen to follow an undulating course, sagging downward as it passes forward to the lens. With the loss of its blood vessels, the vascular capsule disappears, and the lens becomes dependent for nutrition on diffusion via the aqueous and vitreous humours. The lens remains enclosed in the lens capsule, a thickened basal lamina derived from the lens epithelium. Sometimes the pupillary membrane persists at birth, which gives rise to congenital atresia of the pupil.

Vitreous Body

The vitreous body develops between the lens and the optic cup as a transparent, avascular gel of extracellular substance. The precise derivation of the vitreous remains controversial. The lens rudiment and the optic vesicle are in contact at first; they draw apart after closure of the lens vesicle and formation of the optic cup but remain connected by a network of delicate cytoplasmic processes. This network, derived partly from cells of the lens and partly from those of the retina, is the primitive vitreous body. At first, these cytoplasmic processes are connected to the whole of the neuroretinal area of the cup; later, they become limited to the ciliary region, where, by a process of condensation, they form the basis of the suspensory ligaments of the ciliary zonule. The vascular mesenchyme that enters the cup through the choroidal fissure and around the equator of the lens associates locally with this reticular tissue and thus contributes to formation of the vitreous body.

Aqueous Chamber

The aqueous chamber of the eye develops in the space between the surface ectoderm and the lens that is invaded by mesenchymal cells of neural crest origin. The chamber initially appears as a cleft in this mesenchymal tissue. The mesenchyme superficial to the cleft forms the substantia propria of the cornea, and the mesenchyme deep to the cleft forms the mesenchymal stroma of the iris and the pupillary membrane. Tangentially, this early cleft extends as far as the iridocorneal angle, where communications are established with the sinus venosus sclerae. When the pupillary membrane disappears, the cavity continues to form between the iris and the lens capsule as far as the zonular suspensory fibres. In this way, the aqueous chamber is divided by the iris into anterior and posterior chambers that communicate through the pupil. The walls of these chambers furnish both the sites of production of aqueous humour and the channels for its circulation and reabsorption.

Cornea

The cornea is induced in front of the anterior chamber by the lens and optic cup. The corneal epithelium is formed from surface ectoderm, and the epithelium of the anterior chamber is formed from mesenchyme. A regular array of collagen fibres is established between these two layers, and these serve to reduce the scattering of light entering the eye.

Choroid and Sclera

The choroid and sclera differentiate as inner vascular and outer fibrous layers from the mesenchyme that surrounds the optic cup. The blood vessels of the choroid develop from the fifteenth week and include the vasculature of the ciliary body. The choroid is continuous with the internal sheath of the optic nerve, which is pia-arachnoid mater, and the sclera is continuous with the outer sheath of the optic nerve and thus with the dura mater.

Differentiation of Structures around the Eye

Extraocular Muscles

The extrinsic ocular muscles derive from prechordal mesenchyme that ingresses at the primitive node very early in development. The prechordal cells lie at the rostral tip of the notochordal process and remain mesenchymal after the notochordal process becomes epithelial and gains a basal lamina. The prechordal mesenchyme migrates laterally toward the paraxial mesenchyme. Although this is a singular origin for muscle, the early myogenic properties of these cells have been demonstrated experimentally; moreover, if transplanted into limb buds, the cells are able to develop into muscle tissue (Wachtler and Jacob 1986).

Early embryos develop bilateral premandibular, intermediate and caudal cavities in the head, previously described as preotic somites. The walls of the premandibular head cavities are lined by flat or cylindrical cells that do not exhibit the characteristics of a germinal epithelium. As the oculomotor nerve grows down to the level of the head cavity, a condensation of premuscle cells appears at its ventrolateral side, which later subdivides into the blastemata of the different muscles supplied by the nerve. Similar events occur with respect to the intermediate head cavity (trochlear nerve and superior oblique muscle) and the caudal head cavity (abducens nerve and lateral rectus muscle).

There is no doubt that the head cavities are formed by a mesenchymal–epithelial shift similar to that seen in the somites. However, the epithelial plate of the somite is a germinal centre that produces postmitotic myoblasts destined for epaxial regions and migratory premitotic myoblasts destined for the limbs and body wall. The head cavities may serve a similar purpose if a mesenchymal–epithelial shift is part of the maturation process for putative myoblasts. However, there may be no need to provide a centre for cell replication, because premitotic myoblasts differentiated directly from the prechordal mesenchyme may form the premuscular masses.

Eyelids

The eyelids are formed as small cutaneous folds of surface ectoderm and neural crest mesenchyme (see Fig. 3.39C). During the middle of the third month, their edges come together and unite over the cornea to enclose the conjunctival sac, and they usually remain united until about the end of the sixth month. When the eyelids open, the conjunctivae lining their inner surfaces and covering the white (scleral) region of the eye fuse with the corneal epithelium. The eyelashes and the lining cells of the tarsal (meibomian), ciliary and other glands that open onto the margins of the eyelids are all derived from the tarsal plate. Orbicularis oculi develops from skeletal myoblasts that invade the eyelids from the second pharyngeal arch. Levator palpebrae superioris develops from the prechordal mesenchyme and is attached to the upper eyelids by tendons derived from the neural crest. Smooth muscle also develops within the eyelids.

Lacrimal Apparatus

The epithelium of the alveoli and the ducts of the lacrimal gland arise as a series of tubular buds from the ectoderm of the superior conjunctival fornix. These buds are arranged in two groups: one forms the gland proper, and the other forms its palpebral process (de la Cuadra-Blanco, Peces-Peña and Mèrida-Velasco 2003). The lacrimal sac and nasolacrimal duct are derived from ectoderm in the nasomaxillary groove between the lateral nasal process and the maxillary process of the developing face. This thickens to form a solid cord of cells, the nasolacrimal ridge, which sinks into the mesenchyme. During the third month, the cord becomes canalized to form the nasolacrimal duct.

The lacrimal canaliculi arise as buds from the cranial extremity of the cord, which establish openings (puncta lacrimalia) on the margins of the lids. The inferior canaliculus isolates a small part of the lower eyelid to form the lacrimal caruncle and plica semilunaris.

DEVELOPMENT OF THE EAR

Inner Ear

The rudiments of the internal ears appear shortly after those of the eyes as two patches of thickened surface epithelium—the otic placodes—lateral to the hindbrain. The early otic epithelium, which is derived from the otic placode, initiates and then suppresses chondrogenesis in the surrounding periotic mesenchyme. Sonic hedgehog protein, FGFs, and transforming growth factor-β have all been shown to be active in the early stages of otic capsule development in the mouse (Frenz et al 1994).

Each otic placode invaginates as an otic pit while also giving cells to the statoacoustic (vestibulocochlear) ganglion (see Fig. 3.2). The mouth of the pit then closes to form an otocyst (auditory or otic vesicle) (Fig. 3.40). The otocyst is initially piriform, but a vertical infolding of its wall progressively marks off a tubular diverticulum on the medial side, which differentiates into the ductus

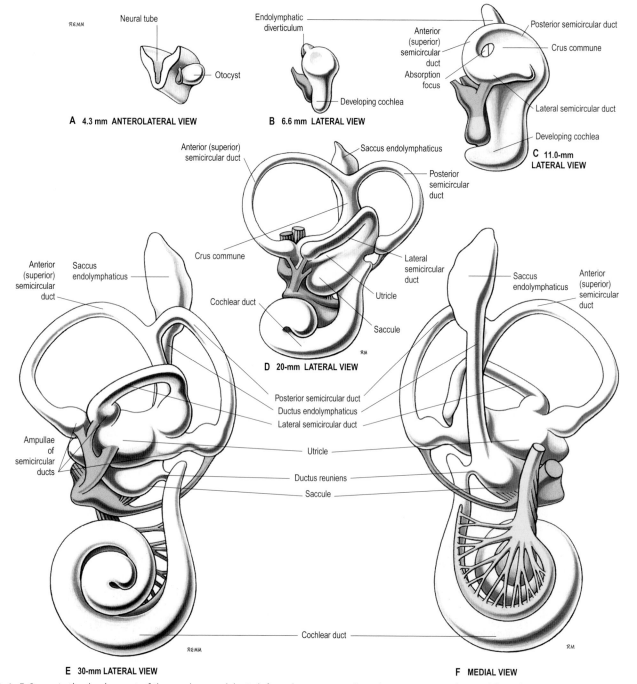

Fig. 3.40 *A–F, Stages in the development of the membranous labyrinth from the otocyst, at the embryonic stages and viewed from the aspects indicated. Note also the relationship of the vestibular* (orange) *and cochlear* (yellow) *parts of the vestibulocochlear nerve.*

and saccus endolymphaticus. The latter both communicate via the ductus with the remainder of the vesicle, the utriculosaccular chamber, which is placed laterally. Three compressed diverticula emerge as disc-like evaginations from the dorsal part of this chamber. The central parts of their walls coalesce and disappear, and their peripheral portions persist as the semicircular ducts. The anterior duct is completed first, and the lateral last. A medially directed evagination arises from the ventral part of the utriculosaccular chamber and coils progressively as the cochlear duct. Its proximal extremity becomes constricted and forms the ductus reuniens.

The central part of the chamber now represents the membranous vestibule, which becomes divided into a small ventral saccule and a larger utricle. This is achieved mainly by horizontal infolding that extends from the lateral wall of the vestibule toward the opening of the ductus endolymphaticus until only a narrow utriculosaccular duct remains between the saccule and the utricle. The duct becomes acutely bent on itself: its apex is continuous with the ductus endolymphaticus. During this period, the membranous labyrinth rotates so that its long axis, which was originally vertical, becomes more or less horizontal.

Cells derived from the otocyst not only contribute placodal cells to the vestibulocochlear ganglion but also differentiate into specialized paraneuronal hair cells of the utricle, saccule, ampullae of the semicircular ducts and organ of Corti; various specialized sustentacular cells and the unique epithelia of the stria vascularis and endolymphatic sac; and cells from which the general epithelial lining of the membranous labyrinth develops.

The periotic mesenchyme surrounding the various parts of the epithelial labyrinth is converted into a cartilaginous otic capsule that ossifies to form most of the bony labyrinth of the internal ear, apart from the modiolus and osseous spiral lamina. For a time, the cartilaginous capsule is incomplete, which means that the cochlear, vestibular and facial ganglia are exposed in the gap between its canalicular and cochlear parts. They are soon covered by an outgrowth of cartilage, and the facial nerve becomes enclosed as cartilage grows from the cochlear to the canalicular part of the capsule. Perilymphatic spaces develop in the embryonic connective tissue between the cartilaginous capsule and the epithelial wall of the labyrinth. The rudiment of the periotic cistern or vestibular perilymphatic space can be seen in an embryo 30 to 40 mm long, in the reticulum between the saccule and the fenestra vestibuli. The scala tympani develops opposite the fenestra cochleae and is followed later by the scala vestibuli. The two scalae gradually extend along each side of the ductus cochlearis, and when they reach the tip of the ductus, a communication—the helicotrema—opens between them. The modiolus and the osseous spiral lamina of the cochlea are not preformed in cartilage but ossify directly from connective tissue.

The rudiment of the eighth nerve appears in the fourth week as the vestibulocochlear ganglion, which lies between the otocyst and the wall of the hindbrain. At first, it is fused with the ganglion of the facial nerve (acousticofacial ganglion); later, the two separate. The cells of the vestibulocochlear ganglion are derived mainly from the placodal ectoderm. The ganglion divides into vestibular and cochlear parts, each associated with the corresponding division of the eighth nerve. Ganglionic neurones, which remain bipolar throughout life, are unusual, in that many of their somata become enveloped in thin myelin sheaths. Their peripheral processes provide the afferent innervation of the labyrinthine hair cells, which also become associated with the outgrowing axons of the olivocochlear bundle—from cells of the superior olivary complexes in the pons.

Middle Ear (Tympanic Cavity) and Pharyngotympanic Tube

The pharyngotympanic tube and tympanic cavity are extensions of the early pharynx and develop from the hollow tubotympanic recess. This lies between the first and third pharyngeal arches and has a floor consisting of the second arch and its limiting pouches. The forward growth of the third arch causes the inner part of the recess to narrow to form the tubal region, and it also excludes the inner part of the second arch from this portion of the floor. The more lateral part of the recess develops into the tympanic cavity, and its floor forms the lateral wall of the tympanic cavity approximately up to the level where the chorda tympani branches off from the facial nerve. The lateral wall of the tympanic cavity contains first and second arch elements. The first arch territory is limited to the part in front of the anterior process of the malleus; the second arch forms the outer wall behind this and also turns on to the posterior wall to include the tympanohyal region.

The tubotympanic recess initially lies inferolateral to the cartilaginous otic capsule, but as the capsule enlarges the spatial relationship alters, and the tympanic cavity becomes anterolateral. A cartilaginous process grows from the lateral part of the capsule to form the tegmen tympani, and it curves caudally to form the lateral wall of the pharyngotympanic tube. In this way, the tympanic cavity and the proximal part of the pharyngotympanic tube become included in the petrous region of the temporal bone. During the sixth or seventh month, the mastoid antrum appears as a dorsal expansion of the tympanic cavity.

The malleus develops from the dorsal end of the ventral mandibular (Meckel's) cartilage, and the incus develops from the dorsal cartilage of the first arch, which is probably homologous to the quadrate bone in birds and reptiles. The stapes stems mainly from the dorsal end of the cartilage of the second (hyoid) arch, first as a ring (anulus stapes) encircling the small stapedial artery. The primordium of the stapedius muscle appears close to the artery and facial nerve at the end of the second month, and at almost the same time, the tensor tympani begins to appear near the extremity of the tubotympanic recess. At first, the ossicles are embedded in the mesenchymal roof of the tympanic cavity; later, they are covered by the mucosa of the middle ear cavity, which becomes filled with air after birth.

External Ear

The external acoustic meatus develops from the dorsal end of the hyomandibular or first pharyngeal groove. Close to its dorsal extremity, this groove extends inward as a funnel-shaped primary meatus, from which the cartilaginous part and a small area of the roof of the osseous meatus are developed. A solid epidermal plug extends inward from the tube along the floor of the tubotympanic recess, and the cells in the centre of the plug subsequently degenerate to produce the inner part of the meatus (secondary meatus). The epidermal stratum of the tympanic membrane is formed from the deepest ectodermal cells of the epidermal plug, and the fibrous stratum is formed from the mesenchyme between the meatal plate and the endodermal floor of the tubotympanic recess.

Development of the auricle is initiated by the appearance of six hillocks that form around the margins of the dorsal portion of the hyomandibular groove at the 4-mm stage. Three of the six are on the caudal edge of the mandibular arch, and three are on the cranial edge of the hyoid arch. These

CASE 1 CHARCOT–MARIE–TOOTH DISEASE (HEREDITARY MOTOR–SENSORY NEUROPATHY)

A 22-year-old man presents following a fall due to bilateral footdrop. He notes that he has always tripped easily and relates difficulty running as a child. His brother has similar problems, and his mother has narrow feet with high arches. On examination, he has distal weakness of the lower extremities, with atrophy and bilateral pes cavus deformity (extremely high arches with hammer toes). There is mild weakness of the interossei in the hands. Sensation is decreased in the lower extremities in a stocking distribution. Reflexes are absent throughout.

Discussion: Charcot–Marie–Tooth disease is the most common hereditary neuropathy, with type 1A being most prevalent. This demyelinating neuropathy is inherited in an autosomal dominant fashion. There is an abnormality on chromosome 17, most commonly a PMP22 duplication. The longest nerves are affected first, resulting in initial signs and symptoms involving the lower extremities distally. Pathologically, myelinated fibres exhibit segmental demyelination with proliferation and onion-bulb formation, resulting in impaired transmission of action potentials. There may be phenotypical variation, with a parent having only mild distal lower extremity changes such as high arches or mild sensory loss. As a result, the diagnosis may be missed. Spontaneous mutations may also produce the genetic defect.

hillocks appear at stage 15; they tend to be less obvious before that stage. Of those on the mandibular arch, only the most ventral, which subsequently forms the tragus, can be identified at earlier stages. The rest of the auricle is formed in the mesenchyme of the hyoid arch, which extends forward around the dorsal end of the remnants of the hyomandibular groove, forming a keel-like elevation that is the forerunner of the helix. The mandibular arch's contribution to the auricle is greatest at the end of the second month, and it becomes relatively reduced as growth continues; eventually, the area of skin supplied by the mandibular nerve extends little above the tragus. The lobule is the last part of the auricle to develop.

References

Allen, M.C., Capute, A.J., 1990. Tone and reflex development before term. J. Pediatr. 85, 393–399. *Provides details of the development of reflexes in extremely premature infants.*

Barkovich, A.J., Kuzniedky, R.I., Jackson, G.D., Guerrini, R., Dobyns, W.B., 2005. A developmental and genetic classification for malformations of cortical development. Neurology 65, 1873–1887.

Begbie, J., Graham, A., 2001. The ectodermal placodes: a dysfunctional family. Phil. Trans. R Soc. Lond. B. Biol. Sci. 356, 1655–1660. *Challenges the view of ectodermal placodes as a coherent group and discusses their early development, induction and evolution.*

Brown, M., Keynes, R., Lumsden, A., 2001. The Developing Brain. Oxford University Press, Oxford. *Covers the main mechanisms of neural development from neurulation to synaptic reorganization.*

de la Cuadra-Blanco, C., Peces-Peña, M.D., Mèrida-Velasco, J.R., 2003. Morphogenesis of the human lacrimal gland. J. Anat. 203, 531–536.

Donoghue, M.J., Rakic, P., 1999. Molecular gradients and compartments in the embryonic primate cerebral cortex. Cereb. Cortex. 9, 586–600. *Presents evidence for the existence of an intrinsic protomap that predicts the functional map of the mature cerebral cortex.*

Frenz, D.A., Liu, W., Williams, J.D., Hatcher, V., Galinovic-Schwartz, V., Flanders, K.C., Van de Water, T.R., 1994. Induction of chondrogenesis: requirement for synergistic interaction of basic fibroblast growth factor and transforming growth factor-beta. Development 120, 415–424.

Gardner, W.J., 1973. The dysraphic states from syringomyelia to anencephaly. Excerpta Medica Amsterdam

Gordon-Weeks, P.R., 2000. Neuronal Growth Cones. Cambridge University Press, Cambridge.

Krumlauf, R., Marshall, H., Studer, M., Nonchev, S., Sham, M.H., Lumsden, A., 1993. Hox homeobox genes and regionalisation of the nervous system. J. Neurobiol. 24, 1328–1340. *Discusses the influence of the* Hox *family of homeobox-containing genes on the patterning of rhombomeres and neural crest.*

Le Douarin, N., Teillet, M., Catala, M., 1998. Neurulation in amniote vertebrates: a novel view deduced from the use of quail–chick chimeras. Int. J. Dev. Biol. 42, 909–916. *Explores the mechanisms that contribute to secondary neurulation using chimeric techniques.*

Muller, F., O'Rahilly, R., 1997. The timing and sequence of appearance of neuromeres and their derivatives in staged human embryos. Acta. Anat. (Basel) 158, 83–99.

Opperman, L.A., Sweeney, T.M., Redmon, J., Persing, J.A., Ogle, R.C., 1993. Tissue interactions with underlying dura mater inhibit osseous obliteration of developing cranial sutures. Dev. Dynam. 198, 312–322. *Examines the role of the dura mater in the development of the skull bones and sutures.*

O'Rahilly, R., 1966. The early development of the eye in staged human embryos. Contrib. Embryol. Carnegie. Inst. 38, 1.

O'Rahilly, R., 1983. The timing and sequence of events in the development of the human eye and ear during the embryonic period proper. Anat. Embryol. 168, 87–99.

O'Rahilly, R., Muller, F., 1986. The meninges in human development. J. Neuropathol. Exp. Neurol. 45, 588–608.

O'Rourke, N.A., Sullivan, D.P., Kaznowski, C.E., Jacobs, A.A., McConnell, S.K., 1995. Tangential migration of neurons in the developing cerebral cortex. Development 121, 2165–2176.

Rakic, P., 1988. Specification of cerebral cortical areas. Science 241, 170–176. *Discusses the radial unit hypothesis as a framework for exploring cerebral evolution and the causes of some cortical disorders in humans.*

Rakic, P., 2003. Developmental and evolutionary adaptations of cortical radial glia. Cereb. Cortex. 13, 541–549. *Discusses cortical development and evolution and the pathogenesis of some genetic and acquired cortical anomalies.*

Saha, M.S., Servetnick, M., Grainger, R.M., 1992. Vertebrate eye development. Curr. Opin. Genet. Dev. 2, 582–588. *Reviews the interactions involved and genes responsible for eye development.*

Volpe, J.J., 2008. Neurology of the Newborn., Unit I, Human Brain Development, fifth ed. Saunders.

Volpe, J.J., 2001. Neurobiology of periventricular leukomalacia in the premature infant. Pediatr. Res. 50, 553–562.

von, Melchner, L., Pallas, S.L., Sur, M., 2000. Visual behaviour mediated by retinal projections directed to the auditory pathway. Nature 404, 820–821. *Describes the consequences of successful routing of visual projections into non-visual structures in the brain.*

Wachtler, F., Jacob, M., 1986. Origin and development of the cranial skeletal muscles. Bibl. Anat. 29, 24–46.

Withington, S., Beddington, R., Cooke, J., 2001. Foregut endoderm is required at head process stage for anteriormost neural patterning in chick. Development 128, 309–320. *Presents evidence for an early system of neuroepithelial patterning by the most rostral endoderm, the region of the prechordal plate.*

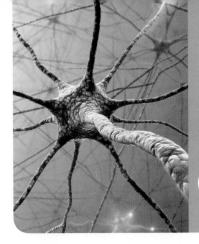

Cranial Meninges

The brain and spinal cord are entirely enveloped by three concentric membranes, the meninges, which provide support and protection. The outermost meningeal layer is the dura mater (pachymeninx). Beneath this lies the arachnoid mater. The innermost layer is the pia mater. The dura is an opaque, tough, fibrous coat. It incompletely divides the cranial cavity into compartments and accommodates the dural venous sinuses. It is separated from the arachnoid by a narrow subdural space. The arachnoid mater and pia mater are sometimes referred to collectively as the leptomeninges, and they share many similarities. The arachnoid is much thinner than the dura and is mostly translucent. It surrounds the brain loosely, spanning depressions and concavities. Beneath the arachnoid lies the subarachnoid space, which contains cerebrospinal fluid (CSF), secreted by the choroid plexuses of the cerebroventricular system. The pia mater is a transparent, microscopically thin membrane that follows the contours of the brain and is closely adherent to its surface. The subarachnoid space varies greatly in depth, and the larger expanses are termed subarachnoid cisterns. CSF circulates within the subarachnoid space and is reabsorbed into the venous system through arachnoid villi and granulations associated with the dural venous sinuses. Cranial and spinal meninges are continuous through the foramen magnum. Only the cranial meninges are described in this chapter.

DURA MATER

The dura mater is a thick, dense, fibrous membrane composed of densely packed fascicles of collagen fibres arranged in laminae. The fascicles run in different directions in adjacent laminae, producing a lattice-like appearance. This is particularly obvious in the tentorium cerebelli and around the defects or perforations that sometimes occur in the anterior portion of the falx cerebri. There is little histological difference between the endosteal and meningeal layers of the dura. The dura is largely acellular, but it contains fibroblasts, which are distributed throughout, and osteoblasts, which are confined to the endosteal layer. Focal calcification may occur in the falx cerebri.

The cranial dura differs from the spinal dura mainly in its relationship to the surrounding bones. The cranial dura lines the cranial cavity. It is composed of two layers: an inner, or meningeal, layer and an outer, or endosteal, layer. They are united except where they separate to enclose the venous sinuses that drain blood from the brain. The dura mater adheres to the internal surfaces of the cranial bones, and fibrous bands pass from it into the bones. Adhesion of the dura to the bones is firmest at the sutures, at the cranial base and around the foramen magnum. In children it is difficult to remove the dura from the suture lines, but in adults the dura becomes separated from the suture lines as they fuse. With increasing age the dura becomes thicker, less pliable and more firmly adherent to the inner surface of the skull, particularly that of the calvaria. The endosteal layer of the dura is continuous with the pericranium through the cranial sutures and foramina and with the orbital periosteum through the superior orbital fissure. The meningeal layer provides tubular sheaths for the cranial nerves as they pass out through the cranial foramina, and these sheaths fuse with the epineurium as the nerves emerge from the skull. The dural sheath of the optic nerve is continuous with the ocular sclera. At sites where major vessels, such as the internal carotid and vertebral arteries, pierce the dura to enter the cranial cavity, the dura is firmly fused with the adventitia of the vessels.

The inner aspect of the dura mater is closely applied to the arachnoid mater over the surface of the brain. They are easily separated, however, and are physically joined only at sites where veins pass from the brain into venous sinuses (e.g. superior sagittal sinus) or where they connect the brain to the dura (e.g. anterior pole of the temporal lobe).

The anatomical organization of the dura and its relationships to the major venous sinuses, sutures and blood vessels have significant pathological implications. In the case of head trauma, separation of the dura from the underlying periosteum requires significant force; consequently, this occurs only when high-pressure arterial bleeding occurs into the virtual space. This can result from damage to any arterial vessel, commonly following skull fracture. The classic site for such injury is along the course of the middle meningeal artery, where a direct blow causing a bone fracture can rupture the artery and cause rapid collection of an extradural haematoma. The haematoma is under considerable pressure due to the arterial blood pressure feeding it and the resistance of the strong adhesion between the dura and the periosteum. As a result of these factors, an extradural haematoma acts as a rapidly expanding intracranial mass lesion and poses a classic medical emergency requiring immediate diagnosis and surgery.

Dural Partitions

The meningeal layer of the dura is reflected inward to form four septa that partially divide the cranial cavity into compartments in which subdivisions of the brain are lodged.

Falx Cerebri

The falx cerebri is a strong, crescent-shaped sheet of dura mater lying in the sagittal plane and occupying the great longitudinal fissure between the two cerebral hemispheres (Figs. 4.2, 4.3). The crescent is narrow in front, where the falx is fixed to the crista galli, and broad behind, where it blends into the midline with the tentorium cerebelli. The anterior part of the falx is thin and may have a number of irregular perforations (see Fig. 4.2). Its convex upper margin is attached to the internal cranial surface on each side of the midline, as far back as the internal occipital protuberance. The superior sagittal sinus runs within the dura along this margin, in a cranial groove, and the falx is attached to the lips of this groove. At its lower edge, the falx is free and concave and contains the inferior sagittal sinus. The straight sinus runs along the line of attachment of the falx to the tentorium cerebelli (see Fig. 4.2).

Tentorium Cerebelli

The tentorium cerebelli (Figs. 4.2–4.4) is a sheet of dura mater with a peaked configuration reminiscent of a single-poled tent, from which its name is derived. It covers the cerebellum and passes under the occipital lobes of the cerebral hemispheres. Its concave anterior edge is free; between it and the dorsum sellae of the sphenoid bone is a large curved hiatus (the tentorial incisure or notch), which is occupied by the midbrain and the anterior part of the superior aspect of the cerebellar vermis. The tentorium divides the cranial cavity into supratentorial and infratentorial compartments that contain the forebrain and hindbrain, respectively. The convex outer limit of the tentorium is attached posteriorly to the lips of the transverse sulci of the occipital bone and the posteroinferior angles of the parietal bones, where it encloses the transverse sinuses. Laterally, the tentorium is attached to the superior borders of the petrous temporal bones, where it contains the superior petrosal sinuses (see Fig. 4.3). Near the apex of the petrous temporal bone, the lower layer of the tentorium is evaginated anterolaterally under the superior petrosal sinus to form a recess between the endosteal and meningeal layers in the middle cranial fossa. This recess is the trigeminal cave (Meckel's cave) and contains the roots and ganglion of the trigeminal nerve. The evaginated meningeal layer fuses in front with the anterior part of the trigeminal ganglion. At the apex of the petrous temporal bone, the free border and attached periphery of the tentorium cross each other (see Fig. 4.4). The anterior ends of the free border are fixed to the anterior clinoid processes, and the attached periphery is fixed to the posterior clinoid processes. The oculomotor nerve lies in the groove between them on each side.

Falx Cerebelli

The falx cerebelli is a small midline fold of dura mater lying below the tentorium cerebelli. It projects forward into the posterior cerebellar notch between the cerebellar hemispheres. Its base is directed upward and attached to the posterior part of the inferior surface of the tentorium cerebelli in the midline. Its posterior margin is attached to the internal occipital crest and contains the occipital sinus. The apex of the falx cerebelli frequently divides

CASE 1 EPIDURAL HAEMATOMA

An 18-year-old boy is involved in a high-speed motor vehicle accident. He is an unrestrained passenger in the front seat. When the paramedics arrive he is awake and conversant but mildly disoriented. He is transported to the local hospital for evaluation. In the emergency department (ED) he becomes progressively lethargic, cannot follow commands and develops a right hemiparesis. He is sent for a computed tomography (CT) scan of the head. On his return to the ED he is unconscious, requiring intubation and mechanical ventilation. The CT scan demonstrates a large epidural haematoma (EDH) on the left, with mass effect on the cerebral hemisphere. He is taken to the operating room for emergent evacuation of the haematoma.

Discussion: EDH occurs most often in adolescents and young adults. The most common cause is closed head injury sustained in a traffic accident, fall or assault. A skull fracture may be present in 75% to 95% of cases. The majority of EDHs are caused by arterial injury, usually the middle meningeal artery; however, they may also be caused by injury to the anterior meningeal artery, dural venous sinuses or vascular malformation.

The presentation of EDH may be variable, depending on the severity of the initial injury. It can range from transient loss of consciousness in mild cases to coma associated with severe head trauma. A commonly observed pattern is the so-called lucid interval: the patient is conscious after the initial injury but deteriorates over the course of a few hours due to increasing intracranial pressure from continued haematoma growth. Associated symptoms may include headache, nausea, vomiting, lethargy, confusion, aphasia, hemiparesis and seizures.

An EDH can readily be seen on an unenhanced head CT scan and typically has a lens-shaped appearance, as it lies in the potential space between the dura and the calvaria (Fig. 4.1). It

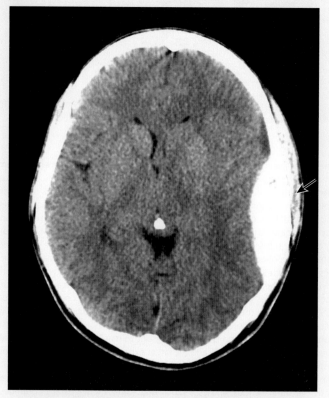

Fig. 4.1 *Epidural haematoma* (arrow). *Computed tomography demonstrates a large acute epidural haematoma.*

does not cross the cranial suture lines because at those locations the dura is tightly adherent to the skull. Emergency surgery is required in most cases to relieve the pressure caused by the haematoma and, if possible, identify the source of bleeding.

into two small folds, which disappear at the sides of the foramen magnum. Frequently the falx is double.

Diaphragma Sellae

The diaphragma sellae (see Fig. 4.2) is a small, circular, horizontal sheet of dura mater that forms a roof to the sella turcica and, in many cases, almost completely covers the pituitary gland (hypophysis). The central opening in the diaphragma allows the infundibulum and pituitary stalk to pass into the pituitary fossa. There is wide individual variation in the size of the central opening. The diaphragma sellae was an important landmark in pituitary surgery in the past—extension of a pituitary tumour above it was an indication for a subfrontal approach through a craniotomy. A transsphenoidal approach is currently preferred, irrespective of whether there is suprasellar extension.

The arrangement of the dura mater in the central part of the middle cranial fossa is complex (see Fig. 4.4). The tentorium cerebelli forms a large part of the floor of the middle cranial fossa and fills much of the gap between the ridges of the petrous temporal bones. On both sides, the rim of the tentorial incisure is attached to the apex of the petrous temporal bone and continues forward as a ridge of dura mater to attach to the anterior clinoid process. This ridge marks the junction of the roof and the lateral part of the cavernous sinus (Figs. 4.5, 4.6). The periphery of the tentorium cerebelli is attached to the superior border of the petrous temporal bone, crosses under the free border of the tentorial incisure and continues forward to the posterior clinoid processes as a rounded, indefinite ridge of the dura mater. Thus, an angular depression exists between the anterior parts of the peripheral attachment of the tentorium and the free border of the tentorial incisure (see Figs. 4.2, 4.4). This depression in the dura mater is part of the roof of the cavernous sinus and is pierced in front by the oculomotor nerve and behind by the

trochlear nerve, which proceed anteroinferiorly into the lateral wall of the cavernous sinus (Fig. 4.7). In the anteromedial part of the middle cranial fossa, the dura mater ascends as the lateral wall of the cavernous sinus. It reaches the ridge produced by the anterior continuation of the free border of the tentorium and runs medially as the roof of the cavernous sinus, where it is pierced by the internal carotid artery (see Figs. 4.2, 4.4). Medially, the roof of the sinus is continuous with the upper layer of the diaphragma sellae. At or just below the opening in the diaphragma for the infundibulum and pituitary stalk, the dura, arachnoid and pia mater blend with one another and with the capsule of the pituitary gland. It is not possible to distinguish the layers of the meninges within the sella turcica, and the subarachnoid space is obliterated.

Through its projections as the falx cerebri and tentorium cerebelli, the dura may act to stabilize the brain within the cranial cavity. However, this arrangement causes problems when there is focal brain swelling or a focal space-occupying lesion within the brain or cranial cavity. Consequently, herniation of the brain may occur under the falx cerebri or, more significantly, through the tentorial incisure, which compresses the oculomotor nerve, midbrain and arteries on the inferomedial surface of the temporal lobe. This process of transtentorial coning is particularly dangerous because of the risk of secondary vascular compression, and it often represents the terminal event in patients with evolving supratentorial space-occupying lesions. Similarly, space-occupying lesions in the small infratentorial compartment may cause upward herniation through the tentorial hiatus or downward herniation through the foramen magnum.

Dural Venous Sinuses

Dural venous sinuses (see Fig. 6.16) are a complex of venous channels that lie between the two layers of dura mater, draining blood from the brain and

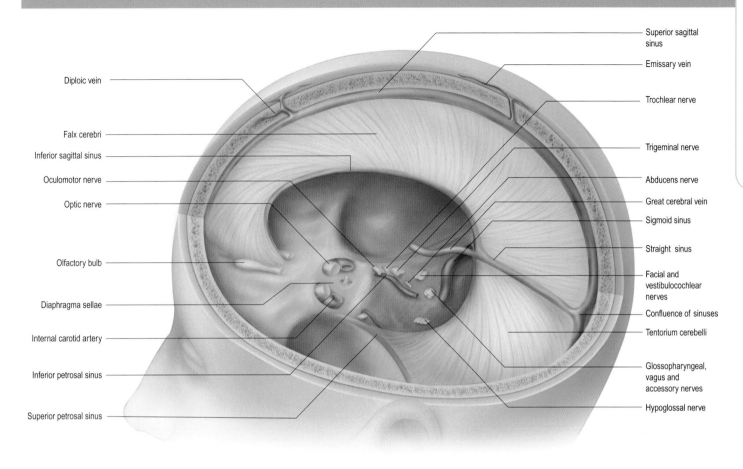

Diploic vein

Falx cerebri

Inferior sagittal sinus

Oculomotor nerve

Optic nerve

Olfactory bulb

Diaphragma sellae

Internal carotid artery

Inferior petrosal sinus

Superior petrosal sinus

Superior sagittal sinus

Emissary vein

Trochlear nerve

Trigeminal nerve

Abducens nerve

Great cerebral vein

Sigmoid sinus

Straight sinus

Facial and vestibulocochlear nerves

Confluence of sinuses

Tentorium cerebelli

Glossopharyngeal, vagus and accessory nerves

Hypoglossal nerve

Fig. 4.2 *The cerebral dura mater, its reflections and major venous sinuses.*

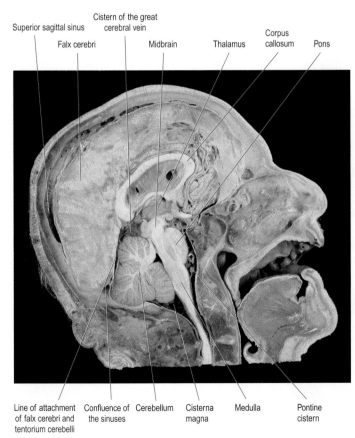

Superior sagittal sinus

Cistern of the great cerebral vein

Falx cerebri

Midbrain

Thalamus

Corpus callosum

Pons

Line of attachment of falx cerebri and tentorium cerebelli

Confluence of the sinuses

Cerebellum

Cisterna magna

Medulla

Pontine cistern

Fig. 4.3 *Parasagittal section of the head showing the disposition of the falx cerebri, together with some of the dural venous sinuses and subarachnoid cisterns. (Figure enhanced by B. Crossman.)*

cranial bones. They are lined by endothelium and have no valves; their walls are devoid of muscular tissue. Developmentally, the venous sinuses emerge as venous plexuses, and most sinuses preserve a plexiform arrangement to a variable degree rather than being simple vessels with a single lumen. Browder and Kaplan (1976) examined human venous sinuses in hundreds of corrosion casts and observed vascular plexuses adjoining the superior and inferior sagittal and straight sinuses and, with a lower incidence, the transverse sinuses. There was much individual variation, and departures from 'average' patterns were frequent in early life; for example, in infancy, the falx cerebelli may contain large plexiform channels and venous lacunae, augmenting the occipital sinus. These variations cannot be detailed in a general text. They must be established on an individual basis by angiography when the clinical necessity arises. However, it is important to emphasize the wide variation possible in the structure of cranial venous sinuses, together with their plexiform nature and wide connections with cerebral and cerebellar veins. Another kind of connection has been shown experimentally. Parts of sinuses (and even diploic veins) can be filled by forcible internal carotid injection, suggesting the existence of arteriovenous shunts (Browder and Kaplan 1976). A connection between the middle meningeal arteries and the superior sagittal sinus has been demonstrated in this way, although the sites of communication are unknown.

Superior Sagittal Sinus

The superior sagittal sinus runs in the attached, convex margin of the falx cerebri; it grooves the internal surface of the frontal bone, the adjacent margins of the two parietal bones and the squamous part of the occipital bone (Fig. 4.8; see also Figs. 4.2, 6.16). It begins near the crista galli, a few millimetres posterior to the foramen caecum, and receives primary tributaries from cortical veins of the frontal lobes, the ascending frontal veins. Narrow anteriorly, the sinus runs backward, gradually widening to approximately 1 cm. Near the internal occipital protuberance it deviates, usually to the right, and continues as a transverse sinus. Triangular in cross-section, the interior of the superior sagittal sinus possesses the openings of superior cerebral veins and projecting arachnoid granulations. It is traversed by many fibrous bands. It also communicates by small orifices with irregular venous lacunae, situated in the dura mater near the sinus. There are usually two or three of these on each side—a small frontal, a large parietal and an intermediate-sized occipital. In the elderly, the lacunae tend to become

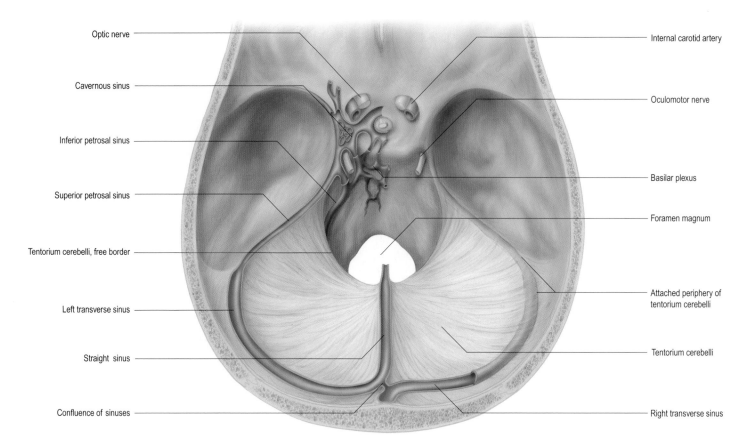

Optic nerve

Cavernous sinus

Inferior petrosal sinus

Superior petrosal sinus

Tentorium cerebelli, free border

Left transverse sinus

Straight sinus

Confluence of sinuses

Internal carotid artery

Oculomotor nerve

Basilar plexus

Foramen magnum

Attached periphery of tentorium cerebelli

Tentorium cerebelli

Right transverse sinus

Fig. 4.4 *Dura mater of the floor of the cranial cavity and the superior aspect of the tentorium cerebelli. Representations of the cavernous sinus and its venous relationships are greatly simplified and are shown on the left only. Note that the trochlear and abducens nerves are not shown (see Fig. 4.6).*

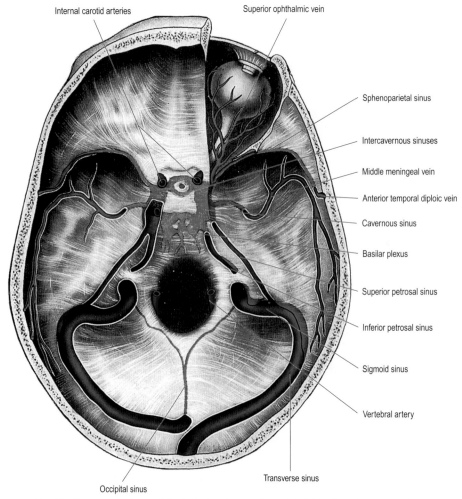

Internal carotid arteries

Superior ophthalmic vein

Sphenoparietal sinus

Intercavernous sinuses

Middle meningeal vein

Anterior temporal diploic vein

Cavernous sinus

Basilar plexus

Superior petrosal sinus

Inferior petrosal sinus

Sigmoid sinus

Vertebral artery

Occipital sinus

Transverse sinus

Fig. 4.5 *Sinuses at the base of the skull. The sinuses coloured dark blue have been opened up.*

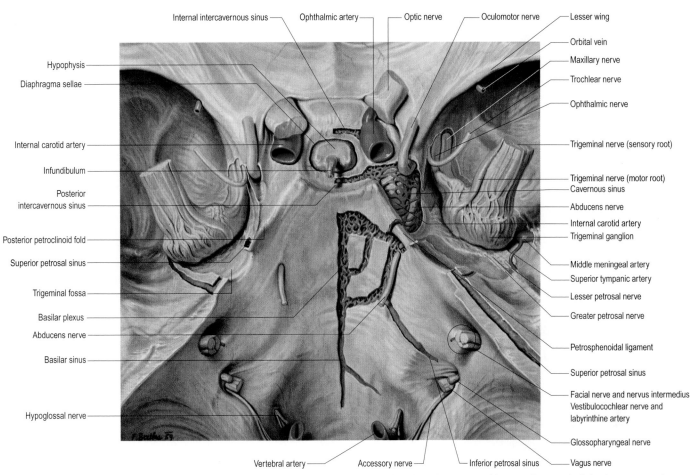

Fig. 4.6 *Middle cranial fossa, viewed from above to show the cavernous and related sinuses. These have been exposed by partial removal of the dura matter. The trigeminal, trochlear and oculomotor nerves have been reflected forward on both sides.*

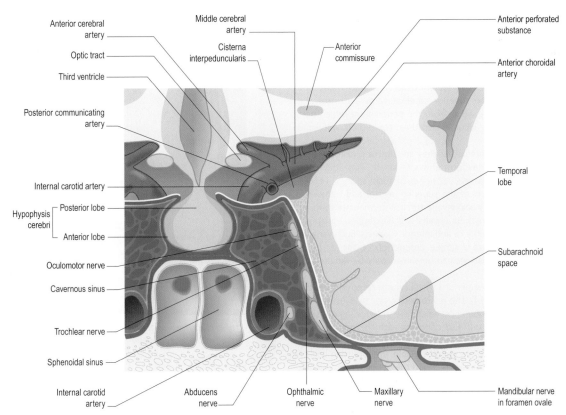

Fig. 4.7 *Coronal, slightly oblique section through the middle cranial fossa, showing the cavernous and cerebral portions of the internal carotid artery and the cavernous sinus. Pia mater, mauve; arachnoid mater, white; layers of dura mater (mesothelium is not indicated), green; endothelium of cavernous sinus, blue.*

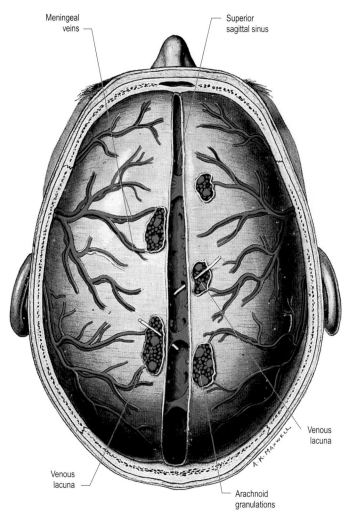

Fig. 4.8 *Superior sagittal sinus laid open after removal of the cranial vault. Some of the fibrous bands that cross the sinus are shown (from two of the venous lacunae). Markers are passed into the sinus.*

confluent, so there is one elongated lacuna on each side. Fine fibrous bands cross them, and numerous arachnoid granulations project into them. The superior sagittal sinus receives the superior cerebral veins and, near the posterior end of the sagittal suture, veins from the pericranium, which pass through the parietal foramina. The lacunae also drain the diploic veins and meningeal veins.

Lateral lacunae are often so complex that they are almost plexiform; they are rarely simple venous spaces. Plexiform arrays of small veins adjoin the sagittal, transverse and straight sinuses, and ridges of such 'spongy' venous tissue often project into the lumina of the superior sagittal and transverse sinuses. The superior sagittal sinus is also invaded, in its intermediate third, by variable bands and projections from its dural walls, which extend as horizontal shelves that divide its lumen into superior and inferior channels. Such variable features make it impossible to give a simple description of this or other venous sinuses, and individual variations can be shown only by radiological investigations.

The dilated posterior end of the superior sagittal sinus is referred to as the confluence of the sinuses (see Fig. 4.4). This is situated to one side (usually the right) of the internal occipital protuberance, where the superior sagittal sinus turns to become a transverse sinus. It also connects with the occipital and contralateral transverse sinus. The size and degree of communication of the channels meeting at the confluence are highly variable. In more than half of subjects, all venous channels that converge toward the occiput interconnect, including the straight and occipital sinuses. In many instances, however, communication is absent or tenuous. Any sinus involved may be duplicated, narrowed or widened near the confluence.

Inferior Sagittal Sinus

The inferior sagittal sinus is located in the posterior half or two-thirds of the free margin of the falx cerebri (see Fig. 4.2). It increases in size posteriorly and ends in the straight sinus. It receives veins from the falx and sometimes from the medial surfaces of the cerebral hemispheres.

A 41-year-old woman, previously well, has purulent frontal sinusitis. She complains of increasingly severe headache and has evidence of increased intracranial pressure, with papilledema but no focal neurological signs. After several days she becomes lethargic and abruptly develops a right hemiparesis with aphasia, with repeated focal seizures involving the left side. She is septic at that juncture. Her spinal fluid contains a moderate pleocytosis and several thousand erythocytes per cubic millimetre, with a normal sugar content.

CT scan of the head demonstrates bilateral venous infarctions involving most prominently the left cerebral hemisphere. Magnetic resonance imaging (MRI) documents obstruction of the superior sagittal sinus (Fig. 4.9).

Discussion: This woman has thrombosis of the superior sagittal sinus secondary to spread of infection from her frontal sinus. (Such infection may also spread from a focus of osteomyelitis.) Non-septic thrombosis may result from invasion of the superior sagittal sinus by tumour, but it has also been associated with a host of systemic and neurological disorders. In some cases, no recognizable cause can be identified. Initially, as in this patient, there may be no focal neurological signs. However, many patients develop occlusion of the draining cerebral veins, with resultant venous infarction (and haemorrhagic spinal fluid) and recurrent focal seizures, along with appropriate neurological signs.

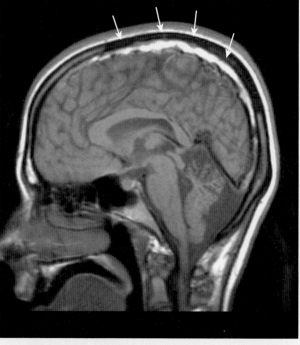

Fig. 4.9 *Superior sagittal sinus thrombosis. T1-weighted sagittal MRI demonstrates acute superior sagittal sinus thrombosis (arrows).*

Straight Sinus

The straight sinus lies in the junction of the falx cerebri and tentorium cerebelli (see Figs. 4.2, 4.4). It runs posteroinferiorly as a continuation of the inferior sagittal sinus into the transverse sinus. It is not continuous (or only tenuously so) with the superior sagittal sinus. Its tributaries include the great cerebral vein (see Figs. 4.2, 6.16) and some superior cerebellar veins. Internally, the straight sinus is triangular in cross-section.

Transverse Sinus

The transverse sinuses begin at the internal occipital protuberance (see Figs. 4.4, 4.5). One of them, usually the right, is directly continuous with the superior sagittal sinus; the other is continuous with the straight sinus. On both sides the sinuses run in the attached margin of the tentorium cerebelli, first on the squama of the occipital bone, then on the mastoid angle of the parietal bone. Each follows a gentle anterolateral curve, increasing in size as it does so, to the posterolateral part of the petrous temporal bone. There it turns down as a sigmoid sinus, which ultimately becomes continuous with the internal jugular vein. Transverse sinuses are triangular in section and usually unequal in size; the one draining the superior sagittal sinus is larger. They receive the inferior cerebral, inferior cerebellar, diploic and inferior anastomotic veins and are joined by the superior petrosal sinuses, where they continue as sigmoid sinuses.

Petrosquamous Sinus

The petrosquamous sinus runs back in a groove (which sometimes becomes a canal posteriorly) along the junction of the squamous and petrous parts of the temporal bone, and it opens behind into the transverse sinus. Anteriorly, it connects with the retromandibular vein through a postglenoid or squamous foramen. The sinus may be absent, or it may drain entirely into the retromandibular vein.

Sigmoid Sinus

The sigmoid sinuses are continuations of the transverse sinuses, beginning where these leave the tentorium cerebelli (Figs. 4.5, 4.10). Each sigmoid sinus curves inferomedially in a groove on the mastoid process of the temporal bone, crosses the jugular process of the occipital bone and turns forward to the superior jugular bulb, lying posterior in the jugular foramen. Anteriorly, a thin plate of bone separates its upper part from the mastoid antrum and air cells. It connects with pericranial veins via mastoid and condylar emissary veins.

Occipital Sinus

The occipital sinus is the smallest of the sinuses. It lies in the attached margin of the falx cerebelli (see Fig. 4.5) and is occasionally paired. It commences near the foramen magnum in several small channels, one joining the end of the

sigmoid sinus, and connects with the internal vertebral plexuses. It ends in the confluence of the sinuses.

Cavernous Sinus

The cavernous sinus is a large venous plexus that lies on both sides of the body of the sphenoid bone (see Figs. 4.5–4.7). The sinus extends from the superior orbital fissure to the apex of the petrous temporal bone, with an average length of 2 cm and a width of 1 cm. The sphenoidal air sinus and pituitary gland are medial to the cavernous sinus. The trigeminal cave is near the inferoposterior part of its lateral wall and extends posteriorly beyond it to enclose the trigeminal ganglion. The uncus of the temporal lobe is also lateral to the sinus.

The internal carotid artery, and its associated sympathetic plexus, passes forward through the sinus together with the abducens nerve, which lies lateral to the artery. The oculomotor and trochlear nerves and the ophthalmic and maxillary divisions of the trigeminal nerve all lie in the lateral wall of the sinus (see Fig. 4.7). Their diameters are such that they project into the lumen and are usually covered medially by little more than endothelium. Propulsion of blood in the cavernous sinus is partly due to pulsation of the internal carotid artery, but it is also influenced by gravity and hence by the position of the head.

Tributaries of the cavernous sinus are the superior ophthalmic vein, a branch from the inferior ophthalmic vein (or sometimes the whole vessel), the superficial middle cerebral vein, inferior cerebral veins and sphenoparietal sinus. The central retinal vein and frontal tributary of the middle meningeal vein sometimes drain into it. The sinus drains to the transverse sinus via the superior petrosal sinus; to the internal jugular vein via the inferior petrosal sinus and a plexus of veins on the internal carotid artery; to the pterygoid plexus by veins traversing the emissary sphenoidal foramen, foramen ovale and foramen lacerum; and to the facial vein via the superior ophthalmic vein.

Carotid cavernous fistula and cavernous sinus thrombosis — The unique location of the internal carotid artery within a venous structure occasionally gives rise to direct communication between the two structures by means of a carotid cavernous fistula (CCF), which is established as a result of either severe head trauma or degenerative or aneurysmal vessel disease (see Chapter 6, Case 3). A CCF causes proptosis, which may be pulsatile, together with vascular dilatation in the tissues of the orbit and globe and combinations of third, fourth and sixth cranial nerve palsies. These changes can cause permanent blindness. CCFs are most commonly treated by passing a catheter up the carotid into the fistula and then occluding it with dilatable balloons or flexible metal coils. Any spreading infection involving the upper nasal cavities, paranasal sinuses, cheek (especially near the medial canthus), upper lip, anterior nares or even upper incisor or canine tooth may rarely lead to septic thrombosis of the cavernous sinuses as infected thrombi pass from the facial vein or pterygoid venous complex into the sinus (via either ophthalmic veins or emissary veins that enter the cranial cavity through the foramen ovale). This is a critical medical emergency with a high risk of disseminated cerebritis and cerebral venous thrombosis (see Case 2).

Intercavernous Sinus

The two cavernous sinuses are connected by anterior and posterior intercavernous sinuses (see Fig. 4.5) and the basilar plexus (see Fig. 4.6). The intercavernous sinuses lie in the anterior and posterior attached borders of the diaphragma sellae, thus forming a complete circular venous sinus (see Fig. 4.6). All connections are valveless, and the direction of flow is reversible. Small irregular sinuses inferior to the pituitary gland drain into the intercavernous sinuses. These inferior intercavernous sinuses are plexiform in nature and are important in a transnasal surgical approach to the pituitary.

Superior Petrosal Sinus

This small, narrow sinus drains the cavernous sinus into the transverse sinus on either side (see Figs. 4.4–4.6). It leaves the posterosuperior part of the cavernous sinus, runs posterolaterally in the attached margin of the tentorium cerebelli and crosses above the trigeminal nerve to lie in a groove on the superior border of the petrous part of the temporal bone. It ends by joining a transverse sinus where this curves down to become the sigmoid. It receives cerebellar, inferior cerebral and tympanic veins and connects with the inferior petrosal sinus and the basilar plexus.

Inferior Petrosal Sinus

The inferior petrosal sinus drains the cavernous sinus into the internal jugular vein (see Figs. 4.5, 6.16). It begins at the posteroinferior aspect of the cavernous sinus and runs back in a groove between the petrous temporal and basilar occipital bones. It traverses the anterior part of the jugular foramen and ends

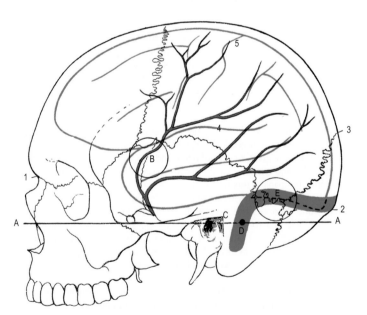

Fig. 4.10 *Relations of the brain, middle meningeal artery and transverse and sigmoid sinuses to the surface of the skull. 1, nasion; 2, inion; 3, lambda; 4, lateral cerebral sulcus; 5, central sulcus; A–A, Frankfurt plane, which traverses the lower margin of the orbital opening and the upper margin of the external acoustic meatus; B, area (including the pterion) for trephining over the frontal branch of the middle meningeal artery and the cerebral Sylvian point; C, suprameatal triangle; D, sigmoid sinus; E, area for trephining over the transverse sinus, exposing the dura mater of both the cerebrum and cerebellum. The outline of the cerebral hemisphere and its major sulci are indicated in blue; the course of the middle meningeal artery is in red. A mental image of this arrangement allows safe planning of craniotomies to avoid injuring major vessels; in trauma patients, it can be used to predict which vessels might be injured when there is an intracranial clot.*

in the superior jugular bulb. It receives labyrinthine veins via the cochlear canaliculus and the vestibular aqueduct and tributaries from the medulla oblongata, pons and inferior cerebellar surface. The sinus is often a plexus and sometimes drains by a vein in the hypoglossal canal to the suboccipital vertebral plexus.

There is a complex relationship among structures in the jugular foramen. The inferior petrosal sinus is anteromedial with a meningeal branch of the ascending pharyngeal artery, and it descends obliquely backward. The sigmoid sinus is situated at the lateral and posterior part of the foramen with a meningeal branch of the occipital artery. Between the sinuses are, in succession posterolaterally, the glossopharyngeal, vagus and accessory nerves.

Sphenoparietal Sinus

The sphenoparietal sinus is located below the periosteum of the lesser wing of the sphenoid bone, near its posterior edge (see Fig. 4.5). It curves medially to open into the anterior part of the cavernous sinus. It receives small veins from the adjacent dura mater and sometimes the frontal ramus of the middle meningeal vein. It may also receive connecting rami, in its middle course, from the superficial middle cerebral vein and veins from the temporal lobe and the anterior temporal diploic vein. When these connections are well developed, the sphenoparietal sinus is a large channel.

Basilar Sinus and Plexus

The basilar sinus and plexus consist of interconnecting channels between layers of dura mater on the clivus (see Fig. 4.6). The basilar venous plexus interconnects the inferior petrosal sinuses and joins with the internal vertebral venous plexus. It also usually connects with the cavernous and superior petrosal sinuses at its anterior end. When veins around the foramen magnum (so-called marginal sinuses) are large, they communicate anteriorly with the plexus, and this produces an almost complete circular venous channel around the foramen magnum, connecting the basilar plexus intracranially to the inferior petrosal, sigmoid and occipital sinuses and extracranially to variable vertebral plexuses in the suboccipital region.

Middle Meningeal Vein (Sinus)

Tributaries of the middle meningeal vein communicate with the superior sagittal sinus through its venous lacunae. Below, they converge and unite as frontal and parietal trunks, which accompany branches of the middle meningeal arteries in grooves on the internal parietal surfaces. The veins lie closer to the bone than the arteries do, and they may occupy separate grooves. This situation makes them particularly liable to tear in cranial fractures. Their termination is variable. The parietal trunk may traverse the foramen spinosum to the pterygoid venous plexus. The frontal trunk may also reach this plexus via the foramen ovale, or it may end in the sphenoparietal or cavernous sinus (see Fig. 4.5). The middle meningeal vein receives meningeal tributaries and small inferior cerebral veins, and it connects with the diploic and superficial middle cerebral veins. It frequently bears arachnoid granulations.

The diploic veins constitute a hypothetical fourth venous tier. However, because they drain into dural veins, they are grouped here with them, following Browder and Kaplan (1976). It should be noted that intracranial veins communicate at many points with extracranial vessels via emissary and other veins.

Emissary Veins

Emissary veins traverse cranial apertures and make connections between intracranial venous sinuses and extracranial veins. Some emissary veins are relatively constant; others are sometimes absent. These connections are of clinical significance in the spread of infection from extracranial foci to venous sinuses. The success of ligature of the internal jugular vein to limit the spread of some oral and pharyngeal pathologies depends on the adequacy of the collateral drainage. The following emissary veins are recognized: a mastoid emissary vein in the mastoid foramen, which unites the sigmoid sinus with the posterior auricular or occipital veins; a parietal emissary vein that traverses the parietal foramen to connect the superior sagittal sinus with the veins of the scalp; the venous plexus of the hypoglossal canal, which is occasionally a single vein and runs between the sigmoid sinus and the internal jugular vein; a (posterior) condylar emissary vein that runs between the sigmoid sinus and veins in the suboccipital triangle via the (posterior) condylar canal; a plexus of emissary veins (venous plexus of the foramen ovale) that links the cavernous sinus to the pterygoid plexus via the foramen ovale; two or three small veins that traverse the foramen lacerum and run between the cavernous sinus and the pharyngeal veins and pterygoid plexus; a vein in the emissary sphenoidal foramen (of Vesalius) that connects the cavernous sinus with the pharyngeal veins and pterygoid plexus; the internal carotid venous plexus, which passes through the carotid canal and connects the cavernous sinus to the

internal jugular vein; and the petrosquamous sinus, which connects the transverse sinus with the external jugular vein. A vein may traverse the foramen caecum (which is patent in approximately 1% of adult skulls) and connect nasal veins with the superior sagittal sinus. An occipital emissary vein usually connects the confluence of sinuses with the occipital vein through the occipital protuberance and also receives the occipital diploic vein. The occipital sinus connects with variably developed veins around the foramen magnum (so-called marginal sinuses) and thus with the vertebral venous plexuses. This is an alternative venous drainage when the jugular vein is blocked or tied. The ophthalmic veins are potentially emissary, because they connect intracranial to extracranial veins. However, parietal emissary veins, included here, are usually minute and do not appear to connect with veins of the scalp in corrosion casts.

Arterial Supply and Venous Drainage of the Cranial Dura Mater

The arterial supply of the dura mater is derived from numerous vessels. In the anterior cranial fossa, the dura is supplied by the anterior meningeal branches of the anterior and posterior ethmoidal and internal carotid arteries and a branch of the middle meningeal artery. In the middle cranial fossa, it is supplied by the middle and accessory meningeal branches of the maxillary artery, a branch of the ascending pharyngeal artery (entering via the foramen lacerum), branches of the internal carotid artery and a recurrent branch of the lacrimal artery. Dura mater in the posterior fossa is supplied by the meningeal branches of the occipital artery (one enters the skull by the jugular foramen and another by the mastoid foramen), the posterior meningeal branches of the vertebral artery and occasional small branches of the ascending pharyngeal artery, which enter by the jugular foramen and hypoglossal canal. The cranial meningeal arteries are chiefly distributed to bone. In contrast to the arterial supply of the spinal dura mater, only very fine arterial branches are distributed to the cranial dura mater per se. The smaller branches of the meningeal vessels are, therefore, mainly in the endosteal layer of dura.

The middle meningeal is the largest of the meningeal arteries. It passes between the roots of the auriculotemporal nerve and may lie lateral to the tensor veli palatini before entering the cranial cavity through the foramen spinosum. It then runs in an anterolateral groove on the squamous part of the temporal bone, dividing into frontal and parietal branches. The larger frontal (anterior) branch crosses the greater wing of the sphenoid, reaches a groove or canal in the sphenoidal angle of the parietal bone and divides into branches between the dura mater and cranium, with some ascending to the vertex and others to the occipital region. One ascending branch grooves the parietal bone approximately 15 mm behind the coronal suture, corresponding approximately to the precentral sulcus (see Fig. 4.10). The parietal (posterior) branch curves back on the squamous temporal bone, reaching the lower border of the parietal bone anterior to its mastoid angle and dividing to supply the posterior parts of the dura mater and cranium. These branches anastomose with their fellows and with the anterior and posterior meningeal arteries.

In the cranial cavity the artery has several branches. Numerous ganglionic branches supply the trigeminal ganglion and roots. A petrosal branch enters the hiatus for the greater petrosal nerve and supplies the facial nerve, geniculate ganglion and tympanic cavity, anastomosing with the stylomastoid artery. A superior tympanic artery runs in the canal for the tensor tympani, supplying both the muscle and the mucosa lining the canal.

Temporal branches traverse minute foramina in the greater wing of the sphenoid and anastomose with deep temporal arteries. An anastomotic branch enters the orbit laterally in the superior orbital fissure and anastomoses with a recurrent branch of the lacrimal artery. Enlargement of this anastomosis explains the occasional origin of the lacrimal from the middle meningeal artery.

Apart from these branches and a supply to the dura mater, the middle meningeal artery is predominantly periosteal and supplies bone and red bone marrow.

The accessory meningeal artery may arise from the maxillary or the middle meningeal artery. It enters the cranial cavity through the foramen ovale and supplies the trigeminal ganglion, dura mater and bone. However, its main distribution is extracranial, principally to the medial pterygoid, lateral pterygoid (upper head), tensor veli palatini, greater wing and pterygoid processes of the sphenoid bone, mandibular nerve and otic ganglion. It is sometimes replaced by separate small arteries.

Meningeal veins begin from plexiform vessels in the dura mater and drain into efferent vessels in the outer dural layer. The latter connect with the lacunae of the superior sagittal sinus and with other cranial sinuses, including those accompanying the middle meningeal arteries, and with diploic veins.

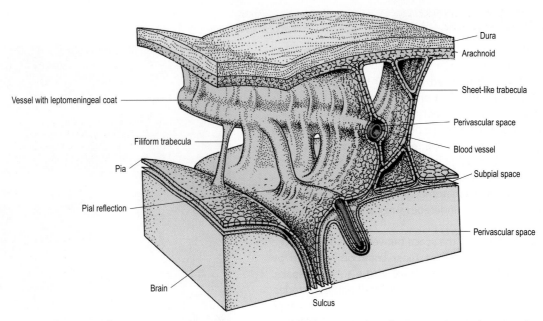

Fig. 4.11 *Relationships of the pia and arachnoid mater to the dura, brain and vessels. (Modified from Alcolado et al, 1988, according to Zhang, E.T., Inman, C.B.E., Weller, R.O. 1990. Interrelationships of the pia mater and the perivascular (Virchow–Robin) spaces in the human cerebrum. J. Anat. 170, 111–123, by permission from Blackwell Science.)*

Innervation of the Cranial Dura Mater

The innervation of the cranial dura mater is derived mainly from the three divisions of the trigeminal nerve, the first three cervical spinal nerves and the cervical sympathetic trunk. Less well-established meningeal branches have been described arising from the vagus and hypoglossal nerves and possibly from the facial and glossopharyngeal nerves.

In the anterior cranial fossa, the dura is innervated by meningeal branches of the anterior and posterior ethmoidal nerves and anterior filaments of the meningeal rami of the maxillary (nervus meningeus medius) and mandibular (nervus spinosus) trigeminal divisions. Nervi meningeus medius and spinosus are, however, largely distributed to the dura of the middle cranial fossa, which also receives filaments from the trigeminal ganglion. The nervus spinosus reenters the cranium through the foramen spinosum with the middle meningeal artery and divides into anterior and posterior branches, which accompany the main divisions of the artery and supply the dura mater in the middle cranial fossa and, to a lesser extent, the anterior fossa and calvaria. The anterior branch communicates with the meningeal branch of the maxillary nerve; the posterior branch also supplies the mucous lining of the mastoid air cells. The nervus spinosus contains sympathetic postganglionic fibres from the middle meningeal plexus. A recurrent tentorial nerve (a branch of the ophthalmic division of the trigeminal) supplies the tentorium cerebelli. The dura in the posterior cranial fossa is innervated by ascending meningeal branches of the upper cervical nerves, which enter through the anterior part of the foramen magnum (second and third cervical nerves) and through the hypoglossal canal and jugular foramen (first and second cervical nerves). Meningeal branches of both the vagus and hypoglossal nerves have been described. Those from the vagus apparently start from the superior vagal ganglion and are distributed to the dura mater in the posterior cranial fossa. Those from the hypoglossal leave the nerve in its canal to supply the diploë of the occipital bone, the dural walls of the occipital and inferior petrosal sinuses and much of the floor and anterior wall of the posterior cranial fossa. These meningeal rami may not contain vagal or hypoglossal fibres but ascending, mixed sensory and sympathetic fibres from the upper cervical nerves and superior cervical sympathetic ganglion. All meningeal nerves contain a postganglionic sympathetic component, either from the superior cervical sympathetic ganglion or by communication with its perivascular intracranial extensions.

The brain itself, the arachnoid mater and the pia mater do not contain sensory nerve endings. These are restricted to the dura mater and cerebral blood vessels. Stimulation of such nerve endings causes pain. The role of the autonomic nerve supply of the cranial dura mater is uncertain.

ARACHNOID MATER

The arachnoid mater and the pia mater together are referred to as the leptomeninges. They share many similarities, including their cellular structure. The arachnoid and pia are composed of the same basic cell type embedded in bundles of collagen. The cells share a common embryological origin from mesenchyme surrounding the developing nervous system. They are flattened or cuboidal and have oval nuclei, usually with a single small but prominent nucleolus. Joined together by desmosomes, gap junctions and, in the outer layer of the arachnoid, tight junctions, these cells are not surrounded by basement membrane, except where they are in contact with collagen in the inner layers of the arachnoid and on the deep aspects of the pia mater.

The outer layer of the arachnoid, the dura–arachnoid interface, is formed from five or six layers of cells joined by numerous desmosomes and tight junctions. This layer forms a barrier that normally prevents the permeation of CSF through the arachnoid into the subdural space. The central portion of the arachnoid is closely apposed to the outer layer and is formed from tightly packed polygonal cells, which are joined by desmosomes and gap junctions. The cells are more loosely packed in the inner layer of the arachnoid, where they intermingle with bundles of collagen continuous with the trabeculae that cross the subarachnoid space.

The arachnoid and pia are separated by the subarachnoid space and joined by trabeculae (Fig. 4.11). The anatomical relationships of the arachnoid and pia differ to some extent in the cerebral and spinal regions.

The cerebral part of the arachnoid mater invests the brain loosely but does not enter the sulci or fissures, except for the great longitudinal fissure between the cerebral hemispheres. The arachnoid also coats the superior surface of the pituitary fossa. In young individuals the arachnoid on the upper surface of the brain is transparent, but in older people it may become white and opaque, particularly near the midline. The arachnoid is thicker on the basal aspect of the brain and is also slightly opaque where it extends between the temporal lobes and the front of the pons, producing a large space between arachnoid and pia mater that is one of the subarachnoid cisterns. The arachnoid is easily separated from the dura over the surface of the brain. However, at sites where the internal carotid and vertebral arteries enter the subarachnoid space, the arachnoid mater is adherent to the adventitia of the vessels. It is then reflected onto the surface of blood vessels in the subarachnoid space and is eventually continuous with the pia mater.

Separation of the arachnoid and dura mater is easily achieved and requires little physical force. Damage to small bridging veins in the space can give rise to a subdural haematoma following even relatively mild head trauma. The characteristics of a subdural haematoma differ from those of the epidural haematoma described earlier. Clinically, the accumulation is often of relatively low pressure and seldom presents as a medical emergency. In many cases there is some predisposing factor, such as cerebral atrophy or increased size of the underlying subarachnoid space, and even sizable accumulations may be tolerated on a chronic basis with mild or no symptoms. The distinction between subdural and extradural haematomas on a neuroimaging scan relies on the anatomical features of the space. Extradural collections tend to be lentiform in shape due to the pressure required to separate the dura and periosteum. They pass deep to any major dural sinuses and cannot extend along the falx cerebri or tentorium cerebelli. Subdural haematomas tend to be biconcave in shape and more extensive, often following the line of the dura along the falx or tentorium and always lying superficial to the deep venous sinuses.

CASE 3   SUBDURAL HAEMATOMA

A 62-year-old woman with chronic renal disease who is on Coumadin for atrial fibrillation stumbles and falls on the sidewalk. She does not hit her head, and other than being bruised, she is not injured. In the ED, a precautionary head CT scan is obtained, which is normal except for age-appropriate cerebral atrophy. Several days later, while bending over, she develops a severe right-sided headache. She returns to the ED, where she is noted to have left facial palsy and mild left-sided weakness. The head CT scan is repeated, this time showing a large subacute right subdural haematoma (SDH). After the effect of Coumadin is reversed, she undergoes surgical evacuation of the haematoma.

Discussion: SDHs arise in the space between the dura and the arachnoid membranes. They are most commonly caused by tearing of the bridging veins that traverse the subdural space. SDH can also be caused by bleeding from small cortical arteries. Symptoms may include headache, nausea, vomiting, lethargy, confusion, aphasia, hemiparesis and seizures. An SDH may present acutely or in a subacute or chronic fashion. Chronic SDH may cause insidious cognitive impairment.

There is a history of antecedent head trauma in most cases of SDH, but they may also arise spontaneously. Falls or "whiplash" injuries without overt head injury can tear bridging veins, leading to SDH. Predisposing factors include cerebral atrophy, as occurs with age or alcohol abuse, and coagulopathy from medications (Coumadin, antiplatelet agents) or medical illness (renal failure, haematological conditions).

SDH can be seen on head CT or MRI; the latter is more sensitive for small SDHs (Fig. 4.12). The accumulated subdural blood typically has a crescent shape, as it can flow freely in the subdural space. Larger SDHs, or those causing neurological dysfunction, require surgical drainage; smaller, asymptomatic SDHs can sometimes be followed expectantly.

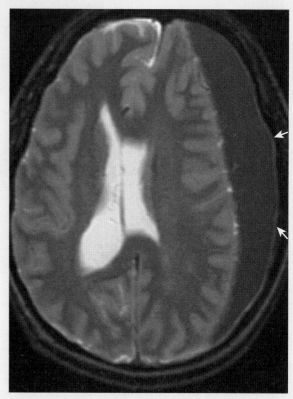

Fig. 4.12 *Chronic subdural haematoma. (arrows). A large haematoma causing mass effect with ventricular shift to the opposite side visualized with MRI.*

Subarachnoid Space

The subarachnoid space lies between the arachnoid and the pia mater. It contains CSF and the larger arteries and veins that traverse the surface of the brain. Arachnoid and pia mater are in close apposition over the convexities of the brain, such as the cortical gyri, whereas concavities are followed by the pia but spanned by the arachnoid. This arrangement produces a subarachnoid space of greatly variable depth that is location dependent. The more expansive spaces are identified as subarachnoid cisterns (Fig. 4.13). Cisterns are continuous with each other through the general subarachnoid space, of which there are dilatations.

The largest cistern, the cisterna magna or cerebellomedullary cistern, is formed where the arachnoid bridges the interval between the medulla oblongata and the inferior surface of the cerebellum. The cistern is continuous above with the lumen of the fourth ventricle through its median aperture—the foramen of Magendie—and below with the subarachnoid space of the spinal cord. The pontine cistern is an extensive space ventral to the pons, continuous below with the spinal subarachnoid space, behind with the cisterna magna and, rostral to the pons, with the interpeduncular cistern. The basilar artery runs through the pontine cistern into the interpeduncular cistern. As the arachnoid mater spans between the two temporal lobes, it is separated from the cerebral peduncles and structures within the interpeduncular fossa by the interpeduncular cistern, which contains the circulus arteriosus (circle of Willis). Anteriorly, the interpeduncular cistern extends to the optic chiasma. The cistern of the lateral fossa is formed by the arachnoid as it bridges the lateral sulcus between the frontal, parietal and temporal opercula, and it contains the middle cerebral artery. The cistern of the great cerebral vein (cisterna ambiens or superior cistern) lies posterior

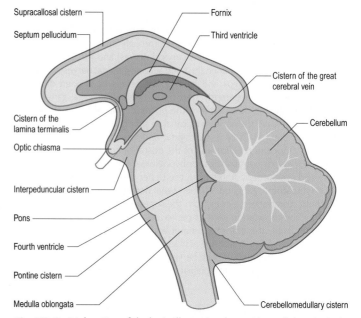

Fig. 4.13 *Sagittal section of the brain illustrating the positions of the principal subarachnoid cisterns. The ventricular system and subarachnoid space are blue.*

to the brain stem and third ventricle and occupies the interval between the splenium of the corpus callosum and the superior cerebellar surface. The great cerebral vein traverses this cistern, and the pineal gland protrudes into it.

Several smaller cisterns have been described, including the prechiasmatic and postchiasmatic cisterns related to the optic chiasma, the cistern of the lamina terminalis and the supracallosal cistern, all of which are extensions of the interpeduncular cistern and contain the anterior cerebral arteries. The subarachnoid space also extends along the optic nerves to the back of the globe, where the dura fuses with the sclera of the eye. There is a connection between the subarachnoid space and the inner ear through the cochlear duct.

The cerebral subarachnoid space is connected with the fourth ventricle of the brain by three openings, through which CSF flows. The median aperture, or foramen of Magendie, lies in the median plane in the inferior part of the roof of the fourth ventricle and provides communication with the cisterna magna. The paired lateral apertures, or foramina of Luschka, are located at the ends of the lateral recesses of the fourth ventricle and open into the subarachnoid space at the cerebellopontine angle, behind the upper roots of the glossopharyngeal nerves (see Fig. 5.10). Occlusion of these foramina in cases of chronic meningitis, such as tuberculous meningitis, may lead to interruption of CSF outflow from the ventricular system, resulting in hydrocephalus.

Trabeculae, in the form of sheets or fine filiform structures, traverse the subarachnoid space from the deep layers of the arachnoid mater to the pia mater and are also attached to large blood vessels within the subarachnoid space (Figs. 4.11, 4.14). Each trabecula has a core of collagen and is coated by leptomeningeal cells. Subarachnoid trabeculae are long and filamentous and cross the subarachnoid cisterns. The topography of trabeculae that cross the subarachnoid space may, in effect, form compartments, particularly in the perivascular regions, enabling directional flow of CSF through the subarachnoid space.

Arteries and veins in the subarachnoid space are coated by a thin layer of leptomeninges, often only one cell thick. The pia mater, the blood vessels and the arachnoid mater are connected by collagenous trabeculae and sheets, which are also coated by leptomeningeal cells (see Fig. 4.11). Cranial and spinal nerves that traverse the subarachnoid space to pass out of cranial or intervertebral foramina are coated by a thin layer of leptomeninges, which fuses with the arachnoid at the exit foramina.

Arachnoid Villi and Granulations

Arachnoid villi and the larger arachnoid granulations represent extensions of the arachnoid mater and subarachnoid space through the wall of the dural venous sinuses. As such, they present an exchange surface to the sinus endothelium (Fig. 4.16), which constitutes the major pathway for the passage of CSF from the subarachnoid space into the blood. They are, therefore, an essential step in the normal circulation and reabsorption of CSF.

These structures are most prominent along the margins of the great longitudinal fissure, where they project into the superior sagittal sinus (see Fig. 4.8). Arachnoid villi are also found in association with other cerebral venous sinuses, such as the transverse sinus. Microscopic villi are present in the superior sagittal sinus of the fetus and newborn infant. These hypertrophy to form granulations that are visible by age 18 months in the parieto-occipital region of the superior sagittal sinus and by 3 years in the laterally located sinuses of the posterior fossa. The arachnoid granulations become more lobulated and complex with increasing age. They may become calcified, when they are known as Pacchionian bodies.

At the base of each arachnoid granulation, a thin neck of arachnoid mater projects through an aperture in the dural lining of the venous sinus and expands to form a core of collagenous trabeculae and interwoven channels (Fig. 4.17). The core is surmounted by an apical cap of arachnoid cells, some 150 µm thick. Channels extend through the cap to reach the subendothelial regions of the granulation. The cap region of each granulation is attached to the endothelium of the sinus over an area some 300 µm in diameter, whereas the rest of the granulation core is separated from the endothelium by a fibrous dural cupola.

PIA MATER

The pia mater is a delicate membrane that closely invests the surface of the brain, from which it is separated by a microscopic subpial space (see Fig. 4.11). It follows the contours of the brain into concavities and into the depths of fissures and sulci. During development, it becomes apposed to the ependyma in the roof of the telencephalon and fourth ventricle to form the stroma of the choroid plexus.

The pia mater shares a common embryological origin and structural similarity with the arachnoid mater. Their common features were previously described under arachnoid mater.

Pia mater is formed from a layer of leptomeningeal cells that is often only one to two cells thick. The cells are joined by desmosomes and gap junctions but few if any tight junctions, and they are continuous with the coating of the subarachnoid trabeculae. They are separated from the basal lamina of the glia limitans by collagen bundles, fibroblast-like cells and arteries and veins lying in the subpial space (see Fig. 4.14).

Despite its delicate and thin nature, the pia mater appears to form a regulatory interface between the subarachnoid space and the brain. In addition to separating the subarachnoid space from the subpial and perivascular spaces,

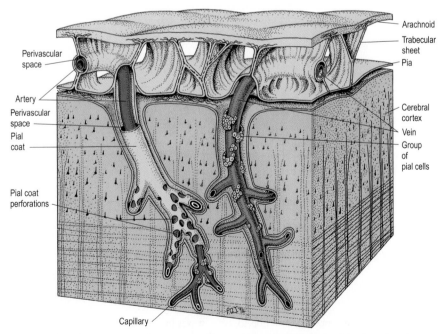

Fig. 4.14 *Interrelationships between leptomeninges and blood vessels entering and leaving the cerebral cortex. The subarachnoid space is divided by trabeculae, and as the artery enters the cortex, a layer of pia mater accompanies the vessel into the brain. With decreasing size of the vessel, the pial coating becomes perforated and finally disappears at the capillary level. The perivascular space between the artery and the pia mater inside the brain is continuous with the perivascular space around the meningeal vessel. Veins do not have a similar coating of pia mater. (Reproduced and modified from Zhang, E.T., Inman, C.B.E., Weller, R.O. 1990. Interrelationships of the pia mater and the perivascular (Virchow–Robin) spaces in the human cerebrum. J. Anat. 170, 111–123, by permission from Blackwell Science.)*

CASE 4   MENINGITIS

A 35-year-old man develops headache, confusion, neck pain and fever. On examination he is sleepy but can be aroused, has poor attention and gets agitated when asked questions. He can follow simple commands intermittently. He is unable to flex or extend his neck because this causes severe pain radiating down his back. He has a diffuse macular rash involving the entire body, including the palms of his hands. A lumbar puncture is performed showing an elevated CSF protein level and white blood cell count (lymphocytic pleocytosis). CSF analysis demonstrates antibodies to *Rickettsia rickettsii,* the agent causing Rocky Mountain spotted fever.

Discussion: This patient has the classic signs of meningitis—fever, altered mental status and a stiff neck. Inflammation of the meninges may be caused by a variety of agents, including infectious (viral, bacterial, fungal) or non-infectious (medications, vasculitis, subarachnoid haemorrhage). Diagnosis of meningitis is by spinal fluid analysis and culture; when CSF cultures are negative, the disease is called aseptic meningitis. Treatment of meningitis is directed by the underlying cause. See Figure 4.15.

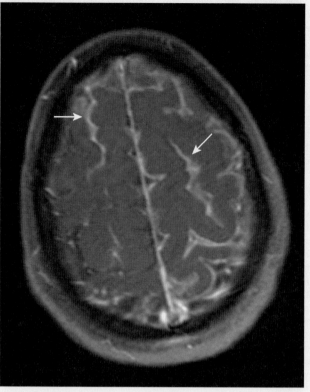

Fig. 4.15 *MRI showing leptomeningeal enhancement* (arrows) *in a case of purulent meningitis.*

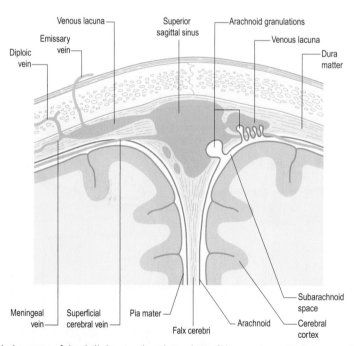

Fig. 4.16 *Coronal section through the vertex of the skull showing the relationships of the superior sagittal sinus, meninges and arachnoid granulations.*

cells of the pia mater exhibit pinocytotic activity and ingest particles up to 1 μm in diameter. They contain enzymes such as catechol-O-methyltransferase and glutamine synthetase, which degrade neurotransmitters. Further evidence of the pia's effectiveness as a barrier is seen in subarachnoid haemorrhages and in subpial haemorrhages in infants—in neither of these situations do red blood cells penetrate the pia mater.

It was long thought that the subarachnoid space connected directly with the perivascular spaces (Virchow–Robin spaces) surrounding blood vessels in the brain. However, it is now recognized that the pia mater is reflected from the surface of the brain onto the surface of blood vessels in the subarachnoid space. Thus, the subarachnoid space is separated by a layer of pia from the subpial and perivascular spaces of the brain (see Figs. 4.11, 4.14).

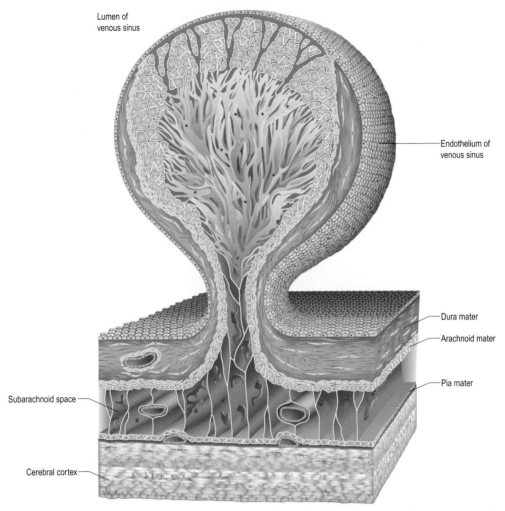

Lumen of
venous sinus

Endothelium of
venous sinus

Dura mater

Arachnoid mater

Pia mater

Subarachnoid space

Cerebral cortex

Fig. 4.17 *Arachnoid granulation. The subarachnoid space between the arachnoid and pia mater is highly trabeculated and is continuous with the channel in the centre of the granulation. Narrow channels traverse the cap region of the granulation to come into contact with the endothelium of the venous sinus. The fluid finally drains through the endothelium. (Modified by permission from Kida, S., Weller, R.O. 1994. Morphology of CSF drainage pathways in man. In: Raimondi, A. (Ed.), Principles of Pediatric Neurosurgery, vol 4. Springer-Verlag, Berlin.)*

References

Browder, J., Kaplan, H.A., 1976. Cerebral Dural Sinuses and Their Tributaries. Springfield, Illinois, Thomas. *Describes variations in the superior sagittal and other venous sinuses.*

Kida, S., Weller, R.O., 1994. Morphology of CSF drainage pathways in man. In: Raimondi, A. (Ed), Principles of Pediatric Neurosurgery, vol 4. Springer, Berlin. *Describes the morphology and relationships of the subarachnoid space, including the structure of arachnoid granulations.*

Klintworth, G.K., 1967. The ontogeny and growth of the human tentorium cerebelli. Anat. Rec. 158, 433–442.

Zhang, E.T., Inman, C.B.E., Weller, R.O., 1990. Interrelationships of the pia mater and the perivascular (Virchow–Robin) spaces in the human cerebrum. J. Anat. 170, 111–123.

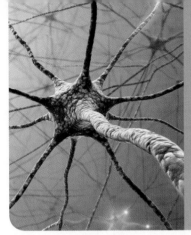

Ventricular System and Cerebrospinal Fluid

The cerebral ventricular system consists of a series of interconnecting spaces and channels within the brain that are derived from the central lumen of the embryonic neural tube and the cerebral vesicles to which it gives rise (Ch. 3). Within each cerebral hemisphere lies a large C-shaped lateral ventricle (Figs. 5.1, 5.2). Near its rostral end the lateral ventricle communicates through the interventricular foramen (foramen of Monro) with the third ventricle, which is a midline, slit-like cavity lying between the right and left halves of the thalamus and hypothalamus. Caudally, the third ventricle is continuous with the cerebral aqueduct, a narrow tube that passes the length of the midbrain; this, in turn, is continuous with the fourth ventricle, a wide, tent-shaped cavity lying between the brain stem and cerebellum. Caudally, the fourth ventricle is continuous with the vestigial central canal of the spinal cord.

The ventricular system contains cerebrospinal fluid (CSF), which is secreted mostly by the choroid plexuses located within the lateral, third and fourth ventricles. CSF flows from the lateral to the third ventricle, through the cerebral aqueduct and into the fourth ventricle. It leaves the fourth ventricle through three apertures to reach the subarachnoid space surrounding the brain.

TOPOGRAPHY AND RELATIONS OF THE VENTRICULAR SYSTEM

Lateral Ventricle

Viewed from its lateral aspect, the lateral ventricle has a roughly C-shaped profile, with an occipital tail (see Fig. 5.1). The shape is a consequence of the developmental expansion of the frontal, parietal and occipital regions of the hemisphere (Ch. 3), which displaces the temporal lobe inferiorly and anteriorly. Both the caudate nucleus and the fornix, which lie in the wall of the ventricle, have adopted a similar morphology, so the tail of the caudate nucleus encircles the thalamus in a C shape, and the fornix traces the outline of the ventricle forward to the interventricular foramen.

The lateral ventricle is customarily divided into a body and anterior, posterior and inferior horns (Figs. 5.1, 5.3). The anterior (frontal) horn lies within the frontal lobe. It is bounded anteriorly by the posterior aspect of the genu and rostrum of the corpus callosum, and its roof is formed by the anterior part of the body of the corpus callosum. The anterior horns of the two ventricles are separated by the septum pellucidum. The coronal profile of the anterior horn is roughly that of a flattened triangle in which the rounded head of the caudate nucleus forms the lateral wall and floor (Fig. 5.4). The anterior horn extends back as far as the interventricular foramen.

The body lies within the frontal and parietal lobes and extends from the interventricular foramen to the splenium of the corpus callosum. The bodies of the lateral ventricles are separated by the septum pellucidum, which contains the columns of the fornices in its lower edge. The coronal profile of the body of the ventricle is a flattened triangle with an inward-bulging lateral wall, formed by the thalamus inferiorly and the tail of the caudate nucleus superiorly. The boundary between the thalamus and caudate nucleus is marked by a groove (see Fig. 5.3), which is occupied by a fascicle of nerve fibres, the stria terminalis, and the thalamostriate vein. The inferior limit of the body of the ventricle and its medial wall are formed by the body of the fornix. The fornix is separated from the thalamus by the choroid fissure. The choroid plexus occludes the choroid fissure and covers part of the thalamus and fornix. The body of the lateral ventricle widens posteriorly to become continuous with the posterior and inferior horns at the collateral trigone or atrium.

The posterior (occipital) horn curves posteromedially into the occipital lobe. It is usually diamond shaped or square in outline, and the two sides are often asymmetric. Fibres of the tapetum of the corpus callosum separate the ventricle from the optic radiation and form the roof and lateral wall of the posterior horn. Fibres of the splenium of the corpus callosum (forceps major) pass medially as they sweep back into the occipital lobe and produce a rounded elevation in the upper medial wall of the posterior horn. Lower

down, a second elevation, the calcar avis, corresponds to the deeply infolded cortex of the anterior part of the calcarine sulcus.

The inferior (temporal) horn is the largest compartment of the lateral ventricle and extends forward into the temporal lobe. It curves around the posterior aspect of the thalamus (pulvinar); at first it passes downward and posterolaterally, and then it curves anteriorly to end within 2.5 cm of the temporal pole, near the uncus. Its position relative to the surface of the hemisphere usually corresponds to the superior temporal sulcus. The roof of the inferior horn is formed mainly by the tapetum of the corpus callosum, but also by the tail of the caudate nucleus and the stria terminalis, which extend forward in the roof to terminate in the amygdala at the anterior end of the ventricle.

The floor of the ventricle consists of the hippocampus medially and the collateral eminence, formed by the infolding of the collateral sulcus, laterally. The inferior part of the choroid fissure lies between the fimbria (a distinct bundle of efferent fibres that leaves the hippocampus) and the stria terminalis in the roof of the temporal horn (Fig. 5.5). The temporal extension of the choroid plexus fills this fissure and covers the outer surface of the hippocampus.

Third Ventricle

The third ventricle is a midline, slit-like cavity derived from the primitive forebrain vesicle (Figs. 5.1, 5.2, 5.6–5.8). The upper part of the lateral wall of the ventricle is formed by the medial surface of the anterior two-thirds of the thalamus, and the lower part is formed by the hypothalamus anteriorly and the subthalamus posteriorly. An indistinct hypothalamic sulcus extends horizontally on the ventricular wall between the interventricular foramen and the cerebral aqueduct, marking the boundary between the thalamus and hypothalamus. Dorsally, the lateral wall is limited by a ridge covering the stria medullaris thalami. The lateral walls of the third ventricle are joined by an interthalamic adhesion, or massa intermedia, a band of grey matter that extends from one thalamus to the other.

Anteriorly, the third ventricle extends to the lamina terminalis (see Fig. 5.8). This thin structure stretches from the optic chiasma to the rostrum of the corpus callosum and represents the rostral boundary of the embryonic neural tube. The lamina terminalis forms the roof of the small virtual cavity lying immediately below the ventricle, called the cistern of the lamina terminalis. This is important because it contains the anterior communicating artery, and aneurysm formation at this site may cause intraventricular haemorrhage through the thin membrane of the lamina terminalis. Above this, the anterior wall is formed by the diverging columns of the fornices and the transversely oriented anterior commissure, which crosses the midline. The anterior and posterior commissures are important neuroradiological landmarks. Before the introduction of modern imaging techniques, the anterior and posterior commissures could be identified by ventriculography. This led to their use as markers of the baseline for stereotactic surgical procedures. This convention is now universal, and the positions of the anterior and posterior commissures are the basic reference points for most surgical atlases of brain anatomy. The narrow interventricular foramen is located immediately posterior to the column of the fornix and separates the fornix from the anterior nucleus of the thalamus.

There is a small, angular, optic recess at the base of the lamina terminalis, just dorsal to and extending into the optic chiasma. Behind it, the anterior part of the floor of the third ventricle is formed mainly by hypothalamic structures. Immediately behind the optic chiasma lies the thin infundibular recess, which extends into the pituitary stalk. Behind this recess, the tuber cinereum and the mammillary bodies form the floor of the ventricle.

The roof of the third ventricle is a thin ependymal layer that extends from its lateral walls to the choroid plexus, which spans the choroid fissure (see Fig. 5.6). Above this is the body of the fornix. The posterior boundary of the ventricle is marked by a suprapineal recess above the pineal gland, by a pineal (epiphyseal) recess that extends into the pineal stalk and by the posterior

A

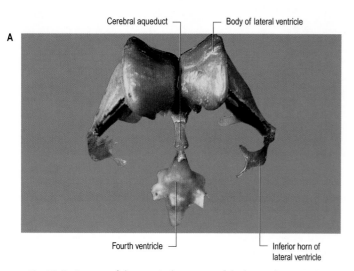

Cerebral aqueduct — | — Body of lateral ventricle

Fourth ventricle — | — Inferior horn of lateral ventricle

B

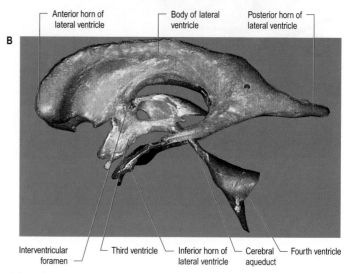

Anterior horn of lateral ventricle — | — Body of lateral ventricle | — Posterior horn of lateral ventricle

Interventricular foramen — | — Third ventricle — | — Inferior horn of lateral ventricle — | — Cerebral aqueduct — | — Fourth ventricle

Fig. 5.1 *Resin casts of the ventricular system of the human brain.* **A,** *Anterior view.* **B,** *Left lateral view.* (*Prepared by D. H. Tompsett, Royal College of Surgeons of England.*)

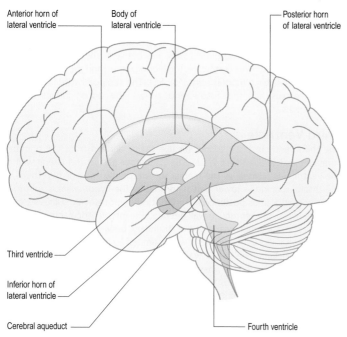

Anterior horn of lateral ventricle — | — Body of lateral ventricle — | — Posterior horn of lateral ventricle

Third ventricle —

Inferior horn of lateral ventricle —

Cerebral aqueduct — | — Fourth ventricle

Fig. 5.2 *Projection of the ventricles onto the left surface of the brain.*

commissure. Below the commissure, the ventricle is continuous with the cerebral aqueduct of the midbrain.

Cerebral Aqueduct

The cerebral aqueduct is a small tube, roughly circular in transverse section and approximately 2 mm in diameter. It extends throughout the dorsal quarter of the midbrain in the midline and is surrounded by the central, periaqueductal grey matter (see Fig. 5.8). Rostrally, it commences immediately behind and below the posterior commissure, where it is continuous with the caudal aspect of the third ventricle. Caudally, it is continuous with the lumen of the fourth ventricle at the junction of the midbrain and pons. The superior and inferior colliculi are dorsal to the aqueduct, and the midbrain tegmentum is ventral.

Fourth Ventricle

The fourth ventricle lies between the brain stem and the cerebellum (Figs. 5.10, 5.11). It is continuous rostrally with the cerebral aqueduct and caudally with the central canal of the spinal cord. In sagittal section, the fourth ventricle has a characteristic triangular profile, and the apex of its tented roof protrudes into the inferior aspect of the cerebellum. The ventricle is at its widest at the level of the pontomedullary junction, where a lateral recess on both sides extends to the lateral border of the brain stem. At this point, the

lateral aperture of the fourth ventricle (foramen of Luschka) provides access to the subarachnoid space at the cerebellopontine angle, and CSF flows through it into the lateral extension of the pontine cistern. Occasionally, a lateral recess may not open.

The floor of the fourth ventricle is a shallow diamond-shaped or rhomboidal depression (rhomboid fossa) on the dorsal surfaces of the pons and the rostral half of the medulla. It consists largely of grey matter and contains important cranial nerve nuclei. The precise location of some nuclei is discernible from surface features. The superior part of the ventricular floor is triangular in shape and is limited laterally by the superior cerebellar peduncles as they converge toward the cerebral aqueduct. Its posterior limit is called the obex. The inferior part of the ventricular floor is also triangular in shape. It is bounded caudally by the gracile and cuneate tubercles, which contain the dorsal column nuclei, and more rostrally by the diverging inferior cerebellar peduncles. A longitudinal median sulcus divides the floor of the fourth ventricle. Each half is itself divided, by an often indistinct sulcus limitans, into a medial region known as the medial eminence and a lateral region known as the vestibular area. The vestibular nuclei lie beneath the vestibular area. In the superior part of the ventricular floor, the medial eminence is represented by the facial colliculus, a small elevation produced by an underlying loop of efferent fibres from the facial nucleus, which covers the abducens nucleus. Between the facial colliculus and the vestibular area, the sulcus limitans widens into a small depression, the superior fovea. In its upper part, the sulcus limitans constitutes the lateral limit of the floor of the fourth ventricle. Here a small region of bluish grey pigmentation denotes the presence of the subjacent locus coeruleus. Inferior to the facial colliculus, at the level of the lateral recess of the ventricle, a variable group of nerve fibre fascicles, known as the striae medullaris, runs transversely across the ventricular floor and passes into the median sulcus. In the inferior area of the floor of the fourth ventricle, the medial eminence is represented by the hypoglossal triangle (trigone), which lies over the hypoglossal nucleus. Laterally, the sulcus limitans widens to produce an indistinct inferior fovea. Caudal to the inferior fovea, between the hypoglossal triangle and the vestibular area, is the vagal triangle (trigone), which covers the dorsal vagal nucleus. The triangle is crossed below by a narrow translucent ridge, the funiculus separans, which is separated from the gracile tubercle by the small area postrema. The funiculus and area postrema are both covered by thickened ependyma containing tanycytes; the area postrema also contains neurones. The blood–brain barrier is modified in both sites.

The roof of the fourth ventricle is formed by the superior and inferior medullary veli. Superiorly, a thin sheet of tissue, the superior medullary velum, stretches across the ventricle between the converging superior cerebellar peduncles (see Fig. 5.10). The superior medullary velum is continuous with the cerebellar white matter and is covered dorsally by the lingula of the superior vermis. The inferior medullary velum is more complex and is composed mostly of a thin sheet, devoid of neural tissue, formed by ventricular ependyma and the pia mater of the tela choroidea, which covers it dorsally. A large median aperture (foramen of Magendie) is present in the roof of the ventricle as a perforation in the posterior medullary velum, just inferior to the nodule of the cerebellum. CSF flows from the ventricle through the foramen into the cerebellomedullary cistern.

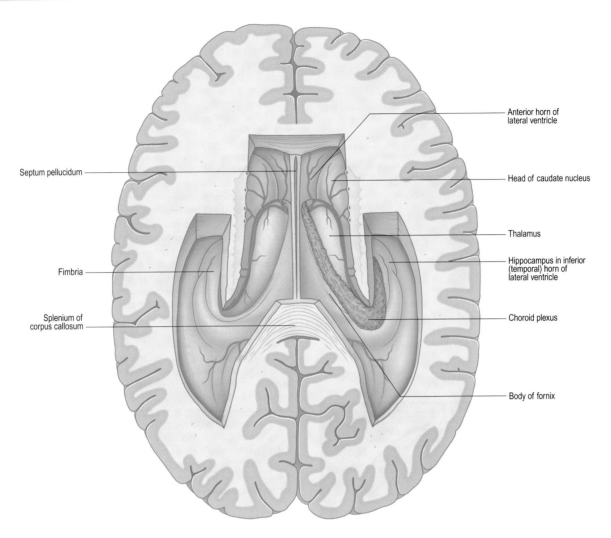

Anterior horn of
lateral ventricle

Septum pellucidum

Head of caudate nucleus

Thalamus

Hippocampus in inferior
(temporal) horn of
lateral ventricle

Fimbria

Splenium of
corpus callosum

Choroid plexus

Body of fornix

Fig. 5.3 *Horizontal section of the cerebrum dissected to remove the roofs of the lateral ventricles.*

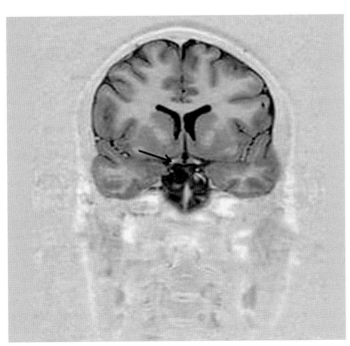

Fig. 5.4 *Transverse MRI scan, at the level of the anterior horn of the lateral ventricle. (Courtesy of Professor Alan Jackson, Department of Neuroradiology, University of Manchester, United Kingdom.)*

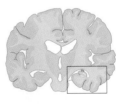

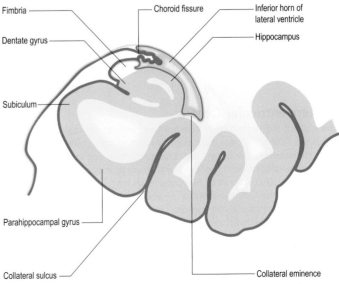

Fimbria

Choroid fissure

Inferior horn of
lateral ventricle

Dentate gyrus

Hippocampus

Subiculum

Parahippocampal gyrus

Collateral sulcus

Collateral eminence

Fig. 5.5 *Coronal section through the inferior horn of the lateral ventricle. Pia mater,* red; *ependyma,* blue.

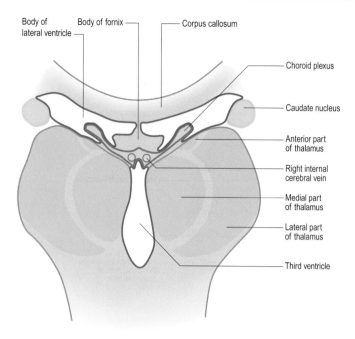

Fig. 5.6 *Coronal section through the lateral and third ventricles. Pia mater of the tela choroidea, red; ependyma, blue.*

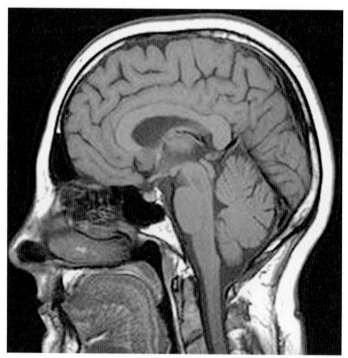

Fig. 5.7 *MRI scan of the head in the sagittal plane. (Courtesy of Professor Alan Jackson, Department of Neuroradiology, University of Manchester, United Kingdom.)*

Circumventricular Organs

The walls of the ventricular system are lined with ependymal cells, beneath which lies a subependymal layer of glia. At certain sites, collectively referred to as circumventricular organs (Fig. 5.12), specialized ependymal cells called tanycytes are also present. Ependyma and tanycytes may be involved in secretion into the CSF; transport of neurochemicals from subjacent neurones, glia or vessels to the CSF; transport of neurochemicals from CSF to the same subjacent structures; and chemoreception. In addition, in the adult, the ependymal and subependymal glial cell layers are the source of undifferentiated stem cells (Mercier, Kitasako, and Hatton 2002), currently under intensive study for their potential neurorestorative properties.

The circumventricular organs are midline sites in the ventricular walls (McKinley et al 2003), where the blood–brain barrier is absent. They include the vascular organ (organum vasculosum), subfornical organ, neurohypophysis, median eminence, subcommissural organ, pineal gland and area postrema.

Vascular organ—The vascular organ lies in the lamina terminalis between the optic chiasma and the anterior commissure. Its external zone contains a rich, fenestrated vascular plexus that covers glia and a network of nerve fibres. The ependymal cells of the vascular organ, like those of other circumventricular organs, are flattened and have few cilia. The major inputs appear to come from the subfornical organ, locus coeruleus and a number of hypothalamic nuclei, and the vascular organ projects to the median preoptic and supraoptic nuclei. The vascular organ is involved in the regulation of fluid balance and may also have neuroendocrine functions.

Subfornical organ—The subfornical organ lies at the level of the interventricular foramen. It contains many neurones, glial cells and a dense fenestrated capillary plexus and is covered by flattened ependyma. It is believed to have widespread hypothalamic interconnections and to function in the regulation of fluid balance and drinking.

Neurohypophysis (posterior pituitary)—The neurohypophysis is the site of termination of neurosecretory projections from the supraoptic and paraventricular nuclei of the hypothalamus. These neurones release vasopressin and oxytocin, respectively, into the capillary bed of the neurohypophysis, where the hormones gain access to the general circulation.

Median eminence—The median eminence contains the terminations of axons of hypothalamic neurosecretory cells. Peptides released from these axons control the hormonal secretions of the anterior pituitary via the pituitary portal system of vessels.

Subcommissural organ—The subcommissural organ lies ventral to and below the posterior commissure (i.e. near the inferior wall of the pineal recess). The ependymal cells on the dorsal aspect of the cerebral aqueduct are tall, columnar and ciliated, with granular basophilic cytoplasm. They may be involved in the secretion of materials into the CSF from adjoining axonal terminals or capillaries.

Pineal gland—The pineal gland is part of the epithalamus, located beneath the splenium of the corpus callosum. It secretes melatonin and is involved in regulation of the circadian rhythm.

Area postrema—The area postrema is a bilaterally paired structure located at the caudal limit of the floor of the fourth ventricle. It is an important chemoreceptive area that triggers vomiting in response to the presence of emetic substances in the blood.

CHOROID PLEXUS AND CEREBROSPINAL FLUID

Choroid Plexus

In the roofs of the third and fourth ventricles and in the medial wall of the lateral ventricle along the line of the choroid fissure, the vascular pia mater lies in close apposition to the ependymal lining of the ventricles, without any intervening brain tissue. It forms the tela choroidea, which gives rise to the highly vascularized choroid plexuses from which CSF is secreted into the ventricles.

Choroid plexuses are located in the lateral ventricles, the third ventricle and the fourth ventricle (see Figs. 5.3, 5.5, 5.6).

In the lateral ventricle, the choroid plexus extends anteriorly as far as the interventricular foramen, through which it is continuous across the third ventricle with the plexus of the opposite lateral ventricle. From the interventricular foramen, the plexus passes posteriorly, in contact with the thalamus, curving around its posterior aspect to enter the inferior horn of the ventricle and reach the hippocampus. Throughout the body of the ventricle, the choroid fissure lies between the fornix superiorly and the thalamus inferiorly (see Fig. 5.6).

From above, the tela choroidea is triangular, with a rounded apex between the interventricular foramina, often indented by the anterior columns of the fornices (see Fig. 5.3). Its lateral edges are irregular and contain choroid vascular fringes. At the posterior basal angles of the tela, these fringes continue and curve into the inferior horn of the ventricle; centrally, the pial layers depart from each other as described earlier. When the tela is removed, a transverse slit (the transverse fissure) is left between the splenium and the junction of the ventricular roof and the tectum. It marks the posterior limit of the extracerebral space enclosed by the posterior extensions of the corpus callosum above the third ventricle. The latter contains the roots of the choroid plexus of the third ventricle and of the lateral ventricles, enclosed between the two layers of pia mater (see Fig. 5.6). The choroid plexus of the third ventricle is attached to the tela choroidea, which is, in effect, the thin roof of the third ventricle as it develops during fetal life. In coronal sections of the cerebral hemispheres, the choroid plexus of the third ventricle can be seen in continuity with the choroid plexus of the lateral ventricles (see Fig. 5.6).

The choroid plexus of the fourth ventricle is similar in structure to that of the lateral and third ventricles. Thus, the roof of the inferior part of the

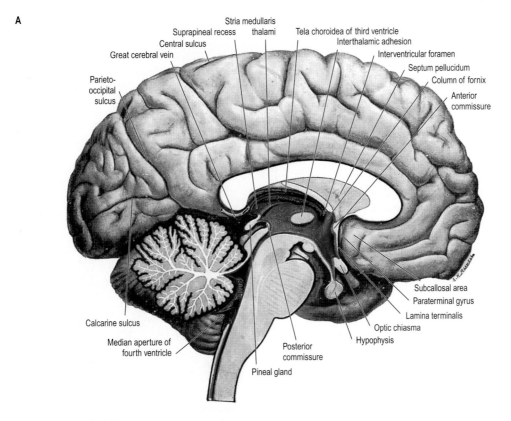

A

Stria medullaris thalami
Suprapineal recess
Central sulcus
Great cerebral vein
Parieto-occipital sulcus
Tela choroidea of third ventricle
Interthalamic adhesion
Interventricular foramen
Septum pellucidum
Column of fornix
Anterior commissure
Calcarine sulcus
Median aperture of fourth ventricle
Pineal gland
Posterior commissure
Hypophysis
Optic chiasma
Lamina terminalis
Paraterminal gyrus
Subcallosal area

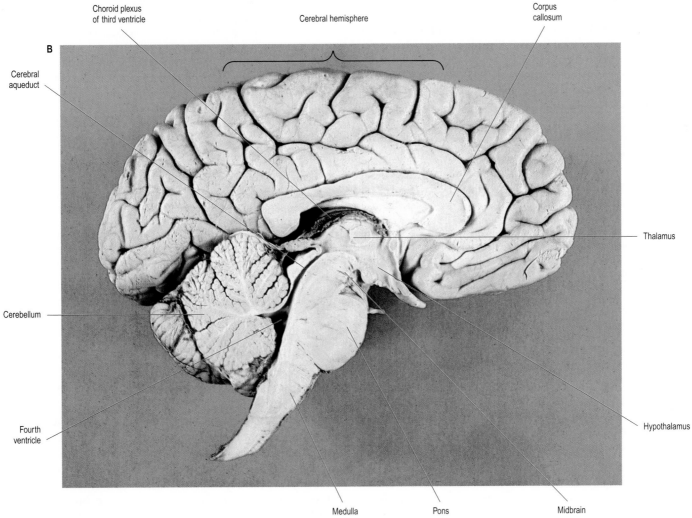

B

Choroid plexus of third ventricle
Cerebral hemisphere
Corpus callosum
Cerebral aqueduct
Thalamus
Cerebellum
Hypothalamus
Fourth ventricle
Medulla
Pons
Midbrain

Fig. 5.8 **A,** *Sagittal hemisection of the brain showing the third and fourth ventricles. Pia mater,* red*; ependyma,* blue. **B,** *Sagittal hemisection through the brain.*
(Hemisection by E. L. Rees; photograph by Kevin Fitzpatrick on behalf of GKT School of Medicine, London.)

CASE 1   AQUEDUCTAL STENOSIS

A middle-aged woman complains of headache of several months' duration; over time she exhibits mental slowing, papilledema with non-specific abducens palsies, spasticity with pyramidal tract signs and limb ataxia. She has a history of presumed viral meningoencephalitis years before but has otherwise been well.

Imaging demonstrates symmetric enlargement of the lateral and third ventricles (Fig. 5.9). The aqueduct is not visualized, and the fourth ventricle and cisterna magna are normal. A diagnosis of aqueductal stenosis is made, and ventricular shunting results in remarkable clinical improvement.

Discussion: Aqueductal stenosis may be congenital or acquired later in life, presumably as a result of viral or bacterial infection with ependymitis and subsequent occlusion of the aqueduct. It is often asymptomatic until adulthood, ultimately presenting with a non-specific syndrome of hydrocephalus involving primarily the anterior ventricular system, as visualized in this case with appropriate neuroimaging.

Differential diagnoses include hydrocephalus secondary to choroid plexus papilloma with overproduction of CSF, pinealoma, invasive tumour of the brain stem or cerebellum, intraventricular tumour such as ependymoma of the fourth ventricle, chronic basilar meningitis obliterating the foramina of Luschka and Magendie, Arnold–Chiari malformation and Dandy–Walker syndrome with enlargement of the fourth ventricle. The syndrome of so-called normal-pressure hydrocephalus is evidenced classically by progressive memory deficits and dementia; ataxia; pyramidal tract signs, especially in the legs; and urinary tract dysfunction. CSF pressure is normal, and there is no papilledema. This disorder is most likely due to obliteration of the cerebral subarachnoid space

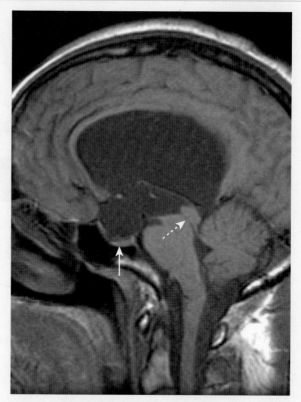

Fig. 5.9 *MRI of aqueductal stenosis* (dashed arrow) *with marked ventricular enlargement. There is an incidental empty sella turcica as well* (solid arrow).

secondary to prior trauma, meningitis, or subarachnoid haemorrhage, and neuroimaging is diagnostic in the majority of cases, many of which respond dramatically to ventricular shunting.

---

fourth ventricle develops as a thin sheet in which the pia mater is in direct contact with the ependymal lining of the ventricle. This thin sheet forms the tela choroidea of the fourth ventricle, lying between the cerebellum and the inferior part of the roof of the ventricle. The choroid plexus of the fourth ventricle is T-shaped, having vertical and horizontal limbs, but this form varies widely. The vertical (longitudinal) limb is double, flanks the midline and is adherent to the roof of the ventricle. The limbs fuse at the superior margin of the median aperture (foramen of Magendie) and are often prolonged on the ventral aspect of the cerebellar vermis. The horizontal limbs of the plexus project into the lateral recesses of the ventricle.

Small tufts of plexus pass through the lateral apertures (foramina of Luschka) and emerge, still covered by ependyma, in the subarachnoid space of the cerebellopontine angle.

The blood supply of the choroid plexus in the tela choroidea of the lateral and third ventricles is usually via a single vessel from the anterior choroidal branch of the internal carotid artery and several choroidal branches of the posterior cerebral artery. The two sets of vessels anastomose to some extent. Capillaries drain into a rich venous plexus served by a single choroidal vein. The blood supply of the fourth ventricular choroid plexus is from the inferior cerebellar arteries.

CASE 2   CHOROID PLEXUS PAPILLOMA

A 14-month-old boy exhibits progressive enlargement of the head, with bulging fontanelles, spreading of the cranial sutures and dilatation of the draining craniocerebral veins. No focal signs are observed, but he demonstrates progressive motor (and cognitive) retardation, spasticity, visual failure with optic atrophy and ataxia, along with occasional seizures.

Imaging demonstrates generalized ventricular dilatation. A large non-invasive tumour mass occupies the choroid plexus on one side.

Discussion: This infant has a tumour involving the choroid plexus, which is responsible for the overproduction of CSF (approaching 2 liters/day in some cases). Most tumours here

are benign papillomas, but they are occasionally malignant, with parenchymal invasion.

When presented with an infant with progressive hydrocephalus, as in this case, other diagnoses to consider include aqueductal stenosis (either congenital atresia of the aqueduct of Sylvius or acquired secondary to chronic infection such as tuberculous meningitis with granular ependymitis); obstruction of draining cerebral veins secondary to vascular events such as infantile subarachnoid haemorrhage or preterm intracerebral haemorrhage, especially in low-birth-weight infants; and colloid cysts of the third ventricle.

Neuroimaging is diagnostic under these circumstances.

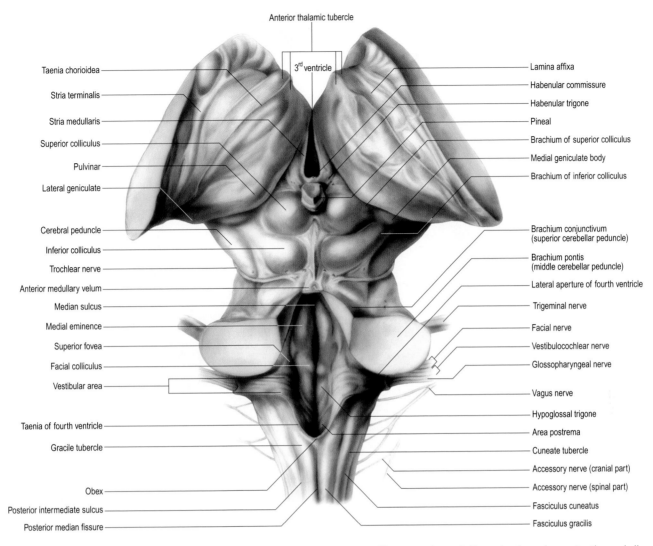

Anterior thalamic tubercle

3rd ventricle

Taenia chorioidea

Stria terminalis

Stria medullaris

Superior colliculus

Pulvinar

Lateral geniculate

Cerebral peduncle

Inferior colliculus

Trochlear nerve

Anterior medullary velum

Median sulcus

Medial eminence

Superior fovea

Facial colliculus

Vestibular area

Taenia of fourth ventricle

Gracile tubercle

Obex

Posterior intermediate sulcus

Posterior median fissure

Lamina affixa

Habenular commissure

Habenular trigone

Pineal

Brachium of superior colliculus

Medial geniculate body

Brachium of inferior colliculus

Brachium conjunctivum (superior cerebellar peduncle)

Brachium pontis (middle cerebellar peduncle)

Lateral aperture of fourth ventricle

Trigeminal nerve

Facial nerve

Vestibulocochlear nerve

Glossopharyngeal nerve

Vagus nerve

Hypoglossal trigone

Area postrema

Cuneate tubercle

Accessory nerve (cranial part)

Accessory nerve (spinal part)

Fasciculus cuneatus

Fasciculus gracilis

Fig. 5.10 *Dorsal aspect of the brain stem. The floor of the fourth ventricle has been exposed by cutting the cerebellar peduncles and removing the cerebellum. (By permission from Mettler, F.A. 1948. Neuroanatomy, 2nd ed. CV Mosby, St. Louis.)*

Cerebrospinal Fluid
Composition and Secretion
CSF is a clear, colourless liquid. In normal individuals, CSF contains a very small amount of protein and differs from blood in its electrolyte content. It is not simply an ultrafiltrate of blood but is actively secreted by the choroid plexus epithelium. Choroid plexus epithelial cells have the characteristics of transport and secretory cells. Their apical surfaces, from which CSF is secreted, possess microvilli, and their basal surfaces exhibit interdigitations and folding. There are tight junctions at the apical ends of the epithelial cells, which are permeable to low-molecular-weight substances. Fenestrated capillaries in the stroma of the choroid plexus lie just beneath the epithelial cells. A blood–CSF barrier is sited at the choroid plexus epithelium.

Circulation and Drainage
Most of the CSF is secreted by the choroid plexuses in the lateral, third and fourth ventricles. However, there is also a small contribution from the ependymal lining of the ventricles and from the extracellular fluid from brain parenchyma.

The total CSF volume is approximately 150 ml, of which 125 ml is intracranial. The ventricles contain approximately 25 ml (almost all of which is in the lateral ventricles), and the remaining 100 ml is located in the cranial subarachnoid space. CSF is secreted at a rate of 0.35 to 0.40 ml per minute, which means that normally, about 50% of the total volume of CSF is replaced every 5 to 6 hours. An effective means of removal from the cranial cavity is thus essential. CSF flows from the lateral ventricles to the third ventricle and then through the cerebral aqueduct to the fourth ventricle. Mixing of CSF from different choroidal sources occurs and is probably assisted by cilia on the ependymal cells lining the ventricles and by arterial pulsations. CSF leaves the fourth ventricle through the medial and lateral apertures to enter the subarachnoid space of the cisterna magna and subarachnoid cisterns over the front of the pons, respectively. The movement of CSF in the extraaxial space is complex and is characterized by a fast-flow component and a much slower bulk-flow component. During systole, the major arteries lying in the basal cisterns and other extraaxial intracranial spaces dilate significantly and exert pressure effects on the CSF, which cause rapid CSF flow around the brain out of the cranial cavity and into the upper cervical spine. The pressure wave that causes this outflow of CSF is dispersed through the spinal CSF space, which acts as a capacitance vessel. As the blood within the major arteries passes into the brain in late systole and diastole, CSF reenters the skull from the spine. This CSF flow occurs at rapid rates and is repeated during every heart cycle. In addition, there is a slow bulk flow of CSF, with a time course measured in hours, which results in circulation of CSF over the cerebral surface in a superolateral direction. CSF is absorbed into the venous system through arachnoid villi associated with the major dural venous sinuses, predominantly the superior sagittal sinus.

Hydrocephalus
Obstruction of the circulation of CSF leads to the accumulation of fluid (hydrocephalus), which causes compression of the brain (Fig. 5.13). Within the brain, critical points at which obstruction may occur correspond to the narrow foramina and passages of the ventricular system. Thus, obstruction of the interventricular foramen, as with an intraventricular tumour, causes enlargement of one or both lateral ventricles. Obstruction of the cerebral aqueduct, which may be congenital, due to atresia of the aqueduct, or acquired, as in ependymitis accompanying chronic infection (e.g. tuberculous meningitis), leads to enlargement of both lateral ventricles and the third ventricle. Obstruction or congenital absence of the apertures of the fourth ventricle leads to enlargement of the entire ventricular system. Obstruction or restriction of CSF circulation can also occur within the subarachnoid space

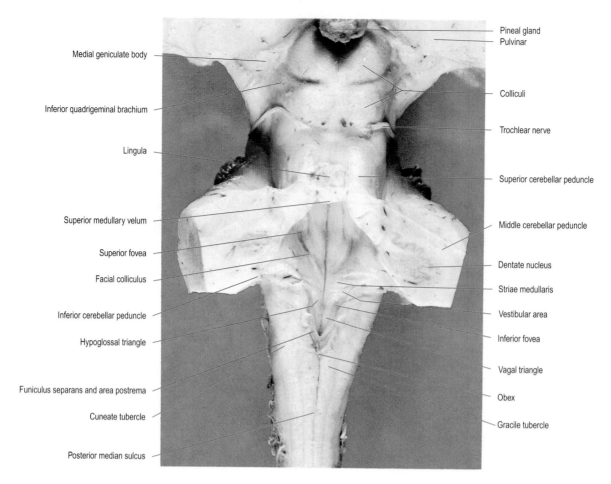

Medial geniculate body

Inferior quadrigeminal brachium

Lingula

Superior medullary velum

Superior fovea

Facial colliculus

Inferior cerebellar peduncle

Hypoglossal triangle

Funiculus separans and area postrema

Cuneate tubercle

Posterior median sulcus

Pineal gland

Pulvinar

Colliculi

Trochlear nerve

Superior cerebellar peduncle

Middle cerebellar peduncle

Dentate nucleus

Striae medullaris

Vestibular area

Inferior fovea

Vagal triangle

Obex

Gracile tubercle

Fig. 5.11 *Dorsal aspect of the brain stem, including the floor of the fourth ventricle.*

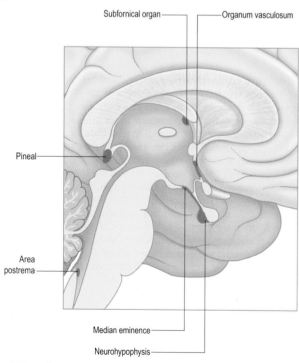

Subfornical organ

Organum vasculosum

Pineal

Area postrema

Median eminence

Neurohypophysis

Fig. 5.12 *Median sagittal section of the brain indicating the locations of the circumventricular organs.*

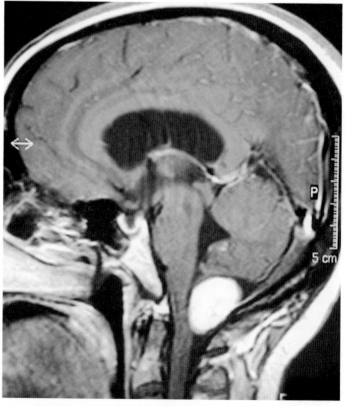

Fig. 5.13 *MRI scan shows an enhancing mass, which is a meningioma growing from the meninges at the edge of the foramen magnum. The tumour is benign but is compressing the brain stem and causing secondary hydrocephalus. (Courtesy of Professor Alan Jackson, Department of Neuroradiology, University of Manchester, United Kingdom.)*

CASE 3 TUBERCULOUS MENINGITIS WITH OBSTRUCTIVE HYDROCEPHALUS

A 16-year-old boy experiences increasing bifrontal headaches for 6 weeks and then develops recurrent vomiting, diplopia and an unsteady gait. Shortly before hospitalization he becomes confused, then stuporous. At the time of admission to the hospital, he exhibits a stiff neck with signs of meningeal irritation, mild facial diplegia, bilateral sixth nerve palsies and papilledema. Cerebellar function cannot be assessed. Reflexes are exaggerated throughout; the plantar responses are silent. He has a low-grade fever, and chest X-ray demonstrates several lesions in both lung fields, consistent with a diagnosis of tuberculosis. Magnetic resonance imaging (MRI) of the head shows enlargement of the lateral third ventricles, along with contrast enhancement of the basal meninges. Spinal fluid is under increased pressure and has a cloudy, opalescent appearance. The CSF clots on standing and contains 125 leukocytes per cubic millimetre, predominantly lymphocytes; it has a protein content of 400 mg% and a sugar content of less than 20 mg%. Within 48 hours, his CSF polymerase chain reaction (PCR) is reported as consistent with tuberculosis, and the CSF culture subsequently yields acid-fast organisms.

Discussion: This is the typical appearance and course of tuberculous meningitis; the CSF findings themselves are characteristic of a subacute to chronic bacterial meningitis. Tuberculous meningitis must be differentiated from other chronic meningitides, such as syphilitic or cryptococcal. Some viral infections, in particular herpes and mumps, may produce a similar set of changes within the spinal fluid. Metastatic leptomeningeal invasion and sarcoid must also be considered in the differential diagnosis. Bacteriological studies are diagnostic.

as a result of meningeal adhesions caused by meningitis. When this occurs at the level of the tentorial notch, passage of CSF from the posterior fossa to its sites of reabsorption is restricted.

References

McKinley, M.J., McAllen, R.M., Davern, P., Giles, M.E., Penschow, J., Sunn, N., Uschakov, A., Oldfield, B.J., 2003. The sensory circumventricular organs of the mammalian brain. Adv. Anat. Embryol. Cell Biol. 172, III–XII, 1–122.

Mercier, F., Kitasako, J.T., Hatton, G.I., 2002. Anatomy of the brain neurogenic zones revisited: fractones and the ?broblast/macrophage network. J. Comp. Neurol. 451, 170–188. Describes the structure and ultrastructure of the basal laminae and subependymal layer.

Paulson, O.B., 2002. Blood–brain barrier, brain metabolism and cerebral blood flow. Eur. Neuropsychopharmacol. 12, 495–501.

Russell, D.S., 1949. Observations on the pathology of hydrocephalus. Medical Research Council.

Strazielle, N., Ghersi-Egea, J.F., 2000. Choroid plexus in the central nervous system: biology and physiopathology. J. Neuropathol. Exp. Neurol. 59, 561–574. Describes choroid plexus functions in brain development, transfer of neurohumoral information, brain–immune system interactions, brain aging and cerebral pharmacotoxicology.

Wolburg, H., Lippoldt, A., 2002. Tight junctions of the blood–brain barrier: development, composition and regulation. Vascul. Pharmacol. 38, 323–337. Reviews the molecular properties of the tight junctions between endothelial cells that constitute the blood–brain barrier.

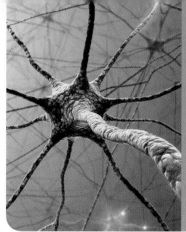

Vascular Supply of the Brain and Spinal Cord

The brain is a highly vascular organ and its profuse blood supply is characterized by a densely branching arterial network (Fig. 6.1). It has high metabolic activity due in part to the energy requirements of constant neural activity. It demands about 15% of the cardiac output and uses 25% of the total oxygen consumed by the body. The brain is supplied by two internal carotid arteries and two vertebral arteries that form a complex anastomosis (circulus arteriosus, or the circle of Willis) on the base of the brain. Vessels diverge from this anastomosis to supply the various cerebral regions. In general, the internal carotid arteries and the vessels arising from them supply the forebrain, with the exception of the occipital lobe of the cerebral hemisphere; the vertebral arteries and their branches supply the occipital lobe, the brain stem and the cerebellum. Venous blood from the brain drains into sinuses within the dura mater. Acute interruption of the blood supply to the brain for more than a few minutes causes permanent neurological damage. Such ischaemic strokes along with intracranial haemorrhages are major sources of morbidity and mortality.

ARTERIAL SUPPLY OF THE BRAIN

The arterial supply of the brain is derived from the internal carotid and vertebral arteries, which lie, together with their proximal branches, within the subarachnoid space at the base of the brain.

Internal Carotid Artery

The internal carotid arteries and their major branches (sometimes referred to as the internal carotid system) essentially supply blood to the forebrain, with the exception of the occipital lobe.

The internal carotid artery (Figs 6.2, 6.3) arises from the bifurcation of the common carotid artery, ascends in the neck and enters the carotid canal of the temporal bone. Its subsequent course is said to have petrous, cavernous and cranial parts.

Petrous Part

The petrous part of the internal carotid artery ascends in the carotid canal and curves anteromedially and then superomedially above the cartilage filling the foramen lacerum, to enter the cranial cavity. It lies at first anterior to the cochlea and tympanic cavity and is separated from the latter and the pharyngotympanic tube by a thin, bony lamella that is cribriform in the young and partly absorbed in old age. Further anteriorly it is separated from the trigeminal ganglion by the thin roof of the carotid canal, although this is often deficient. The artery is surrounded by a venous plexus and the carotid autonomic plexus, which is derived from the internal carotid branch of the superior cervical ganglion. The petrous part of the artery gives rise to two branches. The caroticotympanic artery is a small, occasionally double vessel that enters the tympanic cavity by a foramen in the carotid canal and anastomoses with the anterior tympanic branch of the maxillary artery and the stylomastoid artery. The pterygoid artery is inconsistent. When present, it enters the pterygoid canal with the nerve of the same name and anastomoses with a (recurrent) branch of the greater palatine artery.

Cavernous Part

The cavernous part of the internal carotid artery ascends to the posterior clinoid process. It turns anteriorly to the side of the sphenoid within the cavernous sinus and then curves up medial to the anterior clinoid process to emerge through the dural roof of the sinus. Occasionally, the two clinoid processes form a bony ring around the artery, which is also surrounded by a sympathetic plexus. The oculomotor, trochlear, ophthalmic and abducens nerves are lateral to it.

This part of the artery gives off a number of small vessels. Cavernous branches supply the trigeminal ganglion, the walls of the cavernous and inferior petrosal sinuses and the nerves contained therein. A minute meningeal branch passes over the lesser sphenoid wing to supply the dura mater and bone in the anterior cranial fossa and also anastomoses with a meningeal branch of the posterior ethmoidal artery. Numerous small hypophysial branches supply the neurohypophysis and are of particular importance because they form the pituitary portal system.

Cerebral Part

After piercing the dura mater, the internal carotid artery turns back below the optic nerve to run between the optic and oculomotor nerves. It reaches the anterior perforated substance at the medial end of the lateral cerebral fissure and terminates by dividing into large anterior and middle cerebral arteries.

Several preterminal vessels leave the cerebral portion of the internal carotid. The ophthalmic artery arises from the internal carotid as it leaves the cavernous sinus, often at the point of piercing the dura, and enters the orbit through the optic canal. The posterior communicating artery (Figs 6.4–6.6) runs back from the internal carotid above the oculomotor nerve and anastomoses with the posterior cerebral artery (which is a terminal branch of the basilar artery), thereby contributing to the circulus arteriosus around the interpeduncular fossa. The posterior communicating artery is usually very small. Sometimes, however, it is so large that the posterior cerebral artery is supplied via the posterior communicating artery rather than the basilar artery ('fetal posterior communicating artery'). It is often larger on one side. Small branches from its posterior half pierce the posterior perforated substance, together with branches from the posterior cerebral artery. Collectively, they supply the medial thalamic surface and walls of the third ventricle. The anterior choroidal artery leaves the internal carotid near its posterior communicating branch and passes back above the medial part of the uncus. It crosses the optic tract to reach and supply the crus cerebri of the midbrain; it then turns laterally, recrosses the optic tract and gains the lateral side of the lateral geniculate body, which it supplies with several branches. It finally enters the inferior horn of the lateral ventricle via the choroid fissure and ends in the choroid plexus. This small but important vessel also contributes to the blood supply of the globus pallidus, caudate nucleus, amygdala, hypothalamus, tuber cinereum, red nucleus, substantia nigra, posterior limb of the internal capsule, optic radiation, optic tract, hippocampus and fimbria of the fornix.

Anterior Cerebral Artery

The anterior cerebral artery is the smaller of the two terminal branches of the internal carotid artery (see Figs 6.5, 6.6).

The surgical nomenclature divides the vessel into three parts: A1, from the termination of the internal carotid artery to the junction with the anterior communicating artery; A2, from the junction with the anterior communicating artery to the origin of the callosomarginal artery; A3, distal to the origin of the callosomarginal artery. This segment is also known as the pericallosal artery.

The anterior cerebral artery starts at the medial end of the stem of the lateral cerebral fissure and passes anteromedially above the optic nerve to the great longitudinal fissure, where it connects with its fellow by a short transverse anterior communicating artery. The anterior communicating artery is approximately 4 mm long and may be double. It gives off numerous anteromedial central branches that supply the optic chiasma, lamina terminalis, hypothalamus, para-olfactory areas, anterior columns of the fornix and cingulate gyrus.

The two anterior cerebral arteries travel together in the great longitudinal fissure. They pass around the curve of the genu of the corpus callosum (Fig. 6.7) and then along its upper surface to its posterior end, where they anastomose with posterior cerebral arteries. They give off cortical and central branches.

The cortical branches of the anterior cerebral artery are named by distribution. Two or three orbital branches ramify on the orbital surface of the frontal lobe and supply the olfactory cortex, gyrus rectus and medial orbital gyrus. Frontal branches supply the corpus callosum, cingulate gyrus, medial frontal gyrus and paracentral lobule. Parietal branches supply the precuneus, and the frontal and parietal branches both send twigs over the superomedial border

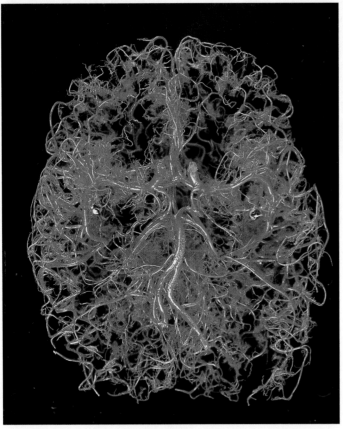

Fig. 6.1 *Resin cast of the arterial supply of the brain. (Photograph by Sarah-Jane Smith.)*

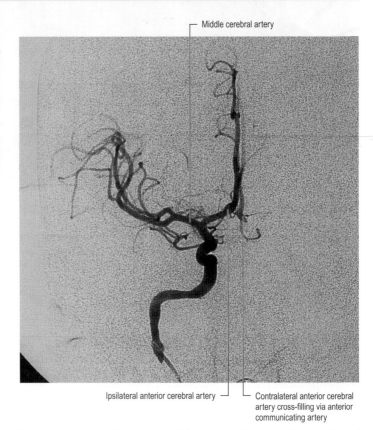

Fig. 6.3 *Internal carotid arteriogram. This image is a Towne's projection obtained by intra-arterial digital subtraction angiography. (Courtesy of Professor P. D. Griffiths, Academic Unit of Radiology, University of Sheffield.)*

Middle cerebral artery

Ipsilateral anterior cerebral artery

Contralateral anterior cerebral artery cross-filling via anterior communicating artery

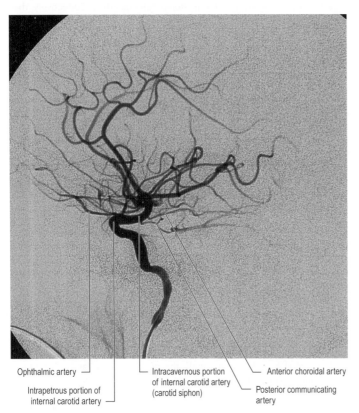

Ophthalmic artery

Intrapetrous portion of internal carotid artery

Intracavernous portion of internal carotid artery (carotid siphon)

Anterior choroidal artery

Posterior communicating artery

Fig. 6.2 *Internal carotid arteriogram. This image is a lateral projection obtained by intra-arterial digital subtraction angiography. (Courtesy of Professor P. D. Griffiths, Academic Unit of Radiology, University of Sheffield.)*

of the hemisphere to supply a strip of territory on the superolateral surface (Fig. 6.8). Cortical branches of the anterior cerebral artery, therefore, supply the areas of the motor and somatosensory cortices that represent the lower limb.

Central branches of the anterior cerebral artery arise from its proximal portion and enter the anterior perforated substance (see Fig. 6.6) and lamina terminalis. Collectively, they supply the rostrum of the corpus callosum, the septum pellucidum, the anterior part of the putamen, the head of the caudate nucleus and adjacent parts of the internal capsule. Immediately proximal or distal to its junction with the anterior communicating artery, the anterior cerebral artery gives rise to the medial striate artery, which supplies the anterior part of the head of the caudate nucleus and adjacent regions of the putamen and internal capsule.

Middle Cerebral Artery

The middle cerebral artery is the larger terminal branch of the internal carotid.

The surgical nomenclature identifies four subdivisions: M1, from the termination of the internal carotid artery to the bi- or trifurcation (also known as the sphenoidal segment); M2, the segment running in the lateral (Sylvian) fissure (also known as the insular segment); M3, coming out of the lateral fissure (also known as the operator segment); and M4, the cortical portions.

The middle cerebral artery runs first in the lateral cerebral fissure, then posterosuperiorly on the insula; it divides into branches distributed to this and the adjacent lateral cerebral surface (see Figs 6.5, 6.6, 6.8). Like the anterior cerebral artery, it has cortical and central branches.

Cortical branches send orbital vessels to the inferior frontal gyrus and the lateral orbital surface of the frontal lobe. Frontal branches supply the precentral, middle and inferior frontal gyri. Two parietal branches are distributed to the postcentral gyrus, the lower part of the superior parietal lobule and the whole inferior parietal lobule. Two or three temporal branches supply the lateral surface of the temporal lobe. Cortical branches of the middle cerebral artery, therefore, supply the motor and somatosensory cortices representing the whole body, with the exception of the lower limb, the auditory area and the insula.

Small central branches of the middle cerebral artery—the lateral striate or lenticulostriate arteries—arise at its commencement and enter the anterior perforated substance together with the medial striate artery. Lateral striate arteries ascend in the external capsule over the lower lateral aspect of the lentiform complex; they then turn medially, traverse the lentiform complex and the internal capsule and extend as far as the caudate nucleus.

Vertebral Artery

The vertebral arteries and their major branches (sometimes referred to as the vertebrobasilar system) essentially supply blood to the upper spinal cord, brain stem, cerebellum and occipital lobe of the cerebrum (Figs 6.9, 6.10). In addition, other branches have a wider distribution.

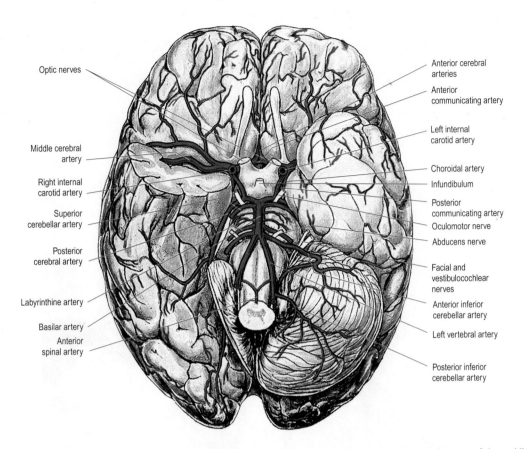

Optic nerves

Middle cerebral
artery

Right internal
carotid artery

Superior
cerebellar artery

Posterior
cerebral artery

Labyrinthine artery

Basilar artery

Anterior
spinal artery

Anterior cerebral
arteries

Anterior
communicating artery

Left internal
carotid artery

Choroidal artery

Infundibulum

Posterior
communicating artery

Oculomotor nerve

Abducens nerve

Facial and
vestibulocochlear
nerves

Anterior inferior
cerebellar artery

Left vertebral artery

Posterior inferior
cerebellar artery

Fig. 6.4 *Arteries at the base of the brain. The anterior part of the right temporal lobe has been removed to display the initial course of the middle cerebral artery within the lateral fissure.*

The vertebral arteries are derived from the subclavian arteries. They ascend through the neck in the foramina transversaria of the upper six cervical vertebrae and enter the cranial cavity through the foramen magnum, close to the anterolateral aspect of the medulla (see Fig. 6.5). They converge medially as they ascend the medulla and unite to form the midline basilar artery at approximately the level of the junction between the medulla and the pons.

One or two meningeal branches arise from the vertebral artery near the foramen magnum. These ramify between the bone and dura mater in the posterior cranial fossa and supply bone, diploë and the falx cerebelli.

A small anterior spinal artery arises near the end of the vertebral artery and descends anterior to the medulla oblongata to unite with its fellow from the opposite side at the mid-medullary level. The single trunk then descends on the ventral midline of the spinal cord and is reinforced sequentially by small spinal rami from the vertebral, ascending cervical, posterior intercostal and first lumbar arteries, which all enter the vertebral canal via intervertebral foramina. Branches from the anterior spinal arteries and the beginning of their common trunk are distributed to the medulla oblongata.

The largest branch of the vertebral artery is the posterior inferior cerebellar artery. It arises near the lower end of the olive, which it curves back around, and then ascends behind the roots of the glossopharyngeal and vagus nerves to reach the inferior border of the pons. There it curves and descends along the inferolateral border of the fourth ventricle before it turns laterally into the cerebellar vallecula between the hemispheres and divides into medial and lateral branches. The medial branch runs back between the cerebellar hemisphere and inferior vermis and supplies both. The lateral branch supplies the inferior cerebellar surface as far as its lateral border and anastomoses with the anterior inferior and superior cerebellar arteries (from the basilar artery). The trunk of the posterior inferior cerebellar artery supplies the medulla oblongata dorsal to the olivary nucleus and lateral to the hypoglossal nucleus and its emerging nerve roots. It also supplies the choroid plexus of the fourth ventricle and sends a branch lateral to the cerebellar tonsil to supply the dentate nucleus. The posterior inferior cerebellar artery is sometimes absent.

A posterior spinal artery usually arises from the posterior inferior cerebellar artery, but it may come directly from the vertebral artery near the medulla oblongata. It passes posteriorly and descends as two branches that lie anterior and posterior to the dorsal roots of the spinal nerves. These are reinforced by spinal twigs from the vertebral, ascending cervical, posterior intercostal and first lumbar arteries, all of which reach the vertebral canal by the intervertebral foramina, thereby sustaining the posterior spinal arteries to the lower spinal levels.

Minute medullary arteries arise from the vertebral artery and its branches and are distributed widely to the medulla oblongata.

Basilar Artery

This large median vessel is formed by the union of the vertebral arteries at the mid-medullary level and extends to the upper border of the pons (see Figs 6.5, 6.6). It lies in the pontine cistern and follows a shallow median groove on the ventral pontine surface. The basilar artery terminates by dividing into two posterior cerebral arteries at a variable level, but most frequently in the interpeduncular cistern, behind the dorsum sellae.

Numerous small pontine branches arise from the front and sides of the basilar artery along its course and supply the pons. The long and slender labyrinthine (internal auditory) artery has a variable origin. It usually arises from the anterior inferior cerebellar artery, but it may originate from the lower part of the basilar artery, the superior cerebellar artery or, occasionally, the posterior inferior cerebellar artery. The labyrinthine artery accompanies the facial and vestibulocochlear nerves into the internal acoustic meatus and is distributed to the internal ear.

The anterior inferior cerebellar artery (see Fig. 6.6) is given off from the lower part of the basilar artery and runs posterolaterally, usually ventral to the abducens, facial and vestibulocochlear nerves. It commonly exhibits a loop into the internal acoustic meatus below the nerves, and when this occurs, the labyrinthine artery may arise from the loop. The anterior inferior cerebellar artery supplies the inferior cerebellar surface anterolaterally and anastomoses with the posterior inferior cerebellar branch of the vertebral artery. A few branches supply the inferolateral parts of the pons and occasionally also supply the upper medulla oblongata.

The superior cerebellar artery (see Fig. 6.6) arises near the distal portion of the basilar artery, immediately before the formation of the posterior cerebral arteries. It passes laterally below the oculomotor nerve, which separates it from the posterior cerebral artery, and curves around the cerebral peduncle below the trochlear nerve to gain the superior cerebellar surface. There it divides into branches that ramify in the pia mater and supply this aspect of the cerebellum and also anastomose with branches of the inferior cerebellar arteries. The superior cerebellar artery supplies the pons, pineal body, superior medullary velum and tela choroidea of the third ventricle.

Posterior Cerebral Artery

The posterior cerebral artery (see Figs 6.5, 6.6) is a terminal branch of the basilar artery.

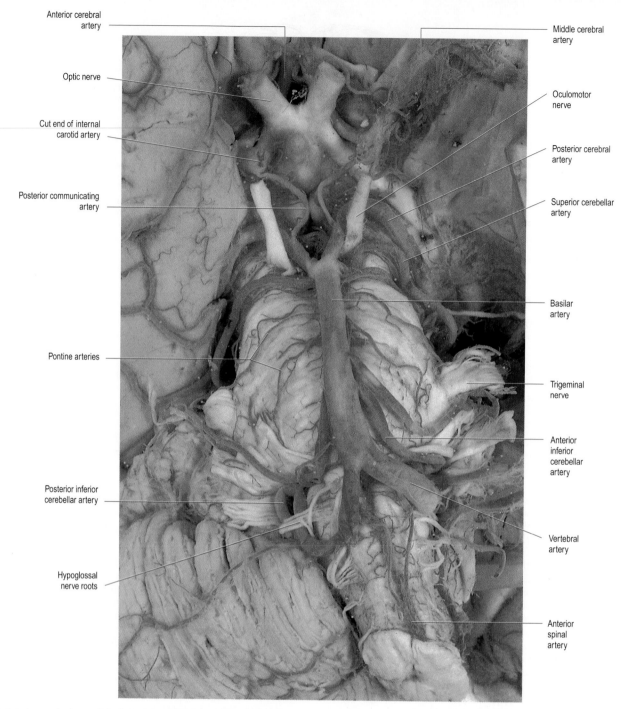

Anterior cerebral artery

Optic nerve

Cut end of internal carotid artery

Posterior communicating artery

Pontine arteries

Posterior inferior cerebellar artery

Hypoglossal nerve roots

Middle cerebral artery

Oculomotor nerve

Posterior cerebral artery

Superior cerebellar artery

Basilar artery

Trigeminal nerve

Anterior inferior cerebellar artery

Vertebral artery

Anterior spinal artery

Fig. 6.5 *Arteries on the base of the brain injected with resin. (By permission from Crossman, A.R., Neary, D. 2000. Neuroanatomy, 2nd ed. Edinburgh, Churchill Livingstone.)*

The surgical nomenclature identifies three segments: P1, from the basilar bifurcation to the junction with the posterior communicating artery; P2, from the junction with the posterior communicating artery to the portion in the perimesencephalic cistern; and P3, the portion running in the calcarine fissure.

The posterior cerebral artery is larger than the superior cerebellar artery, from which it is separated near its origin by the oculomotor nerve and, lateral to the midbrain, by the trochlear nerve. It passes laterally, parallel with the superior cerebellar artery, and receives the posterior communicating artery. It then winds around the cerebral peduncle and reaches the tentorial cerebral surface, where it supplies the temporal and occipital lobes. Like the anterior and middle cerebral arteries, the posterior cerebral artery has cortical and central branches.

The cortical branches of the posterior cerebral artery are named by distribution. Temporal branches, usually two, are distributed to the uncus and the parahippocampal, medial and lateral occipitotemporal gyri. Occipital branches supply the cuneus, lingual gyrus and posterolateral surface of the occipital lobe. Parieto-occipital branches supply the cuneus and precuneus. The posterior cerebral artery supplies the visual areas of the cerebral cortex and other structures in the visual pathway.

The central branches supply subcortical structures. Several small posteromedial central branches arise from the beginning of the posterior cerebral artery (see Fig. 6.6) and, together with similar branches from the posterior communicating artery, pierce the posterior perforated substance and supply the anterior thalamus, subthalamus, lateral wall of the third ventricle and globus pallidus. One or more posterior choroidal branches pass over the lateral geniculate body and supply it before entering the posterior part of the inferior horn of the lateral ventricle via the lower part of the choroid fissure. Branches also curl around the posterior end of the thalamus and pass through the transverse fissure, go to the choroid plexus of the third ventricle or traverse the upper choroid fissure. Collectively, these supply the choroid plexuses of the third and lateral ventricles and the fornix. Small posterolateral central branches arise from the posterior cerebral artery beyond the cerebral peduncle and supply the peduncle and the posterior thalamus, superior and inferior colliculi, pineal gland and medial geniculate body.

Circulus Arteriosus

The circulus arteriosus (circle of Willis) is a large arterial anastomosis that unites the internal carotid and vertebrobasilar systems (see Figs 6.5, 6.6). It lies

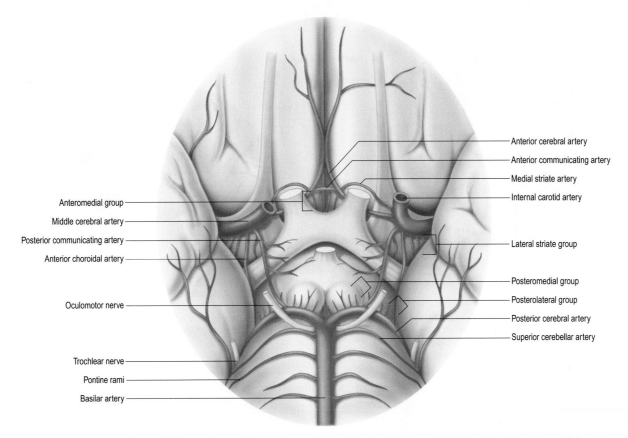

Fig. 6.6 *Circulus arteriosus at the base of the brain showing the distribution of central (perforating or ganglionic) branches. The anteromedial, posteromedial, posterolateral and anterolateral (lateral striate) vessels are shown. The medial striate and anterior choroidal arteries are also shown.*

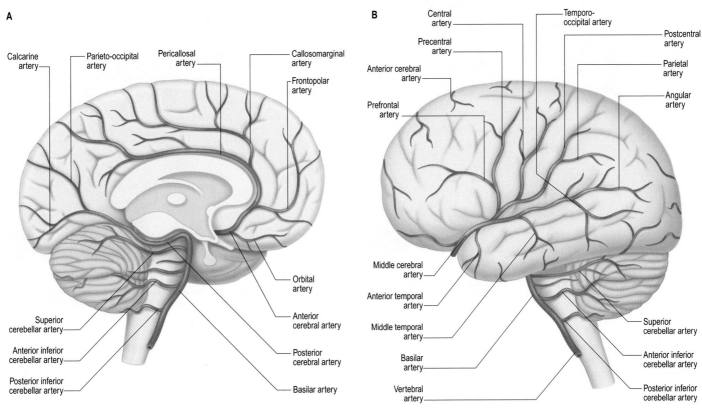

Fig. 6.7 *Major arteries of the brain.* **A,** *Medial aspect.* **B,** *Lateral aspect.*

in the subarachnoid space within the deep interpeduncular cistern and surrounds the optic chiasma, the infundibulum and other structures of the interpeduncular fossa. Anteriorly, the anterior cerebral arteries, which are derived from the internal carotid arteries, are joined by the small anterior communicating artery. Posteriorly, the two posterior cerebral arteries, which are formed by the division of the basilar artery, are joined to the ipsilateral internal carotid artery by a posterior communicating artery. In the majority of

cases, the posterior communicating arteries are very small; however, a limited flow is possible between the anterior and posterior circulations. This is important because the primary purpose of the vascular circle is to provide anastomotic channels if one vessel is occluded. The normal-sized posterior communicating artery usually cannot fulfill this role.

There are considerable individual variations in the pattern and calibre of vessels that make up the circulus arteriosus. Although a complete circular

A

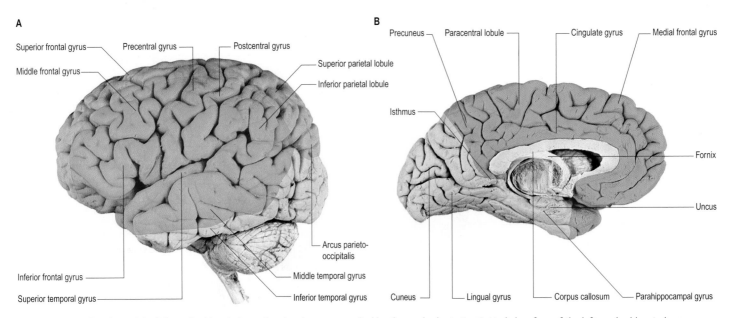

Superior frontal gyrus — Precentral gyrus — Postcentral gyrus
Middle frontal gyrus —
— Superior parietal lobule
— Inferior parietal lobule

Inferior frontal gyrus —
— Arcus parieto-occipitalis
Superior temporal gyrus —
— Middle temporal gyrus
— Inferior temporal gyrus

B

Precuneus — Paracentral lobule — Cingulate gyrus — Medial frontal gyrus
Isthmus —
— Fornix
— Uncus
Cuneus — Lingual gyrus — Corpus callosum — Parahippocampal gyrus

Fig. 6.8 *A, Lateral surface of the left cerebral hemisphere, showing the areas supplied by the cerebral arteries. B, Medial surface of the left cerebral hemisphere, showing the areas supplied by the cerebral arteries. In these figures, the area supplied by the anterior cerebral artery is coloured blue, that by the middle cerebral artery is pink and that by the posterior cerebral artery is yellow.*

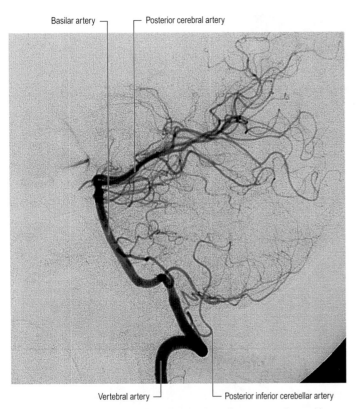

Basilar artery — Posterior cerebral artery

Vertebral artery — Posterior inferior cerebellar artery

Fig. 6.9 *Vertebral arteriogram. This image is a lateral projection obtained by intra-arterial digital subtraction angiography. (Courtesy of Professor P. D. Griffiths, Academic Unit of Radiology, University of Sheffield.)*

Right posterior cerebral artery — Superior cerebellar artery

Anterior inferior cerebellar artery — Basilar artery — Left vertebral artery

Fig. 6.10 *Vertebral arteriogram. This image is a Towne's projection obtained by intra-arterial digital subtraction angiography. (Courtesy of Professor P. D. Griffiths, Academic Unit of Radiology, University of Sheffield.)*

channel almost always exists, one vessel is usually sufficiently narrowed to reduce its role as a collateral route. Cerebral and communicating arteries may be absent, variably hypoplastic, double or even triple. The circle is rarely functionally complete.

The haemodynamics of the circle is influenced by variations in the calibre of communicating arteries and in the segments of the anterior and posterior cerebral arteries that lie between their origins and their junctions with the corresponding communicating arteries. The greatest individual variation in calibre occurs in the posterior communicating artery. Commonly, the diameter of the precommunicating part of the posterior cerebral artery is larger than that of the posterior communicating artery, in which case the blood supply to the occipital lobes is mainly from the vertebrobasilar system. Sometimes, however, the diameter of the precommunicating part of the posterior cerebral artery is smaller than that of the posterior communicating artery, in which case the blood supply to the occipital lobes is mainly from

the internal carotids via the posterior communicating arteries. Agenesis or hypoplasia of the initial segment of the anterior cerebral artery is more frequent than anomalies in the anterior communicating artery and contributes to defective circulation in about one third of individuals.

Central or Perforating Arteries

Numerous small central (perforating or ganglionic) arteries arise from the circulus arteriosus or from vessels near it (see Fig. 6.6). Many of these enter the brain through the anterior and posterior perforated substances (see Fig. 15.9). Central branches supply nearby structures on or near the base of the brain, along with the interior of the cerebral hemisphere, including the internal capsule, basal ganglia and thalamus. They form four principal groups. The anteromedial group arises from the anterior cerebral and anterior communicating arteries and passes through the medial part of the anterior perforated substance. These arteries supply the optic chiasma; lamina terminalis; anterior,

CASE 1   SUBARACHNOID HAEMORRHAGE

A 42-year-old woman develops neck pain followed by a severe headache after lifting a laundry basket. She has a history of poorly controlled hypertension and smokes a pack of cigarettes daily. She is initially awake and alert, but within an hour she becomes somnolent. On examination, she can be aroused briefly, can answer simple questions and can follow one-step commands. She has no weakness. A head computed tomography (CT) scan shows diffuse subarachnoid blood with hydrocephalus (Fig. 6.11). Emergent angiography demonstrates a left middle cerebral artery aneurysm, which is treated by endovascular coiling.

Discussion: Bleeding into the subarachnoid space is frequently caused by a ruptured cerebral aneurysm (Fig. 6.12). The circle of Willis and cerebral arteries lie within the subarachnoid space. It also contains CSF. Blood in the subarachnoid space disrupts the circulation of CSF and frequently leads to hydrocephalus.

The clinical presentation of subarachnoid haemorrhage (SAH) can range from a mild headache to lethargy, hemiparesis, coma or even sudden death. Patients frequently complain of having the worst headache of their life. Risk factors for developing a cerebral aneurysm include hypertension, smoking and a family history of aneurysm.

Other causes of SAH include head trauma, cerebrovascular malformations and vasculopathies. Diagnosis of SAH is made by CT scan, but an arteriogram is usually required to identify its cause. A lumbar puncture demonstrates a large number of red blood cells in the CSF. Cerebral aneurysm may be treated surgically by craniotomy and clipping of the aneurysm or, in certain cases, by placing coils in the aneurysm via an endovascular approach. Hydrocephalus may require placement of a ventriculostomy to externally drain CSF to control intracranial pressure.

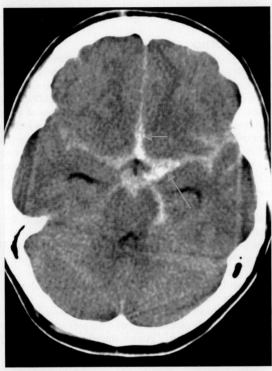

Fig. 6.11 *CT scan demonstrates diffuse subarachnoid haemorrhage (arrows) secondary to rupture of a middle cerebral artery aneurysm. (© 2010 Thomas Jefferson University. All rights reserved. Reproduced with the permission of Thomas Jefferson University.)*

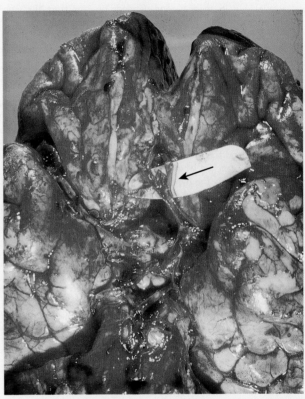

Fig. 6.12 *Ruptured anterior communicating artery aneurysm (arrow).*

preoptic and supraoptic areas of the hypothalamus; septum pellucidum; paraolfactory areas; anterior columns of the fornix; cingulate gyrus; rostrum of the corpus callosum; anterior part of the putamen and head of the caudate nucleus. The posteromedial group comes from the entire length of the posterior communicating artery and from the proximal portion of the posterior cerebral artery. Anteriorly, these arteries supply the hypothalamus and pituitary and the anterior and medial parts of the thalamus via thalamoperforating arteries. Caudally, branches of the posteromedial group supply the mammillary bodies, subthalamus, lateral wall of the third ventricle, including the medial thalamus, and globus pallidus. The anterolateral group comprises mostly branches from the proximal part of the middle cerebral artery; they are also known as striate, lateral striate or lenticulostriate arteries. They enter the brain through the anterior perforated substance and supply the posterior striatum, lateral globus pallidus and anterior limb, genu and posterior limb of the internal capsule. The medial striate artery, which is derived from the middle or anterior cerebral arteries, supplies the rostral part of the caudate nucleus and putamen and the anterior limb and genu of the internal

capsule. The posterolateral group is derived from the posterior cerebral artery distal to its junction with the posterior communicating artery and supplies the cerebral peduncle, colliculi, pineal gland and, via thalamogeniculate branches, posterior thalamus and medial geniculate body.

Regional Arterial Supply of the Brain
Brain Stem

The medulla oblongata is supplied by the branches of the vertebral, anterior and posterior spinal arteries, posterior inferior cerebellar arteries and basilar arteries, which enter along the anterior median fissure and the posterior median sulcus. Vessels that supply the central substance enter along the rootlets of the glossopharyngeal, vagus, accessory and hypoglossal nerves. There is an additional supply via a pial plexus from the same main arteries.

The pons is supplied by the basilar artery and the anterior inferior and superior cerebellar arteries. Direct branches from the basilar artery enter the pons along the ventral medial groove (basilar sulcus). Other vessels enter along the trigeminal, abducens, facial and vestibulocochlear nerves and from the pial plexus.

The midbrain is supplied by the posterior cerebral, superior cerebellar and basilar arteries. The crura cerebri are supplied by vessels entering on their medial and lateral sides. The medial vessels enter the medial side of the crus and also supply the superomedial part of the tegmentum, including the oculomotor nucleus; lateral vessels supply the lateral part of the crus and the tegmentum. The colliculi are supplied by three vessels on each side from the posterior cerebral and superior cerebellar arteries. An additional supply to the crura and the colliculi and their penduncles comes from the posterolateral group of central branches of the posterior cerebral artery.

Cerebellum

The cerebellum is supplied by the posterior inferior, anterior inferior and superior cerebellar arteries. The cerebellar arteries form superficial anastomoses on the cortical surface. Anastomoses between deeper, subcortical branches have been postulated.

The choroid plexus of the fourth ventricle is supplied by the posterior inferior cerebellar arteries.

Optic Chiasma, Tract and Radiation

The blood supplies of the optic chiasma, tract and radiation are of considerable clinical importance. The chiasma is supplied in part by the anterior cerebral arteries, but its median zone depends on rami from the internal carotid arteries reaching it via the stalk of the hypophysis. The anterior choroidal and posterior communicating arteries supply the optic tract, and the optic radiation receives blood through deep branches of the middle and posterior cerebral arteries.

Diencephalon

The thalamus is supplied chiefly by branches of the posterior communicating, posterior cerebral and basilar arteries. A contribution from the anterior choroidal artery is often noted, but this has been disputed. The medial branch of the posterior choroidal artery supplies the posterior commissure, habenular region, pineal gland and medial parts of the thalamus, including the pulvinar. Small central branches, which arise from the circulus arteriosus and its associated vessels, supply the hypothalamus. The pituitary gland is supplied by hypophysial arteries derived from the internal carotid artery, and the anterior cerebral and anterior communicating arteries supply the lamina terminalis.

The choroid plexuses of the third and lateral ventricles are supplied by branches of the internal carotid and posterior cerebral arteries.

Basal Ganglia

The majority of the arterial supply to the basal ganglia comes from the striate arteries, which are branches from the roots of the anterior and middle cerebral arteries (Fig. 6.13). They enter the brain through the anterior perforated substance and also supply the internal capsule. The caudate nucleus

receives blood additionally from the anterior and posterior choroidal arteries. The posteroinferior part of the lentiform complex is supplied by the thalamostriate branches of the posterior cerebral artery. The anterior choroidal artery, a preterminal branch of the internal carotid artery, contributes to the blood supply of both segments of the globus pallidus and the caudate nucleus. In a well known case, ligation of this vessel during a neurosurgical procedure on a patient suffering from Parkinson's disease led to the alleviation of Parkinsonian symptoms, presumably as a consequence of infarction of the globus pallidus. This chance observation led to the initiation of pallidal surgery (pallidotomy) for this condition.

Internal Capsule

The internal capsule is supplied by central, or perforating, arteries that arise from the circulus arteriosus and its associated vessels (see Fig. 6.13). These include the lateral and medial striate arteries, which come from the middle and anterior cerebral arteries and also supply the basal ganglia. The lateral striate arteries supply the anterior limb, genu and much of the posterior limb of the internal capsule and are commonly involved in ischaemic and haemorrhagic strokes. One of the larger striate branches of the middle cerebral artery is known as Charcot's artery of cerebral haemorrhage.

The medial striate artery, a branch of the proximal part of the middle or anterior cerebral, supplies the anterior limb and genu of the internal capsule and the basal ganglia. The anterior choroidal artery also contributes to the supply of the ventral part of the posterior limb and the retrolenticular (retrolentiform) part of the internal capsule.

Cerebral Cortex

The entire blood supply of the cerebral cortex comes from cortical branches of the anterior, middle and posterior cerebral arteries. In general, long branches traverse the cortex and penetrate the subjacent white matter for 3 or 4 cm without communicating. Short branches are confined to the cerebral cortex and form a compact network in the middle zone of the grey matter, whereas the outer and inner zones are sparingly supplied. Although adjacent vessels anastomose on the surface of the brain, they become end-arteries as soon as they enter it. In general, superficial anastomoses occur only between microscopic branches of the cerebral arteries, and there is little evidence that they can provide an effective alternative circulation after the occlusion of larger vessels.

The lateral surface of the hemisphere is supplied mainly by the middle cerebral artery (see Fig. 6.8). This includes the territories of the motor and somatosensory cortices, which represent the whole body except for the lower limb and also the auditory cortex and language areas. The anterior cerebral artery supplies a strip next to the superomedial border of the hemisphere, as far back as the parieto-occipital sulcus. The occipital lobe and most of the inferior temporal gyrus (excluding the temporal pole) are supplied by the posterior cerebral artery.

Medial and inferior surfaces of the hemisphere are supplied by the anterior, middle and posterior cerebral arteries. The area supplied by the anterior cerebral artery is the largest; it extends almost to the parieto-occipital sulcus and includes the medial part of the orbital surface. The rest of the orbital surface and the temporal pole are supplied by the middle cerebral artery, and the remaining medial and inferior surfaces are supplied by the posterior cerebral artery.

Near the occipital pole, the junctional zone between the territories of the middle and posterior cerebral arteries corresponds to the visual (striate) cortex, which receives information from the macula. When the posterior cerebral artery is occluded, a phenomenon known as macular sparing may occur, in which vision involving the central part of the retina is preserved. Collateral circulation of blood from branches of the middle cerebral artery into those of the posterior cerebral artery may account for this phenomenon. Indeed, in some individuals, the middle cerebral artery may itself supply the macular area.

Cerebral Bloodflow

The brain is devoid of either glucose stores or a means of storing oxygen and is therefore dependent, minute by minute, on an adequate blood supply. It has a high metabolic rate in comparison with other organs, which reflects the metabolic demands of constant neural activity. The blood supply of grey matter is more copious than that of white matter.

Cerebral bloodflow in the human brain is approximately 50 ml/g/min. Global cerebral bloodflow is autoregulated—that is, it remains constant in normal individuals despite variations in mean arterial blood pressure over a range of approximately 8.7 to 18.7 kPa (65 to 140 mm Hg). If the blood pressure falls below this range, cerebral bloodflow decreases. Alternatively, if the pressure rises above this range, cerebral bloodflow may increase. Arterial and arteriolar intraluminal pressures directly control the contraction of intramural

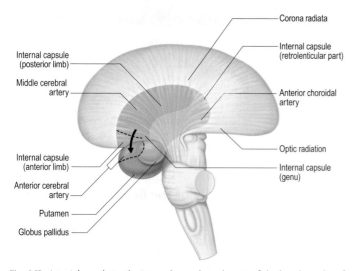

Corona radiata

Internal capsule (retrolenticular part)

Internal capsule (posterior limb)

Middle cerebral artery

Anterior choroidal artery

Optic radiation

Internal capsule (anterior limb)

Internal capsule (genu)

Anterior cerebral artery

Putamen

Globus pallidus

Fig. 6.13 *Arterial supply to the internal capsule and parts of the basal ganglia of the left cerebral hemisphere. The outer layers of the hemisphere have been removed to reveal these structures. The putamen and globus pallidus are displaced downward to display the internal capsule. Territory supplied by branches of the anterior and middle cerebral arteries is shown in red. Territory supplied by the anterior choroidal artery is shown in green.*

CASE 2   CEREBROVASCULAR DISEASE

A 68-year-old man with hypertension, diabetes mellitus, and a long history of cigarette smoking suddenly collapses at work. He is unable to speak or move his right side. He is taken to the local emergency department, where he is found to be lethargic and to have a dense right hemiparesis, left gaze preference and global aphasia. His head CT scan is unremarkable. He is diagnosed with an acute ischaemic stroke; intravenous recombinant tissue plasminogen activator (rtPA) is administered. The following day his magnetic resonance imaging (MRI) scan reveals extensive infarction of the left middle cerebral artery territory. Three months later, he is awake, has dysarthric speech but no aphasia and is able to walk with the assistance of a cane.

Discussion: Cerebrovascular disease may be broadly categorized as ischaemic or haemorrhagic. Ischaemic cerebrovascular disease, or stroke, occurs when there is a lack of bloodflow to a region of the brain. The symptoms of stroke are variable and are determined by the blood vessels and area of the brain affected. Patients with anterior cerebral artery strokes may present with contralateral leg weakness greater than arm weakness. Middle cerebral artery strokes are usually associated with a dense contralateral hemiparesis, whereas posterior cerebral artery strokes may cause homonymous visual field loss. Strokes affecting the dominant hemisphere often result in an aphasia; non-dominant hemisphere strokes can cause neglect syndromes such as anosognosia (patient's lack of recognition of any deficits).

Ischaemic strokes are frequently defined by their cause. They may be cardioembolic, such as from atrial fibrillation or intracardiac pathology, or the cause may be artery-to-artery emboli, such as from carotid artery disease, or thrombosis of small perforating arteries, called lacunar strokes. Acute strokes are frequently not seen on initial CT scanning. Treatment in the first several hours after a stroke occurs may include intravenous rtPA or endovascular procedures to remove the arterial blockage.

Haemorrhagic stroke occurs when a cerebral blood vessel ruptures. Depending on the location of the vessel, bleeding may be epidural, subdural, intraparenchymal, intraventricular or subarachnoid (Fig. 6.14). The most common cause of intracerebral haemorrhage is hypertension; other causes include cerebral aneurysms, vascular malformations and amyloid angiopathy. Treatment options for intracerebral haemorrhage are limited and are largely directed toward preventing secondary damage from the haemorrhage mass.

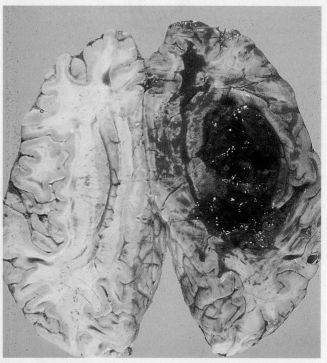

Fig. 6.14 *Massive acute hypertensive intracerebral haemorrhage.*

muscle, so an increase in arterial pressure, for example, causes arterial constriction, and bloodflow remains constant.

Although autoregulation normally ensures that global cerebral bloodflow remains constant, regional bloodflow varies in response to the level of neural activity and, thus, to local metabolic demand. This has been demonstrated in many brain areas, including the motor and sensory cortical regions, areas involved in convulsive activity and even cortical areas involved in complex thought processes. The principal local factors affecting regional bloodflow are the local hydrogen ion (H^+) or carbon dioxide concentration, which causes arterial dilatation.

Not all substances circulating in arterial blood have access to the brain parenchyma. Particulate matter, such as bacteria, is excluded. In general, lipophilic molecules and small molecules, such as oxygen and carbon dioxide, can cross the blood–brain barrier, but hydrophilic ones (excluding glucose) cannot. The cellular basis for the blood–brain barrier is discussed in Chapter 2.

VENOUS DRAINAGE OF THE BRAIN

The venous drainage of the brain occurs through a complex system of deep and superficial veins. These veins possess no valves and have thin walls devoid of muscular tissue. They pierce the arachnoid mater and the inner layer of the dura mater to open into the dural venous sinuses.

Veins of the Brain Stem

The veins of the brain stem form a superficial venous plexus deep to the arteries.

Veins of the medulla oblongata drain into the veins of the spinal cord or the adjacent dural venous sinuses or into variable radicular veins that accompany the last four cranial nerves either to the inferior petrosal or occipital sinuses or to the superior bulb of the jugular vein. Anterior and posterior median medullary veins may run along the anterior median fissure and posterior median sulcus to become continuous with the spinal veins in corresponding positions. Pontine veins, which may include a median vein and a lateral vein on each side, drain into the basal vein, cerebellar veins, petrosal sinuses, transverse sinus or venous plexus of the foramen ovale. Veins of the midbrain join the great cerebral vein or basal vein.

Veins of the Cerebellum

The veins of the cerebellum drain mainly into sinuses adjacent to them or, from the superior surface, into the great cerebral vein. The cerebellar veins course on the cerebellar surface and constitute superior and inferior groups. Superior cerebellar veins either run anteromedially across the superior vermis to the straight sinus or great cerebral vein or run laterally to the transverse and superior petrosal sinuses. Inferior cerebellar veins include a small median vessel running backward on the inferior vermis to enter the straight or sigmoid sinus. Laterally coursing vessels join the inferior petrosal and occipital sinuses.

Veins of the Cerebral Hemisphere

External and internal cerebral veins (Figs 6.15–6.19) drain the surfaces and the interior of the cerebral hemisphere. External cerebral veins may be divided into three groups: superior, middle and inferior.

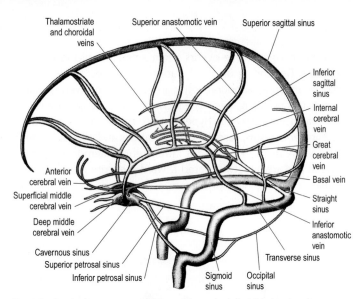

Fig. 6.15 *Cerebral venous system* (viewed from the left side) *showing the principal superficial and deep veins of the brain and their relationship to the dural venous sinuses. The more deeply placed veins are shown in* blue *and those inside the brain are shown in* interrupted blue.

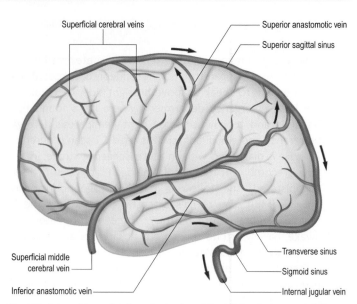

Fig. 6.16 *External (superficial) cerebral veins of the left hemisphere and their relationship to the dural venous sinuses.*

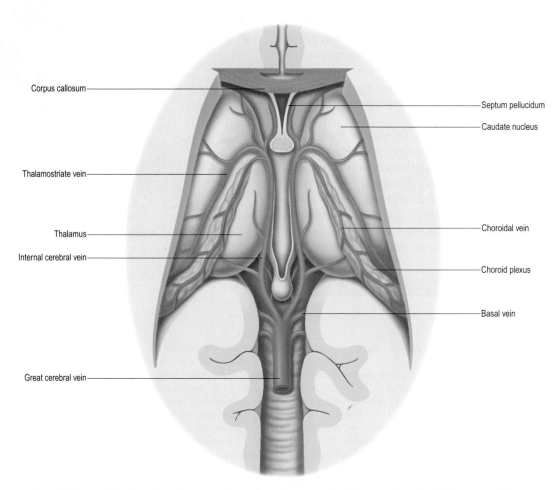

Fig. 6.17 *Internal (deep) cerebral veins, viewed from above after removal of the central portion of the corpus callosum.*

Eight to 12 superior cerebral veins drain the superolateral and medial surfaces of each hemisphere. They mainly follow the sulci, although some do pass across gyri. They ascend to the superomedial border of the hemisphere, where they receive small veins from the medial surface, and then open into the superior sagittal sinus. Superior cerebral veins in the anterior part of the hemisphere join the sinus almost at right angles. The larger posterior veins are directed obliquely forward, against the direction of flow in the sinus, an arrangement that may resist their collapse when intracranial pressure is raised.

The superficial middle cerebral vein drains most of the lateral surface of the hemisphere and follows the lateral fissure to end in the cavernous sinus.

A superior anastomotic vein runs posterosuperiorly between the superficial middle cerebral vein and the superior sagittal sinus, thus connecting the superior sagittal and cavernous sinuses. An inferior anastomotic vein courses over the temporal lobe and connects the superficial middle cerebral vein to the transverse sinus. The deep middle cerebral vein drains the insular region and joins the anterior cerebral and striate veins to form a basal vein. Regions drained by the anterior cerebral and striate veins correspond approximately to those supplied by the anterior cerebral artery and the central branches that enter the anterior perforated substance. The basal veins pass back alongside the interpeduncular fossa and midbrain, receive tributaries from this vicinity and join the great cerebral vein.

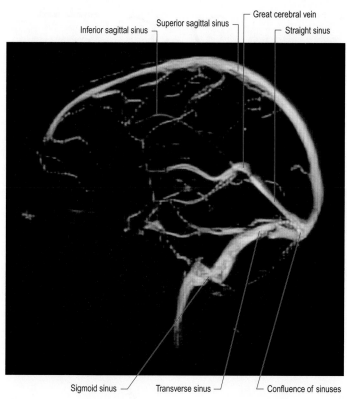

Fig. 6.18 *Lateral projection from a magnetic resonance venogram using time-of-flight methods. (Courtesy of Professor P. D. Griffiths, Academic Unit of Radiology, University of Sheffield.)*

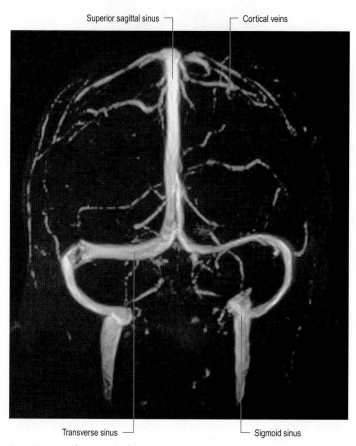

Fig. 6.19 *Frontal projection from a magnetic resonance venogram using time-of-flight methods. (Courtesy of Professor P. D. Griffiths, Academic Unit of Radiology, University of Sheffield.)*

Inferior cerebral veins on the orbital surface of the frontal lobe join the superior cerebral veins and thus drain to the superior sagittal sinus. Those on the temporal lobe anastomose with basal veins and middle cerebral veins and drain to the cavernous, superior petrosal and transverse sinuses.

The basal vein begins at the anterior perforated substance by the union of a small anterior cerebral vein, which accompanies the anterior cerebral artery;

a deep middle cerebral vein, which receives tributaries from the insula and neighbouring gyri and runs in the lateral cerebral fissure; and striate veins, which emerge from the anterior perforated substance. The basal vein passes back around the cerebral peduncle to the great cerebral vein (see Fig. 6.15) and receives tributaries from the interpeduncular fossa, inferior horn of the lateral ventricle, parahippocampal gyrus and midbrain.

The internal cerebral vein drains the deep parts of the hemisphere and the choroid plexuses of the third and lateral ventricles. It is formed near the interventricular foramen, behind the column of the fornix, primarily by union of the thalamostriate and choroidal veins, although numerous smaller veins from surrounding structures also converge there. The thalamostriate vein runs anteriorly, between the caudate nucleus and thalamus, and receives many tributaries from both. The choroidal vein runs a convoluted course along the whole choroid plexus and receives veins from the hippocampus, fornix, corpus callosum and adjacent structures. After their formation, the two internal cerebral veins travel back parallel to each other, beneath the splenium of the corpus callosum, where they unite to form the great cerebral vein. The great cerebral vein is a short median vessel that curves sharply up around the splenium of the corpus callosum and opens into the anterior end of the straight sinus after receiving the right and left basal veins.

Vascular Supply of the Spine (see also Crock 1996)

Arteries

The vertebral column, its contents and its associated soft tissues all receive their arterial supply from derivatives of dorsal branches of the embryonic intersegmental somatic arteries (Fig. 6.21). The relevant named artery depends on the level of the column. These intersegmental vessels persist in the thoracic and lumbar regions as the posterior intercostal and lumbar arteries. In the cervical and sacral regions, longitudinal anastomoses between the intersegmental vessels persist as longitudinal vessels, which themselves give spinal branches to the vertebral column. In the neck, the postcostal anastomosis becomes most of the vertebral artery, whereas the post-transverse anastomosis forms most of the deep cervical artery. The ascending cervical artery and the lateral sacral artery are persistent parts of the precostal anastomosis.

In the thorax and abdomen, the primitive arterial pattern is retained by the paired branches of the descending aorta, which supply the vertebral column (see Fig. 6.21A). On each side, the main trunk of the artery (posterior intercostal or lumbar) passes around the vertebral body, giving off primary periosteal and equatorial branches to the body and then a major dorsal branch. The dorsal branch gives off a spinal branch, which enters the intervertebral foramen before supplying the facet joints, posterior surfaces of the laminae and overlying muscles and skin. There is free anastomosis between these dorsal articular and soft tissue branches, extending over several segments (Crock and Yoshizawa 1976; Boelderl et al 2002). At cervical and sacral levels, the longitudinally running arteries described earlier have direct spinal branches. The spinal branches are the main arteries of supply to all bony elements of the vertebrae and to the dura and epidural tissues; they also contribute to the supply of the spinal cord and nerve roots via radicular branches (see later). As they enter the vertebral canal, the spinal arteries divide into postcentral, prelaminar and radicular branches. The postcentral branches, which are the main nutrient arteries to the vertebral bodies and to the periphery of the intervertebral discs, anastomose beneath the posterior longitudinal ligament with their fellows above and below, as well as across the midline (see Fig. 6.21). This anastomosis also supplies the anterior epidural tissues and dura. The majority of the vertebral arch, the posterior epidural tissues and dura and the ligamentum flavum are supplied by the prelaminar branches and their anastomotic plexus on the posterior wall of the vertebral canal.

Veins

Veins of the vertebral column form intricate plexuses along the entire column, external and internal to the vertebral canal (Fig. 6.22). Both groups are devoid of valves, anastomose freely with each other and join the intervertebral veins. Interconnections are widely established between these plexuses and longitudinal veins early in fetal life. When development is complete, the plexuses drain into the caval and azygos ascending lumbar systems via named veins that accompany the arteries described earlier.

The veins also communicate with cranial dural venous sinuses and with the deep veins of the neck and pelvis. The venous complexes associated with the vertebral column can dilate considerably and can form alternative routes of venous return in patients with major venous obstruction in the neck, chest or abdomen. The absence of valves allows pathways for the wide and sometimes paradoxical spread of malignant disease and sepsis. Pressure changes in the body cavities are transmitted to these venous plexuses and thus to the CSF,

CASE 3   CAROTID CAVERNOUS FISTULA

A 45-year-old man sustains a minor head injury with fleeting loss of consciousness but no immediate sequelae. Several days later he notes increasing pain in and around the left eye, along with double vision, lid ptosis and protrusion of the affected eye. On examination, he demonstrates unilateral exophthalmos, ptosis, ophthalmoparesis, orbital oedema and papilloedema with retinal haemorrhages. A loud bruit is audible over the left eye. The exophthalmos is pulsatile in character.

Discussion: This man has developed a carotid cavernous fistula secondary to head trauma, with laceration of the carotid artery within the cavernous sinus (Fig. 6.20). In a small proportion of cases the lesion is spontaneous, secondary to rupture of a previously unrecognized carotid aneurysm. Several structures within the cavernous sinus are variously affected, along with the pulsatile exophthalmos, orbital congestion and oedema secondary to involvement of the carotid artery within the sinus itself. The differential diagnosis includes, most importantly, cavernous sinus thrombosis secondary to spread of sepsis from infection in the sinuses or the upper face. Under these circumstances, the patient is generally febrile and acutely ill; physical findings are otherwise much the same as in a traumatic carotid cavernous fistula, as observed in this patient.

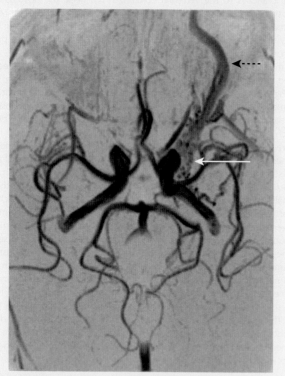

Fig. 6.20 *Magnetic resonance imaging of a carotid cavernous fistula, demonstrating blood in the cavernous sinus* (solid arrow) *and dilatation of the ipsilateral superior ophthalmic vein* (dashed arrow).

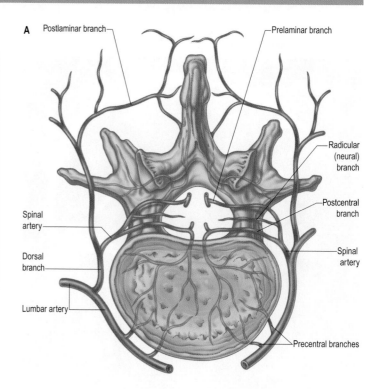

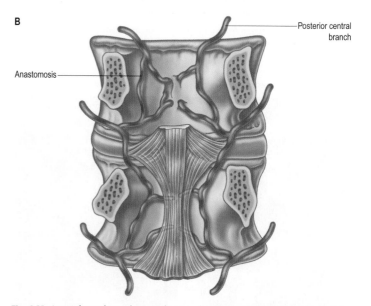

Fig. 6.21 *Arterial supply to the vertebrae and contents of the vertebral canal.* **A,** *Branching pattern of lumbar segmental arteries.* **B,** *Arterial anastomoses between postcentral branches of spinal arteries within the vertebral canal.* (© *Thomas Jefferson University. All rights reserved. Reproduced with the permission of Thomas Jefferson University.*)

processes. They anastomose with the internal plexuses and join the vertebral, posterior intercostal and lumbar veins.

Internal Vertebral Venous Plexuses — The internal vertebral venous plexuses occur between the dura mater and vertebrae and receive tributaries from the bones, red bone marrow and spinal cord. They form a denser network than the external plexuses and are arranged vertically as four interconnecting longitudinal vessels, two anterior and two posterior.

The anterior internal plexuses are large plexiform veins on the posterior surfaces of the vertebral bodies and intervertebral discs. They flank the posterior longitudinal ligament, beneath which they are connected by transverse branches into which the large basivertebral veins open. The posterior internal plexuses, on each side in front of the vertebral arches and ligamenta flava, anastomose with the posterior external plexuses via veins that pass through and between the ligaments. The internal plexuses interconnect by venous rings near each vertebra. Around the foramen magnum they form a dense network connecting with vertebral veins, occipital and sigmoid sinuses, the basilar plexus, the venous plexus of the hypoglossal canal and the condylar emissary veins.

Basivertebral Veins — The basivertebral veins emerge from the posterior foramina of the vertebral bodies. They are large and tortuous channels in

although the cord itself may be protected from such congestion by valves in the small veins that drain from the cord into the internal vertebral plexus.

External Vertebral Venous Plexuses — The external vertebral venous plexuses are anterior and posterior. They anastomose freely and are most developed in the cervical region. Anterior external plexuses are anterior to the vertebral bodies, communicate with basivertebral and intervertebral veins and receive tributaries from vertebral bodies. Posterior external plexuses lie posterior to the vertebral laminae and around spinous, transverse and articular

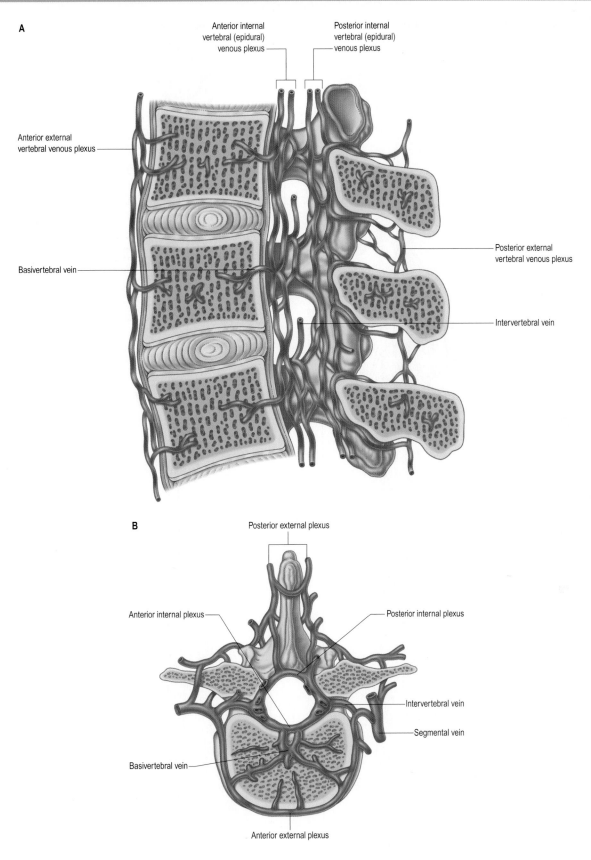

A

Anterior internal vertebral (epidural) venous plexus

Posterior internal vertebral (epidural) venous plexus

Anterior external vertebral venous plexus

Basivertebral vein

Posterior external vertebral venous plexus

Intervertebral vein

B

Posterior external plexus

Anterior internal plexus

Posterior internal plexus

Intervertebral vein

Segmental vein

Basivertebral vein

Anterior external plexus

Fig. 6.22 *A and B, Venous drainage of the vertebral column.*

bone, like those in the cranial diploë. The basivertebral veins also drain into the anterior external vertebral plexuses through small openings in the vertebral bodies. Posteriorly, they form one or two short trunks that open into the transverse branches and unite the anterior internal vertebral plexuses. They enlarge in advanced age.

Intervertebral Veins — The intervertebral veins accompany the spinal nerves through intervertebral foramina, draining the spinal cord and internal and external vertebral plexuses and ending in the vertebral, posterior intercostal, lumbar and lateral sacral veins. Upper posterior intercostal veins may drain into the caval system via brachiocephalic veins, whereas the lower

intercostals drain into the azygos system. Lumbar veins are joined longitudinally in front of the transverse processes by the ascending lumbar veins, in which they may terminate. Alternatively, they may proceed around the vertebral bodies to drain into the inferior vena cava. Whether the basivertebral or intervertebral veins contain effective valves is uncertain, but experimental evidence strongly suggests that their bloodflow can be reversed (Batson 1957). This may explain how pelvic neoplasms (e.g. prostate carcinoma) may metastasize in vertebral bodies: the cells spread into the internal vertebral plexuses via their connections with the pelvic veins when bloodflow is temporarily reversed by raised intra-abdominal pressure or postural alterations.

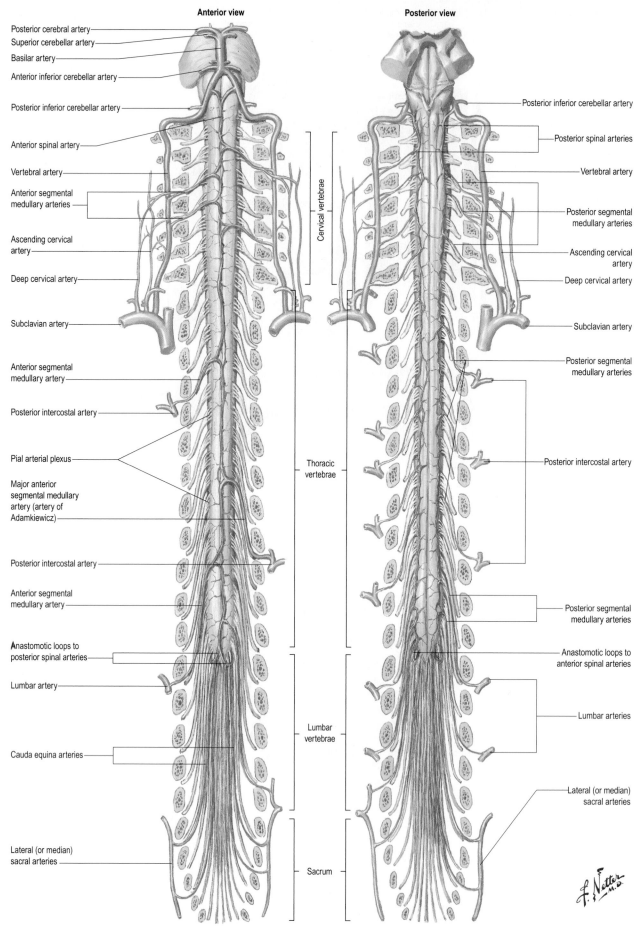

Anterior view

Posterior cerebral artery

Superior cerebellar artery

Basilar artery

Anterior inferior cerebellar artery

Posterior inferior cerebellar artery

Anterior spinal artery

Vertebral artery

Anterior segmental
medullary arteries

Ascending cervical
artery

Deep cervical artery

Subclavian artery

Anterior segmental
medullary artery

Posterior intercostal artery

Pial arterial plexus

Major anterior
segmental medullary
artery (artery of
Adamkiewicz)

Posterior intercostal artery

Anterior segmental
medullary artery

Anastomotic loops to
posterior spinal arteries

Lumbar artery

Cauda equina arteries

Lateral (or median)
sacral arteries

Posterior view

Posterior inferior cerebellar artery

Posterior spinal arteries

Vertebral artery

Posterior segmental
medullary arteries

Ascending cervical
artery

Deep cervical artery

Subclavian artery

Posterior segmental
medullary arteries

Posterior intercostal artery

Posterior segmental
medullary arteries

Anastomotic loops to
anterior spinal arteries

Lumbar arteries

Lateral (or median)
sacral arteries

Cervical vertebrae

Thoracic
vertebrae

Lumbar
vertebrae

Sacrum

Fig. 6.23 *Arteries of the spinal cord. (Netter illustration from www.netterimages.com. © Elsevier Inc. All rights reserved.)*

Vascular Supply of Spinal Cord, Roots and Nerves

Arteries

The spinal cord, its roots and nerves are supplied with blood by both longitudinal and segmental vessels. Three major longitudinal vessels—a single anterior and two posterior spinal arteries (each of which is sometimes doubled to pass on either side of the dorsal rootlets)—originate intracranially from the vertebral artery and terminate in a plexus around the conus medullaris (Fig. 6.23). The anterior spinal artery forms from the fused anterior spinal branches of the vertebral artery and descends in the anterior median fissure of the cord. Each posterior spinal artery originates either directly from the ipsilateral vertebral artery or from its posterior inferior cerebellar branch and descends in a posterolateral sulcus of the cord. The segmental arteries are derived in craniocaudal sequence from spinal branches of the vertebral, deep cervical, intercostal and lumbar arteries. These vessels enter the vertebral canal through the intervertebral foramina and anastomose with branches of the longitudinal vessels to form a pial plexus on the surface of the cord. The segmental spinal arteries send anterior and posterior radicular branches to the spinal cord along the ventral and dorsal roots. Most anterior radicular arteries are small and end in the ventral nerve roots or in the pial plexus of the cord. The small posterior radicular arteries also supply the dorsal root ganglia; branches enter at both ganglionic poles to be distributed around ganglion cells and nerve fibres.

Segmental Medullary Feeder Arteries — Some radicular arteries, mainly situated in the lower cervical, lower thoracic and upper lumbar regions, are large enough to reach the anterior median sulcus, where they divide into slender ascending and large descending branches. These are the anterior medullary feeder arteries (Dommisse 1975). They anastomose with the anterior spinal arteries to form a single or partly double longitudinal vessel of uneven calibre along the anterior median sulcus. The largest anterior medullary feeder, the great anterior segmental medullary artery of Adamkiewicz, varies in level, arising from a spinal branch of one of the lower posterior intercostal arteries (T9–11) or subcostal artery (T12) or, less frequently, a spinal branch of the upper lumbar arteries (L1 and L2). It most often arises on the left side (Carmichael and Gloviczki 1999). Reaching the spinal cord, it sends a branch to the anterior spinal artery below and another to anastomose with the ramus of the posterior spinal artery, which lies anterior to the dorsal roots. It may be the main supply to the lower two-thirds of the cord. Central branches of the anterior spinal artery enter the anterior median fissure and then turn right or left to supply the ventral grey column, the base of the dorsal grey column, including the dorsal nucleus, and the adjacent white matter (Fig. 6.24).

Each posterior spinal artery contributes to a pair of longitudinal anastomotic channels, anterior and posterior to the dorsal spinal roots. These are reinforced by posterior medullary feeders from the posterior radicular arteries. The latter are variable in number and size but are smaller, more numerous and more evenly distributed than the anterior medullary feeders. The anterior channel is joined by a ramus from the descending branch of the great anterior

segmental medullary artery of Adamkiewicz. In all longitudinal spinal arteries, the width of the lumen is uneven, and complete interruptions may occur. At the conus medullaris, they communicate by anastomotic loops. Anastomoses other than those between the pial or peripheral spinal arterial branches may be important, such as a posterior spinal series of anastomoses between rami of the dorsal divisions of segmental arteries near the spinous processes.

Intramedullary Arteries — The central branches of the anterior spinal artery supply about two-thirds of the cross-sectional area of the cord. The rest of the dorsal grey and white columns and peripheral parts of the lateral and ventral white columns are supplied by numerous small radial vessels that branch from posterior spinal arteries and the pial plexus. In a microangiographic study of the human cervical spinal cord, up to six anterior and eight posterior radicular spinal arteries were described, and up to eight central branches arose from each centimetre of the anterior spinal artery (Turnbull, Brieg and Hassler 1966).

Spinal Cord Ischaemia — The spinal cord cannot rely entirely on the longitudinal arteries for either its transverse or its longitudinal blood supply. The anterior longitudinal artery and the intramedullary arteries are functional end-arteries, although overlapping territories of supply have been described. Damage to the anterior longitudinal artery can result in loss of function of the anterior two-thirds of the cord. The longitudinal arteries cannot supply the whole length of the cord, and the input of the segmental medullary feeder vessels is essential. This is especially true of the artery of Adamkiewicz (great

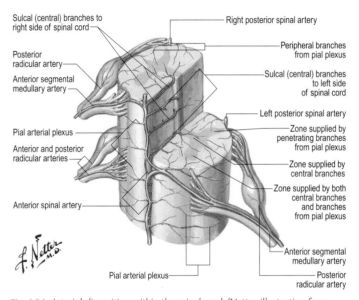

Sulcal (central) branches to right side of spinal cord

Posterior radicular artery

Anterior segmental medullary artery

Pial arterial plexus

Anterior and posterior radicular arteries

Anterior spinal artery

Right posterior spinal artery

Peripheral branches from pial plexus

Sulcal (central) branches to left side of spinal cord

Left posterior spinal artery

Zone supplied by penetrating branches from pial plexus

Zone supplied by central branches

Zone supplied by both central branches and branches from pial plexus

Anterior segmental medullary artery

Pial arterial plexus

Posterior radicular artery

Fig. 6.24 *Arterial disposition within the spinal cord. (Netter illustration from www.netterimages.com. © Elsevier Inc. All rights reserved.)*

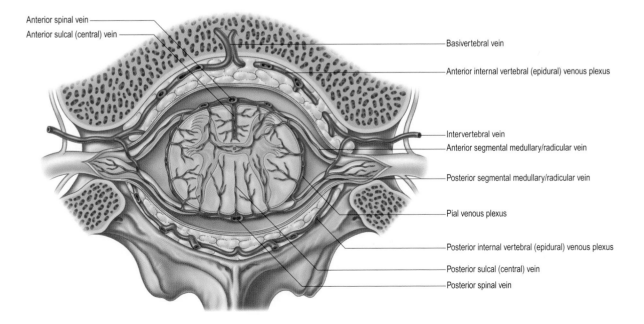

Anterior spinal vein

Anterior sulcal (central) vein

Basivertebral vein

Anterior internal vertebral (epidural) venous plexus

Intervertebral vein

Anterior segmental medullary/radicular vein

Posterior segmental medullary/radicular vein

Pial venous plexus

Posterior internal vertebral (epidural) venous plexus

Posterior sulcal (central) vein

Posterior spinal vein

Fig. 6.25 *Venous disposition within the spinal cord.*

anterior segmental medullary artery), which may effectively carry the major supply for the lower cord. The midthoracic cord, distant from the main anterior medullary feeders, is particularly liable to become ischaemic after periods of hypotension.

Veins

The venous drainage of the spinal cord (Fig. 6.25) follows a similar pattern to that of its arterial supply (Gillilan 1970). Intramedullary veins within the substance of the cord drain into a plexus of surface veins, the coronal plexus. There are six tortuous longitudinal channels within this plexus—one in each of the anterior and posterior median fissures, and four others that run on either side of the ventral and dorsal nerve roots. Only the anterior median vein, which drains the central grey matter, is consistently complete. These vessels connect freely. They drain superiorly into the cerebellar veins and cranial sinuses and segmentally into mainly the medullary veins. These segmental veins drain into the intervertebral veins and then into the external vertebral venous plexuses, the caval and azygos systems.

Segmental Veins — Anterior and posterior medullary veins run along some of the ventral and dorsal roots. They are larger than radicular veins and drain the cord but not the roots themselves. Like the medullary feeder arteries, they are largest in the cervical and lumbar regions of the cord but do not necessarily occur in the same segments as the medullary feeders. Anterior and posterior great medullary veins may arise in the lower thoracic or upper lumbar cord segments. There are 8 to 14 anterior medullary veins. Posterior medullary veins are more numerous.

Very small anterior and posterior radicular veins occur in most spinal segments, accompanying and draining the ventral and dorsal roots and some of the cord at the points of entry and exit of the rootlets. They usually drain into the intervertebral veins.

References

Batson, O.V., 1957. The vertebral vein system. AJR Am. J. Roentgenol. 78, 195–212. *A pioneering study of the venous plexuses of the vertebral column that has become the standard reference in its field.*

Boelderl, A., Daniaux, H., Kathrein, A., Maurer, H., 2002. Danger of damaging the medial branches of the posterior rami of spinal nerves during a dorsomedian approach to the spine. Clin. Anat. 15, 77–81. *Detailed descriptions of the vascular supply and innervation of the posterior elements of the thoracolumbar spine and the overlying muscles.*

Carmichael, S.W., Gloviczki, P., 1999. Anatomy of the blood supply to the spinal cord: the artery of Adamkiewicz revisited. Perspect. Vasc. Surg. 12, 113–122.

Crock, H.V., 1996. Atlas of Vascular Anatomy of the Skeleton and Spinal Cord. Martin Dunitz, London.

Crock, H.V., Yoshizawa, H., 1976. The blood supply of the lumbar vertebral column. Clin. Orthop. 115, 6–21.

Dommisse, G.F., 1975. The Arteries and Veins of the Human Spinal Cord from Birth. Churchill Livingstone, Edinburgh.

Duvernoy, H.M., Delon, S., Vannson, J.L., 1981. Cortical blood vessels of the human brain. Brain Res. Bull. 7, 519–579.

Duvernoy, H., Delon, S., Vannson, J.L., 1983. The vascularization of the human cerebellar cortex. Brain Res. Bull. 11, 419–480.

Gillilan, L.A., 1970. Veins of the spinal cord: anatomic details, suggested clinical applications. Neurology 20, 860–868.

Kaplan, H.A., Ford, D.H., 1966. The Brain Vascular System. Elsevier, Amsterdam.

Plets, C., De Reuck, J., Vander Eecken, H., Van den Bergh, R., 1970. The vascularization of the human thalamus. Acta. Neurol. Belg. 70, 687–770.

Puchades-Orts, A., Nombela-Gomez, M., Ortuño-Pacheco, G., 1976. Variation in form of the circle of Willis: some anatomical and embryological considerations. Anat. Rec. 185, 119–123.

Sengupta, R.P., McAllister, V.L. (Eds.), 1986. Subarachnoid Haemorrhage. Springer-Verlag, Berlin, pp. 9–31. *Includes details on variations of the circle of Willis.*

Turnbull, I.M., Brieg, A., Hassler, O., 1966. Blood supply of cervical spinal cord in man: a microangiographic cadaver study. J. Neurosurg. 24, 951–965.

Section II

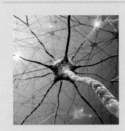

The Spine

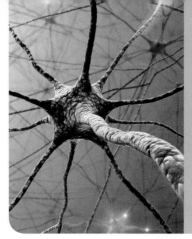

Spinal Column

Chapter 7

SPINAL CORD AND ITS COVERINGS

The surface relationships of the spinal cord and its coverings are of great clinical importance throughout life (Fig. 7.1).

During development the vertebral column elongates more rapidly than the spinal cord, which leads to an increasing discrepancy between the anatomical level of spinal cord segments and their corresponding vertebrae. At stage 23, the vertebral column and spinal cord are the same length, and the cord ends at the last coccygeal vertebra; this arrangement continues until the third fetal month. At birth the spinal cord terminates at the lower border of the second lumbar vertebra and may sometimes reach the third lumbar vertebra. In the adult the spinal cord is said to terminate at the level of the disc between the first and second lumbar vertebral bodies, which lies a little above the level of the elbow joint when the arm is by the side and also lies approximately in the transpyloric plane. However, there is considerable variation in the level at which the spinal cord ends. It may end below this level in as many as 40% of subjects, or opposite the body of either the first or second lumbar vertebra; occasionally, it ends opposite the twelfth thoracic or even the third lumbar vertebra.

The dural sac (theca), and thus the subarachnoid space and its contained cerebrospinal fluid (CSF), usually extends to the level of the second segment of the sacrum. This corresponds to the line joining the sacral dimples located in the skin over the posterior superior iliac spines. Occasionally, the dural sac ends as high as the fifth lumbar vertebra, and very rarely it may extend to the third part of the sacrum, in which case it is occasionally possible to enter the subarachnoid space inadvertently during the course of a sacral nerve block.

CLINICAL EXAMINATION

Clinical examination of the back of the trunk and neck best follows the order of inspection, palpation and movement. The examination is determined by the presentation and by the history, and it may include musculoskeletal, neurological and vascular observations. Information relevant to the neurological and vascular examination of the skin and material relating to spinal movements and deeper innervation are presented later. Palpation of the region involves careful assessment of the bony and musculotendinous landmarks described earlier, looking in particular for asymmetry, deformity and tenderness. Note that, apart from the spines, most of the bony elements of the vertebrae and almost all the intervertebral joints are not palpable from behind. In regions of lordosis (sagittal plane curves of the spine with anterior convexity, such as mid-cervical and mid and lower lumbar), parts of the vertebral column can often be palpated anteriorly with care in well-relaxed, thin subjects.

CLINICAL PROCEDURES

Access to Cerebrospinal Fluid

The safest approach to the CSF is to enter the lumbar cistern of the subarachnoid space in the midline, well below the level at which the spinal cord normally terminates (see Fig. 7.1). The fine needle employed is unlikely to damage the mobile nerve roots of the cauda equina. This procedure is called lumbar puncture. It is also possible to access the CSF by midline puncture of the cerebellomedullary cistern (cisterna magna); this is called cisternal puncture.

Lumbar Puncture: Adult

Lumbar puncture in the adult may be performed with the patient either sitting or lying on the side on a firm, flat surface. In each position, the lumbar spine must be flexed as far as possible to separate the vertebral spines maximally and expose the ligamentum flavum in the interlaminar window (Fig. 7.2). A line between the highest points of the iliac crests intersects the vertebral column just above the palpable spine of L4. With the spines now identified, the skin is anaesthetized and a needle is inserted between the spines of L3 and L4 (or L4 and L5). Exact identification of the level by palpation is difficult (Broadbent et al 2000). The soft tissues the needle will ultimately traverse should also be anaesthetized, but care should be taken to avoid injection of an excessive amount of local anaesthetic, which can compromise one's appreciation of the structures being traversed. These include the subcutaneous fat and supraspinous and interspinous ligaments down to the ligamentum flavum itself. The lumbar puncture needle is then inserted in the midline or just to one side and angled in the horizontal and sagittal planes sufficiently to pierce the ligamentum flavum in or very near the midline (Fig. 7.3).There is a slight loss of resistance as the needle enters the epidural space, and careful advancement pierces the dura and arachnoid to release CSF.

Lumbar Puncture: Neonate and Infant

At full term (40 weeks) the spinal cord usually terminates somewhat lower than the adult level, sometimes reaching the body of L3. The supracristal plane intersects the vertebral column slightly higher (L3–4). By the second postnatal month, the level of cord termination has usually reached its permanent position, level with the body of the first lumbar vertebra. The lower end of the subarachnoid spine is found at sacral level 1 or 2. These differences must be borne in mind when identifying landmarks before undertaking lumbar puncture in neonates and infants.

A lumbar puncture is performed by placing the baby in a position, either lying or 'sitting,' that gives maximum convex curvature to the lumbar spine. A needle with trocar is inserted into the back between the spines of the third and fourth lumbar vertebrae and into the subarachnoid space below the level of the conus medullaris. The space between L3 and L4 is approximately level with the iliac crests, and the needle and trocar are usually inserted into the intervertebral space immediately above or below the iliac crests.

Cisternal Puncture

In cisternal puncture, the cisterna magna is entered by midline puncture through the posterior atlanto-occipital membrane. Further details of this difficult specialist technique are beyond the scope of this book.

Access to the Epidural Space

The epidural 'space' lies between the spinal dura and the wall of the vertebral canal. It contains epidural fat and a venous plexus. Access to this space, usually in the lumbar region, is required for the administration of anaesthetic and analgesic drugs and for endoscopy. The caudal route is used mainly for analgesic injections.

Lumbar Epidural

For access to the lumbar epidural space, the approach is as for lumbar puncture. The intention in epidural injection is to avoid dural puncture, so it is best to enter the epidural space in the midline posteriorly, where the depth of the space is greatest. Techniques for entering the epidural space rely on the appreciation of loss of resistance to injection of the chosen medium (usually air or saline) as the space is entered. There is very little distance between the ligamentum flavum and the underlying dura on either side of the median plane.

Caudal Epidural

The route of access to the caudal epidural space is via the sacral hiatus. The space is thus entered below the level of termination of the dural sac (S2). With the patient in the lateral position or lying prone over a pelvic pillow, the sacral hiatus is identified by palpation of the sacral cornua (Fig. 7.4). These are felt at the upper end of the natal cleft approximately 5 cm above the tip of the coccyx. Alternatively, the sacral hiatus may be identified by constructing an equilateral triangle based on a line joining the posterior superior iliac spines: the inferior apex of this triangle overlies the hiatus. After local anaesthetic infiltration, a needle is introduced at a 45-degree angle to the skin to

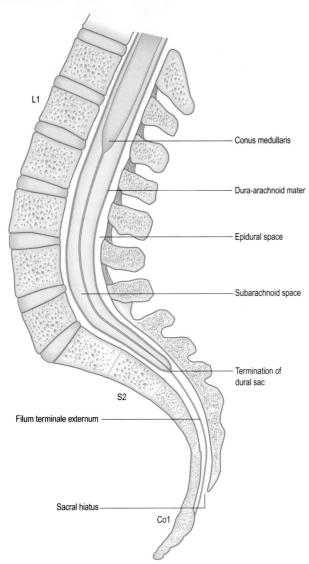

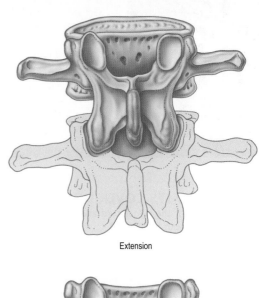

Extension

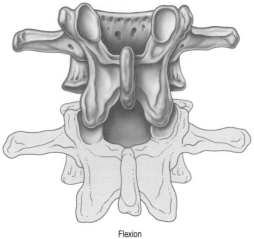

Flexion

Fig. 7.2 *Lumbar interlaminar window in extension and flexion.*

Fig. 7.1 *Contents of the vertebral canal in the lumbosacral region. (Modified with permission from Mackintosh, R.R. 1951. Lumbar Puncture and Spinal Analgesia. E&S Livingstone, Edinburgh.)*

penetrate the posterior sacrococcygeal ligament and enter the sacral canal. Once the canal is entered, the hub of the needle is lowered so that the needle may pass along the canal (Fig. 7.5). If the needle is angled too obliquely it will strike bone; if it is placed too superficially it will lie outside the canal. The latter malposition can be confirmed by careful injection of air while palpating the skin over the lower sacrum.

Thoracic and Cervical Epidurals

It is possible to access the epidural space at the thoracic and cervical levels, but the specialist techniques required are outside the scope of this book. The principles are the same as those for lumbar epidurals, but the special anatomy of the vertebral spines at the other levels requires the angle of approach to be modified.

VERTEBRAL COLUMN

The vertebral column is a curved linkage of individual bones or vertebrae (Figs 7.6, 7.7). A continuous series of vertebral foramina runs through the articulated vertebrae posterior to their bodies and collectively constitutes the vertebral canal, which transmits and protects the spinal cord and nerve roots, their coverings and vasculature. A series of paired lateral intervertebral foramina transmit the spinal nerves and their associated vessels between adjacent vertebrae. The linkages between the vertebrae include cartilaginous interbody joints and paired synovial facet (zygapophyseal) joints (Fig. 7.8), together with a complex of ligaments and overlying muscles and fasciae. The muscles directly concerned with vertebral movements and attached to the column lie mainly posteriorly. Several large muscles producing major spinal movements lie distant from the column and have no direct attachment to it, such as the anterolateral abdominal wall musculature. The column as a whole receives its vascular supply and innervation according to the general anatomical principles considered later in this chapter.

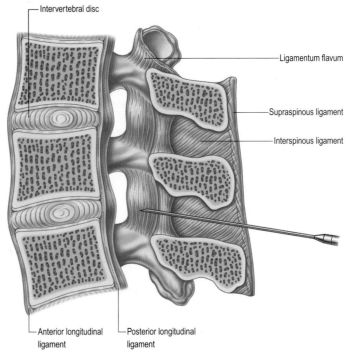

Fig. 7.3 *Position of the needle in lumbar puncture.*

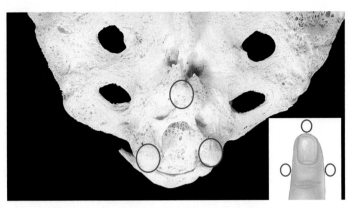

Fig. 7.4 *Palpation of the sacral cornua for caudal epidural injection. (With permission from Ellis, H., Feldman, S.A. 1997. Anatomy for Anaesthetists, 7th ed. Blackwell Science, Oxford.)*

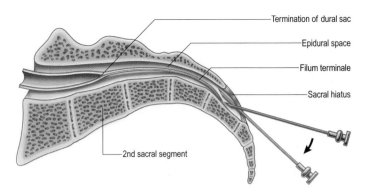

Termination of dural sac

Epidural space

Filum terminale

Sacral hiatus

2nd sacral segment

Fig. 7.5 *Position of the needle in caudal epidural injection.*

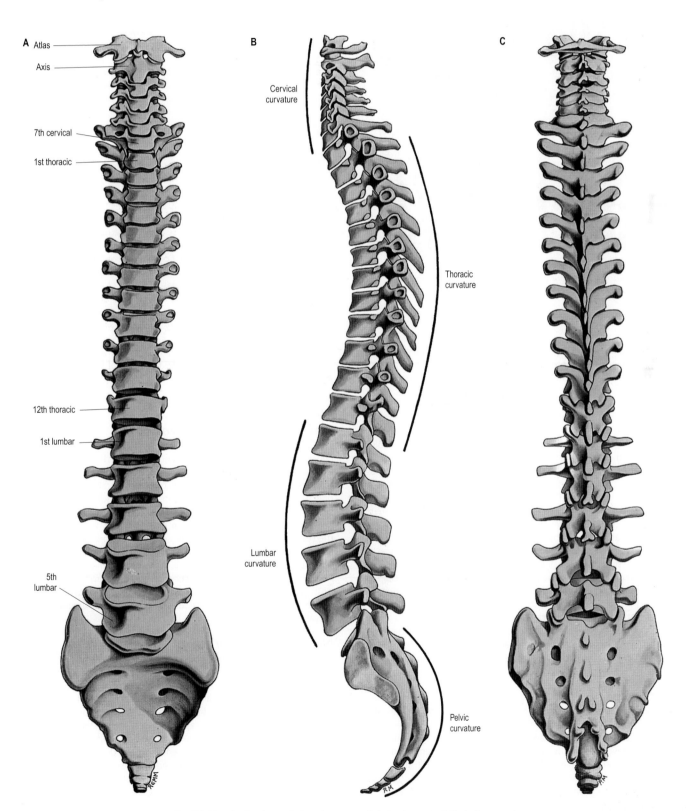

A Atlas

Axis

7th cervical

1st thoracic

12th thoracic

1st lumbar

5th lumbar

B Cervical curvature

Thoracic curvature

Lumbar curvature

Pelvic curvature

C

Fig. 7.6 *Vertebral column. A, Anterior aspect. B, Lateral aspect. C, Posterior aspect.*

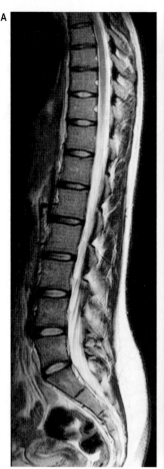
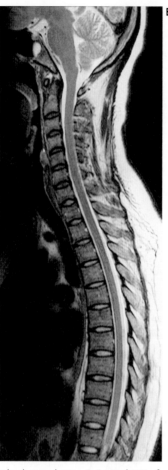

A

B

Fig. 7.7 *A, Sagittal MRI of the thoracolumbosacral spine. B, Sagittal MRI of the cervicothoracic spine. (Courtesy of Dr. Justin Lee, Chelsea and Westminster Hospital, London.)*

Vertebral column morphology is influenced externally by mechanical and environmental factors and internally by genetic, metabolic and hormonal factors. These all affect its ability to react to the dynamic forces of everyday life, such as compression, traction and shear. These dynamic forces can vary in magnitude and are influenced by occupation, locomotion and posture.

The adult vertebral column usually consists of 33 vertebral segments. Each presacral segment (except the first two cervical) is separated from its neighbour by a fibrocartilaginous intervertebral disc. The functions of the column are to support the trunk, protect the spinal cord and nerves and provide attachments for muscles. It is also an important site of haemopoiesis throughout life. The total length of the vertebral column is approximately 70 cm in males and 60 cm in females. The intervertebral discs contribute about one-quarter of this length in young adults, although there is some diurnal variation in this contribution. Approximately 8% of overall body length is accounted for by the cervical spine, 20% by the thoracic, 12% by the lumbar and 8% by the sacrococcygeal regions. Although the usual number of vertebrae is 7 cervical, 12 thoracic, 5 lumbar, 5 sacral and 4 coccygeal, this total is often variable, with reports of between 32 and 35 bones. The demarcation of groups by their morphological characteristics may be blurred. Thus, there may be thoracic costal facets on the seventh cervical vertebra, giving it the appearance of an extra thoracic vertebra; lumbar-like articular processes may be found on the lowest thoracic vertebra or the fifth lumbar vertebra may be wholly or partially incorporated into the sacrum. As a result of these changes in transition between vertebral types, there may be 23 to 25 mobile presacral vertebrae.

Anterior Aspect

The anterior aspect of the column is formed by the anterior surfaces of the vertebral bodies and of the intervertebral discs (see Fig. 7.6A). It has important anatomical relations at all levels and should be considered in continuity. It forms part of several clinically significant junctional or transitional zones, including the prevertebral–retropharyngeal zone of the neck, the thoracic inlet, the diaphragm and the pelvic inlet. The anterior aspect of the column is covered centrally by the anterior longitudinal ligament, which forms a

fascial plane with the prevertebral and endothoracic fascia and with the subperitoneal areolar tissue of the posterior abdominal wall. Infection and other pathological processes may spread along this fascial plane.

Lateral Aspect

The lateral aspect of the vertebral column is arbitrarily separated from the posterior by articular processes in the cervical and lumbar regions and by transverse processes in the thoracic region (see Fig. 7.6B). Anteriorly, it is formed by the sides of vertebral bodies and intervertebral discs. The oval intervertebral foramina, behind the bodies and between the pedicles, are smallest at the cervical and upper thoracic levels and progressively increase in size in the thoracic and upper lumbar regions. The lumbosacral (L5–S1) intervertebral foramen is the smallest of the lumbar foramina. The foramina permit communication between the lumen of the vertebral canal and the paravertebral soft tissues (a 'paravertebral space' is sometimes described), which may be important in the spread of tumours and other pathological processes. The lateral aspects of the column have important anatomical relations, some of which vary considerably between the two sides.

Posterior Aspect

The posterior aspect of the column is formed by the posterior surfaces of the laminae and spinous processes, their associated ligaments and the facet joints (see Fig. 7.6C). It is covered by the deep muscles of the back.

Structural Defects of the Posterior Bony Elements

Deformity and bony deficiency may occur at several sites within the posterior elements. The laminae may be wholly or partially absent, or the spinous process alone may be affected, even without overlying soft tissue signs (spina bifida occulta). A defect may occur in the part of the lamina between the superior and inferior articular processes (pars interarticularis); this condition is called spondylolysis, and it may be developmental or result from acute or fatigue fracture. If such defects are bilateral, the column becomes unstable at that level, and forward displacement of that part of the column above (cranial to) the defects may occur; this is called spondylolisthesis. Abnormality of the laminar bone or degenerative changes in the facet joints may lead to similar displacement in the absence of pars defects. The deformity of the vertebral canal, resulting from severe spondylolisthesis, may lead to neural damage. Much more rarely, bony defects may occur elsewhere in the posterior elements, such as in the pedicles.

Detailed anatomical relations of all aspects of the vertebral column at the various levels are best appreciated by the study of horizontal (axial) sections and images.

Curvatures
Embryonic and Fetal Curvatures

The embryonic body appears flexed. It has primary thoracic and pelvic curves that are convex dorsally. Functional muscle development leads to the early appearance of secondary cervical and lumbar spinal curvatures in the sagittal plane. The cervical curvature appears at the end of the embryonic period and reflects the development of function in the muscles responsible for head extension, an important component of the 'grasp reflex.' Radiographic examination of human fetuses aged 8 to 23 weeks shows that the secondary cervical curvature is almost always present. Lumbar flattening has also been identified as early as the eighth week. Ultrasound investigations support the role of movement in the development of these curvatures. The early appearance of the secondary curves is probably accentuated by postnatal muscular and nervous system development at a time when the vertebral column is highly flexible and is capable of assuming almost any curvature.

Neonatal Curvatures

In the neonate the vertebral column has no fixed curvatures. It is particularly flexible and, if dissected free from the body, can easily be bent (flexed or extended) into a perfect half circle. A slight sacral curvature may develop as the sacral vertebrae ossify and fuse. The thoracic part of the column is the first to develop a relatively fixed curvature, which is concave anteriorly. An infant can support its head at approximately 3 or 4 months, can sit upright at 9 months and commences walking between 12 and 15 months. These functional changes exert a major influence on the development of secondary curvatures in the vertebral column and changes in the proportional size of the vertebrae, particularly in the lumbar region. The secondary lumbar curvature becomes important in maintaining the centre of gravity of the trunk

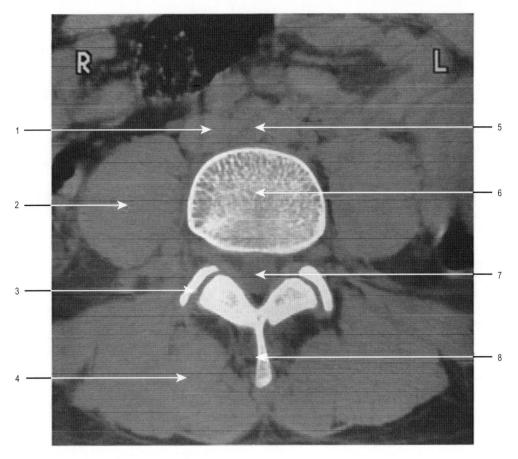

1. Inferior vena cava.
2. Psoas major.
3. Facet synovial joint between L4 and 5.
4. Erector spinae muscle mass.
5. Bifurcation of aorta.
6. Fourth lumbar vertebral body.
7. Thecal sac.
8. Spinous process.

Fig. 7.8 *High-resolution computed tomogram through the posterior abdominal wall at the level of the body of the fourth lumbar vertebra, showing zygapophyseal joints between the fourth and fifth lumbar vertebrae.*

over the legs when walking starts; thus, changes in body proportions exert a major influence on the subsequent shape of curvatures in the vertebral column.

Adult Curvatures

In adults, the cervical curve is a lordosis (convex forward) and is the least marked. It extends from the atlas to the second thoracic vertebra, with its apex between the fourth and fifth cervical vertebrae. Sexual dimorphism has been described in cervical curvatures. The thoracic curve is a kyphosis (convex dorsally). It extends between the second and the eleventh or twelfth thoracic vertebrae, and its apex lies between the sixth and ninth thoracic vertebrae. This curvature is caused by the increased posterior depth of the thoracic vertebral bodies. The lumbar curve is also a lordosis. It has a greater magnitude in females and extends from the twelfth thoracic vertebra to the lumbosacral angle; there is increased convexity of the last three segments as a result of the greater anterior depth of the intervertebral discs and some posterior wedging of the vertebral bodies. Its apex is at the level of the third lumbar vertebra. The pelvic curve is concave anteroinferiorly and involves the sacrum and coccygeal vertebrae. It extends from the lumbosacral junction to the apex of the coccyx.

The presence of these curvatures means that the cross-sectional profile of the trunk changes with the spinal level. The anteroposterior diameter of the thorax is much greater than that of the lower abdomen. In the normal vertebral column there are well-marked curvatures in the sagittal plane and no lateral curvatures other than in the upper thoracic region, where there is often a slight lateral curvature that is convex to the right in right-handed persons and to the left in left-handed persons. Compensatory lateral curvature may

also develop to cope with pelvic obliquity, such as that imposed by unequal leg lengths. The sagittal curvatures are present in the cervical, thoracic, lumbar and pelvic regions (see Fig. 7.6). These curvatures developed with rounding of the thorax and pelvis as an adaptation to bipedal gait.

Vertebral Column in the Elderly

In older people, age-related changes in the structure of bone lead to broadening and loss of height of the vertebral bodies. These changes are more severe in females. The bony changes in the vertebral column are accompanied by changes in the collagen content of the discs and by decline in the activity of the spinal muscles. This leads to progressive decline in vertebral column mobility, particularly in the lumbar spine. The development of a 'dowager's hump' in the midthoracic region in females, caused by age-related osteoporosis, increases the thoracic kyphosis and cervical lordosis. Overall, these changes in the vertebral column lead directly to loss of total height in the individual.

In the mid-lumbar region, the width of the vertebral body increases with age. In men, there is a relative decrease of posterior-to-anterior body height; in both sexes anterior height decreases relative to width. Twomey and coworkers (1983) observed a reduction in bone density of lumbar vertebral bodies with age, principally as a result of a reduction in transverse trabeculae (more marked in females owing to postmenopausal osteoporosis); this was associated with increased diameter and increasing concavity in the juxtadiscal surfaces (end-plates).

Other changes affect the vertebral bodies. Osteophytes (bony spurs) may form from the compact cortical bone on the anterior and lateral surfaces of the bodies. Although individual variations occur, these changes appear in most

CASE 1   ACUTE LUMBAR DISC HERNIATION

A healthy 58-year-old man sneezes violently and immediately develops sharp pain in his right lower back, radiating over the right buttock and down the posterolateral aspect of the right thigh and calf. Because of acute paravertebral muscle spasm, he cannot stand erect. Pain is increased with coughing or straining or with attempted back movement and is accompanied by pins and needles paraesthesia down the lateral calf to the ankle.

Examination demonstrates paravertebral muscle spasm, impaired pain appreciation along the right lateral calf, weakness of the extensor hallucis longus muscle and loss of the right Achilles tendon reflex.

Discussion: This is a classic presentation of radicular pain (i.e. sciatica) secondary to an acute lateral intervertebral disc protrusion at L5–S1 (Fig. 7.9). Typically, there is narrowing of the intervertebral disc space at the involved segment. The herniated disc fragment can be identified by magnetic resonance imaging (MRI).

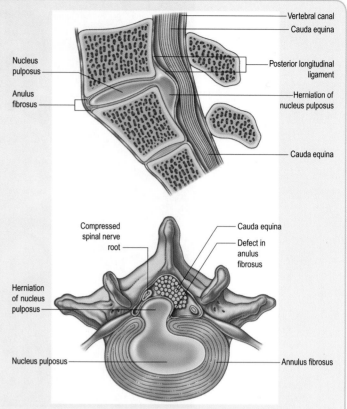

Fig. 7.9 *Posterolateral disc prolapse. (By permission from Moore, K., Agur, A.M.R. 2002. Essential Clinical Anatomy, 2nd ed. Lippincott Williams and Wilkins, Philadelphia.)*

individuals from about age 20 years onward. They are most common on the anterior aspect of the body and never involve the ring epiphysis. Osteophytic spurs are frequently asymptomatic but may result in diminished movements within the spine.

References

Adams, M.A., Bogduk, N., Burton, K., Dolan, P., 2002. The Biomechanics of Back Pain. Churchill Livingstone, Edinburgh. *A comprehensive and detailed source of information on the functional anatomy, tissue biology and biomechanics of the lumbar spine.*

Bogduk, N., 1997. Clinical Anatomy of the Lumbar Spine and Sacrum, third ed. Churchill Livingstone, Edinburgh.

Broadbent, C.R., Maxwell, W.E., Ferrie, R., Wilson, D.J., Gawne-Cain, M., Russell, R., 2000. Ability of anaesthetists to identify a marked lumbar interspace. Anaesthesia 55, 1122–1126.

Denis, F., 1983. The three column spine and its significance in the classification of acute thoraco-lumbar spinal injuries. Spine 8, 817–831. *Seminal paper for the understanding and classification of spinal instability.*

Dvorák, J., Vajda, E.G., Grob, D., Panjabi, M.M., 1995. Normal motion of the lumbar spine related to age and gender. Eur. Spine J. 4, 18–23.

Frobin, W., Leivseth, G., Biggeman, M., Brinckmann, P., 2002. Sagittal plane segmental motion of the cervical spine: a new precision measurement protocol and normal motion data of healthy adults. Clin. Biomech. 17, 21–31.

MacLaughlin, S.M., Oldale, K.N.M., 1992. Vertebral body diameters and sex prediction. Ann. Hum. Biol. 19, 285–293. *Describes the archaeological and forensic examination of skeletal material.*

MacNab, I., McCulloch, J., 1990. Backache, second ed. Williams and Wilkins, Baltimore, Chapter 1. *Functional anatomy of the lumbar spine, described as a basis for the clinical management of low back pain.*

McGregor, A.H., McCarthy, I.D., Hughes, S.P.F., 1995. Motion characteristics of the lumbar spine in the normal population. Spine 20 (22), 2421–2428.

Newell, R.L.M., 1999. The spinal epidural space. Clin. Anat. 12, 375–379. *Review of the morphological, developmental and topographical aspects of the spinal epidural space.*

Ordway, N.R., Seymour, R., Donelson, R.G., Hojnowski, L., Lee, E., Edwards, T., 1997. Cervical sagittal range of motion using three methods. Spine 22, 501–508.

Pearcy, M., Protek, I., Shepherd, J., 1984. Three-dimensional X-ray analysis of normal movement in the lumbar spine. Spine 9, 294–297.

Pearcy, M., Tibrewal, S.B., 1984. Axial rotation and lateral bending in the normal lumbar spine. Spine 9, 582–587.

Taylor, J.R., Twomey, L.T., 1984. Sexual dimorphism in human vertebral shape. J. Anat. 138, 281–286. *Anthropometric and radiological studies of children and adolescents.*

Trott, P.H., Pearcy, M.J., Ruston, S.A., Fulton, I., Brien, C., 1996. Three-dimensional analysis of active cervical motion: the effect of age and gender. Clin. Biomech. 11, 201–206.

Twomey, L.T., Taylor, J.R., Furniss, B., 1983. Age changes in the bone density and structure of the lumbar vertebral column. J. Anat. 136, 15–25.

White, A.A., Panjabi, M.M., 1990. Clinical Biomechanics of the Spine, second ed. JB Lippincott, Philadelphia.

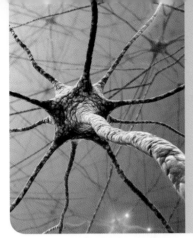

Spinal Cord and Nerve Roots

The spinal cord provides innervation for the trunk and limbs through the paired spinal nerves and their peripheral ramifications. Through them it receives primary afferent fibres from peripheral receptors located in widespread somatic and visceral structures. It also sends motor axons to skeletal muscle and provides autonomic innervation of cardiac and smooth muscle and secretory glands. Many functions are regulated by intraspinal reflex connections. Profuse ascending and descending pathways link the spinal cord with the brain. They allow higher centres to monitor and perceive external and internal stimuli and modulate and control spinal efferent activity.

The spinal cord is essentially a segmental structure. It gives rise to 31 pairs of segmentally arranged spinal nerves, which are attached to the cord by a linear series of dorsal and ventral rootlets. Dorsal rootlets contain afferent nerve fibres, and ventral rootlets contain efferent fibres (see Fig. 1.5). Groups of adjacent rootlets coalesce to form dorsal or ventral nerve roots. These cross the subarachnoid space and unite to form functionally mixed spinal nerves as they pass through the intervertebral foramina. The dorsal roots bear dorsal root ganglia, which contain the cell bodies of primary afferent neurones.

TOPOGRAPHICAL ANATOMY OF THE SPINAL CORD

Macroscopic Anatomy of the Spinal Cord and Spinal Nerves

The gross anatomy of the structures that lie within the vertebral canal and its extensions through the intervertebral foramina, the spinal nerve or radicular ('root') canals is the subject of this chapter. The spinal cord, its blood vessels and nerve roots lie within a meningeal sheath, the theca, which occupies the central zone of the vertebral canal and extends from the foramen magnum, where it is in continuity with the meningeal coverings of the brain, to the level of the second sacral vertebra in the adult. Distal to this level the dura extends as a fine cord, the filum terminale externum, which fuses with the posterior periosteum of the first coccygeal segment. Tubular prolongations of the dural sheath extend around the spinal roots and nerves into the lateral zones of the vertebral canal and out into the 'root' canals, eventually fusing with the epineurium of the spinal nerves. Between the theca and the walls of the vertebral canal is the epidural (spinal extradural) space (Ch. 4), which is loosely filled with fat, connective tissue containing small arteries and lymphatics and an important venous plexus. Three-dimensional appreciation of the anatomy of the spinal theca and its surroundings is essential for the efficient management of spinal pain, spinal injuries, tumours and infections. Equally significant clinically is the anatomy of the often precarious blood supply of the spinal cord and its associated structures. The increasing application and refinement of diagnostic imaging and endoscopic procedures lend new importance to topographical detail here.

SPINAL CORD (MEDULLA)

The spinal cord is an elongated, approximately cylindrical part of the central nervous system, occupying the superior two-thirds of the vertebral canal (Figs 8.1–8.6). Its average length in European males is 45 cm; its weight is approximately 30 g (for dimensional data, consult Barson and Sands 1977). It extends from the upper border of the atlas to the junction between the first and second lumbar vertebrae; this lower level varies, and there is some correlation with the length of the trunk, especially in females. The termination may be as high as the caudal third of the twelfth thoracic vertebra or as low as the disc between the second and third lumbar vertebrae, and its position rises slightly in vertebral flexion. The spinal cord is enclosed in the dura, arachnoid and pia mater, separated from each other by the subdural and subarachnoid spaces, respectively. The former is a potential space, whereas the latter contains cerebrospinal fluid (CSF). The cord is continuous cranially with the medulla oblongata and narrows caudally to the conus medullaris, from whose apex a connective tissue filament, the filum terminale, descends to the dorsum of

the first coccygeal vertebral segment. The spinal cord varies in transverse width, gradually tapering craniocaudally, except at the levels of the cervical and lumbosacral enlargements. It is not cylindrical, being wider transversely at all levels, especially in the cervical segments.

The cervical enlargement is the source of the spinal nerves that supply the upper limbs. It extends from the third cervical to the second thoracic segments; its maximal circumference (approximately 38 mm) is in the sixth cervical segment. (A spinal cord segment provides the attachment of the rootlets of a pair of spinal nerves.)

The lumbar enlargement corresponds to the innervation of the lower limbs and extends from the first lumbar to the third sacral segments, the equivalent vertebral levels being the ninth to twelfth thoracic vertebrae. The greatest circumference (apprpoximately 35 mm) is near the lower part of the body of the twelfth thoracic vertebra, below which it rapidly dwindles into the conus medullaris.

Fissures and sulci extend along most of the external surface of the cord. An anterior median fissure and a posterior median sulcus and septum almost completely separate the cord into right and left halves, but they are joined by a commissural band of nervous tissue that contains a central canal.

The anterior median fissure extends along the whole ventral surface with an average depth of 3 mm, although it is deeper at caudal levels. It contains a reticulum of pia mater. Dorsal to it is the anterior white commissure. Perforating branches of the spinal vessels pass from the fissure to the commissure to supply the central spinal region. The posterior median sulcus is shallower, and from it a posterior median septum of neuroglia penetrates more than halfway into the cord, almost to the central canal. The septum varies in anteroposterior extent from 4 to 6 mm, and it diminishes caudally as the canal becomes more dorsally placed and the cord contracts.

A posterolateral sulcus exists from 1.5 to 2.5 mm lateral to each side of the posterior median sulcus. Dorsal roots (strictly rootlets) of spinal nerves enter the cord along this sulcus. The white substance between the posterior median and posterolateral sulcus on each side is the posterior funiculus. In cervical and upper thoracic segments, a longitudinal posterointermediate sulcus marks a septum dividing each posterior funiculus into two large tracts: the fasciculus gracilis (medial) and the fasciculus cuneatus (lateral). Between the posterolateral sulcus and anterior median fissure is the anterolateral funiculus. This is subdivided into anterior and lateral funiculi by ventral spinal roots that pass through its substance to issue from the surface of the cord. The anterior funiculus is medial to, and includes, the emerging ventral roots; the lateral funiculus lies between the roots and the posterolateral sulcus. In upper cervical segments, nerve rootlets emerge through each lateral funiculus to form the spinal accessory nerve (cranial nerve XI), which ascends in the vertebral canal lateral to the spinal cord and enters the posterior cranial fossa via the foramen magnum (Fig. 8.7).

The filum terminale, a filament of connective tissue approximately 20 cm long, descends from the apex of the conus medullaris. Its upper 15 cm, the filum terminale internum, is continued within extensions of the dural and arachnoid meninges and reaches the caudal border of the second sacral vertebra. Its final 5 cm, the filum terminale externum, fuses with the investing dura mater and then descends to the dorsum of the first coccygeal vertebral segment. The filum is continuous above with the spinal pia mater. A few strands of nerve fibres, which probably represent roots of rudimentary second and third coccygeal spinal nerves, adhere to its upper part. The central canal is continued into the filum for 5 to 6 mm. A capacious part of the subarachnoid space surrounds the filum terminale internum and is the usual access site for lumbar puncture.

DORSAL AND VENTRAL ROOTS

The paired dorsal and ventral roots of the spinal nerves are continuous with the spinal cord (see Figs 8.6 and 8.10). They cross the subarachnoid space and traverse the dura mater separately, uniting in or close to their intervertebral foramina to form the (mixed) spinal nerves. Because the spinal cord is shorter

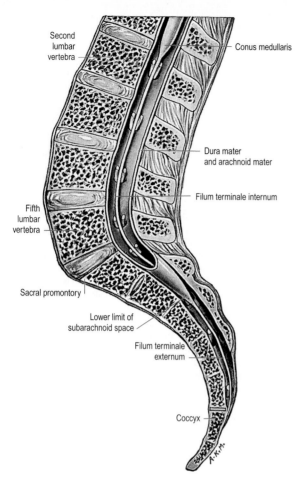

Fig. 8.1 *Median sagittal section of the lumbosacral part of the vertebral column showing the conus medullaris and filum terminale. The section has opened up the subarachnoid space as far as the first sacral vertebra. Note the difference in levels between the inferior limits of the spinal cord and meninges. Note that there are two inaccuracies in this figure: the epidural space is not shown, and the fibres of interspinous ligaments should slope dorsocranially.*

than the vertebral column, the more caudal spinal roots descend for varying distances around and beyond the cord to reach their corresponding foramina. In so doing they form, mostly distal to the apex of the cord, a divergent sheaf of spinal nerve roots, the cauda equina, which is gathered around the filum terminale in the spinal theca.

Ventral spinal roots contain efferent somatic and, at some levels, efferent sympathetic nerve fibres that emerge from their spinal sources. There are also afferent nerve fibres in these roots. The rootlets constituting each ventral root emerge from the anterolateral sulcus over an elongated vertical elliptical area. Dorsal spinal roots bear ovoid swellings, the spinal ganglia, one on each root proximal to its junction with the corresponding ventral root in an intervertebral foramen. Each root fans out into six to eight rootlets before entering the cord in a vertical row in the posterolateral sulcus. Dorsal roots are usually said to contain only afferent axons (both somatic and visceral) from unipolar neurones in spinal root ganglia, but they may also contain a small number (3%) of efferent fibres and autonomic vasodilator fibres.

Each ganglionic neurone has a single short stem that divides into a medial branch, which enters the spinal cord via a dorsal root, and a lateral branch, which passes peripherally to a sensory end-organ. The central branch is an axon, whereas the peripheral one is an elongated dendrite (but when traversing a peripheral nerve it is, in general structural terms, indistinguishable from an axon). The region of spinal cord associated with the emergence of a pair of nerves is a spinal segment, but there is no actual surface indication of segmentation. Moreover, the deep neural sources or destinations of radicular fibres may lie far beyond the confines of the 'segment' so defined.

MENINGES

Dura Mater

The single layer of dura that lines the cranial cavity divides into two layers as it passes downward through the foramen magnum, although it is still a single layer as it forms the anterior and posterior atlanto-occipital membranes. Within the vertebral column, it has been suggested that the outer endosteal

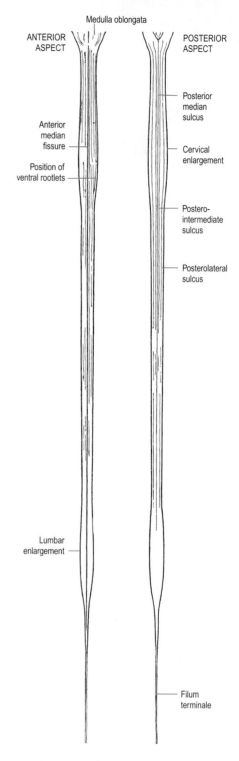

Fig. 8.2 *Main features of the spinal cord.*

layer becomes the periosteum of the vertebral canal, which is separated from the spinal dura mater by an extradural (epidural) space (see later). This interpretation, which would make the epidural space 'intradural,' is not generally agreed on (Newell 1999). The spinal dura mater forms a tube whose upper end is attached to the edge of the foramen magnum and to the posterior surfaces of the second and third cervical vertebral bodies, as well as to the posterior longitudinal ligament by fibrous bands, especially toward the caudal end of the vertebral canal. The dural tube narrows at the lower border of the second sacral vertebra. It invests the thin spinal filum terminale, descends to the back of the coccyx, and blends with the periosteum. The meningeal coverings of the spinal roots and nerves are described later in this chapter.

Epidural Space

The epidural space lies between the spinal dura mater and the tissues that line the vertebral canal (Fig. 8.8). It is closed above by fusion of the spinal dura with the edge of the foramen magnum, and below by the posterior

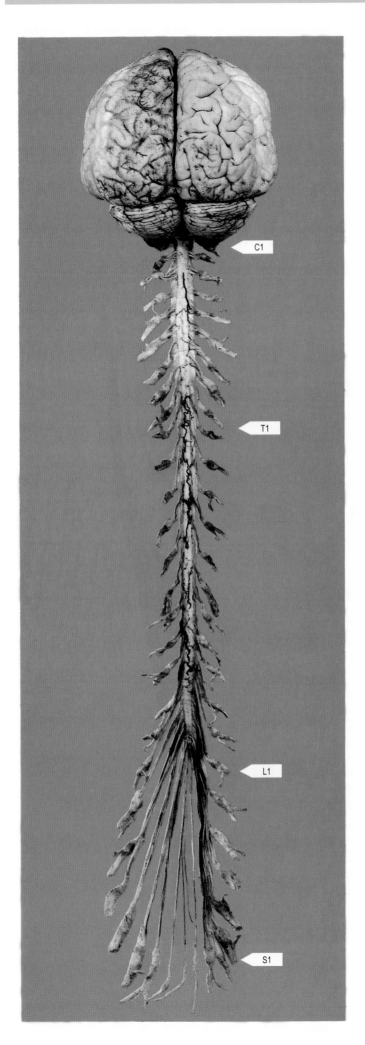

C1

T1

L1

S1

Fig. 8.3 *Brain and spinal cord with attached spinal nerve roots and dorsal root ganglia, photographed from the dorsal aspect. Note the fusiform cervical and lumbar enlargements of the cord and the changing obliquity of the spinal nerve roots as the cord is descended. The cauda equina is undisturbed on the right but has been spread out on the left to show its individual components. (Dissection by M. C. E. Hutchinson, GKT School of Medicine; photograph by Kevin Fitzpatrick on behalf of GKT School of Medicine, London.)*

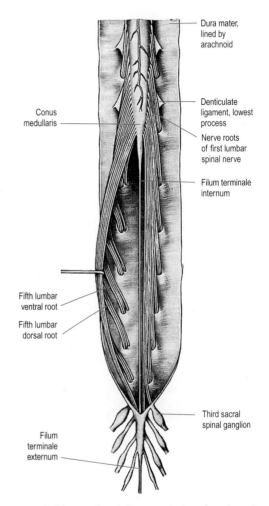

Dura mater, lined by arachnoid

Conus medullaris

Denticulate ligament, lowest process

Nerve roots of first lumbar spinal nerve

Filum terminale internum

Fifth lumbar ventral root

Fifth lumbar dorsal root

Third sacral spinal ganglion

Filum terminale externum

Fig. 8.4 *Lower end of the spinal cord, filum terminale and cauda equina exposed from behind. The dura mater and the arachnoid have been opened and spread out.*

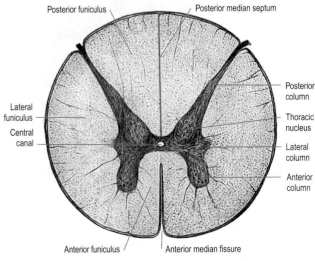

Posterior funiculus

Posterior median septum

Posterior column

Thoracic nucleus

Lateral column

Anterior column

Lateral funiculus

Central canal

Anterior funiculus

Anterior median fissure

Fig. 8.5 *Transverse section of the spinal cord at a midthoracic level.*

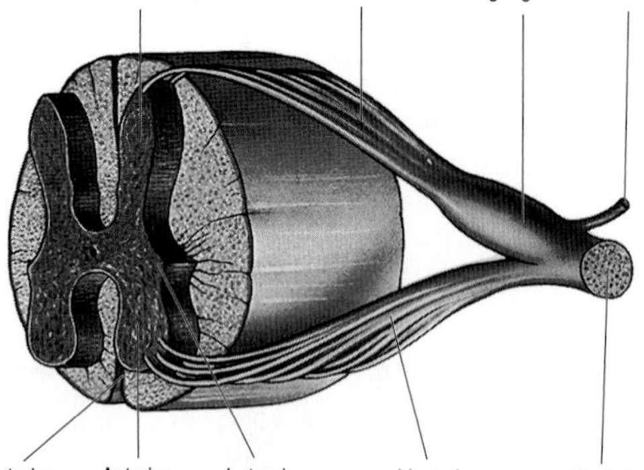
Posterior grey column
Dorsal nerve root
Spinal ganglion
Dorsal ramus
Anterior median fissure
Anterior grey column
Lateral grey column
Ventral nerve root
Ventral ramus

Fig. 8.6 *Diagram of a spinal cord segment showing the formation of a typical spinal nerve and the gross relationships of the grey and white matter. Note the dorsal nerve rootlets in a single linear row, and the ventral rootlets in three or more rows.*

sacrococcygeal ligament, which closes the sacral hiatus. It contains loosely packed connective tissue, fat, a venous plexus, small arterial branches, lymphatics and fine fibrous bands that connect the theca with the lining tissue of the vertebral canal. These bands, the meningovertebral ligaments, are best developed anteriorly and laterally. Similar bands tether the nerve root sheaths or 'sleeves' within their canals. There is also a midline attachment from the posterior spinal dura to the ligamentum nuchae at the atlanto-occipital and atlanto-axial levels (Dean and Mitchell 2002). The venous plexus consists of longitudinally arranged chains of vessels connected by circumdural venous 'rings.' The vertebral venous plexus is commonly known as Batson's plexus. The anteriorly placed vessels receive the basivertebral veins.

The shape of the space within each spinal segment is not uniform, although the segmental pattern is metamerically repeated. It is difficult to define the true shape of the 'space' because it changes with the introduction of fluid or as a result of preservation techniques. In the lumbar region, the dura mater is apposed to the walls of the vertebral canal anteriorly and attached by connective tissue in a manner that permits displacement of the dural sac during movement and venous engorgement. Adipose tissue is present posteriorly in recesses between the ligamentum flavum and the dura. The connective tissue extends for a short distance through the intervertebral foramina along the sheaths of the spinal nerves. Like the main thecal sac, the root sheaths are partially tethered to the walls of the foramina by fine meningovertebral

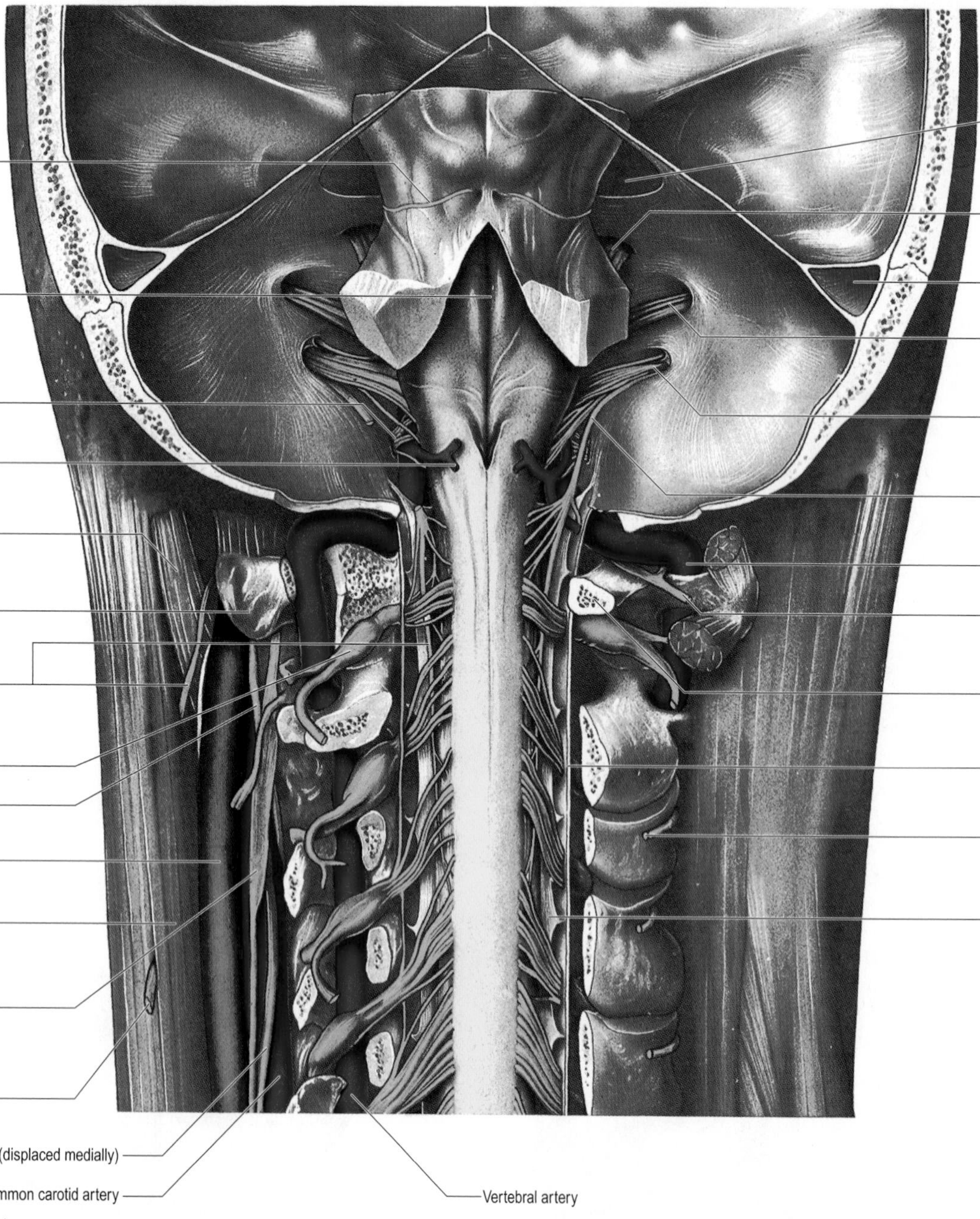
Trochlear nerve
Median sulcus of fourth ventricle
Hypoglossal nerve
Posterior spinal artery
Digastric, posterior belly
Atlas, transverse process
Spinal accessory nerve
Second cervical spinal ganglion
Vagus nerve
Internal jugular vein
Sternocleido-mastoid
Superior cervical sympathetic ganglion
Spinal accessory nerve
Vagus nerve (displaced medially)
Common carotid artery
Vertebral artery
Tentorial notch
Trigeminal nerve
Transverse dural venous sinus
Facial and vestibulocochlear nerves
Glossopharyngeal, vagus and accessory nerves
Accessory nerve, spinal root
Vertebral artery
First cervical (suboccipital) nerve
Atlas, posterior arch
Dura mater
Third cervical dorsal ramus
Denticulate ligament

Fig. 8.7 *Dissection showing the brain stem and upper five cervical spinal segments after the removal of large portions of the occipital and parietal bones, cerebellum and roof of the fourth ventricle. On the left, the foramina transversaria of the atlas and of the third, fourth and fifth cervical vertebrae have been opened to expose the vertebral artery.* On the right, *the posterior arch of the atlas and the laminae of the succeeding cervical vertebrae have been removed.*

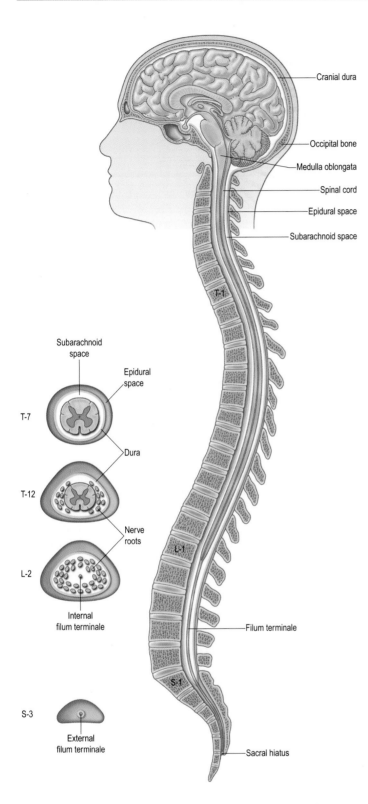

Fig. 8.8 *Epidural space. (Adapted with permission from Rosse, C., Gaddum-Rosse, P., 1997. Hollinshead's Textbook of Anatomy, 5th ed. Lippincott-Raven, Philadelphia, Fig. 13-3.)*

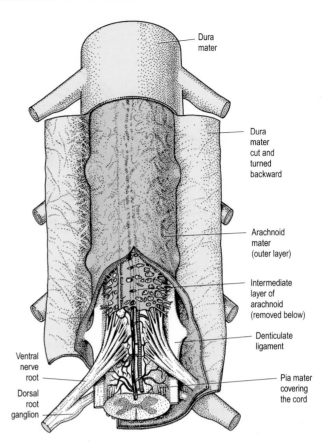

Fig. 8.9 *Part of the spinal cord exposed from the anterior aspect to show meningeal coverings.*

catheterization may occur during extradural injections. Injection of fluid into the subdural space may damage the cord either by direct toxic effects or by compression of the vasculature.

Arachnoid Mater

The arachnoid mater that surrounds the spinal cord is continuous with the cranial arachnoid mater (Figs 8.9, 8.10). It is closely applied to the deep aspect of the dura mater. At sites where vessels and nerves enter or leave the subarachnoid space, the arachnoid mater is reflected on to the surface of these structures and forms a thin coating of leptomeningeal cells over the surface of both vessels and nerves. Thus, a subarachnoid angle is formed as nerves pass through the dura into the intervertebral foramina. At this point, the layers of leptomeninges fuse and become continuous with the perineurium. The epineurium is in continuity with the dura. Such an arrangement seals the subarachnoid space so that particulate matter does not pass directly from the subarachnoid space into nerves. The existence of a pathway of lymphatic drainage from the CSF is controversial.

Pia Mater

The spinal pia mater closely invests the surface of the spinal cord and passes into the anterior median fissure (see Figs 8.9, 8.10). As in the cranial region, there is a subpial 'space'; however, over the surface of the spinal cord the subpial collagenous layer is thicker than in the cerebral region, and it is continuous with the collagenous core of the ligamentum denticulatum.

The ligamentum denticulatum is a flat, fibrous sheet that lies on each side of the spinal cord between the ventral and dorsal spinal roots. Its medial border is continuous with the subpial connective tissue of the cord, and its lateral border forms a series of triangular processes, the apices of which are fixed at intervals to the dura mater. There are usually 21 processes on each side. The first crosses behind the vertebral artery, where it is attached to the dura mater, and is separated by the artery from the first cervical ventral root. Its site of attachment to the dura mater is above the rim of the foramen magnum, just behind the hypoglossal nerve; the spinal accessory nerve ascends on its posterior aspect (see Fig. 8.7). The last of the dentate ligaments lies between the exiting twelfth thoracic and first lumbar spinal nerves and is a narrow, oblique band that descends laterally from the conus medullaris. Changes in the form and position of the dentate ligaments during spinal movements have been demonstrated by cineradiography.

Beyond the conus medullaris, the pia mater continues as a coating of the filum terminale.

ligaments. Contrast media and other fluids injected into the epidural space at the sacral level can spread up to the cranial base. Local anaesthetics injected near the spinal nerves, just outside the intervertebral foramina, may spread up or down the epidural space to affect the adjacent spinal nerves or may pass to the opposite side. The paravertebral spaces of each side communicate via the epidural space, particularly at the lumbar levels.

Subdural Space

The subdural space is a potential space in the normal spine because the arachnoid and dura are closely apposed (Haines, Harkey and Al-Mefty 1993). It does not connect with the subarachnoid space but continues for a short distance along the cranial and spinal nerves. Accidental subdural

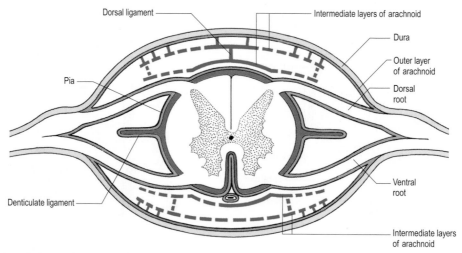

Fig. 8.10 *Transverse section through the spinal cord and meninges showing the relationships of the meninges and ligaments with the spinal cord and roots: dura mater* (yellow), *outer layer of arachnoid mater* (pale blue), *intermediate layer of arachnoid mater* (dark blue), *pia mater* (pink), *and subpial connective tissue* (green).

Intermediate Layer

In addition to the well-defined coats of arachnoid and pia mater, the cord is surrounded by an extensive intermediate layer of leptomeninges (see Fig. 8.10). This layer is concentrated in the dorsal and ventral regions and forms a highly perforated, almost lace-like structure that is focally compacted to form the dorsal, dorsolateral and ventral ligaments of the spinal cord. Dorsally, the intermediate layer is adherent to the deep aspect of the arachnoid mater and forms a discontinuous series of dorsal ligaments that attach the spinal cord to the arachnoid. The dorsolateral ligaments are more delicate and fenestrated, and they extend from the dorsal roots to the parietal arachnoid. As the intermediate layer spreads laterally over the dorsal surface of the dorsal roots, it becomes increasingly perforated and eventually disappears. A similar arrangement is seen over the ventral aspect of the spinal cord, but the intermediate layer is less substantial.

The intermediate layer is structurally similar to the trabeculae that cross the cranial subarachnoid space, in that a collagenous core is coated by leptomeningeal cells. The intermediate layers of leptomeninges around the spinal cord may act as a baffle within the subarachnoid space to dampen waves of CSF in the spinal column. Inflammation within the spinal subarachnoid space may result in extensive fibrosis within the intermediate layer and the complications of chronic arachnoiditis.

SPINAL NERVES

In those body segments that largely retain a metameric (segmental) structure (e.g. the thoracic region), spinal nerves exhibit a common plan (Fig. 8.11). The dorsal, epaxial ramus passes back, lateral to the articular processes, and divides into medial and lateral branches that penetrate the deeper muscles of the back; both branches innervate the adjacent muscles and supply a band of skin from the posterior median line to the scapular line. The ventral, hypaxial ramus is connected to a corresponding sympathetic ganglion by white and grey rami communicantes. It innervates the prevertebral muscles and curves around in the body wall to supply the lateral muscles of the trunk. Near the mid-axillary line it gives off a lateral branch that pierces the muscles and divides into anterior and posterior cutaneous branches. The main nerve advances in the body wall, where it supplies the ventral muscles, and terminates in branches to the skin.

Spinal nerves are united ventral and dorsal spinal roots, attached in series to the sides of the spinal cord. Strictly speaking, the term 'spinal nerve' applies only to the short segment after union of the roots and before branching occurs. This segment, the spinal nerve proper, lies in the intervertebral foramen; in clinical practice it is often loosely termed the 'nerve root.' There are 31 pairs of spinal nerves: 8 cervical, 12 thoracic, 5 lumbar, 5 sacral and 1 coccygeal. The abbreviations C, T, L, S and Co, with corresponding numerals, are commonly applied to individual nerves. The nerves emerge through intervertebral foramina. At the thoracic, lumbar, sacral and coccygeal levels, the numbered nerve exits the vertebral canal by passing below the pedicle of the corresponding vertebra: for example, the L4 nerve exits the intervertebral foramen between L4 and L5. However, in the cervical region, nerves C1 to C7 pass above their corresponding vertebrae. C1 leaves the vertebral canal between the occipital bone and atlas and hence is often termed the 'suboccipital nerve'. The last pair of cervical nerves does not have a correspondingly numbered vertebra, and C8 passes between the seventh cervical and first thoracic vertebrae. Each nerve is continuous with the spinal cord by ventral and dorsal roots; each of the latter bears a spinal ganglion (dorsal root ganglion).

Spinal Roots and Ganglia
Ventral (Anterior) Roots

Ventral roots contain axons of neurones in the anterior and lateral spinal grey columns. Each emerges as a series of rootlets in two or three irregular rows in an area approximately 3 mm in horizontal width.

Dorsal (Posterior) Roots

Dorsal roots contain centripetal processes of neurones located in the spinal ganglia. Each consists of medial and lateral fascicles that diverge into rootlets and enter along the posterolateral sulcus. The rootlets of adjacent dorsal roots are often connected by oblique filaments, especially in the lower cervical and lumbosacral regions.

Little is known about the regions of entry and emergence of afferent and efferent rootlets in humans, but these zones of transition between the central and peripheral nervous systems have been extensively described in rodents (Fraher 2000).

Appearance and Orientation of Roots at Each Spinal Level

The size and direction of spinal nerve roots vary. The upper four cervical roots are small; the lower four are large. The thickness ratio of cervical dorsal roots to ventral roots is 3:1, which is greater than in the other regions. The first dorsal root is an exception, being smaller than the ventral root, and it is occasionally absent. The conventional view is that the first and second

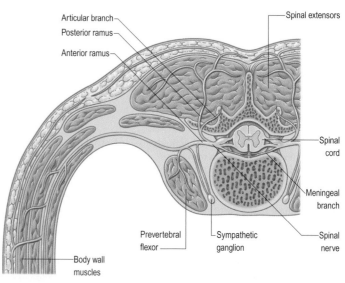

Fig. 8.11 *Formation and branching pattern of a typical spinal nerve.*

cervical spinal roots are short, running almost horizontally to their exits from the vertebral canal, and from the third to eighth cervical levels, the roots slope obliquely down. Obliquity and length increase successively, although the distance between spinal attachment and vertebral exit never exceeds the height of one vertebra. An alternative view is that upper cervical roots descend, the fifth is horizontal, the sixth to eighth ascend, the first two thoracic roots are horizontal, the next three ascend, the sixth is horizontal and the rest descend (Kubik and Müntener 1969). This view is based on the observation that the cervicothoracic part of the spinal cord grows more in length than the other parts do.

Thoracic roots, except the first, are small, and the dorsal root only slightly exceeds the ventral in thickness. They increase successively in length. In the lower thoracic region, the roots descend in contact with the spinal cord for at least two vertebrae before emerging from the vertebral canal.

Lower lumbar and upper sacral roots are the largest, and their rootlets are most numerous. Coccygeal roots are the smallest. Kubik and Müntener (1969) confirm that lumbar, sacral and coccygeal roots descend with increasing obliquity to their exits. The spinal cord ends near the lower border of the first lumbar vertebra, and the lengths of successive roots rapidly increase; the consequent collection of roots is the cauda equina (see Fig. 8.3). The largest roots, and hence the largest spinal nerves, are continuous with the spinal cervical and lumbar swellings and innervate the upper and lower limbs.

Spinal Ganglia (Dorsal Root Ganglia)

Spinal ganglia are large groups of neurones on the dorsal spinal roots. Each is oval and reddish; its size is related to that of its root. A ganglion is bifid medially where the two fascicles of the dorsal root emerge to enter the cord. Ganglia are usually located in the intervertebral foramina, immediately lateral to the perforation of the dura mater by the roots (see Fig. 8.4). However, the first and second cervical ganglia lie on the vertebral arches of the atlas and axis, the sacral lies inside the vertebral canal, and the coccygeal ganglion usually lies within the dura mater. The first cervical ganglion may be absent. Small aberrant ganglia sometimes occur on the upper cervical dorsal roots between the spinal ganglia and the cord.

Spinal Nerves Proper

Immediately distal to the spinal ganglia, ventral and dorsal roots unite to form spinal nerves (Figs 8.11, 8.12). These soon divide into dorsal and ventral rami, both of which receive fibres from both roots. At all levels above the sacral, this division occurs within the intervertebral foramen. Division of the sacral spinal nerves occurs within the sacral vertebral canal, and the dorsal and ventral rami exit separately through posterior and anterior sacral foramina at each level. Spinal nerves trifurcate at some cervical and thoracic levels, and the third branch is called a ramus intermedius. At or distal to its origin, each ventral ramus gives off recurrent meningeal (sinuvertebral) branches and receives a grey ramus communicans from the corresponding sympathetic ganglion. The thoracic and first and second lumbar ventral rami each contributes a white ramus communicans to the corresponding sympathetic ganglia. The second, third and fourth sacral nerves also supply visceral branches, unconnected with sympathetic ganglia, that carry a parasympathetic outflow directly to the pelvic plexuses.

Cervical spinal nerves enlarge from the first to the sixth nerve. The seventh and eighth cervical and the first thoracic nerves are similar in size to the sixth cervical nerve. The remaining thoracic nerves are relatively small. Lumbar nerves are large, increasing in size from the first to the fifth. The first sacral is the largest spinal nerve; thereafter, the sacral nerves decrease in size. The coccygeal nerves are the smallest spinal nerves.

Meningeal Branches

The recurrent meningeal or sinuvertebral nerves number two to four filaments on each side and occur at all vertebral levels. Each receives one or more rami from a nearby grey ramus communicans or directly from a thoracic sympathetic ganglion; most then pursue a recurrent (often perivascular) course into the vertebral canal through the intervertebral foramen ventral to the dorsal root ganglion. Here these mixed sensory and sympathetic nerves divide into transverse, ascending and descending branches that are distributed to the dura mater, walls of blood vessels, periosteum, ligaments and intervertebral discs in the anterolateral region of the vertebral canal. Fine meningeal branches occasionally pass dorsal to reach the spinal ganglia to innervate the dorsal dura, periosteum and ligaments; others pass ventrally to the posterior longitudinal ligament. Ascending branches of the upper three cervical meningeal nerves are large and are distributed to the dura mater in the posterior cranial fossa. Meningeal nerves are clinically important in relation to referred pain, which is characteristic of many spinal disorders and occipital headache.

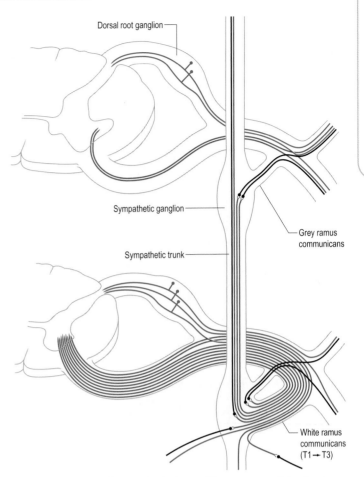

Fig. 8.12 *Constitution of a typical spinal nerve. The* upper part *of the diagram shows the somatic components of the spinal nerve roots; the* lower part *shows the visceral components: somatic efferent and preganglionic sympathetic fibres* (red), *somatic and visceral afferent fibres* (blue) *and postganglionic sympathetic fibres* (black).

Coverings and Relations of the Spinal Roots and Nerves in the Radicular Canal

Tubular prolongations of the spinal dura mater, closely lined by the arachnoid, extend around the spinal roots and nerves as they pass through the lateral zone of the vertebral canal and through the intervertebral foramina (Figs 8.9, 8.10, 8.13). These prolongations, the spinal nerve sheaths (root sheaths), gradually lengthen as the spinal roots become increasingly oblique. Each individual dorsal and ventral root runs in the subarachnoid space with its own covering of pia mater. Each root pierces the dura separately, taking a sleeve of arachnoid with it, before joining within the dural prolongation just distal to the spinal ganglion. The dural sheaths of the spinal nerves fuse with the epineurium, within or slightly beyond the intervertebral foramina. The arachnoid prolongations within the sheaths do not extend as far distally as their dural coverings, but the subarachnoid space and its contained CSF extend sufficiently distally to form a radiologically demonstrable 'root sleeve' for each nerve. Shortening or obstruction of this sleeve seen on myelography indicates compression of the spinal nerve. At the cervical level, where the nerves are short and the vertebral movement is greatest, the dural sheaths are tethered to the periosteum of the adjacent transverse processes. In the lumbosacral region there is less tethering of the dura to the periosteum, although there may be an attachment posteriorly to the facet joint capsule.

In the radicular ('root') canal and intervertebral foramen, the spinal nerve is related to the spinal artery of that level and its radicular branch, as well as to a small plexus of veins. At the outer end of the foramen, the nerve may lie above or below transforaminal ligaments.

The size of the spinal nerve and its associated structures within the intervertebral foramen is not in direct relation to the size of the foramen. At lumbar levels, although L5 is the largest nerve, its foramen is smaller than those of L1–4, which renders this nerve particularly vulnerable to compression.

Functional Components of Spinal Nerves

Each typical spinal nerve contains somatic and visceral (autonomic) fibres.

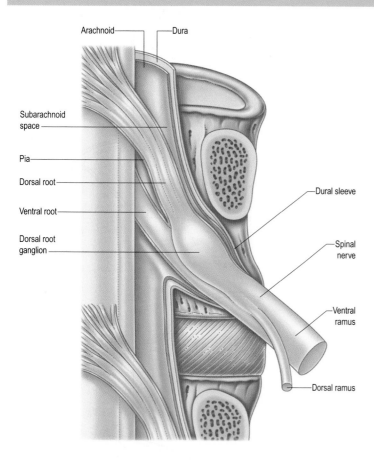

Fig. 8.13 *Lumbar spinal nerve and its roots and meningeal coverings.*

Somatic components — Somatic components are efferent and afferent. Somatic efferent fibres that innervate skeletal muscles are axons of α, β and γ neurones in the spinal anterior grey column. Somatic afferent fibres convey impulses into the central nervous system from receptors in the skin, subcutaneous tissues, muscles, tendons, fasciae and joints; they are peripheral processes of unipolar neurones in the spinal ganglia.

Visceral components — Visceral components are also afferent and efferent and belong to the autonomic nervous system. They include sympathetic or parasympathetic fibres at different spinal levels. Preganglionic visceral efferent sympathetic fibres are axons of neurones in the spinal lateral grey column in the thoracic and upper two or three lumbar segments; they join the sympathetic trunk along corresponding white rami communicantes and synapse with postganglionic neurones distributed to non-striated muscle or glands. The preganglionic visceral efferent parasympathetic fibres are axons of neurones in the spinal lateral grey column of the second to fourth sacral segments; they leave the ventral rami of corresponding sacral nerves and synapse in pelvic ganglia. The postganglionic axons are distributed mainly to muscle or glands in the walls of the pelvic viscera. Visceral afferent fibres have cell bodies in the spinal ganglia. Their peripheral processes pass through white rami communicantes and, without synapsing, through one or more sympathetic ganglia to end in viscera. Some visceral afferent fibres may enter the spinal cord in the ventral roots.

Central processes of ganglionic unipolar neurones enter the spinal cord by posterior roots and synapse on somatic or sympathetic efferent neurones, usually through interneurones, completing reflex paths. Alternatively, they may synapse with other neurones in the spinal or brain stem grey matter, which gives origin to a variety of ascending tracts.

Variations of Spinal Roots and Nerves

The courses of spinal roots and nerves in relation to the thecal sac and vertebral and radicular canals may be aberrant. An individual intervertebral foramen may contain a duplicated sheath, nerve and roots, which are then absent at an adjacent level. Abnormal communications between roots may occur within the vertebral canal. These anomalies have been described and classified for the lumbosacral spine by Neidre and Macnab (1983).

Rami of the Spinal Nerves

Ventral (anterior primary) rami supply the limbs and the anterolateral aspects of the trunk; in general, they are larger than the dorsal rami. Thoracic ventral rami run independently and retain a largely segmental distribution. Cervical,

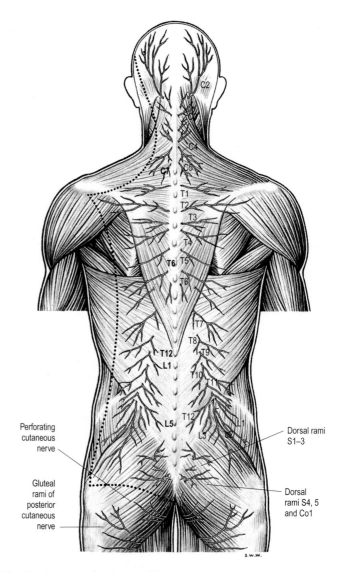

Fig. 8.14 *Cutaneous distribution of the dorsal rami of the spinal nerves. The nerves are shown lying on the superficial muscles; on the left side, the limit of the skin area supplied by these nerves is indicated by the* dotted line. *The nerves are numbered on the right side; the spines of the seventh cervical, sixth and twelfth thoracic and first and fifth lumbar vertebrae are labelled in* bold *on the left side.*

lumbar and sacral ventral rami connect near their origins to form plexuses. Dorsal rami do not join these plexuses.

Dorsal (posterior primary) rami of spinal nerves are usually smaller than the ventral rami and are directed posteriorly. Retaining a segmental distribution, they all (except for the first cervical, fourth and fifth sacral and coccygeal) divide into medial and lateral branches that supply the muscles and skin of the posterior regions of the neck and trunk (Fig. 8.14).

Cervical dorsal spinal rami — Each cervical spinal dorsal ramus, except the first, divides into medial and lateral branches that innervate muscles. In general, only medial branches of the second to fourth, and usually the fifth, supply the skin. Except for the first and second, each dorsal ramus passes back, medial to a posterior intertransverse muscle, and curves around the articular process into the interval between semispinalis capitis and semispinalis cervicis.

The first cervical dorsal ramus, the suboccipital nerve (see Fig. 8.7), is larger than the ventral. It emerges superior to the posterior arch of the atlas and inferior to the vertebral artery and enters the suboccipital triangle to supply the rectus capitis posterior major and minor, obliquus capitis superior and inferior and semispinalis capitis. A filament from the branch to the inferior oblique joins the second dorsal ramus. The suboccipital nerve occasionally has a cutaneous branch that accompanies the occipital artery to the scalp and connects with the greater and lesser occipital nerves. It may also communicate with the accessory nerve.

The second cervical dorsal ramus is slightly larger than the ventral and all the other cervical dorsal rami (see Figs 8.7, 11.10B). It emerges between the posterior arch of the atlas and the lamina of the axis, below the inferior oblique, which it supplies. It receives a connection from the first cervical dorsal ramus and divides into a large medial and smaller lateral branch. The medial branch, termed the 'greater occipital nerve', ascends between the inferior oblique and semispinalis capitis, pierces the latter and trapezius near their occipital attachments and is joined by a filament from the medial branch of the third dorsal ramus. It ascends with the occipital artery, divides into branches that connect with the lesser occipital nerve and supplies the skin of the scalp as far forward as the vertex. It supplies the semispinalis capitis and, occasionally, the back of the auricle. The lateral branch supplies the splenius capitis, longissimus capitis and semispinalis capitis and is often joined by the corresponding third cervical branch.

Greater occipital neuralgia is a syndrome of pain and paraesthesia felt in the distribution of the greater occipital nerve. It is usually due to an entrapment neuropathy as the nerve pierces the attachment of the neck extensors to the occiput. A similar syndrome may be caused by upper facet joint arthritis involving the second cervical root.

The third cervical dorsal ramus is intermediate in size between the second and fourth. It courses back around the articular pillar of the third cervical vertebra, medial to the posterior intertransverse muscle, and divides into medial and lateral branches. Its medial branch runs between spinalis capitis and semispinalis cervicis and pierces splenius and trapezius to end in the skin. Deep to trapezius it gives rise to a branch, the third occipital nerve, that pierces trapezius and ends in the skin of the lower occipital region, medial to the greater occipital nerve and connected to it. The lateral branch often joins a branch of the second cervical dorsal ramus. The dorsal ramus of the suboccipital nerve and medial branches of the dorsal rami of the second and third cervical nerves are sometimes joined by loops to form the posterior cervical plexus.

The dorsal rami of the lower five cervical nerves curve back around the vertebral articular pillars and divide into medial and lateral branches. Medial branches of the fourth and fifth cervical nerves run between semispinalis cervicis and semispinalis capitis, reach the vertebral spines and pierce splenius and trapezius to end in the skin. The fifth medial branch may not reach the skin. The medial branches of the lowest three cervical nerves are small and end in semispinalis cervicis, semispinalis capitis, multifidus and interspinales. The lateral branches supply iliocostalis cervicis, longissimus cervicis and longissimus capitis.

Thoracic dorsal spinal rami — Thoracic dorsal rami pass backward close to the vertebral facet joints to divide into medial and lateral branches. Each medial branch emerges between a joint and the medial edges of the superior costotransverse ligament and intertransverse muscle. Each lateral branch runs in the interval between the ligament and the muscle before inclining posteriorly on the medial side of levator costae.

Medial branches of the upper six thoracic dorsal rami pass between and supply semispinalis thoracis and multifidus, then pierce rhomboids and trapezius and reach the skin near the vertebral spines.

Medial branches of the lower six thoracic dorsal rami mainly supply multifidus and longissimus thoracis and occasionally the skin in the median region. Lateral branches increase inferiorly in size and run through, or deep to, longissimus thoracis to the interval between it and iliocostalis cervicis, supplying these muscles and levatores costarum. The lower five or six also have cutaneous branches and pierce serratus posterior inferior and latissimus dorsi in line with the costal angles. Some upper thoracic lateral branches supply the skin. The twelfth thoracic lateral branch sends a filament medially along the iliac crest, then passes down to the anterior gluteal skin. Medial cutaneous branches of the thoracic dorsal rami descend close to the vertebral spines before reaching the skin; lateral branches descend across as many as four ribs before becoming superficial. The branch of the twelfth thoracic reaches the skin a little above the iliac crest.

Lumbar dorsal spinal rami — Lumbar dorsal rami pass back, medial to the medial intertransverse muscles, and divide into medial and lateral branches. Medial branches run near the vertebral articular processes to end in multifidus. They are related to the bone between the accessory and mammillary processes and may groove it, crossing a distinct notch or even a foramen. Lateral branches supply erector spinae. In addition, the upper three rami give rise to cutaneous nerves that pierce the aponeurosis of latissimus dorsi at the lateral border of erector spinae and cross the iliac crest posteriorly to reach the gluteal skin, some extending as far as the level of the greater trochanter.

Sacral dorsal spinal rami — Sacral dorsal rami are small, diminishing downward. Other than the fifth, they all emerge though the dorsal sacral foramina. The upper three are covered at their exit by multifidus and divide into medial and lateral branches. Medial branches are small and end in multifidus. Lateral branches join together and with lateral branches of the last lumbar and fourth sacral dorsal rami, forming loops dorsal to the sacrum. Branches from these loops run dorsal to the sacrotuberous ligament and form a second series of

loops under gluteus maximus. From these, two or three gluteal branches pierce the gluteus maximus (along a line from the posterior superior iliac spine to the coccygeal apex) to supply the posterior gluteal skin.

The dorsal rami of the fourth and fifth sacral nerves are small and lie below multifidus. They unite with each other and with the coccygeal dorsal ramus to form loops dorsal to the sacrum; filaments from these supply the skin over the coccyx.

Coccygeal dorsal spinal ramus — The coccygeal dorsal spinal ramus does not divide into medial and lateral branches. Its connections and distribution were noted earlier.

DERMATOMES

The cutaneous area supplied by one spinal nerve, through both rami, is a dermatome (Fig. 8.15). Typically, dermatomes extend around the body from the posterior to the anterior median line. The upper half of each zone is supplemented by the nerve above, and the lower half by the nerve below. The area supplied by dorsal rami is limited laterally by the dorsolateral line, which descends laterally from the occiput to the medial end of the acromion, continues to the posterior aspect of the greater trochanter and curves medially to the coccyx. Cutaneous strips supplied by dorsal rami do not correspond exactly to those served by ventral rami and differ in both breadth and position. Dermatomes of adjacent spinal nerves overlap markedly, particularly in the segments least affected by development of the limbs (i.e. second thoracic to first lumbar). In some regions (e.g. upper anterior thoracic wall), cutaneous nerves supplying adjoining areas are not from consecutive spinal nerves, and the overlap is minimal. When the second thoracic spinal ramus is severed, anaesthesia is sharply demarcated, but some overlap for awareness of painful and thermal stimuli may exist. Likewise, after section of a peripheral nerve (e.g. ulnar nerve at the wrist), the area of tactile loss is always greater than that of lost pain and temperature sensation. Hence, the area of total anaesthesia and analgesia following section of peripheral nerves is always less than might be anticipated from their anatomical distribution.

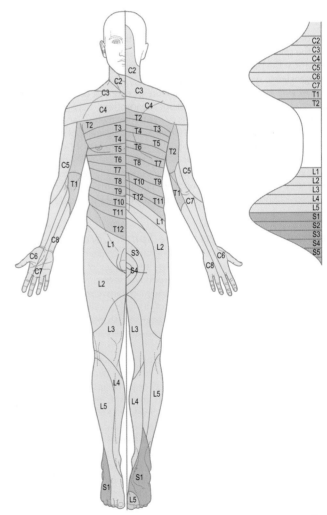

Fig. 8.15 *Dermatomes. The small diagram* shows the regular arrangement of dermatomes in the upper and lower limbs of the embryo. (By permission from Moffat, D.B., 1993. Lecture Notes on Anatomy, 2nd ed. Blackwell Scientific, Oxford.)

INTERNAL ORGANIZATION

In transverse section, the spinal cord is incompletely divided into symmetric halves by a dorsal (posterior) median septum and a ventral (anterior) median sulcus (see Fig. 8.5). It consists of an outer layer of white matter and an inner core of grey matter. The dimensions and relative volumes of white matter and centrally aggregated neurone cell bodies vary according to the level (Fig. 8.16). The amount of grey matter at any level is a function of the amount of muscle, skin and other tissues innervated by neurones at that level. It is therefore largest by proportion in the cervical and lumbar enlargements, because neurones in these segments of the cord innervate the limbs; it is attenuated at thoracic levels. The absolute amount of white matter is greatest at cervical levels and decreases progressively at lower levels; this is the case because descending tracts shed fibres as they descend, and ascending tracts accumulate fibres as they ascend.

In the centre of the spinal grey matter, the central canal extends the whole length of the spinal cord. Rostrally, the central canal extends into the caudal half of the medulla oblongata, where it opens into the fourth ventricle. Caudally, in the conus medullaris, it expands as a fusiform 'terminal ventricle' that is 8 to 10 mm long, contains CSF and is lined by columnar, ciliated epithelium (ependyma). The terminal ventricle is obliterated at approximately 40 years of age.

Spinal Grey Matter

In three dimensions, the spinal grey matter is shaped like a fluted column (see Fig. 8.6). In transverse section (see Fig. 8.16) the column is often described as being 'butterfly shaped' or resembling the letter 'H.' It consists of four cellular masses, referred to as the dorsal and ventral horns (or columns), which project dorsolaterally and ventrolaterally toward the surface. The grey matter that immediately surrounds the central canal and unites the two sides is termed the dorsal and ventral grey commissure. The dorsal horns are the site of termination of primary afferent fibres, which enter via the dorsal roots of spinal nerves. The tip of the dorsal horn is separated from the surface of the cord by a thin dorsolateral tract (tract of Lissauer) in which primary afferents ascend and descend for a short distance before terminating in the subjacent grey matter (Figs 8.17, 8.18). The dorsal horn may be described in terms of a head, neck and base, the individual constituents of which are described in more detail later. The ventral horns contain efferent neurones whose axons leave the spinal cord in ventral nerve roots. A small intermediate lateral horn is present at the thoracic and upper lumbar levels and contains the cell bodies of preganglionic sympathetic neurones.

Spinal grey matter is a complex mixture of neuronal cell bodies (somata), their processes (neurites) and synaptic connections, neuroglia and blood vessels (Fig. 8.19). Neurones in the grey matter are multipolar and vary in size and other features, particularly the length and arrangement of their axons and dendrites. Many are Golgi types I and II neurones. Axons of Golgi type I neurones pass out of the grey matter into ventral spinal roots or spinal tracts. Axons and dendrites of Golgi type II neurones are largely confined to the nearby grey matter. The distribution of neurones may be intrasegmental—deployed within a single segment—or intersegmental—spread through several segments.

Neuronal Cell Groups of the Spinal Cord

Viewed from the perspective of its longitudinal columnar organization, the grey matter of the spinal cord consists of a series of discontinuous cell groupings associated with their corresponding segmentally arranged spinal nerves. At any particular spinal level (as seen in transverse section), the spinal grey matter is considered to consist of 10 layers, called Rexed's laminae, which are defined on the basis of neuronal size, shape, cytological features and density. The laminae are numbered sequentially in a dorsoventral sequence (Fig. 8.22).

Laminae I to IV correspond to the head of the dorsal horn and are the main receiving areas for cutaneous primary afferent terminals and collateral branches. Many complex polysynaptic reflex paths (ipsilateral, contralateral, intrasegmental and intersegmental) start from this region, and many long ascending tract fibres that pass to higher levels arise from it. Lamina I (lamina marginalis) is a very thin layer with an ill-defined boundary at the dorsolateral tip of the dorsal horn. It has a reticular appearance, reflecting its content of intermingling bundles of coarse and fine nerve fibres. It contains small, intermediate and large neuronal somata, many of which are fusiform in shape. Lamina II occupies most of the head of the dorsal horn and consists of densely packed small neurones, accounting for its dark appearance in Nissl-stained sections. With myelin stains, lamina II is characteristically distinguished from adjacent laminae by the almost total lack of myelinated fibres. Lamina II corresponds to the substantia gelatinosa. Lamina III consists of somata that are mostly larger, more variable and less closely packed than those in lamina II. It also contains many myelinated fibres. Some workers believe that the

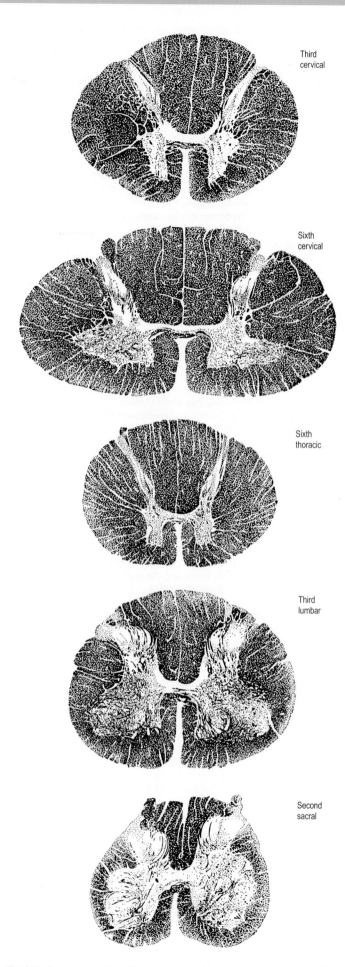

Third cervical

Sixth cervical

Sixth thoracic

Third lumbar

Second sacral

Fig. 8.16 *Transverse sections through the spinal cord at representative levels. Note the changes in overall profile and the relative changes in grey and white regions, their shapes, sizes and proportions (magnification ×5).*

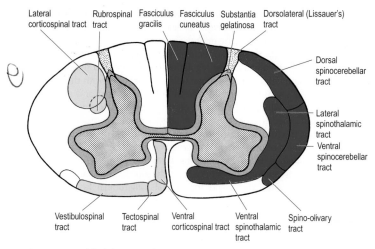

Fig. 8.17 *Simplified diagram of the main tracts of the spinal cord. The ascending tracts are shown in red on the right side of the figure; the descending tracts are shown in yellow on the left side; the 'intersegmental' tracts are shown in orange on both sides. Many tracts are omitted (see Fig. 8.18).*

substantia gelatinosa contains part or all of lamina III as well as lamina II. The ill-defined nucleus proprius of the dorsal horn corresponds to some of the cell constituents of laminae III and IV. Lamina IV is a thick, loosely packed, heterogeneous zone permeated by fibres. Its neuronal somata vary considerably in size and shape: small and round, intermediate and triangular, very large and stellate.

Laminae V and VI receive most of the terminals of proprioceptive primary afferents and profuse corticospinal projections from the motor and sensory cortex and subcortical levels, which suggests their intimate involvement in the regulation of movement. Lamina V is a thick layer that includes the neck of the dorsal horn. It is divisible into a lateral third and medial two thirds. Both have a mixed cell population, but the former contains many prominent well-staining somata interlaced by numerous bundles of transverse, dorsoventral and longitudinal fibres. Lamina VI is most prominent in the limb enlargements. It has a densely staining medial third of small, densely packed neurones and a lateral two-thirds containing larger, more loosely packed, triangular or stellate somata. Lamina VI corresponds approximately to the base of the dorsal horn.

Laminae VII to IX show a variety of complex forms in the limb enlargements (see Fig. 8.22). Lamina VII includes much of the intermediate (lateral) horn. It contains prominent neurones of Clarke's column (nucleus dorsalis, nucleus

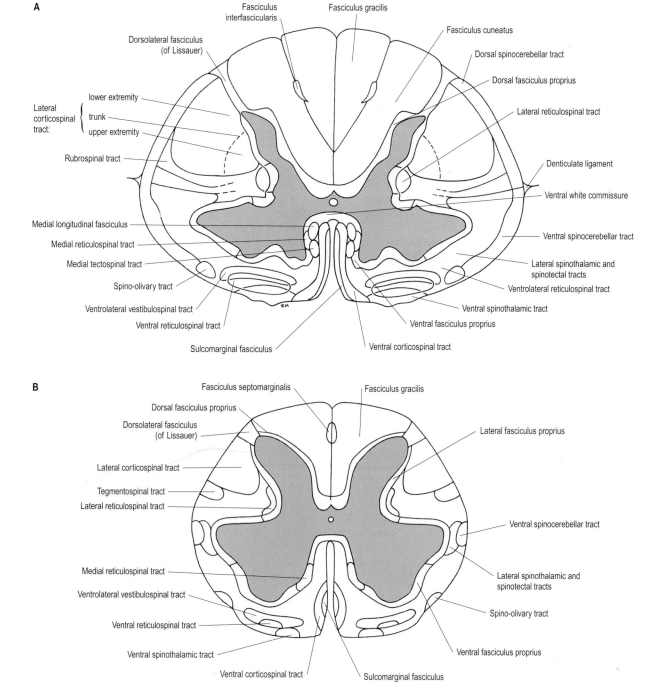

Fig. 8.18 *Approximate relative positions of nerve fibre tracts of the human spinal cord at the mid-cervical (A) and lumbar (B) levels. (Adapted from Crosby et al: Correlative Anatomy of the Nervous System, New York, Macmillan, 1962.)*

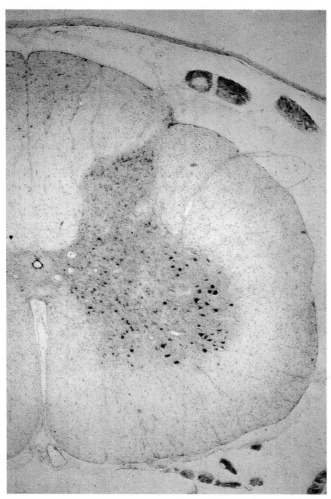

thoracicus, thoracic nucleus) and intermediomedial and intermediolateral cell groupings (Fig. 8.23). The lateral part of lamina VII has extensive ascending and descending connections with the midbrain and cerebellum (via the spinocerebellar, spinotectal, spinoreticular, tectospinal, reticulospinal and rubrospinal tracts) and is thus involved in the regulation of posture and movement. Its medial part has numerous propriospinal reflex connections with the adjacent grey matter and segments concerned with both movement and autonomic functions. Lamina VIII spans the base of the thoracic ventral horn but is restricted to its medial aspect in limb enlargements. Its neurones display a heterogeneous mixture of sizes and shapes from small to moderately large. Lamina VIII is a mass of propriospinal interneurones. It receives terminals from the adjacent laminae, many commissural terminals from the contralateral lamina VIII and descending connections from the interstitiospinal, reticulospinal and vestibulospinal tracts and the medial longitudinal fasciculus. The axons from these interneurones influence motor neurones bilaterally, perhaps directly but more probably by excitation of small neurones supplying γ-efferent fibres to muscle spindles. Lamina IX is a complex array of cells (Fig. 8.24) consisting of α and γ motor neurones and many interneurones. The large α motor neurones supply motor end-plates of extrafusal muscle fibres in striated muscle. Recording techniques have demonstrated tonic and phasic α motor neurones. The former have a lower rate of firing and lower conduction velocity and tend to innervate type S muscle units. The latter have higher conduction velocity and tend to supply fast twitch (type FR, FF) muscle units. The smaller γ motor neurones give rise to small-diameter efferent axons (fusimotor fibres), which innervate the intrafusal muscle fibres in muscle spindles. There are several functionally distinct types of γ motor neurone. The 'static' and 'dynamic' responses of muscle spindles have separate controls mediated by static and dynamic fusimotor fibres, which are distributed variously to nuclear chain and nuclear bag fibres.

Lamina X surrounds the central canal and consists of the dorsal and ventral grey commissures.

Dorsal Horn

The dorsal horn is a major receptive zone (zone of termination) of primary afferent fibres, which enter the spinal cord through the dorsal roots of spinal nerves. Dorsal root fibres contain numerous molecules that are either known or suspected to fulfill a neurotransmitter or neuromodulator role. These include glutamate, substance P, calcitonin gene–related peptide, bombesin, vasoactive intestinal polypeptide, cholecystokinin (CCK), somatostatin, dynorphin and angiotensin II. Dorsal root afferents carry exteroceptive,

Fig. 8.19 *Transverse section of the left half of a human spinal cord at a mid-lumbar level. Note the dorsal and ventral grey columns and commissural grey mass. The larger motor neurones in the ventral grey column are visibly grouped (cresyl fast violet stain).*

CASE 1 POSTPOLIO SYNDROME

A 64-year-old man develops progressive weakness and fatigue. At age 4 years he had acute poliomyelitis, characterized by profound weakness of both lower extremities and less severe weakness of the upper extremities. Upper extremity strength improved significantly thereafter, but he had persistent weakness in the lower extremities, which gradually improved. After 2 years he continued to exhibit weakness and significant atrophy of all muscles in the right lower extremity, particularly the gastrocnemius. He was unchanged thereafter until age 60, when he began to experience increased weakness in the lower extremities, particularly on the right side, ultimately necessitating the use of a leg brace. He also complains of pain in the right lower extremity, especially in the knee and ankle, and notes global fatigue. There are no symptoms of a sphincter disorder.

Neurological examination demonstrates mild weakness in the left lower extremity and marked weakness of all muscle groups in the right lower extremity, particularly the dorsiflexors and plantar flexors of the right foot. Patellar and Achilles reflexes are absent in both lower extremities. There are no sensory abnormalities.

An electromyogram with a nerve conduction study of the lower extremities shows denervation in all muscles tested. There is mild slowing of the right peroneal and posterior tibial motor responses.

Discussion: A diagnosis of postpolio syndrome is established. This is a poorly understood disorder that may be caused by a gradual dropout of motor units or muscle fibres as a result of aging superimposed on residual anterior horn cells that were previously depleted as a result of the original poliomyelitis (Fig. 8.20). Increased metabolic demand on the maximally reinnervated motor units may also play a significant role.

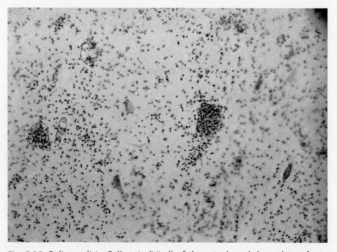

Fig. 8.20 *Poliomyelitis. Cell stain (Nissl) of the spinal cord shows loss of anterior horn cells. Phagocytic neuronophagic (microglial) clusters mark the site of dying motor neurones.*

CASE 2 AMYOTROPHIC LATERAL SCLEROSIS

A 62-year-old, right-handed man presents with a 6-month history of weakness in the lower extremities and easy fatigability. He has noted increasing difficulty jogging and has had several falls as a result of catching his foot on a curb. He finds it increasingly difficult to climb stairs in his home. He also reports deterioration in his penmanship and trouble typing on his computer keyboard. He has observed increased 'twitching' of his muscles and muscular pain after jogging. There is no history of a sensory disturbance. He denies symptoms referable to bulbar function and has experienced no sphincter disturbances.

Neurological examination demonstrates mild diffuse weakness in both lower extremities, weakness of the distal muscles of the right upper extremity, atrophy of the dorsal interosseous and thenar eminence muscles of the right hand, generalized hyperreflexia in all four extremities, bilateral extensor plantar responses (Babinski's sign) and fasciculations throughout both lower extremities and in the right upper extremity,

including the pectoralis major. The remainder of the examination is normal.

Discussion: Although a combination of upper and lower motor neurone symptoms and signs can be found in a variety of clinical conditions, this patient's progressive history of motor symptoms over 6 months, with upper and lower motor neurone signs in three extremities in the absence of sensory and autonomic disturbances, points to a progressive motor neurone disorder—in this case, amyotrophic lateral sclerosis (Lou Gehrig's disease, motor system disease). Some afflicted patients develop signs of frontotemporal degeneration as well. Pathologically, degeneration is observed primarily in the anterior horns of the spinal cord, in motor cranial nerve nuclei, and in the lateral corticospinal tracts. Although it begins at spinal levels, the disease generally spreads to involve motor cranial nerve nuclei, with resultant dysarthria, dysphagia and impaired respiratory function. See Figure 8.21.

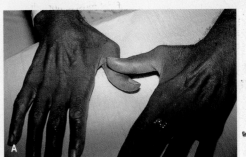 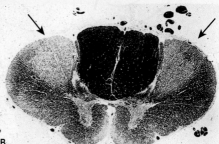 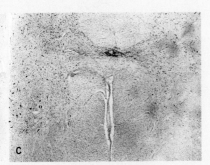

*Fig. 8.21 Amyotrophic lateral sclerosis. **A**, Atrophy of intrinsic hand muscles. **B**, Spinal cord. Cross-section stained for myelin sheaths demonstrates degeneration of the lateral (corticospinal) pathways (arrows); less marked changes reflect loss of recurrent anterior horn cell collateral fibres. **C**, Spinal cord. Cell stain demonstrates asymmetric loss of anterior horn cells. (**B** and **C**, Courtesy of C. S. Kubik Laboratory of Neuropathology, Massachusetts General Hospital, Tessa Hedley-White, Director.)*

proprioceptive and interoceptive information. Laminae I to IV are the main cutaneous receptive areas; lamina V receives fine afferents from the skin, muscle and viscera; and lamina VI receives proprioceptive and some cutaneous afferents. Most if not all primary afferent fibres divide into ascending and descending branches on entering the cord. These then travel for variable distances in the tract of Lissauer, near the surface of the cord, and send collaterals into the subjacent grey matter. The formation, topography and division of dorsal spinal roots have all been confirmed in humans.

At the dorsolateral tip of the dorsal horn, deep to the tract of Lissauer, lies a thin lamina of neurones, the lamina marginalis. Beneath this lies the substantia gelatinosa (laminae II and III), which is present at all levels and consists mostly of small Golgi type II neurones, together with some larger neurones. It receives afferents via the dorsal roots and is the site of origin of the spinothalamic tract complex. The large cells of the nucleus proprius lie ventral to the substantia gelatinosa (see Fig. 8.23). These propriospinal neurones link segments for the mediation of intraspinal coordination.

Clarke's column lies at the base of the dorsal horn. At most levels, it is near the dorsal white funiculus and may project into it. In the human spinal cord, it can usually be identified from the eighth cervical to the third or fourth lumbar segments. Neurones of Clarke's column vary in size, but most are large, especially in the lower thoracic and lumbar segments. Some send axons into the dorsal spinocerebellar tracts, and others are interneurones.

Lateral Horn

The lateral horn is a small lateral projection of grey matter located between the dorsal and ventral horns. It is present from the eighth cervical or first thoracic segment to the second or third lumbar segment. It contains the cell bodies of preganglionic sympathetic neurones. These develop in the embryonic cord dorsolateral to the central canal and migrate laterally, forming intermediomedial and intermediolateral cell columns. Their axons travel via ventral spinal roots and white rami communicantes to the sympathetic trunk.

A similar cell group is found in the second to fourth sacral segments, but unlike the thoracolumbar lateral cell column, it does not form a visible lateral projection. It is the source of the sacral outflow of parasympathetic preganglionic nerve fibres.

Ventral Horn

Neurones in the ventral horn vary in size. The largest cell bodies, which may exceed 25 μm in diameter, are those of α motor neurones whose axons emerge in ventral roots to innervate extrafusal fibres in striated skeletal muscles. Large numbers of smaller neurones, 15 to 25 mm in diameter, are also present. Some of these are γ motor neurones, which innervate intrafusal fibres of muscle spindles, and the rest are interneurones. The motor neurones utilize acetylcholine as their neurotransmitter.

Considered longitudinally, ventral horn neurones are arranged in elongated groups and form a number of separate columns that extend through several segments. These are seen most easily in transverse sections (see Fig. 8.19). The ventral horn is essentially divided into medial, central and lateral cell columns, all of which are subdivided at certain levels, usually into dorsal and ventral parts. As can be seen in Figure 8.23, the medial group extends throughout the cord but may be absent in the fifth lumbar and first sacral segments. In the thoracic and the upper four lumbar segments, it is subdivided into ventromedial and dorsomedial groups. In segments cranial and caudal to this region, the medial group has only a ventromedial moiety, except in the first cervical segment, where only the dorsomedial group exists.

The central group of cells is the least extensive and is found only in some cervical and lumbosacral segments. The third to seventh cervical segments contain the centrally situated phrenic nucleus; abundant experimental and clinical evidence shows that its neurones innervate the diaphragm. Neurones whose axons are thought to enter the spinal accessory nerve form an irregular accessory group in the upper five or six cervical segments at the ventral border of the ventral horn (see Fig. 8.23).

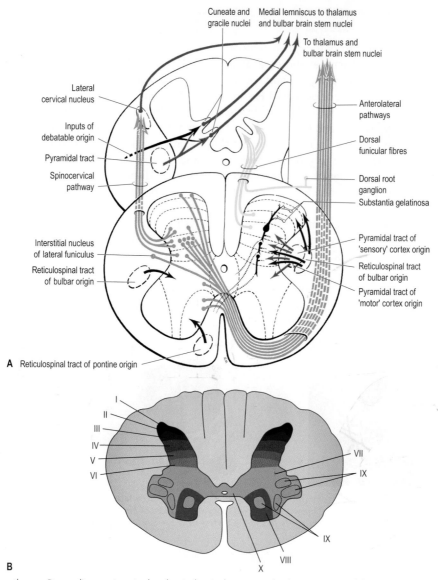

Cuneate and Medial lemniscus to thalamus
gracile nuclei and bulbar brain stem nuclei

To thalamus and
bulbar brain stem nuclei

Lateral
cervical nucleus

Inputs of
debatable origin

Pyramidal tract

Spinocervical
pathway

Anterolateral
pathways

Dorsal
funicular fibres

Dorsal root
ganglion

Substantia gelatinosa

Interstitial nucleus
of lateral funiculus

Reticulospinal tract
of bulbar origin

Pyramidal tract of
'sensory' cortex origin

Reticulospinal tract
of bulbar origin

Pyramidal tract of
'motor' cortex origin

A Reticulospinal tract of pontine origin

I
II
III
IV
V
VI
VII
IX
IX
B
VIII
X

Fig. 8.22 *Principal somaesthetic pathways. Descending corticospinal and reticulospinal tracts involved in sensory modulation are also indicated. (Modified from data provided by K. E. Webster, GKT School of Medicine, London.)*

The lateral group of cells in the ventral horn is subdivided into ventral, dorsal and retrodorsal groups, largely confined to the spinal segments that innervate the limbs. Their extents are indicated in Figure 8.23. The nucleus of Onuf, which is thought to innervate the perineal striated muscles, is a ventrolateral group of cells in the first and second sacral segments.

The motor neurones of the ventral horn are somatotopically organized. The basic arrangement is that medial cell groups innervate the axial musculature, and lateral cell groups innervate the limbs. The basic building block of the somatic motor neuronal populations is represented by a longitudinally disposed group of neurones that innervate a given muscle and in which the α and γ motor neurones are intermixed. The various groups innervating different muscles are aggregated into two major longitudinal columns: medial and lateral. In transverse section these form the medial and lateral cell groups in the ventral horn (Figs 8.24, 8.25).

The medial longitudinal motor column extends throughout the length of the spinal cord. Its neurones innervate epaxial and hypaxial muscle groups. Basically, epaxial muscles include the erector spinae group (which extend the head and vertebral column), and hypaxial muscles include prevertebral muscles of the neck, intercostal and anterior abdominal wall muscles (which flex the neck and the trunk). The epaxial muscles are innervated by branches of the dorsal primary rami of the spinal nerves, and the hypaxial muscles are innervated by branches of the ventral primary rami. In the medial column, motor neurones supplying epaxial muscles are sited ventral to those supplying hypaxial muscles.

The lateral longitudinal motor column is found only in the enlargements of the spinal cord. The motor neurones in this column in the cervical and lumbar enlargements innervate muscles of the upper and lower limbs, respectively. In the cervical enlargement, motor neurones that supply muscles intrinsic to the upper limb are situated dorsally in the ventral grey column,

and those innervating the most distal (hand) muscles are located farther dorsally. Motor neurones of the girdle muscles lie in the ventrolateral part of the ventral horn (see Fig. 8.25). There is a further somatotopic organization, in that the proximal muscles of the limb are supplied from motor cell groups located more rostrally in the enlargement than those supplying the distal muscles. For example, motor neurones innervating intrinsic muscles of the hand are sited in segments C8 and T1, whereas motor neurones of shoulder muscles are in segments C5 and C6. A similar overall arrangement of motor neurones innervating lower limb muscles applies in the lumbosacral cord (Fig. 8.26).

The main afferent connections to motor neurones are direct monosynaptic connections from proprioceptive dorsal root afferents in the same or nearby segments, connections from axonal collaterals of dorsal horn and other interneurones and direct monosynaptic connections from the vestibulospinal and corticospinal tracts.

Spinal Reflexes

The intrinsic connections of the spinal cord and brain stem subserve a number of reflexes by which the functions of peripheral structures are modulated in response to afferent information in a relatively automatic or autonomous fashion. The fundamental components of such reflex 'arcs' are thus an afferent and an efferent neurone. However, in all but the simplest of reflexes, interneurones intervene between the afferent and efferent components and confer the capacity to increase the versatility and complexity of reflex responses. Reflexes, by their very nature, are relatively fixed and stereotyped in form. Nevertheless, they are strongly influenced and modulated by descending connections. In the case of spinal reflexes, these descending controls come from both the brain stem and the cerebral cortex. Pathology of descending supraspinal pathways commonly causes abnormalities of spinal

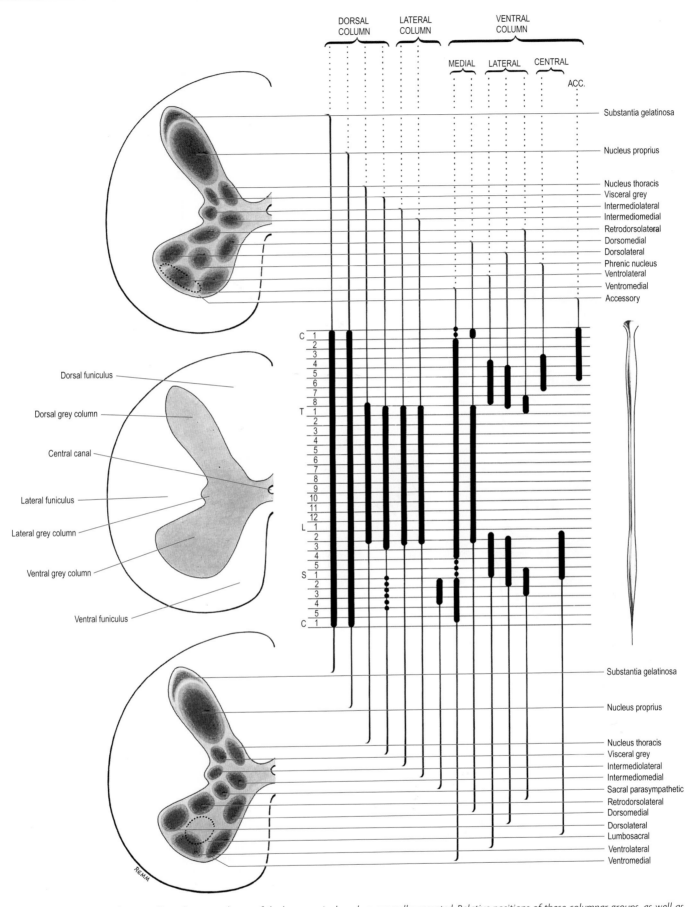

Fig. 8.23 *Groups or nuclei of nerve cells in the grey columns of the human spinal cord, as generally accepted. Relative positions of these columnar groups, as well as their extension through varying series of spinal segments, are indicated. ACC, accessory group. (Modified with permission of Simon and Schuster from Crosby, E., Humphrey, T., Lauer, E., 1962. Correlative Anatomy of the Nervous System. Macmillan. Copyright 1962 Macmillan Publishing Company.)*

reflex activity, which are routinely tested for during neurological examination. During development, descending control mechanisms suppress what may be regarded as 'primitive' reflex responses. However, these may be released or uncovered in certain pathological conditions, such as the plantar (Babinski's) and grasp reflexes.

Stretch reflex — The stretch reflex is the mechanism by which stretch applied to a muscle elicits its reflex contraction. It is essential for the maintenance of both muscle tone and an upright stance (via innervation of the postural muscles of the neck, back and lower limbs). Anatomically, it is the simplest of reflexes—it consists of one afferent and one efferent neurone.

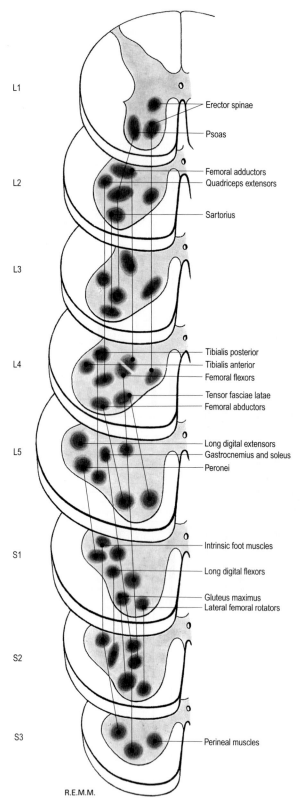

Fig. 8.24 *Approximate location in the transverse plane and longitudinal extent of the nerve cell groups innervating muscles, chiefly in the leg, in the lumbosacral segments of the human spinal cord. Based on clinicopathological studies of poliomyelitis. (Reproduced by permission and copyright © of the British Editorial Society of Bone and Joint Surgery. [From Sharrard, W.J.W., 1955. The distribution of the permanent paralysis in the lower limb in poliomyelitis. J. Bone Joint Surg. 37, B: 540–558.])*

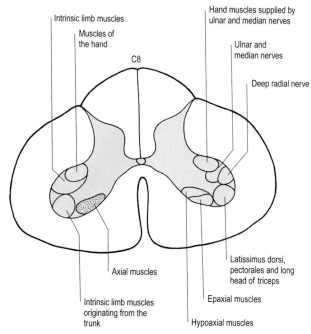

Fig. 8.25 *Schematic overview of the location of motor cell groups at the C8 segmental level of the spinal cord. The left side of the figure shows the subdivision of the lateral and medial longitudinal motor columns; the right side depicts these in more detail. (Redrawn and modified from Holstege, G., 1991. Descending motor pathways and the spinal motor system: limbic and non-limbic components. Prog. Brain Res. 87, 307–421 with permission from Elsevier.)*

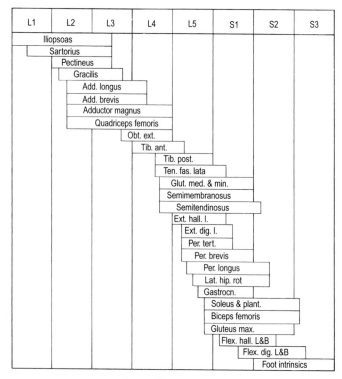

Fig. 8.26 *Segmental arrangement of innervation of the lower limb muscles. (Reproduced with permission and copyright © of the British Editorial Society of Bone and Joint Surgery [From Sharrard 1964. Sharrard WJ. Posterior iliopsoas transplantation in the treatment of paralytic dislocation of the hip. J Bone Joint Surg BR. 1964 Aug; 46: 426–444, Fig. 2.].)*

The afferent component arises from stretch receptors associated with intrafusal muscle fibres located within muscle spindles; their primary or anulospiral endings give rise to primary afferent fibres, which enter the spinal cord and make excitatory synaptic contact directly on α motor neurones innervating the same muscle (Fig. 8.27). The α motor neurones of antagonistic muscles are simultaneously inhibited via collateral connections to inhibitory interneurones.

Gamma reflex — In addition to α motor neurones innervating extrafusal muscle fibres, muscles receive γ motor neurones that innervate intrafusal muscle fibres. Activation of γ motor neurones increases the sensitivity of the intrafusal fibres to stretch (Fig. 8.28). Therefore, changes in γ activity have a profound effect on the stretch reflex and on muscle tone. Like α motor neurones, γ motor neurones are under the influence of descending pathways from the brain stem and cerebral cortex. Changes in the activity of the stretch reflex

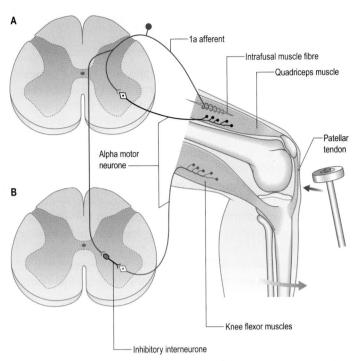

Fig. 8.27 *Stretch reflex. (By permission from Crossman, A.R., Neary, D., 2000. Neuroanatomy, 2nd ed. Churchill Livingstone, Edinburgh.)*

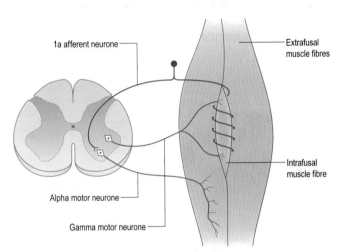

Fig. 8.28 *Gamma reflex. (By permission from Crossman, A.R., Neary, D., 2000. Neuroanatomy, 2nd ed. Churchill Livingstone, Edinburgh.)*

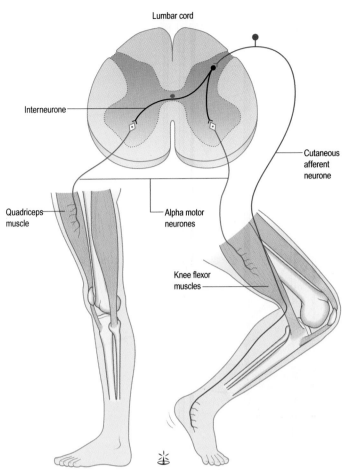

Fig. 8.29 *Flexor reflex and crossed extensor reflex. (By permission from Crossman, A.R., Neary, D., 2000. Neuroanatomy, 2nd ed. Churchill Livingstone, Edinburgh.)*

and of muscle tone are commonly found in disorders of both the central and peripheral nervous systems.

Flexor reflex — Painful stimulation of the limbs leads to reflex flexion withdrawal mediated by a polysynaptic reflex in which interneurones are interposed between afferent and efferent elements (Fig. 8.29). Thus, activation of nociceptive primary afferents indirectly causes activation of limb flexor motor neurones. Collateralization of fibres to nearby spinal segments mediates flexion of a limb at several joints, depending on the intensity of the stimulus. Decussating connections to the contralateral side of the cord activate α motor neurones innervating corresponding extensor muscles, which produces the so-called 'crossed extensor reflex'. In principle, virtually any cutaneous stimulus has the potential to induce a flexor reflex, but with the exception of noxious stimuli, this response is normally inhibited by descending pathways. When descending influences are lost, even harmless cutaneous stimulation can elicit flexion of the limbs. The Babinski (extensor plantar) reflex, which is generally regarded as pathognomonic of damage to the corticospinal tract, at least in adults, is part of a flexion withdrawal of the lower limb in response to stimulation of the sole of the foot.

Spinal White Matter

The spinal white matter surrounds the central core of grey matter. It contains nerve fibres, neuroglia and blood vessels. Most of the nerve fibres run longitudinally. They are arranged in three large masses—the dorsal, lateral and ventral funiculi—on either side of the cord (see Fig. 8.5). Fibres of related function and those with common origins or destinations are grouped to form ascending and descending tracts within the funiculi. Narrow dorsal and ventral white commissures run between the two halves of the cord. Here, the tracts are considered under three main headings: ascending, descending and propriospinal. Ascending tracts contain primary afferent fibres, which enter by dorsal roots, and fibres derived from intrinsic spinal neurones, which carry afferent impulses to supraspinal levels. Descending tracts contain long fibres, which descend from various supraspinal sources to synapse with spinal neurones. Propriospinal tracts, both ascending and descending, contain the axons of neurones that are localized entirely to the spinal cord and link nearby and distant spinal segments. They mediate intrasegmental and intersegmental coordination.

Fibres in the white matter vary in calibre. Many are small and lightly or non-myelinated. Most regions contain a wide spectrum of fibre diameters, from 1 mm or less to 10 mm. Some tracts, including the dorsolateral tract, fasciculus gracilis and central part of the lateral funiculus, typically contain only small fibres. The fasciculus cuneatus, anterior funiculus and peripheral zone of the lateral funiculus contain many large-diameter fibres.

Although the ascending and descending tracts are to a large extent discrete and regularly located, significant overlap between adjacent tracts occurs. The following account of spinal tracts is concerned with the human cord; findings in animals are discussed only when adequate clinicopathological data are unavailable in humans. The general disposition of the major tracts is shown in Figure 8.17 and is depicted in greater detail at two transverse levels in Figure 8.18. Other features are summarized in Figures 8.22 and 8.30.

Ascending Tracts

Dorsal columns — The dorsal funiculus on each side of the cord consists of two large ascending tracts—the fasciculus gracilis and fasciculus cuneatus (Fig. 8.32)—separated by a posterointermediate septum. They are also known as the dorsal columns. The dorsal columns contain a high proportion of myelinated fibres carrying proprioception (position sense and kinaesthesia) and exteroceptive (touch-pressure) information, including vibratory sensation, to higher levels. These fibres come from several sources: long primary afferent

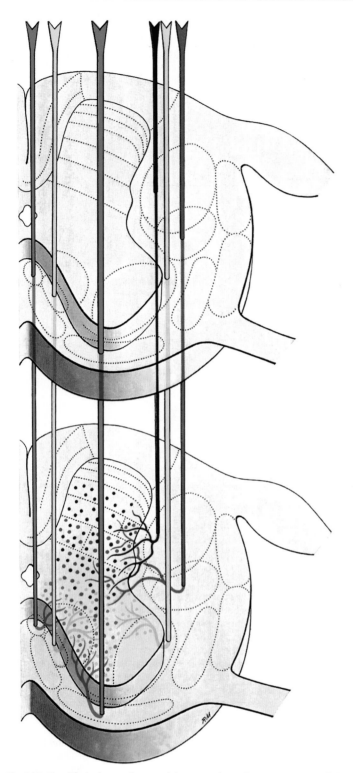

Fig. 8.30 *Simplified scheme of some of the major descending tract systems of the spinal cord, including their overlapping zones of termination in the grey matter. Within the grey matter, the dotted lines show the laminar pattern; within the white matter, they are an approximate guide to the topography of the tracts: corticospinal tract (mauve), rubrospinal tract (magenta), reticulospinal tracts (yellow), and vestibulospinal tracts (blue).*

fibres that enter the cord in the dorsal roots of spinal nerves and ascend to the dorsal column nuclei in the medulla oblongata, shorter primary afferent fibres projecting to neurones of Clarke's column and other spinal neurones and axons from secondary neurones of the spinal cord ascending to the dorsal column nuclei. The dorsal columns also contain axons of propriospinal neurones.

The fasciculus gracilis begins at the caudal end of the spinal cord. It contains long ascending branches of primary afferents, which enter the cord through ipsilateral dorsal spinal roots and ascending axons of secondary neurones in laminae IV to VI of the ipsilateral dorsal horn. As the fibres ascend, they are joined by axons of successive dorsal roots. Fibres entering in coccygeal and

CASE 3 SUBACUTE COMBINED DEGENERATION

A 58-year-old woman develops pins and needles paraesthesia in both feet, gradually ascending over several weeks to the mid-calf level. She notes difficulty walking, especially in the dark. Weakness and stiffness of both legs ensue.

Examination demonstrates weakness distally in both lower extremities, with spasticity and a spastic gait. Reflexes are exaggerated, more so in the legs than in the arms. The plantar responses are extensor. Sensory examination demonstrates striking impairment of vibratory sense and proprioception in both feet, with mild shading impairment of pain appreciation distally in the legs.

Discussion: Weakness, spasticity and hyperreflexia in the legs suggest involvement of the corticospinal tracts within the spinal cord (Fig. 8.31). Impaired vibratory and position sense indicates involvement of the posterior columns, with relative sparing of the spinothalamic sensory pathways. This is a typical clinical presentation of subacute combined degeneration of the cord due to vitamin B_{12} deficiency, documented with appropriate testing. The mild impairment of cutaneous sensibility indicates the coexistence of a polyneuropathy, similarly due to vitamin B_{12} deficiency. Dementia and visual impairment due to involvement of the optic nerves and cerebral white matter may occur.

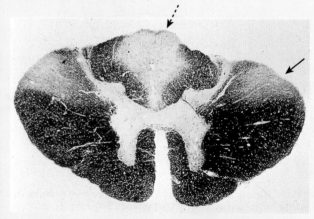

Fig. 8.31 *Subacute combined degeneration. Spinal cord stained for myelin sheaths exhibits degenerative changes in the posterior (dashed arrow) and lateral columns (solid arrow) in an individual with vitamin B_{12} deficiency.*

lower sacral regions are shifted medially by successive additions of fibres entering at higher levels.

The fasciculus gracilis lies medial to the fasciculus cuneatus in the upper spinal cord (see Fig. 8.18). At upper cervical levels, the fasciculus gracilis contains a larger proportion of afferents from cutaneous receptors than from deep proprioceptors because many of the latter leave the fasciculus at lower segments to synapse in Clarke's column. Indeed, proprioception from the lower limb reaches the thalamus mostly by relaying in Clarke's column and again in the nucleus Z. Axons of the fasciculus gracilis, from both primary and secondary neurones, terminate in the nucleus gracilis of the dorsal medulla.

The fasciculus cuneatus (see Fig. 8.32) begins at mid-thoracic level and lies lateral to the fasciculus gracilis. It is composed mostly of primary afferent fibres of the upper thoracic and cervical dorsal roots. At upper cervical levels, it contains a large population of afferents from both deep and cutaneous receptors of the upper limb. In addition, some of its axons arise from secondary neurones in laminae IV to VI of the ipsilateral dorsal horn. Many axons

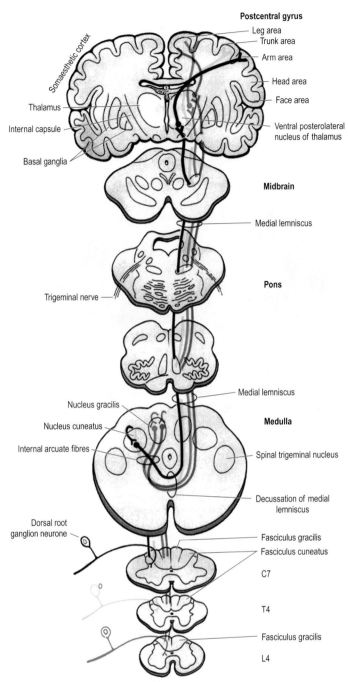

Fig. 8.32 *Dorsal column system. Primary afferent fibres from different levels and their associated second- and third-order neurones are depicted in different colours: sacral (red), lumbar (blue), thoracic (yellow), and cervical (black). (Reprinted by permission from Carpenter, M.B., 1991. Core Text of Neuroanatomy, 4th ed. Baltimore, Williams and Wilkins.)*

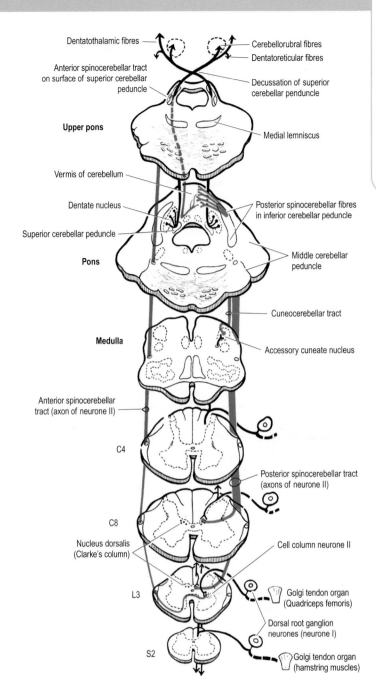

Fig. 8.33 *Spinocerebellar tracts. The cells of the dorsal spinocerebellar tract and cuneocerebellar tract are shown in blue; the cells of the ventral spinocerebellar tract are shown in red. (Reprinted by permission from Carpenter, M.B., 1991. Core Text of Neuroanatomy, 4th ed. Baltimore, Williams and Wilkins.)*

(both primary and secondary) that ascend in the fasciculus cuneatus terminate in the nucleus cuneatus of the dorsal medulla. Some also end in the lateral (external or accessory) cuneate nucleus, whose neurones project to the cerebellum via the cuneocerebellar pathway.

Many ascending fibres of the fasciculus gracilis and fasciculus cuneatus terminate by synapsing on neurones of the dorsal column nuclei (nucleus gracilis and nucleus cuneatus, respectively) in the medulla oblongata. (The connections of the dorsal column nuclei are described further with the medulla oblongata in Chapter 10.) Axons arising from neurones in the dorsal column nuclei arch ventromedially around the central grey matter of the medulla as internal arcuate fibres (see Fig. 10.6) and decussate in the sensory or lemniscal decussation. At the medial lemniscus, they ascend to the ventral posterolateral nucleus of the thalamus; from there, neurones project to the somatosensory cortex in the postcentral gyrus of the parietal lobe (areas 3, 1 and 2). Some neurones of the dorsal column nuclei form posterior external arcuate fibres, which enter the cerebellum.

The high degree of somatotopic organization present in the dorsal columns is preserved as the pathways ascend through the dorsal column nuclei and

thalamus to reach the primary somatosensory cortex. In the dorsal column nuclei, the lower limb is represented in the nucleus gracilis, the upper limb in the nucleus cuneatus and the trunk in between them. Fibres are also segregated by modality in the dorsal columns. Fibres from hair receptors are most superficial; those from tactile and vibratory receptors lie in deeper layers.

Spinocerebellar tracts — There are two principal spinocerebellar tracts: dorsal or posterior, and ventral or anterior. They occupy the periphery of the lateral aspect of the spinal white matter and carry proprioceptive and cutaneous information to the cerebellum for the coordination of movement (Fig. 8.33). Both tracts contain large-diameter myelinated fibres, but there are more in the posterior tract. Finer-calibre fibres are associated with the anterior tract.

The dorsal spinocerebellar tract lies lateral to the lateral corticospinal tract (see Fig. 8.17). It begins at about the level of the second or third lumbar segment and enlarges as it ascends. Axons of the tract originate ipsilaterally from the larger neurones of Clarke's column, in lamina VII throughout spinal segments T1 to L2. Clarke's column receives input from collaterals of long ascending primary afferents of the doral columns and terminals of shorter ascending primary afferents of the dorsal columns. Many of these afferent fibres ascend from segments caudal to L2. In the medulla, the dorsal

CASE 4   FRIEDREICH'S ATAXIA

At age 15 years, a young man develops increasing ataxia of the trunk and subsequently of the limbs. In addition to the ataxia, examination demonstrates nystagmus; dysarthria; areflexia primarily in the legs, along with extensor plantar responses; scoliosis; and impaired vibratory sense and proprioception in the legs. Ophthalmological evaluation demonstrates optic atrophy and ocular dysmetria. In addition, he has prominent scoliosis and bilateral pes cavus deformities, and he is subsequently found to have cardiomyopathy. He becomes increasingly incapacitated by virtue of the ataxic disorder and dies at age 32 years, primarily due to cardiac dysfunction.

Discussion: As with all the so-called spinocerebellar ataxias, the core clinical deficit in Friedreich's ataxia is a progressively incapacitating cerebellar deficit. Sensory changes involving especially proprioception are important and contribute to, if not actually causing, the ataxia (so-called sensory ataxia). The disease is clearly not confined to the cerebellar proprioceptive pathways, given the widespread clinical deficits such as areflexia, extensor plantar responses, optic atrophy and occasional deafness, along with non-neurological issues such as scoliosis, pes cavus and cardiomyopathy. Neuropathological changes include marked degeneration in Clarke's column of the spinal cord as well as in the posterior columns, often with gross shrinkage of the spinal cord, degeneration in the corticospinal tracts and variable changes in other ascending and descending pathways (Fig. 8.34). The cerebellum itself is often normal. Generally inherited as an autosomal recessive trait, Friedreich's ataxia is characterized by expanded trinucleotide (GAA) repeats.

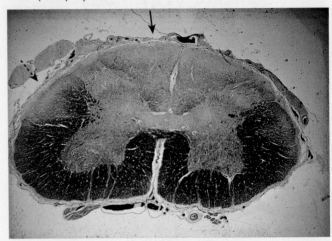

Fig. 8.34 *Friedreich's ataxia. Myelin sheath–stained section of spinal cord demonstrates marked symmetric degeneration in the posterior columns (solid arrow), with less prominent changes in the corticospinal tracts (dashed arrow). Atrophy of Clarke's column is not evident with this preparation. There is minimal degeneration of the spinocerebellar pathways.*

---

spinocerebellar tract passes through the inferior cerebellar peduncle to terminate ipsilaterally in the rostral and caudal parts of the cerebellar vermis.

The ventral spinocerebellar tract (see Fig. 8.33) lies immediately ventral to the dorsal spinocerebellar tract (see Fig. 8.17). The cells of origin are in laminae V to VII of the lumbosacral cord, and the tract carries information from the lower limb. Axons forming the tract mostly decussate; a few remain ipsilateral. The tract begins in the upper lumbar region and ascends through the medulla oblongata to reach the upper pontine level; it then descends in the dorsal part of the superior cerebellar peduncle and terminates, mainly contralaterally, in the anterior cerebellar vermis.

The spinocerebellar tracts are laminated, such that fibres from lower segments are superficial. Both tracts convey proprioceptive and exteroceptive information, but they are functionally different. Neurones of Clarke's column are excited monosynaptically by group Ia and Ib primary afferent fibres (from muscle spindles and tendon organs, respectively), as well as by group II muscle afferents and cutaneous touch and pressure afferents. The proprioceptive impulses often arise from a single muscle or from synergistic muscles acting at a common joint. Thus, the dorsal spinocerebellar tract transmits modality-specific and space-specific information used in the fine coordination of individual limb muscles. In contrast, the cells of the ventral tract are activated monosynaptically by Ib afferents and transmit information from large receptive fields that include different segments of a limb. The ventral tract lacks subdivisions for different modalities and transmits information for the coordinated movement and posture of the entire lower limb.

Because Clarke's column diminishes rostrally (see Fig. 8.23) and does not extend above the lowest cervical segment, it follows that the dorsal spinocerebellar tract carries information from the trunk and lower limb. Proprioceptive and exteroceptive information from the upper limb travels in primary afferent fibres of the fasciculus cuneatus. These fibres end somatotopically in the accessory (external or lateral) cuneate nucleus and the adjoining part of the cuneate nucleus situated in the medulla oblongata. Cells of these nuclei give rise to the posterior external arcuate fibres that form the cuneocerebellar tract (see Fig. 8.33), which enters the cerebellum via the ipsilateral inferior cerebellar peduncle. The accessory cuneate nucleus and the lateral part of the cuneate nucleus are considered homologous to the cells of Clarke's column. The cuneocerebellar tract is therefore functionally allied to the dorsal spinocerebellar tract and is its upper limb equivalent.

Axons of all the spinocerebellar tracts and the cuneocerebellar tract form part of the 'mossy-fibre' system. They end in the cerebellar cortex in a highly organized, somatotopic and functional pattern (Ch. 13).

Spinothalamic tracts — The spinothalamic tracts consist of second-order neurones that convey pain, temperature, coarse (non-discriminative) touch and pressure information to the somatosensory region of the thalamus. Axons arise from neurones in diverse laminae in all segments of the cord. Tract fibres decussate in the ventral white commissure. Pain and temperature fibres do so promptly, within about one segment of their origin, whereas fibres carrying other modalities may ascend for several segments before crossing. Spinothalamic fibres mostly ascend in the white matter ventrolateral to the ventral horn, partly intermingled with ascending spinoreticular fibres and descending reticulospinal fibres. Some authorities describe two spinothalamic tracts (lateral and ventral) with more or less distinct anatomical locations and functions. However, it should be noted that physiological studies in animals support the notion that these tracts are best considered a structural and functional continuum.

The lateral spinothalamic tract (Fig. 8.35) is sited in the lateral funiculus, lying medial to the ventral spinocerebellar tract (see Fig. 8.17). Clinical evidence indicates that it subserves pain and temperature sensations. The ventral spinothalamic tract (Fig. 8.36) lies in the anterior funiculus medial to the point of exit of the ventral nerve roots and dorsal to the vestibulospinal tract (see Fig. 8.17), which it overlaps. On the basis of clinical evidence, it subserves coarse tactile and pressure modalities.

A dorsolateral spinothalamic tract has been described in animals, arising mainly from lamina I neurones whose axons cross to ascend in the contralateral dorsolateral funiculus. These neurones respond maximally to noxious, mechanical and thermal cutaneous stimuli. That such a projection exists in humans is suggested by examples of clinical pain relief following dorsolateral cordotomy.

On reaching the lower brain stem, spinothalamic tract axons separate. Axons in the ventral tract join the medial lemniscus. Axons in the lateral tract continue as the spinal lemniscus.

There is clear somatotopic organization of the fibres in the spinothalamic tracts throughout their extent. Fibres crossing at any cord level join the deep aspect of those that have already crossed, which means that both tracts are segmentally laminated (Fig. 8.37). Somatotopy is maintained throughout the medulla oblongata and pons. In the midbrain, fibres in the spinal lemniscus conveying pain and temperature sensation from the lower limb extend dorsally, whereas those from the trunk and upper limb are more ventrally placed. Both lemnisci ascend to end in the thalamus (see Figs 8.35, 8.36). The major spinothalamic projections in humans are to the ventral posterolateral nucleus and to the centrolateral intralaminar nucleus of the thalamus.

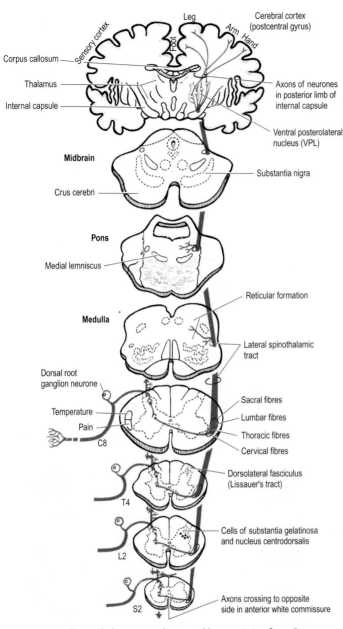

Fig. 8.35 *Lateral spinothalamic tract. (Reprinted by permission from Carpenter, M.B., 1991. Core Text of Neuroanatomy, 4th ed. Baltimore, Williams and Wilkins.)*

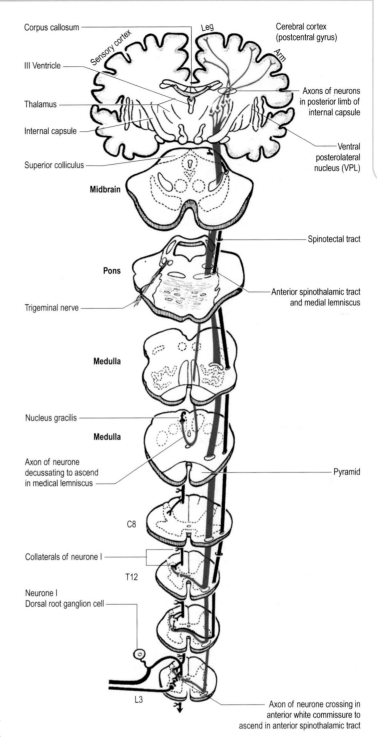

Fig. 8.36 *Ventral (anterior) spinothalamic tract. (Reprinted by permission from Carpenter, M.B., 1991. Core Text of Neuroanatomy, 4th ed. Baltimore, Williams and Wilkins.)*

Neurones of the spinothalamic tract — The specific localization of spinothalamic tract cell bodies in humans is poorly documented. In animal studies, about one third are localized to the upper three cervical segments, about 20% are located in lower cervical segments, 20% in the thoracic region (mostly segments T1–3), 20% in the lumbar region and 10% in the sacrococcygeal cord. Cells are located in laminae I and IV to VIII, with the greatest concentration in laminae VI and VII. Cell bodies giving rise to spinothalamic tract axons are predominantly contralateral. A relatively small number (10%) are ipsilateral, with the majority in the upper three cervical segments.

Neurones of the spinothalamic tract have very different receptive fields. The specificity of separate channels, which exists in the dorsal column nuclei, is absent in the laminae of the cord. Convergence of different functional types of afferent fibres onto an individual tract cell is a common feature in the cord. On the basis of laminar site, functional properties and specific thalamic termination of their axons, spinothalamic tract neurones can be divided into three separate groups: apical cells of the dorsal grey column (lamina I), deep dorsal column cells (laminae IV to VI) and cells in the ventral grey column (laminae VII and VIII). There are species differences, and the following data are found in the monkey.

Lamina I cells that project to the thalamus respond maximally to noxious or thermal cutaneous stimulation and consist mainly of high-threshold units as well as some wide dynamic range units. Their receptive fields are usually small, representing a part of a digit or a small area of skin involving several digits. Lamina I spinothalamic tract neurones receive input from Aδ and C

fibres, and some respond to convergent input from deep somatic and visceral receptors. Spinothalamic tract cells in the thoracic cord display marked viscerosomatic convergence. Lamina I spinothalamic tract neurones project preferentially to the ventral posterolateral nucleus of the thalamus, with limited projections to the centrolateral and mediodorsal thalamic nuclei.

The population of deep dorsal column (laminae IV to VI) spinothalamic neurones of the lumbar cord contains wide dynamic range (60%), high-threshold (30%) and low-threshold (10%) units. They can accurately code both innocuous and noxious cutaneous stimuli. Some cells also respond to input from deep somatic and visceral receptors. In the lumbar cord their receptive fields are small or medium-sized—larger than the area of the foot but smaller than the entire leg. In the thoracic cord the fields of these laminar cells are larger and often include the entire upper limb plus part of the chest. Many of the deep dorsal column spinothalamic tract neurones in the thoracic segments receive convergent input from sympathetic afferent fibres. Laminae IV to VI spinothalamic tract units project to either the ventral posterolateral

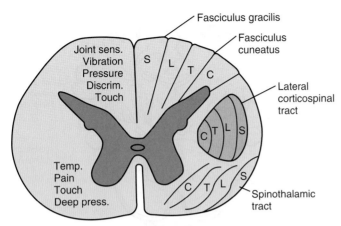

Fasciculus gracilis

Fasciculus cuneatus

Joint sens.
Vibration
Pressure
Discrim.
Touch

Lateral
corticospinal
tract

Temp.
Pain
Touch
Deep press.

Spinothalamic
tract

Fig. 8.37 *Segmental arrangement of nerve fibers in major clinically relevant tracts within the spinal cord is demonstrated. Specific sensory modalities mediated respectively by the two principle ascending pathways (spinothalmic and posterior columns) are labeled, as is the segmental distribution of motor fibers within the descending lateral corticospinal (pyramidal) tract. C: cervical; T: thoracic; L: lumbar; S: sacral (Modified from Brodal A: Neurological Anatomy, 2e. New York, Oxford Univ. Press, 1969, Figure 2-8. By permission of Oxford University Press.)*

nucleus or the centrolateral nucleus of the thalamus, and sometimes to both. Units projecting to the ventral posterolateral nucleus receive input from all classes (Aβ, Aδ and C) of cutaneous fibres.

Ventral grey column (laminae VII and VIII) spinothalamic tract cells respond mainly to deep somatic (muscle and joint) stimuli but also to innocuous or noxious cutaneous stimuli. In the thoracic regions of the spinal cord they also receive convergent input from visceral sources. The majority of laminae VII and VIII spinothalamic tract neurones have large, complex receptive fields (often bilateral) that encompass widespread areas of the body. Cells of this group, which project exclusively to the medial thalamus, receive input from Aβ, Aδ and C classes of afferent fibres, and many respond to convergent input from receptors of deep structures. This population of neurones contains wide dynamic range (25%), high-threshold (63%) and low-threshold or deep (12%) units. Most of the spinothalamic tract cells in the ventral grey column project to the intralaminar nuclei of the thalamus. Wide dynamic range–type neurones are particularly effective for discriminating between different intensities of painful stimulation. It has been suggested that the spinothalamic projection to the ventral posterolateral nucleus is concerned with the discriminative aspects of pain perception, whereas the projection to other thalamic regions, particularly the intralaminar nuclei, may be involved in arousal or aversive behaviour.

The activity of spinothalamic tract neurones may be selectively modulated by pathways descending from the brain to the spinal cord. Many studies show that the response of spinothalamic tract cells to noxious stimuli is inhibited by the stimulation of certain regions of the brain. This is obviously of considerable clinical interest in the treatment of chronic, intractable pain. In the brain stem these regions include the nucleus raphe magnus, the periaqueductal grey matter and parts of the mesencephalic and medullary reticular formation, including the parabrachial region. These neuronal groups and their connections constitute the endogenous analgesic system. Forebrain sites, which inhibit spinothalamic tract cells on stimulation, include the periventricular grey matter, ventral posterolateral nucleus of the thalamus and primary sensory and posterior parietal cortices. Inhibition of spinothalamic tract neurones is also produced by electrical stimulation of peripheral nerves, the most effective being volleys from Aδ fibres. In contrast, some spinothalamic tract cells are excited by stimulation of the medullary reticular formation and the primary motor cortex (the latter effect is probably mediated by the corticospinal tract).

Spinoreticular pathway — Spinoreticular fibres are intermingled with those of the spinothalamic tracts and ascend in the ventrolateral quadrant of the spinal cord (Fig. 8.39). Evidence from animal studies suggests that the cells of origin occur at all levels of the spinal cord, particularly in the upper cervical segments. Most neurones are in lamina VII, some are in lamina VIII, and others are in the dorsal horn, especially lamina V. Most axons in the lumbar and cervical enlargements cross the midline, but there is a large uncrossed component in cervical regions. Most axons are myelinated. The pattern of anterograde degeneration, in both human postmortem studies and experimental animals following anterolateral cordotomy, indicates spinoreticular projections to many nuclei of the medial pontomedullary reticular formation. There is also a projection to the lateral reticular nucleus (a precerebellar relay nucleus). No somatotopic arrangement has been reported. Spinoreticular neurones respond

CASE 5   SYRINGOMYELIA

A 32-year-old woman burns her hand while cooking but experiences no pain. She denies other symptoms. Examination demonstrates modest weakness and wasting of the musculature of the right hand, with impairment of pain and thermal sensibilities in that limb. Vibratory and position senses are intact. Pain appreciation is reduced in a shawl-like distribution over both shoulders and the upper torso. Sensation is otherwise preserved. Reflex activity is reduced in the involved limb but preserved elsewhere. A right-sided Horner's syndrome is noted.

Discussion: The disassociated sensory loss, of which the patient was originally unaware, along with unilateral muscular atrophy and loss of reflexes is the classic expression of syringomyelia. Early lesions are typically found within the cervical cord. The cyst generally appears at the base of the posterior horn and extends into the central grey and anterior commissure of the cord, thus involving the decussating spinothalamic fibres (Fig. 8.38). When the cyst extends into the anterior horn, lower motor neurone signs such as atrophy, weakness and reflex loss appear. Horner's syndrome indicates spread of the lesion into the intermediolateral column. With the passage of time, the cystic lesion enlarges and may involve much of the remainder of the cord, with widespread motor and sensory deficits. The lesion commonly extends inferiorly in the cord and superiorly into the lower brain stem (syringobulbia).

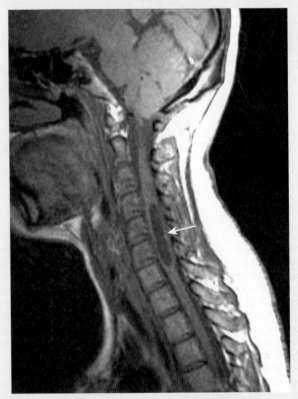

Fig. 8.38 *Syringomyelia. MRI of the cervical cord demonstrates a typical cystic lesion (arrow). (© 2010 Thomas Jefferson University. All rights reserved. Reproduced with the permission of Thomas Jefferson University.)*

to inputs from the skin or deep tissues. Innocuous cutaneous stimuli may inhibit or excite a particular cell, whereas noxious stimuli are often excitatory. A spinoreticulothalamocortical pathway has been proposed as an important route serving pain perception. Like other ascending pathways, the tract cells are influenced by descending control. For example, electrical stimulation of

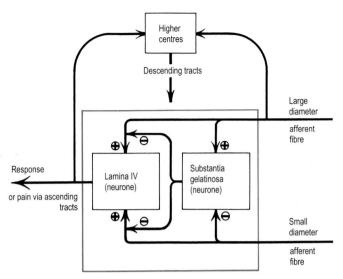

Fig. 8.40 Basic arrangement of the sensory 'gate' mechanism in the dorsal laminae of the grey matter of the spinal cord. (Redrawn with permission from Melzack, R., Wall, P.D. 1965. Pain mechanisms: a new theory. Science 150, 971–979. Copyright 1965 American Association for the Advancement of Science. Reprinted with permission from AAAS.)

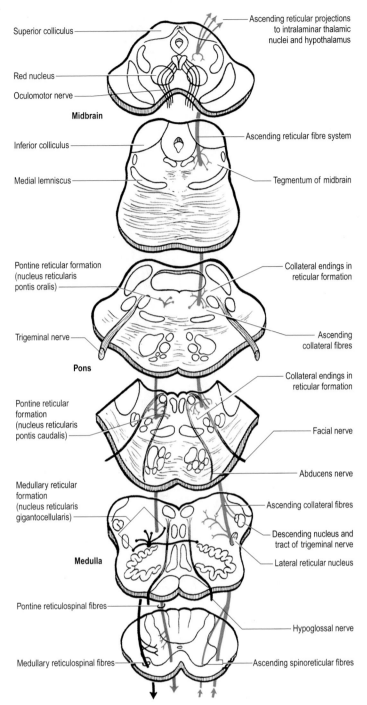

Fig. 8.39 Reticular tracts: ascending (blue), descending (red), and medullary (black). (Reprinted by permission from Carpenter, M.B., 1991. Core Text of Neuroanatomy, 4th ed. Baltimore, Williams and Wilkins.)

the periaqueductal grey matter inhibits the responses of certain spinoreticular cells to input from cardiopulmonary afferents. Stimulation of the reticular formation also alters the activity of spinoreticular neurones.

Spinocervicothalamic pathway — The lateral cervical nucleus is small in humans. It lies in the lateral funiculus, ventrolateral to the dorsal horn in the upper two cervical segments. In some human cord specimens the nucleus is not distinctly defined and may be incorporated into the dorsal horn. It receives axons from the spinocervical tract, which ascends in the dorsolateral funiculus. The tract cells are found in laminae III to V at all levels of the spinal cord, ipsilateral to the nucleus. Most neurones of the nucleus project to the contralateral thalamus via the medial lemniscus, and some project to the contralateral midbrain. Specific thalamic targets include the ventral posterolateral nucleus and part of the posterior complex. Spinocervical tract neurones respond to hair movement, pressure, pinch and thermal stimuli and to high-threshold muscle input; many also respond to noxious stimuli. Like tract cells of other ascending pathways, they are under tonic descending inhibitory control.

Spinomesencephalic pathway — The spinomesencephalic pathway consists of a number of tracts ascending from the spinal cord to various regions of

the midbrain. It includes the spinotectal tract projecting to the superior colliculus, neurones synapsing in the periaqueductal grey matter and other spinal cord projections that terminate in the parabrachial nucleus, pretectal nuclei and Darkshevich's nucleus. Cells of origin are located throughout the length of the spinal cord, particularly in the cervical segments and the lumbosacral enlargement, mostly in lamina I; however, they are also present in laminae IV to VIII, where they are concentrated in lamina V. Most are contralateral, but a prominent ipsilateral group is also found at upper cervical levels. Fibres of the spinomesencephalic tract are mostly myelinated and ascend in the white matter of the ventrolateral quadrant of the spinal cord, in association with the spinothalamic and spinoreticular tracts.

Spinomesencephalic tract neurones are of low-threshold, wide dynamic range, or high-threshold classes. Their receptive fields may be small, or they may be very complex and encompass large surface areas of the body. Many spinomesencephalic tract cells are nociceptive and are likely to be involved in the motivational-affective component of pain. Electrical stimulation of their site of termination in the periaqueductal grey matter results in severe pain in humans. Furthermore, the cells of the deeper layers of the superior colliculus, where spinotectal fibres synapse, are activated by noxious stimuli.

Spino-olivary tract — The spino-olivary tract is described in animals as arising from neurones in the deeper laminae of grey matter. Axons forming the tract cross and then ascend superficially at the junction of the anterior and lateral white funiculi, ending in the 'spinal' regions of the dorsal and medial accessory olivary nuclei. The tract carries information from muscle and tendon proprioceptors and from cutaneous receptors. A functionally similar route, the dorsal spino-olivary tract, ascends in the dorsal white funiculi and relays in the dorsal column nuclei to the contralateral inferior olive. Information on these tracts in primates is scant, but postmortem evidence following cordotomies in humans reveals degenerating axonal terminals in the inferior olive.

Pain mechanisms — The ascending connections through which sensory information reaches higher centres should not be regarded as simple relays because it is known that they are subject to modulation by complex intraspinal influences and by descending pathways from the brain stem and cerebral cortex. This is particularly important in relation to the spinothalamic and spinoreticular pathways and the perception of pain.

Presynaptic inhibition influences many, and possibly all, primary afferent terminals. A much-investigated site of presynaptic effects is the substantia gelatinosa. It has been proposed that impulses from cutaneous (and other) afferents are subjected there to tonic control by presynaptic modulation of primary afferent terminals, mediated by small neurones of the substantia gelatinosa.

The gate control theory (Melzack and Wall 1965) defined a possible mechanism for modulating the inflow of information along nociceptive and other afferent pathways (Fig. 8.40). The proposition was that large-diameter afferents (e.g. from hairs and touch corpuscles) are excitatory to the large neurones of lamina IV, from which spinothalamic fibres arise, and to interneurones in the substantia gelatinosa. In contrast, fine non-myelinated afferents are excitatory to tract cells but inhibitory to interneurones. The axons of substantia gelatinosa interneurones are presumed to presynaptically inhibit the terminals of all afferents that synapse with tract cells. In such a system, low activity in the fine afferents inhibits the interneurones and thus prevents them from inhibiting tract cells; hence the 'gate' to T cells in lamina IV is open to transmit intermittent small volleys of impulses from the large fibres. A prolonged high-frequency volley of impulses in the large-diameter afferents would be transmitted to lamina IV tract cells initially, but this would soon cease as activity in the interneurones closed the gate. Conversely, persistent high activity in the fine afferents would open the gate, resulting in massive bombardment of neurones of lamina IV (which include some high-threshold neurones that are activated only by such bombardment). It was assumed that onward transmission in the lateral spinothalamic tract would evoke pain at supraspinal centres. Pain would therefore result from an imbalance between the varieties of afferent impulses when there was disproportionately large traffic along the fine afferents.

The overall sensitivity of the gate may be varied by descending supraspinal control systems. These originate within three principal, interconnected regions in the midbrain, hindbrain and spinal cord, each of which receives a variety of afferents and contains an array of neuromediators.

The midbrain regions are the periaqueductal grey matter, dorsal raphe nucleus and part of the cuneiform nucleus. Neurones in these sites contain serotonin (5-HT), γ-aminobutyric acid (GABA), substance P, CCK, neurotensin, enkephalin and dynorphin. The periaqueductal grey matter receives afferents from the frontal somatosensory and cingulate neocortex, the amygdala, numerous local reticular nuclei and the hypothalamus. Afferents from the last are separate bundles that carry histamine, luteinizing hormone-releasing hormone, vasopressin, oxytocin, adrenocorticotrophic hormone, melanocyte-stimulating hormone, endorphin and angiotensin II. Some fibres descend from the periaqueductal grey matter to rhombencephalic centres; others pass directly to the spinal cord.

In the rhombencephalon, the raphe magnus nucleus and medial reticular column constitute an important multineuromediator centre. Neurones in these sites contain serotonin, substance P, CCK, thyrotropin-releasing hormone, enkephalin and dynorphin. Some neurones contain two or even three neuromediators. Descending bulbospinal fibres pass to the nucleus of the spinal tract of the trigeminal nerve and its continuation, the substantia gelatinosa. The latter extends throughout the length of the cord and contains populations of neurones expressing many different neuromediators (e.g. GABA, substance P, neurotensin, enkephalin, dynorphin). There is abundant physiological and pharmacological evidence that all these regions are intimately concerned with the control of nociceptive (and probably other modality) inputs.

Descending Tracts

Descending pathways to the spinal cord originate primarily in the cerebral cortex and in numerous sites within the brain stem (Figs 8.39, 8.41, 8.42). They are concerned with the control of movement, muscle tone and posture; the modulation of spinal reflex mechanisms; and the transmission of afferent information to higher levels. They also mediate control over spinal autonomic neurones.

Corticospinal tract — Corticospinal fibres arise from neurones of the cerebral cortex. They project, in a somatotopically organized fashion, to neurones that are located mostly in the contralateral side of the spinal cord (see Fig. 8.41). The majority of corticospinal fibres arise from cells situated in the upper two-thirds of the precentral motor cortex (area 4) and from the premotor cortex (area 6). A small contribution of fibres comes from cells of the postcentral gyrus (somatosensory cortex, areas 1, 2, and 3) and the adjacent parietal cortex (area 5). In the monkey, 30% of corticospinal fibres arise from area 4, 30% from area 6 and 40% from the parietal regions. Cells of origin of corticospinal fibres vary in size in the different cortical areas and are clustered into groups or strips. The largest cells (giant pyramidal neurones, or Betz cells) are in the precentral cortex.

Corticospinal fibres descend first through the subcortical white matter and enter the posterior limb of the internal capsule. They then pass through the ventral part of the midbrain in the cerebral peduncle or crus cerebri. As they continue caudally through the pons, they are separated from its ventral surface by transversely running pontocerebellar fibres. In the medulla oblongata they form a discrete bundle, the pyramid (see Fig. 10.3), which forms a prominent longitudinal column on the ventral surface of the medulla. Thus, the corticospinal tracts are also referred to as the pyramidal tracts. However, this term is often used to denote not only corticospinal fibres but also corticobulbar fibres, which diverge above this level and end in association with cranial motor nuclei. Each pyramid contains about a million axons of varying diameters. The majority (70%) are myelinated; most (90%) have a diameter of 1 to 4 mm, 9% have diameters of 5 to 10 mm and less than 2%

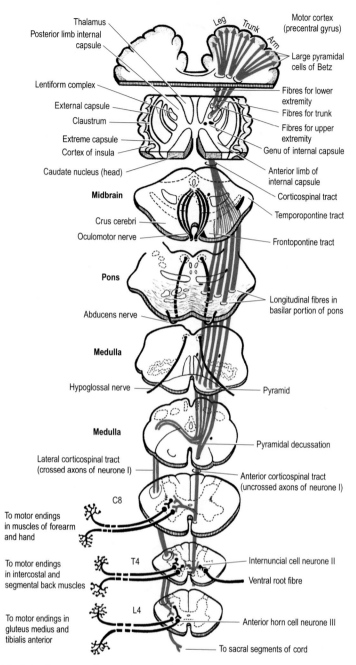

Fig. 8.41 *Corticospinal tracts. (Reprinted by permission from Carpenter, M.B., 1991. Core Text of Neuroanatomy, 4th ed. Baltimore, Williams and Wilkins.)*

have diameters of 11 to 22 mm. The largest-diameter axons arise from the giant Betz cells.

Just rostral to the level of the spinomedullary junction, approximately 75% to 90% of the corticospinal fibres in the pyramid cross the median plane in the pyramidal decussation (decussation of the pyramids) and continue caudally as the lateral corticospinal tract. The rest of the fibres continue uncrossed as the ventral corticospinal tract. The lateral tract also contains some uncrossed corticospinal fibres. The lateral corticospinal tract (see Fig. 8.41) descends in the lateral funiculus throughout most of the length of the spinal cord. It occupies an oval area, ventrolateral to the dorsal horn and medial to the dorsal spinocerebellar tract (see Fig. 8.18). In the lumbar and sacral regions, where the dorsal spinocerebellar tract is absent, the lateral corticospinal tract reaches the dorsolateral surface of the cord. As it descends, the lateral corticospinal tract progressively diminishes in size until about the fourth sacral spinal segment. Its axons terminate on ipsilateral spinal neurones.

The smaller ventral corticospinal tract (see Fig. 8.41) descends in the ventral funiculus. It lies close to the ventral median fissure and is separated from it by the sulcomarginal fasciculus (see Fig. 8.18). The ventral corticospinal tract diminishes as it descends and usually disappears completely at mid-thoracic cord levels. It may be absent or, very rarely, contain almost all the corticospinal fibres. Near their termination, most fibres of the tract cross the median plane in the ventral white commissure to synapse with contralateral neurones.

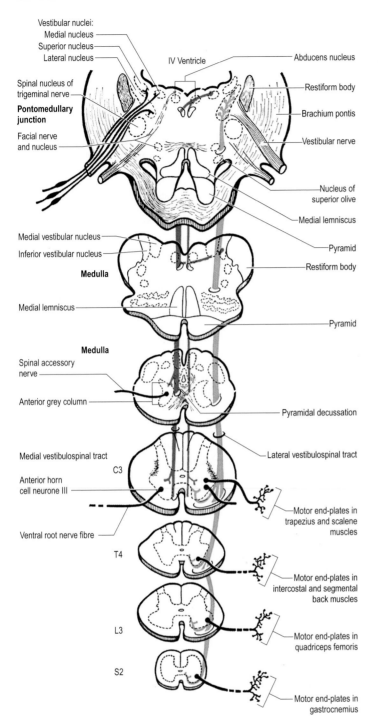

Vestibular nuclei:
Medial nucleus
Superior nucleus
Lateral nucleus

IV Ventricle

Abducens nucleus

Spinal nucleus of
trigeminal nerve

**Pontomedullary
junction**

Facial nerve
and nucleus

Restiform body

Brachium pontis

Vestibular nerve

Nucleus of
superior olive

Medial lemniscus

Medial vestibular nucleus

Inferior vestibular nucleus

Medulla

Pyramid

Restiform body

Medial lemniscus

Pyramid

Medulla

Spinal accessory
nerve

Anterior grey column

Pyramidal decussation

Medial vestibulospinal tract

C3

Anterior horn
cell neurone III

Ventral root nerve fibre

Lateral vestibulospinal tract

Motor end-plates in
trapezius and scalene
muscles

T4

Motor end-plates in
intercostal and segmental
back muscles

L3

Motor end-plates in
quadriceps femoris

S2

Motor end-plates in
gastrocnemius

Fig. 8.42 *Vestibulospinal tracts. (Reprinted by permission from Carpenter, M.B., 1991. Core Text of Neuroanatomy, 4th ed. Baltimore, Williams and Wilkins.)*

The vast majority of corticospinal fibres, irrespective of the tract in which they descend, terminate in the spinal cord on the side contralateral to their cortical origin.

Knowledge of the detailed termination of corticospinal fibres is based largely on animal studies but is supplemented by data from postmortem studies on human brains using anterograde degeneration methods. Most corticospinal fibres are believed to terminate contralaterally on interneurones in the lateral parts of laminae IV to VI and both lateral and medial parts of lamina VII. Some are also distributed to lamina VIII bilaterally. Terminals are associated with contralateral motor neuronal cell groups in lamina IX, in the dorsolateral group and in the lateral parts of both the central and ventrolateral groups (see Fig. 8.30).

Corticospinal fibres from the frontal cortex, including motor and premotor areas 4 and 6, terminate mostly on interneurones in laminae V to VIII, with the densest concentration laterally in lamina VI. They influence α and γ motor neurones of lamina IX via these interneurones. Because the widespread dendrites of multipolar neurones in lamina IX penetrate lamina VII, direct monosynaptic axodendritic contacts also occur on large α motor

neurones. Direct termination on motor neurones is most abundant in the spinal enlargements.

Experimental evidence shows that precentral corticospinal axons influence the activities of both α and γ motor neurones, facilitating flexor muscles and inhibiting extensors—opposite of the effects mediated by lateral vestibulospinal fibres. Evidence from animal studies shows that direct projections from the precentral cortical areas to spinal motor neurones are concerned with highly fractionated, precision movements of the limbs. Accordingly, in primates, precentral corticospinal fibres are distributed mainly to motor neurones supplying the distal limb muscles. Corticospinal projections may use glutamate or aspartate, often co-localized, as excitatory neurotransmitters.

Corticospinal fibres from parietal sources end mainly in the contralateral dorsal horn, in the lateral parts of laminae IV to VI and VII. Phylogenetically, these fibres represent the oldest part of the corticospinal system. Axons from the sensory cortex terminate chiefly in laminae IV and V. They are concerned with the supraspinal modulation of the transmission of afferent impulses to higher centres, including the motor cortex.

Experimental studies in primates indicate that isolated transection of corticospinal fibres at the level of the pyramid (pyramidotomy) results in flaccid paralysis or paresis of the contralateral limbs and loss of independent hand and finger movements. Destruction of corticospinal fibres at the level of the internal capsule, commonly caused by a cerebrovascular accident or 'stroke,' results in a contralateral hemiplegia. The paralysis is initially flaccid but later becomes spastic; it is most marked in the distal muscles of the extremities, especially those concerned with individual movements of the fingers and hand. Associated signs on the paralysed side are hyperactive deep tendon reflexes, hypertonicity, loss of superficial abdominal and cremasteric reflexes and dorsiflexion of the toes (Babinski's sign) in response to stroking the sole of the foot. The last is usually interpreted as pathognomonic of corticospinal damage, but it is not always present in patients with confirmed corticospinal lesions. Moreover, Babinski's sign is normally present in human children up to about 2 years of age. Its subsequent disappearance may reflect the completion of myelination of the corticospinal fibres or the establishment of direct cortical connections to lower motor neurones.

Some of the sequelae of stroke damage in the internal capsule, in particular hyperreflexia and hypertonia, are due to the involvement of other pathways in addition to the corticospinal tract. These include descending cortical fibres to brain stem nuclei, such as the vestibular and reticular nuclei, which themselves give rise to descending projections that influence motor neurone activity.

Rubrospinal tract — The rubrospinal tract arises from neurones in the caudal magnocellular part of the red nucleus, an ovoid mass of cells situated centrally in the midbrain tegmentum (Ch. 10). This part of the nucleus contains some 150 to 200 large neurones, interspersed with smaller neurones.

The origin, localization, termination and functions of rubrospinal connections are poorly defined in humans, and the tract appears to be rudimentary. Rubrospinal fibres cross in the ventral tegmental decussation and descend in the lateral funiculus of the cord, where they lie ventral to, and intermingled with, fibres of the lateral corticospinal tract (see Fig. 8.18). In animals, the tract descends as far as lumbosacral levels, whereas in humans it appears to project only to the upper three cervical cord segments. Rubrospinal fibres are distributed to the lateral parts of laminae V and VI and the dorsal part of lamina VII of the spinal grey matter. The terminal zones of the tract correspond to those of corticospinal fibres from the motor cortex. Animal studies demonstrate that the effects of rubrospinal fibres on α and γ motor neurones are similar to those of corticospinal fibres.

Tectospinal tract — The tectospinal tract arises from neurones in the intermediate and deep layers of the superior colliculus of the midbrain. It crosses ventral to the periaqueductal grey matter in the dorsal tegmental decussation and descends in the medial part of the ventral funiculus of the spinal cord (see Fig. 8.17). Fibres of the tract project only to the upper cervical cord segments, ending in laminae VI to VIII. They make polysynaptic connections with motor neurones serving muscles in the neck, facilitating those that innervate contralateral muscles and inhibiting those that innervate ipsilateral ones. In animals, turning of the head to the contralateral side results from unilateral electrical stimulation of the superior colliculus and is effected mainly through the tectospinal tract.

Vestibulospinal tracts — The large vestibular nuclear complex lies in the lateral part of the floor of the fourth ventricle around the pontomedullary junction of the brain stem. It gives rise to the lateral and ventral vestibulospinal tracts, which are functionally and topographically distinct (see Fig. 8.42).

The lateral vestibulospinal tract arises from small and large neurones of the lateral vestibular nucleus (Deiters' nucleus). It descends ipsilaterally, initially in the periphery of the ventrolateral spinal white matter but subsequently shifting into the medial part of the ventral funiculus at lower spinal levels. Fibres of this tract are somatotopically organized. Thus, fibres projecting to the cervical, thoracic and lumbosacral segments of the cord arise from neurones in the rostroventral, central and dorsocaudal parts, respectively, of the lateral vestibular nucleus. Lateral vestibulospinal fibres end ipsilaterally, mostly in the medial part of the ventral horn in lamina VIII and the medial part of lamina VII. Axons of the lateral vestibulospinal tract excite, through mono- and polysynaptic connections, motor neurones of extensor muscles of the neck, back and limbs; γ motor neurones are probably facilitated as well. Lateral vestibulospinal tract axons also inhibit, disynaptically, motor neurones of flexor limb muscles via 1a inhibitory interneurones.

The medial vestibulospinal tract arises mainly from neurones in the medial vestibular nucleus, but some are also located in the inferior and lateral vestibular nuclei. The medial vestibulospinal tract (see Fig. 8.42) descends in the medial longitudinal fasciculus into the ventral funiculus of the spinal cord, where it lies close to the midline in the so-called sulcomarginal fasciculus (see Fig. 8.18). Unlike the lateral tract, it contains both crossed and uncrossed fibres and does not extend beyond the mid-thoracic cord level. Fibres of the medial tract project mainly to the cervical cord segments, ending in lamina VIII and the adjacent dorsal part of lamina VII. Data from stimulation of the vestibular nuclei in animals indicate that axons of the medial tract monosynaptically inhibit the motor neurones that innervate axial muscles of the neck and upper part of the back.

Reticulospinal tracts — The reticulospinal tracts pass from the brain stem reticular formation to the spinal cord. Detailed knowledge of their origins and connections has been obtained mainly from studies in animals.

The medial reticulospinal tract (see Fig. 8.39) originates from the medial tegmental fields of the pons and medulla. The main sources are the oral and caudal pontine reticular nuclei and the gigantocellular reticular nucleus in the medulla. Pontine fibres descend, mainly ipsilaterally, in the ventral funiculus of the cord. Medullary fibres descend, both ipsilaterally and contralaterally, in the ventral funiculus and ventral part of the lateral funiculus. These fibres have many collaterals, and two-thirds of the reticulospinal neurones that reach the cervical cord also descend to lumbosacral levels. The terminals of reticulospinal fibres are distributed to lamina VIII and the central and medial parts of lamina VII. The medullary reticulospinal terminals are more widely distributed, ending additionally in the lateral parts of laminae VI and VII and directly on motor neurones. From animal studies, it appears that terminations of reticulospinal fibres that originate in the medulla are, in general, more dorsally placed than those that originate in the pons, although there is considerable overlap.

Both α and γ motor neurones are influenced by reticulospinal fibres through polysynaptic and monosynaptic connections. Physiological evidence shows that reticulospinal fibres from pontine sources excite motor neurones of axial and limb muscles, whereas medullary fibres excite or inhibit motor neurones of cervical muscles and excite motor neurones of axial muscles. Functionally, the medial reticulospinal tract is concerned with posture, the steering of head and trunk movements in response to external stimuli and crude stereotyped movements of the limbs.

The lateral reticulospinal tract lies in the lateral funiculus of the spinal cord, closely associated with the rubrospinal and lateral corticospinal tracts (see Fig. 8.18). Its fibres arise from neurones of the ventrolateral tegmental field of the pons. The fibres cross in the rostral medulla oblongata and project, with a high degree of collateralization, throughout the length of the spinal cord. Axons of this tract terminate in laminae I, V and VI and also bilaterally in the lateral cervical nucleus. Evidence suggests that this pathway is involved in the control of pain perception and in motor functions.

Interstitiospinal tract — The interstitiospinal tract arises from neurones in the interstitial nucleus (of Cajal) and the immediate surrounding area and descends via the medial longitudinal fasciculus into the ventral funiculus of the spinal cord. Its fibres project, mainly ipsilaterally, as far as lumbosacral levels and are distributed mostly to the dorsal part of lamina VIII and the dorsally adjoining part of lamina VII. They establish some monosynaptic connections with motor neurones supplying neck muscles, but their main connections are disynaptic with motor neurones supplying limb muscles.

Solitariospinal tract — The solitariospinal tract is a small group of mostly crossed fibres that arise from neurones in the ventrolateral part of the nucleus solitarius of the medulla. Descending in the ventral funiculus and ventral part of the lateral funiculus of the cord, these axons terminate on phrenic motor neurones supplying the diaphragm and thoracic motor neurones that innervate intercostal muscles. A pathway with a somewhat similar course and terminations originates from the nucleus retroambiguus. Both pathways subserve respiratory activities by driving inspiratory muscles, and some descending axons from the nucleus retroambiguus facilitate expiratory motor neurones. There is clinical evidence that bilateral ventrolateral cordotomy at high cervical levels abolishes rhythmic ventilatory movements.

Hypothalamospinal fibres — Hypothalamospinal fibres exist in animals. They arise from the paraventricular nucleus and other areas of the

hypothalamus and descend ipsilaterally, mainly in the dorsolateral region of the cord, to be distributed to sympathetic and parasympathetic preganglionic neurones in the intermediolateral column. Fibres from the paraventricular nucleus show oxytocin and vasopressin immunoreactivity. They are also distributed to laminae I and X. Descending fibres from the dopaminergic cell group (A11) situated in the caudal hypothalamus innervate sympathetic preganglionic neurones and neurones in the dorsal horn. That similar pathways exist in humans can be inferred from ipsilateral sympathetic deficits (e.g. Horner's syndrome) that follow lesions of the hypothalamus, the lateral tegmental brain stem or the lateral funiculus of the cord.

Monoaminergic spinal pathways — Monoaminergic cell groups utilize dopamine, adrenaline (epinephrine), noradrenaline (norepinephrine) and 5-HT as neurotransmitters. They occur widely throughout the brain stem and in the hypothalamus. They project rostrally to many forebrain areas and caudally to the spinal cord and appear to be concerned with the modulation of sensory transmission and the control of autonomic and somatic motor neuronal activities.

The projections to the spinal cord arise from several sources. Coeruleospinal projections originate from noradrenergic cell groups A4 and A6 in the locus coeruleus complex in the pons and descend via the ventrolateral white matter to innervate all cord segments bilaterally. They end in the dorsal grey matter (laminae IV to VI) and the intermediate and ventral horns. They also project extensively to preganglionic parasympathetic neurones in the sacral cord. Descending noradrenergic fibres, which arise from lateral tegmental cell groups A5 and A7 of the pons, travel in the dorsolateral white matter. They are distributed to laminae I to III and particularly to the intermediate grey horn. Descending fibres from adrenergic cell groups C1 and C3 of the medulla oblongata have been traced into the anterior funiculus of the cord and are extensively distributed to the intermediolateral column. Dopaminergic fibres projecting to the spinal cord travel in the hypothalamospinal pathway.

The raphe nuclei pallidus (B1), obscurus (B2) and magnus (B3) in the brain stem give rise to two serotoninergic descending bundles. The lateral raphe spinal bundle, from B3 neurones, is concerned with the control of nociception. It descends close to the lateral corticospinal tract and ends in the dorsal horn (laminae I, II and V). The ventral bundle, composed mainly of axons from B1 neurones, travels in the medial part of the ventral white column and ends in the ventral horn (laminae VIII and IX). It facilitates extensor and flexor motor neurones. Some descending serotoninergic fibres project to sympathetic preganglionic neurones and are concerned with the central control of cardiovascular function.

Summary of major descending brain stem tracts — In an analysis of the descending tracts in mammals, Kuypers (1981) subdivided the descending brain stem pathways into groups A and B, on the basis of their terminal distribution and functional attributes.

Group A (ventromedial brain stem pathways) consists of both vestibulospinal tracts, together with the medial reticulospinal, tectospinal and interstitiospinal tracts, all of which pass through the medial and ventral parts of the lower brain stem tegmentum to descend in the ventral and ventrolateral funiculi of the spinal cord. Fibres of these tracts end, often with a bilateral distribution, in the ventromedial part of the intermediate zone (laminae V to VII) of the spinal grey matter. The fibres of most of these tracts are highly collateralized. Some make monosynaptic connections with motor neurones innervating muscles of the limbs. The neurones from which group A axons arise receive cortical projections mainly from areas rostral to the precentral gyrus. Functionally, this system is concerned with the maintenance of posture, the integration of movements of the body and limbs and synergistic whole-limb movements, but it also subserves the orientation movements of the body and head.

Group B (lateral brain stem pathways) consists of the rubrospinal tract and the lateral reticulospinal tract. These tracts descend through the ventrolateral part of the lower brain stem tegmentum and continue in the dorsolateral funiculus of the spinal cord. They terminate, mainly ipsilaterally, in the dorsal and lateral parts of the intermediate zone of spinal grey matter (laminae V to VII). Rubrospinal fibres in non-human primates also establish monosynaptic connections with motor neurones innervating distal limb muscles. Rubrospinal neurones receive cortical afferent fibres mainly from the precentral gyrus. Group B pathways provide the capacity for independent, flexion-biased movements of the limbs and shoulders, and especially of the elbows and hands. They supplement the motor control mediated by group A pathways. The termination of the two groups of brain stem pathways is largely overlapped by that of the corticospinal pathway arising from motor areas of the frontal lobe. Functionally, this part of the corticospinal system enhances the brain stem controls. In addition, it provides the capacity for fractionation of movements, as exemplified by individual finger movements, which are probably executed through direct corticospinal connections with motor neurones.

Propriospinal Tracts

Propriospinal pathways, or tracts, are sometimes referred to as the fasciculi proprii. Propriospinal neurones are confined to the spinal cord; that is, their ascending and descending fibres begin and end within the spinal grey matter. They connect neurones within the same segment or other neurones in more distant segments of the spinal cord and thus subserve intrasegmental and intersegmental integration and coordination. The majority of spinal neurones are propriospinal neurones, most of which lie in laminae V to VIII. Propriospinal fibres are concentrated mainly around the margins of the grey matter (see Fig. 8.17) but are also dispersed diffusely in the white funiculi.

The propriospinal system plays important roles in spinal functions. Descending pathways end on specific subgroups of propriospinal neurones, and these in turn relay to motor neurones and other spinal neurones. The system mediates all those automatic functions that continue after transection of the spinal cord, including sudomotor and vasomotor activities and bowel and bladder functions.

Some propriospinal axons are very short and span only one segment; others run the entire length of the cord. The shortest axons lie immediately adjacent to the grey matter, and the longer ones are situated more peripherally. Propriospinal neurones can be categorized according to the length of their axons as long, intermediate or short. Long propriospinal neurones distribute their axons throughout the length of the cord, mainly via the ventral and lateral funiculi; their cell bodies are in lamina VIII and the dorsally adjoining part of lamina VII. Axons from the long propriospinal neurones of the cervical cord descend bilaterally, whereas those from the corresponding lumbosacral neurones ascend mainly contralaterally. Most of the fibres are fine (<3 mm in diameter). Some are the first spinal tract axons to become myelinated. Intermediate propriospinal neurones occupy the central and medial parts of lamina VII and project mainly ipsilaterally. Short propriospinal neurones are found in the lateral parts of laminae V to VIII, and their axons run ipsilaterally in the lateral funiculus.

Propriospinal fibres in the different parts of the white funiculi are distributed preferentially to specific regions of the spinal grey matter. In the spinal enlargements, the propriospinal fibres in the dorsolateral funiculus project to the dorsal and lateral parts of the intermediate zone and also to spinal motor neurones that supply distal limb muscles, especially those of the hands and feet. The propriospinal fibres in the ventral part of the ventrolateral funiculus are distributed to the central and medial parts of lamina VII and to motor neurones of proximal limb and girdle muscles. Other propriospinal fibres run in the medial part of the ventral funiculus and travel mainly to the ventromedial part of the intermediate zone, which characteristically contains long propriospinal neurones, and to motor neurones innervating axial and girdle muscles.

Tract of Lissauer

The tract of Lissauer, or the dorsolateral tract, lies between the apex of the dorsal horn and the surface of the spinal cord, where it surrounds the incoming dorsal root fibres. It is present throughout the spinal cord and is most developed in the upper cervical regions.

The tract consists of fine myelinated and non-myelinated axons. Many are the branches of axons in the lateral bundles of the dorsal roots. These axons bifurcate into ascending and descending branches as they enter the cord. The branches travel in the tract of Lissauer for one or two segments and give off collaterals, which end on and around neurones in the dorsal horn. The tract also contains propriospinal fibres, some of which are short axons of small substantia gelatinosa neurones, which reenter the dorsal horn.

CASE 6   ACUTE TRANSVERSE MYELITIS

A 50-year-old woman presents to the emergency department with acute paraparesis. She had experienced some tingling paraesthesia in the feet before going to bed but had no other neurological complaints. She awoke unable to move her legs. She reports having had a viral respiratory illness 1 week ago.

On examination, her cranial nerves are intact. Motor power is normal in the upper extremities but absent in the legs. Reflexes are preserved throughout, and the plantar responses are silent. All sensory modalities are lost below T6. She is unable to void. MRI reveals swelling of the spinal cord from T5 to T7. Lumbar puncture yields CSF with an elevated protein content and 30 white cells per cubic millimetre, predominantly lymphocytes. A diagnosis of acute transverse myelitis is made, and she is given a course of corticosteroids.

At follow-up 3 months later, she is walking with a walker and exhibits severe spasticity in the legs, with exaggerated reflexes and extensor plantar responses. She continues to require intermittent bladder catheterization.

Discussion: Acute transverse myelitis is an acute or subacutely evolving idiopathic inflammatory disorder of the spinal cord, usually presenting as an acute sensorimotor segmental myelopathy. The lesions often involve several adjacent segments of the spinal cord; both grey and white matter are affected. The diagnosis is confirmed by MRI and spinal fluid analysis (Fig. 8.43).

The cause of acute transverse myelitis is variable. It may occur after systemic infection; multiple sclerosis, vasculitis and other autoimmune conditions have also been implicated. High-dose corticosteroid treatment may be of some benefit, but many patients experience permanent disability.

Sometimes a patient with transverse myelitis also develops acute optic neuritis. This combination, referred to as neuromyelitis optica, or Devic's disease, was previously thought

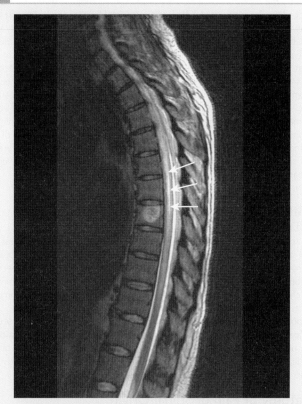

Fig. 8.43 *MRI of the thoracic spine demonstrates the changes of acute transverse myelitis (arrows). (© 2010 Thomas Jefferson University. All rights reserved. Reproduced with the permission of Thomas Jefferson University.)*

to be a type of multiple sclerosis. However, the recent identification of a specific serum autoantibody (NMO-Ig) in such cases, but not in more traditional forms of multiple sclerosis, indicates that this unitary hypothesis is no longer tenable.

SPINAL CORD INJURY AND VERTEBRAL COLUMN INJURY

In the assessment of a patient with spinal injury and neurological damage, it is important to remember that the level of cord and root injury does not coincide with that of the skeletal damage to the vertebral column.

In estimating the vertebral levels of cord segments in the adult, a useful approximation is that in the cervical region, the tip of a vertebral spinous process corresponds to the succeeding cord segment (e.g. the sixth cervical spine is opposite the seventh spinal segment); at upper thoracic levels, the tip of a vertebral spine corresponds to the cord two segments lower (e.g. the fourth thoracic spine is level with the sixth segment); and in the lower thoracic region, there is a difference of three segments (e.g. the tenth thoracic spine is level with the first lumbar segment). The eleventh thoracic spine overlies the third lumbar segment, and the twelfth is opposite the first sacral segment. When making this estimate by palpation of the vertebral spines, the relationship of the individual spines to their vertebral bodies should be remembered.

Complete division above the fourth cervical segment causes respiratory failure because of the loss of activity in the phrenic and intercostal nerves. Lesions between C5 and T1 paralyse all four limbs (quadriplegia), but the effects in the upper limbs vary with the site of injury: at the fifth cervical segment, paralysis is complete; at the sixth, each arm is positioned in abduction and lateral rotation, with the elbow flexed and the forearm supinated, due to unopposed activity in the deltoid, supraspinatus, rhomboid and brachial flexors (all supplied by the fifth cervical spinal nerves). In lower cervical lesions, upper limb paralysis is less marked. Lesions of the first thoracic segment paralyse small muscles in the hand and damage the sympathetic outflow, resulting in contraction of the pupil, recession of the eyeball, narrowing of the palpebral fissure and loss of sweating in the face and neck (Horner's syndrome). However, sensation is retained in areas innervated by segments above the lesion; thus, cutaneous sensation is retained in the neck and chest down to the second intercostal space, because this area is innervated by the supraclavicular nerves (C3 and C4). At thoracic levels, division of the cord paralyses the trunk below the segmental level of the lesion and both lower limbs (paraplegia). The first sacral neural segment is approximately level with the thoracolumbar vertebral junction; injury here, which is common, paralyses the urinary bladder, the rectum and the muscles supplied by the sacral segments, and cutaneous sensibility is lost in the perineum, buttocks, backs of the thighs and legs and soles of the feet. The roots of lumbar nerves descending to join the cauda equina may be damaged at this level, causing complete paralysis of both lower limbs. Lesions below the first lumbar vertebra may divide or damage the cauda equina, but severe nerve damage is uncommon and is usually confined to the spinal roots at the level of the trauma. Neurological symptoms may also occur as a result of interference with the spinal blood supply, particularly in the lower thoracic and upper lumbar segments.

LESIONS OF THE SPINAL ROOTS, NERVES AND GANGLIA

The spinal roots, nerves and ganglia may be damaged in the vertebral and 'root' canals and at the intervertebral foramina. Neurofibromas may occur on the roots and nerves in the root canals, and as they enlarge, they become dumbbell shaped, with both intra- and extraspinal components in continuity. The clinical picture may thus include paradoxical features as this asymmetric space-occupying lesion grows.

Root compression usually presents acutely with pain, which may be severe. The pain, paraesthesia and numbness occur in a dermatomal distribution. It may be difficult to demonstrate sensory loss on the trunk because of the overlap of the dermatomes. Severe traction injuries of the upper limbs may cause avulsion of spinal roots from the cord in the cervical region.

Anatomy of Pain of Spinal Origin

In the diagnosis and description of pain of spinal origin, it is particularly important to distinguish anatomically among radicular ('nerve root') pain, referred pain and radiating pain. The second and third terms are often used imprecisely, and their meanings can be confused.

Radicular pain occurs in a spinal nerve (dermatomal) distribution, is well localized and results from involvement of the spinal nerve in the pathological process, such as when it is compressed by a disc prolapse.

Referred pain is not strictly of spinal origin. The source of the pain is usually a visceral structure whose afferent innervation shares an interneuronal pool in the posterior horn of the spinal cord with the somatic structure where the pain is felt. The pain may be felt in a dermatome; however, the pain-producing lesion is not in the spinal nerve.

CASE 7   BROWN–SÉQUARD SYNDROME

A 30-year-old man is involved in a street brawl and is stabbed in the neck, with the knife penetrating at approximately the C4 level. Examination in the emergency room demonstrates a flaccid paralysis of the right arm and leg, with loss of reflexes; loss of vibratory and position sense below and ipsilateral to the level of the injury; and contralateral loss of pain and temperature sensation, also below the level of the lesion. MRI imaging demonstrates the wound penetrating the substance of the spinal cord (Fig. 8.44).

Discussion: This patient presents with typical Brown–Séquard syndrome as a manifestation of hemisection of the spinal cord at approximately the C4–5 level. The clinical syndrome reflects the level of the lesion, affecting the corticospinal tracts and posterior columns and being responsible for the ipsilateral paralysis and loss of proprioception and vibratory senses below the lesion. Involvement of the spinothalamic tract is responsible for the contralateral loss of pain and temperature sensations. Brown–Séquard syndrome is frequently of traumatic origin but may be encountered with demyelinating diseases such as multiple sclerosis, tumour, or other focal myelopathic disorders. Incomplete forms of the syndrome are common.

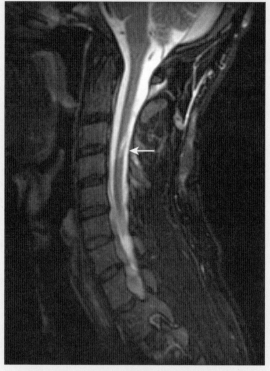

Fig. 8.44 MR image showing the residual cavity in the spinal cord from a stab wound at C4 (arrow).

Radiating pain does not adopt any particular anatomical distribution. It is often vaguely localized, and the patient may use the whole hand to indicate the affected area. The extent of its area of distribution often relates directly to the severity of the pain. Spinal pain of this type commonly radiates around the hip and down into the thigh.

Spinal Cord Lesions

Mechanical compression and secondary ischaemic damage to underlying nervous tissue cause surgically relevant spinal cord disease (myelopathy). The

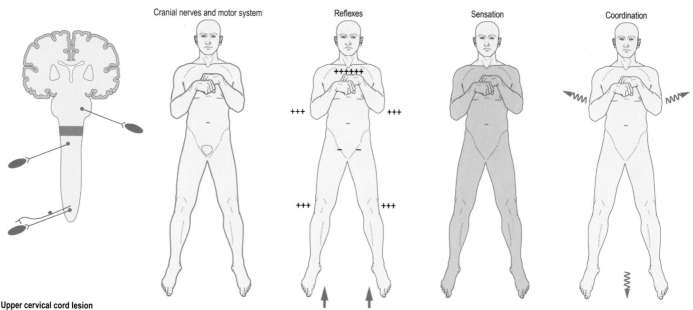

Upper cervical cord lesion
A high cervical cord lesion causes spastic tetraplegia with hyperreflexia, extensor plantar responses (upper motor neurone lesion), incontinence, sensory loss below the level of the lesion and 'sensory' ataxia.

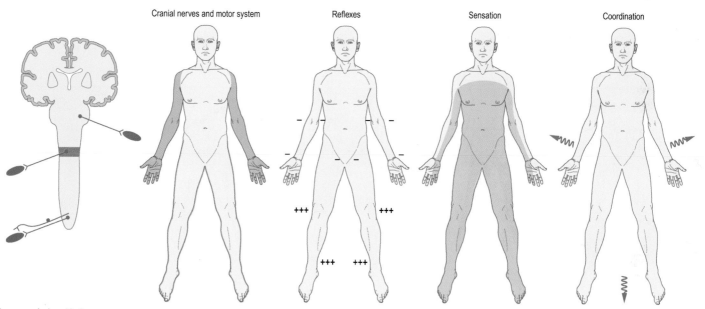

Lower cervical cord lesion
A lower cervical cord lesion causes weakness, wasting and fasciculation of muscles and areflexia of the upper limbs (lower motor neurone lesion). In addition, there is spastic paraparesis, hyperreflexia and extensor plantar responses (upper motor neurone lesion) in the lower limbs, incontinence, sensory loss below the level of the lesion and 'sensory' ataxia.

Fig. 8.45 *Lesions of the spinal cord. (By permission from Crossman, A.R., Neary, D., 2000. Neuroanatomy, 2nd ed. Churchill Livingstone, Edinburgh.)*

site and the level of cord damage determine the particular clinical syndrome—for example, whether the lesion involves the upper or lower cervical, thoracic or lumbosacral spinal cord. At each of these levels, symptoms and signs are determined by direct destruction of segmental tissue, or transversely distributed damage, and by disconnection of suprasegmental ascending and descending tracts above and below the level of a lesion, or longitudinally distributed damage (Fig. 8.45). For example, a lower cervical spinal cord lesion damages the segmental sensory and motor contributions to the nerve roots and brachial plexus, causing sensory loss, weakness and wasting of the muscles and loss of tendon reflexes in the upper limbs. Disruption of the ascending sensory pathways in the lateral and dorsal columns of the cervical spinal cord leads to loss of pain and temperature sensation (lateral spinothalamic tracts) and touch and proprioception (dorsal fasciculi) below the 'sensory level' corresponding to the spinal cord segment. Damage to the descending corticospinal tracts in the lateral columns of the spinal cord produces a spastic paraparesis, with increased muscle tone, weakness of flexion movements, exaggerated tendon reflexes and abnormal superficial reflexes (e.g. extensor plantar responses, absent abdominal reflexes). Descending pathways to the bladder are interrupted, producing a 'neurogenic bladder.' The same principles apply to lesions at other levels of the spinal cord, as illustrated in Figure 8.45.

The precise clinical syndrome is determined by anatomical site alone, not by pathology. However, it is of practical use to classify lesions on the basis of their anatomical relationship to the spinal cord and meninges—that is, whether they are extradural, intradural or intramedullary (Table 8.1). This anatomical classification provides a guide to the diagnostic probabilities as well as an aid to neuroradiological interpretation before neurosurgical intervention. For example, neurofibromas are common in the cervical spinal canal, meningiomas in the thoracic spinal canal and ependymomas in the lumbosacral spinal canal. Degenerative disease of the vertebral column is common in the cervical and lumbosacral vertebrae but rare in the thoracic vertebrae. Discrete anterior and central intramedullary lesions, such as those due to syringomyelia and angioma, respectively, preferentially destroy the spinothalamic pathways in the anterolateral columns and central areas of the spinal cord. This leads to a characteristic 'dissociated' sensory loss, with loss of pain and temperature sensation but preservation of touch sensation and proprioception at and below the level of the lesion.

Lesions of the Conus and Cauda Equina
Lesions of the conus and cauda equina, such as tumours, cause bilateral deficits, often with pain in the back extending into the sacral segments and to the legs. Loss of bladder and erectile function can be early features. There are

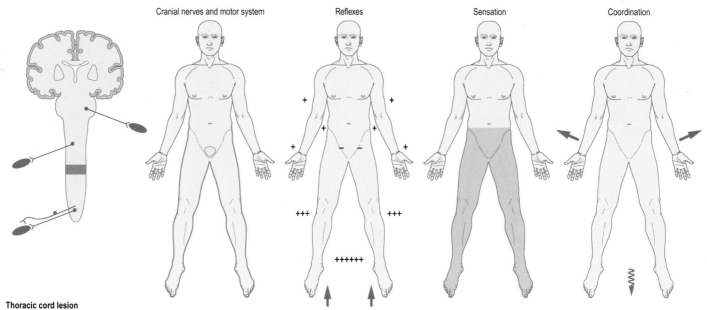

Thoracic cord lesion
A thoracic cord lesion causes a spastic paraparesis, hyperreflexia and extensor plantar responses (upper motor neurone lesion), incontinence, sensory loss below the level of the lesion and 'sensory' ataxia.

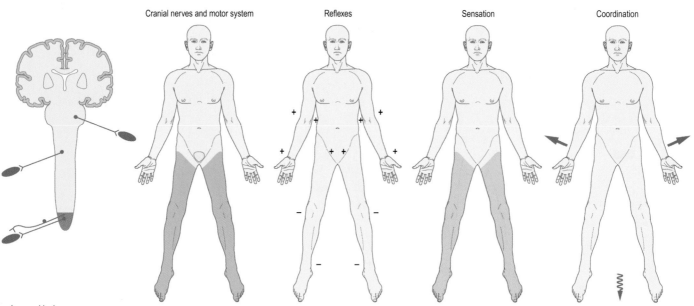

Lumbar cord lesion
A lumbar cord lesion causes weakness, wasting and fasciculation of muscles, areflexia of the lower limbs (lower motor neurone lesion), incontinence, sensory loss below the level of the lesion and 'sensory' ataxia.

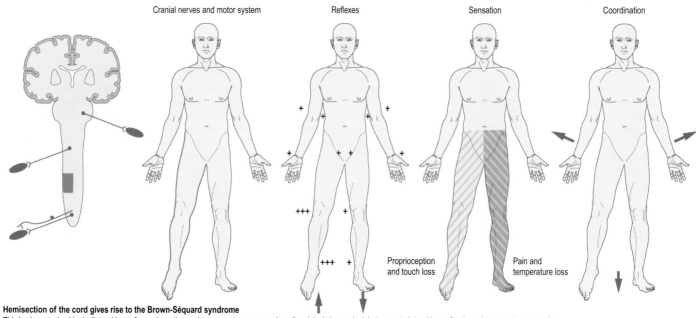

Hemisection of the cord gives rise to the Brown-Séquard syndrome
This is characterised by ipsilateral loss of proprioception and upper motor neurone signs (hemiplegia/monoplegia) plus contralateral loss of pain and temperature sensation.

Fig. 8.45, cont'd *Lesions of the spinal cord. (By permission from Crossman, A.R., Neary, D., 2000. Neuroanatomy, 2nd ed. Churchill Livingstone, Edinburgh.)*

CASE 8   SPINAL CORD INFARCTION

Patient 1: An elderly man with coronary artery disease and an abdominal aortic aneurysm develops acute midthoracic back pain, followed by flaccid paraparesis with impaired pain and temperature sensation at T8; proprioception is relatively spared. There is loss of bladder and bowel function. Magnetic resonance imaging (MRI) of the spine demonstrates signal change from T8 through the conus medullaris, consistent with infarction in the distribution of the artery of Adamkiewicz.

Patient 2: An 18-year-old boy experiences acute low back pain after a session of strenuous weightlifting. He cannot stand. Examination demonstrates a flaccid paraparesis with a sensory level at T12. Spinal MRI shows an L1–2 disc herniation and infarction of the conus medullaris. The clinical and radiographic findings suggest spinal cord infarction from fibrocartilaginous embolization.

Patient 3: A 69-year-old woman with cervical arthritis is involved in a minor automobile accident in which she suffers a 'whiplash' injury. Thereafter she has intermittent neck pain and then develops acute quadriparesis, with impairment of pain and temperature sensation at the level of C5 but sparing of position and vibratory sense. MRI shows cord swelling with signal change at C5–6. The diagnosis is anterior spinal cord infarction due to injury to the cervical anterior spinal artery.

Discussion: The anterior spinal artery supplies the anterior two-thirds of the spinal cord. Arising from the vertebral artery in the cervical region, it receives contributions from the medullary segmental arteries, the largest of which, the artery of Adamkiewicz, is in the thoracic region. Because there is little collateral circulation in the spinal cord, it is particularly sensitive to ischaemia; because the posterior one-third of the cord receives its blood supply from the posterior spinal arteries, posterior column function (e.g. proprioception) is often intact in the setting of anterior spinal artery disease. Spinal cord infarcts, which are most common in the thoracic region, may be due to systemic hypotension, with infarction at 'border zones' between vascular territories; surgery, particularly in the thoracic region, which may compromise the aorta or medullary arteries; direct injury to the anterior spinal artery with extension injury of the neck; rarely, fibrocartilaginous embolization in patients with preexisting spinal disc disease; or after relatively minor spinal trauma. See Figure 8.46.

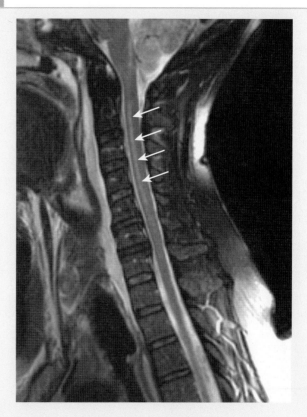

Fig. 8.46 *Anterior spinal artery occlusion. MRI shows infarction of the ventral cord* (arrows). (© 2010 Thomas Jefferson University. All rights reserved. Reproduced with the permission of Thomas Jefferson University.)

Table 8.1 *Classification of lesions based on anatomical relationship to the spinal cord and meninges*

Extradural Lesions

Disorder of the vertebral column
  Degenerative osteoarthritis (osteophytes and prolapsed intervertebral disc)
  Infection (tuberculosis)
  Tumour (chordoma, sarcoma, metastatic tumour, carcinoma, myeloma, lymphoma)
Abscess (complication of bleeding diathesis or anticoagulation)
Haematoma

Intradural Lesions

Meningioma, neurofibroma, lipoma, angioma

Intramedullary Lesions

Syringomyelia (Arnold-Chiari malformation), angioma, glioma, ependymoma, epidermoid tumour

---

lower motor neurone signs in the legs, with fasciculation and muscle atrophy. Sensory loss usually involves the perineal or 'saddle area' as well as other lumbar and sacral dermatomes. There may be congenital abnormalities, including spina bifida, lipoma or diastematomyelia, and the conus may extend below the lower border of L1, often with a tethered filum terminale. Extramedullary lesions include prolapsed intervertebral discs. A midline (central) disc protrusion in the lumbar region may present with involvement of only the sacral segments.

References

Barson, A.J., Sands, J., 1977. Regional and segmental characteristics of the human adult spinal cord. J. Anat. 123, 797–803.

Bogduk, N., 1997. Clinical Anatomy of the Lumbar Spine and Sacrum, third ed. Churchill Livingstone, Edinburgh.

Dean, N.A., Mitchell, B.S., 2002. Anatomic relation between the nuchal ligament (ligamentum nuchae) and the spinal dura mater in the craniocervical region. Clin. Anat. 15, 182–185.

Fraher, J.P., 2000. The transitional zone and CNS regeneration. J. Anat. 196, 137–158.

Gordon, P.H., Cheng, B., Katz, I.B., et al, 2006. The natural history of primary lateral sclerosis. Neurology 66, 647-653.

Haines, D.E., Harkey, H.L., Al-Mefty, O., 1993. The 'subdural' space: a new look at an outdated concept. Neurosurgery 32, 111–120. *Proposes that the subdural 'space' is a pathological cleavage plane rather than a normal anatomical element.*

Kubik, S., Müntener, M., 1969. Zur Topographie der spinalen Nervenwurzeln. II Der Einfluss des Wachstums des Duralsackes, sowie der Krümmagen und der Bewegungen der spinalen Nervenwurzeln. Acta. Anat. 74, 149–168. *An alternative view of the obliquity of the cervicothoracic spinal nerve roots based on observations of differential cord growth.*

Kuypers, H.G.J.M., 1981. Anatomy of descending pathways. In: Brookhart, J.M., Mountcastle, V.B., et al, (Eds.), Handbook of Physiology, vol. 2 Motor Control, pt 1. American Physiological Society, Bethesda, MD, pp. 597–666.

Mancall, E.L., Rosales, R.K., 1964. Necrotizing myelopathy associated with visceral carcinoma. Brain 87, 639–656.

Melzack, R., Wall, P.D., 1965. Pain mechanisms: a new theory. Science 150, 971–979.

Neidre, A., Macnab, I., 1983. Anomalies of the lumbosacral nerve roots. Spine 8, 294–299.

Newell, R.L.M., 1999. The spinal epidural space. Clin. Anat. 12, 375–379.

Rothstein, J.D., 2009. Current hypotheses for the underlying biology of amyotrophic lateral sclerosis. Ann. Neurol. 65, S3–S9.

Steele, J.C., McGeer, P.L., 2008. The ALS/PDS syndrome of Guam and the cycad hypothesis. Neurology 70, 1984–1990.

Section III

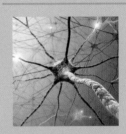

The Brain Stem and Cranial Nerves

Skull

The skull is the bony skeleton of the head and is the most complex osseous structure in the body. It is protective, shielding the brain, the organs of special sense and the cranial parts of the respiratory and digestive systems. It also provides attachments for many of the muscles of the head and neck, thus allowing for movement. Of particular importance is movement of the lower jaw (mandible), which occurs at the temporomandibular joint. The marrow within the skull bones is a site of haemopoiesis, at least in the young skull.

The skull is composed of 28 separate bones, most of which are paired; however, some bones in the median plane are single. Many of the bones are flat bones, consisting of two thin plates of compact bone enclosing a narrow layer of cancellous bone containing bone marrow. In terms of shape, however, the bones are far from flat and can exhibit pronounced curvatures. The term diploë is used to describe the cancellous bone within the flat bones of the skull. The inner table is thinner and more brittle; the outer table is generally very resilient. Many bones are so thin that the tables are fused, for example, the vomer and pterygoid plates. The skull bones vary in thickness in different regions but tend to be thinner where they are covered by muscles, such as in the temporal and posterior cranial fossae. The skull is thicker in some races, but there is no relationship between skull thickness and cranial capacity, which averages approximately 1400 ml. In all races the bone is thinner in women and children than in adult males.

The majority of bones in the skull are held firmly together by fibrous joints termed sutures. In the developing skull, sutures allow for growth. There are three main arrangements: the margins of adjacent bones of a suture may be smooth and meet end to end, resulting in a simple (butt-end) suture (e.g. median palatine suture); the margins of adjacent bones may be bevelled, so that the border of one bone overlaps the other (e.g. zygomaticomaxillary suture); or the margins of adjacent bones may present numerous projections that interlock, giving a serrated appearance (e.g. sagittal suture). The complexity of serrated sutures increases from the inner to the outer surface. Fusion across sutures (synostosis) commences at approximately 30 years of age, but the variability of this process precludes its use to determine the age of skulls. Fusion commences on the internal surface of the cranium, and the sagittal suture is one of the first affected. At approximately 40 years of age the sphenofrontal, lambdoid and occipitomastoid sutures close. In the facial region the posterior part of the median palatine suture starts to close at about 30 years, followed by the sutures around the nose. The squamosal, zygomaticofrontal and anterior parts of the intermaxillary suture rarely exhibit synostosis. Premature fusion of sutures during the early growth phase of the skull results in various cranial abnormalities.

The bones forming the base of the skull develop endochondrally and play an important part in growth. In this region, therefore, primary cartilaginous joints are encountered during growth; one of the most important is the spheno-occipital synchondrosis, which disappears at approximately 14 to 16 years of age. The skull articulates with the first cervical vertebra at the synovial atlanto-occipital joints. These joints allow flexion and extension of the skull. Rotation of the skull does not directly involve any joints of the skull but occurs at the atlanto-axial joint between the first and second cervical vertebrae.

Many important nerves and vessels pass in and out of the skull via openings termed foramina. The skull is a prime site for fractures resulting from trauma, and these structures can be damaged as a result of head injury. Detailed clinical examination should reveal signs and symptoms that, together with radiological examination, provide information regarding the extent and seriousness of a traumatic incident. In addition to the main foramina, irregular emissary foramina allow veins situated externally on the face and scalp to communicate with those lying intracranially. Spread of infection along these routes can have serious clinical consequences.

For ease of navigation, the skull can be divided into the cranium and the mandible, based on the fact that the mandible is easily detached, whereas most of the bones of the skull articulate by relatively fixed joints. The cranium can then be subdivided into a number of regions: the cranial vault, which is the upper, dome-like part of the skull and includes the skullcap or calvaria; the cranial base, which consists of the inferior surface of the skull extracranially and the floor of the cranial cavity intracranially; the facial skeleton, which includes the orbital cavities and the nasal fossae; the tooth-bearing bones or jaws; the acoustic cavities, which contain the middle and inner ears; and the cranial cavity, which houses the brain. Alternatively, the skull can be divided into the neurocranium and viscerocranium. The neurocranium is defined as that part of the skull that houses and protects the brain and the organs of special sense, whereas the viscerocranium is associated with the cranial parts of the respiratory and digestive tracts.

INFERIOR (BASAL) SURFACE

The inferior surface of the skull, the base of the cranium, is complex and extends from the upper incisor teeth in front to the superior nuchal lines of the occipital bone behind (Fig. 9.1). The region contains many of the foramina through which structures enter and exit the cranial cavity. The inferior surface can be conveniently divided into anterior, middle, posterior and lateral parts. The anterior part contains the hard palate and the dentition of the upper jaw, and it lies at a lower level than the rest of the cranial base. The middle and posterior parts can be arbitrarily divided by a transverse plane passing through the anterior margin of the foramen magnum. The middle part is occupied mainly by the base of the sphenoid bone, the petrous processes of the temporal bones and the basilar part of the occipital bone. The lateral part contains the zygomatic arches and the mastoid and styloid processes. Whereas the middle and posterior parts are directly related to the cranial cavity (the middle and posterior cranial fossae), the anterior part (the palate) is some distance from the anterior cranial fossa, being separated from it by the nasal cavities.

Anterior Part of the Cranial Base

The bony palate within the superior alveolar arch is formed by the palatine processes of the maxillae and the horizontal plates of the palatine bones, which meet at a cruciform system of sutures. The median palatine suture runs anteroposteriorly and divides the palate into right and left halves. This suture is continuous with the intermaxillary suture between the maxillary central incisor teeth. The transverse palatine (palatomaxillary) sutures run transversely across the palate between the maxillary and the palatine bones. The palate is arched sagittally and transversely; its depth and breadth are variable but are always greatest in the molar region, with the average width between the maxillary first molars being approximately 50 mm. The incisive fossa lies behind the central incisor teeth, and the lateral incisive foramina, through which incisive canals pass to the nasal cavity, lie in its lateral walls. Median incisive foramina, present in some skulls, open on the anterior and posterior walls of the fossa. The incisive fossa transmits the nasopalatine nerve and the termination of the greater palatine vessels. When median incisive foramina occur, the left nasopalatine nerve traverses the anterior foramen, and the right nerve traverses the posterior foramen. The greater palatine foramen lies near the lateral palatal border of the transverse palatine suture, and a vascular groove that is deep posteriorly leads forward from it. The lesser palatine foramina (usually two) lie behind the greater palatine foramen and pierce the pyramidal process of the palatine bone, which is wedged between the lower ends of the medial and lateral pterygoid plates. The palate is pierced by many other small foramina and is marked by pits for palatine glands. Variably prominent palatine crests extend medially from behind the greater palatine foramina. The posterior border projects back as a median posterior nasal spine. The alveolar arch has 16 sockets or alveoli for teeth, varying in size and depth; some are single, and some are divided by septa in adaptation to tooth roots.

The nasal fossae, separated in the midline by the nasal septum, lie above the hard palate. The two posterior nasal apertures (choanae) are located where the nasal fossae end. The posterior part of the septum is formed by the vomer. The upper border of the vomer is applied to the inferior aspect of the body of the sphenoid, where it expands into an ala on each side. The

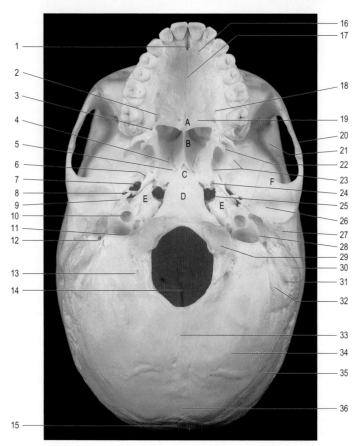

Fig. 9.1 *Inferior view of the skull. (By permission from Berkovitz, B.K.B., Moxham, B.J., 1994. Color Atlas of the Skull. Mosby-Wolfe, London.)*

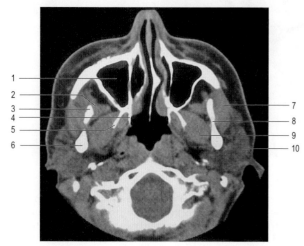

Fig. 9.2 *Horizontal computed tomography scan at the level of the upper part of the ramus of the mandible shows the relationships of the pterygoid plates. (By permission from Berkovitz, B.K.B., Moxham, B.J., 1994. Color Atlas of the Skull. Mosby-Wolfe, London.)*

lateral border of each ala reaches a thin vaginal process that projects medially from the medial pterygoid plate. The two may touch, or the vaginal process may overlap the ala of the vomer inferiorly. The inferior surface of the vaginal process bears an anteroposterior groove, which is converted into a canal anteriorly by the superior aspect of the sphenoidal process of the palatine bone. This palatovaginal canal opens anteriorly into the pterygopalatine fossa and transmits a pharyngeal branch of the pterygopalatine ganglion and a pharyngeal branch from the third part of the maxillary artery. An inconstant vomerovaginal canal may lie between the ala of the vomer and the vaginal process of the sphenoid bone, medial to the palatovaginal canal, and lead into the anterior end of the palatovaginal canal. It transmits the pharyngeal branch of the third part of the maxillary artery.

Middle Part of the Cranial Base

The middle part of the cranial base is made up of the occipital, sphenoid and temporal bones. The body of the sphenoid bone lies anteriorly, and the basilar part of the occipital bone lies posteriorly, just in front of the foramen magnum. Where these two bones meet in the growing skull, the junction between them is a primary cartilaginous joint, the spheno-occipital synchondrosis. This joint is important for growth of the skull in an anteroposterior direction and ossifies at approximately 14 to 16 years of age. The basilar part of the occipital bone bears a small midline pharyngeal tubercle, which provides an attachment to the pharyngeal raphe and the highest attachment of the superior pharyngeal constrictor.

The middle part of the cranial base is completed by the petrous processes of the two temporal bones, which pass from the lateral sides of the base of the skull toward the site of union of the sphenoid and occipital bones. Each petrous process meets the basilar part of the occipital bone at a petro-occipital suture, which is deficient posteriorly at the jugular foramen. The petrosphenoidal suture and the groove for the pharyngotympanic tube lie between the petrous process and the infratemporal surface of the greater wing of the sphenoid. The apex of the petrous process does not meet the spheno-occipital suture, and the deficit produced is called the foramen lacerum.

Each pterygoid process of the sphenoid bone bears medial and lateral pterygoid plates separated by a pterygoid fossa. Anteriorly, the plates are fused, except below, where they are separated by the pyramidal process of the palatine bone. Sutures are usually discernible at this site. Laterally, the pterygoid plates are separated from the posterior maxillary surface by the

pterygomaxillary fissure, which leads into the pterygopalatine fossa. The posterior border of the medial pterygoid plate is sharp and bears a small projection near the midpoint, above which it is curved and attached to the pharyngeal end of the pharyngotympanic tube. Above, the medial pterygoid plate divides to enclose the scaphoid fossa; below, it projects as a slender pterygoid hamulus, which curves laterally and is grooved anteriorly by the tendon of tensor veli palatini. The pterygoid hamulus gives origin to the pterygomandibular raphe. The lateral pterygoid plate projects posterolaterally, and its lateral surface forms the medial wall of the infratemporal fossa. Superiorly and laterally, the pterygoid process is continuous with the infratemporal surface of the greater wing of the sphenoid bone, which forms part of the roof of the infratemporal fossa. This surface forms the posterolateral border of the inferior orbital fissure and bears an infratemporal crest associated with the origin of the upper part of the lateral pterygoid. The infraorbital and zygomatic branches of the maxillary nerve and accompanying vessels pass through the inferior orbital fissure. Laterally, the greater wing of the sphenoid bone articulates with the squamous part of the temporal bone. Features associated with the pterygoid plate region can be assessed radiographically (Fig. 9.2).

A thin-walled depression in the temporal bone, the mandibular fossa, can be inspected when the mandible is removed; in front of this, the zygomatic arch extends laterally. A distinct ridge, the articular eminence, is anterior to the fossa, and three fissures can be distinguished behind it. The squamotympanic fissure extends from the spine of the sphenoid, between the mandibular fossa and the tympanic plate of the temporal bone, and curves up the anterior margin of the external acoustic meatus. A thin wedge of bone forming the inferior margin of the tegmen tympani lies within the fissure and divides the squamotympanic fissure into petrotympanic and petrosquamous fissures. The petrotympanic fissure transmits the chorda tympani branch of the facial nerve from the skull into the infratemporal fossa.

The foramen lacerum is bounded in front by the body and adjoining roots of the pterygoid process and greater wing of the sphenoid bone, posterolaterally by the apex of the petrous part of the temporal bone and medially by the basilar part of the occipital bone. Although it is nearly 1 cm long, no large structure completely traverses it. A large, almost circular foramen, the carotid canal, lies behind and posterolateral to the foramen lacerum in the petrous part of the temporal bone. The internal carotid artery enters the skull through this foramen, ascends in the carotid canal and turns anteromedially to reach the posterior wall of the foramen lacerum. It ascends through the upper end of the foramen lacerum with its venous and sympathetic nerve plexuses. Meningeal branches of the ascending pharyngeal artery and emissary veins from the cavernous sinus also traverse the foramen lacerum. In life, the lower part of the foramen lacerum is partially occluded by cartilaginous remnants of the developmental chondrocranium. The pterygoid canal can be seen on the base of the skull at the anterior margin of the foramen lacerum, above and between the pterygoid plates of the sphenoid bone. It leads into the pterygopalatine fossa and contains the nerve of the pterygoid canal and accompanying blood vessels.

The foramen ovale and foramen spinosum lie lateral to the foramen lacerum on the infratemporal surface of the greater wing of the sphenoid bone. The foramen ovale, near the posterior margin of the lateral pterygoid plate, transmits the mandibular nerve as well as the lesser petrosal nerve, the accessory meningeal branch of the maxillary artery and an emissary vein that connects the cavernous venous sinus to the pterygoid venous plexus in the infratemporal fossa. Posterolaterally, the smaller and rounder foramen spinosum transmits the middle meningeal artery and a meningeal branch of the mandibular nerve. The irregular spine of the sphenoid projects posterolateral to the foramen spinosum. The medial surface of the spine is flat and forms, with the adjoining posterior border of the greater wing of the sphenoid, the anterolateral wall of a groove that is completed posteromedially by the petrous part of the temporal bone. This groove contains the cartilaginous pharyngotympanic (auditory) tube and leads posterolaterally into the bony portion of the tube lying within the petrous part of the temporal bone. Occasionally, the foramen ovale and foramen spinosum are confluent. The posterior edge of the foramen spinosum may be defective. A small foramen, the sphenoidal emissary foramen (of Vesalius), is sometimes found between the foramen ovale and scaphoid fossa. When present, it contains an emissary vein linking the pterygoid venous plexus in the infratemporal fossa with the cavernous sinus in the middle cranial fossa.

The zygomaticotemporal foramen passes up and backward from the posterior surface of the zygomatic bone in the anterior wall of the infratemporal fossa. It transmits the zygomaticotemporal nerve and a small accompanying artery.

Posterior Part of the Cranial Base

The posterior part of the cranial base is formed by the occipital and temporal bones. Prominent features are the foramen magnum and associated occipital condyles, jugular foramen, mastoid and styloid processes of the temporal bone, stylomastoid foramen, mastoid notch and squamous part of the occipital bone up to the external occipital protuberance and the superior nuchal lines, hypoglossal canals (anterior condylar canals) and condylar canals (posterior condylar canals).

The foramen magnum lies in an anteromedian position. It is oval and wider behind, with its greatest diameter being anteroposterior. It contains the lower end of the medulla oblongata, the vertebral arteries and the spinal accessory nerve. Anteriorly, the margin of the foramen magnum is slightly overlapped by the occipital condyles, which project down to articulate with the superior articular facets on the lateral masses of the atlas. Each occipital condyle is oval in outline and oriented obliquely so that its anterior end lies nearer the midline. It is markedly convex anteroposteriorly and less so transversely; its medial aspect is roughened by ligamentous attachments. The hypoglossal canal, directed laterally and slightly forward, traverses each condyle and transmits the hypoglossal nerve, a meningeal branch of the ascending pharyngeal artery and an emissary vein from the basilar plexus. A depression, the condylar fossa, lies immediately posterior to the condyle and sometimes contains a (posterior) condylar canal for an emissary vein from the sigmoid sinus. A jugular process joins the petrous part of the temporal bone lateral to each condyle, and its anterior border forms the posterior boundary of the jugular foramen.

Laterally, the occipital bone joins the petrous part of the temporal bone anteriorly, at the petro-occipital suture, and the mastoid process of the temporal bone more posteriorly, at the petromastoid suture. The jugular foramen, a large irregular hiatus, lies at the posterior end of the petro-occipital suture between the jugular process of the occipital bone and the jugular fossa of the petrous part of the temporal bone. A number of important structures pass through this foramen: inferior petrosal sinus (anterior); glossopharyngeal, vagus and accessory nerves (midway); internal jugular vein (posterior). A mastoid canaliculus runs through the lateral wall of the jugular fossa and transmits the auricular branch of the vagus nerve. The canaliculus for the tympanic nerve—a branch of the glossopharyngeal nerve in the cavity of the middle ear—lies on the ridge between the jugular fossa and the opening of the carotid canal. A small notch, related to the inferior glossopharyngeal ganglion, may be found medially, on the upper boundary of the jugular foramen (it is more easily identified internally). The orifice of the cochlear canaliculus may be found at the apex of the notch.

The stylomastoid foramen lies between the mastoid and styloid processes of the temporal bone on the lateral aspect. It transmits the facial nerve and the stylomastoid artery. A groove, the mastoid notch, lies medial to the mastoid process and gives origin to the posterior belly of the digastric. A groove related to the occipital artery often lies medial to the mastoid notch. A mastoid foramen may be present near or in the occipitomastoid suture; when present, it transmits an emissary vein from the sigmoid sinus. The external acoustic meatus lies in front of the mastoid process. It is surrounded inferiorly by the tympanic plate, which partly ensheaths the base of the styloid process.

The squamous part of the occipital bone exhibits the external occipital protuberance; supreme, superior and inferior nuchal lines; and the external

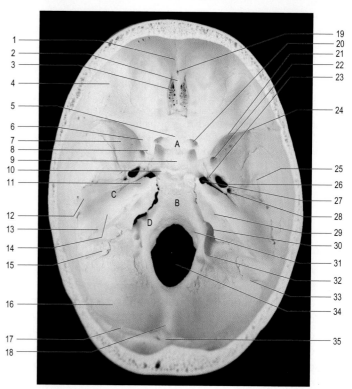

Fig. 9.3 *Floor of the cranial cavity showing the cranial fossae. (By permission from Berkovitz, B.K.B., Moxham, B.J., 1994. Color Atlas of the Skull. Mosby-Wolfe, London.)*

occipital crest, all of which lie in the midline, posterior to the foramen magnum. The region is roughened for the attachment of muscles whose primary function is extension of the skull.

CRANIAL FOSSAE

The base of the cranial cavity is divided into three distinct fossae: anterior, middle and posterior (Fig. 9.3). The floor of the anterior cranial fossa is at the highest level and the floor of the posterior fossa is at the lowest.

Anterior Cranial Fossa

The anterior cranial fossa is formed at the front and sides by the frontal bone. Its floor contains the orbital plate of the frontal bone, the cribriform plate and crista galli of the ethmoid bone and the lesser wings and anterior part of the body of the sphenoid. Unlike the other cranial fossae, it does not directly communicate with the inferior surface of the cranium; instead, it is related to the roofs of the orbits and the nasal fossae.

A perforated plate of bone, the cribriform plate of the ethmoid bone, spreads across the midline between the orbital plates of the frontal bone and is depressed below them, forming part of the roof of the nasal cavity. Olfactory nerves pass from the nasal mucosa to the olfactory bulb of the brain through numerous small foramina in the cribriform plate. Anteriorly, a spur of bone, the crista galli, projects upward between the cerebral hemispheres. A depression between the crista galli and the crest of the frontal bone is crossed by the frontoethmoidal suture and bears the foramen caecum, which is usually a small blind-ended depression but occasionally accommodates a vein draining from the nasal mucosa to the superior sagittal sinus. The anterior ethmoidal nerve enters the cranial cavity where the cribriform plate meets the orbital part of the frontal bone and then passes into the roof of the nose via a small foramen by the side of the crista galli; the nerve grooves the crista galli. The anterior ethmoidal vessels accompany the nerve. The posterior ethmoidal canal, which transmits the posterior ethmoidal nerve and vessels, opens at the posterolateral corner of the cribriform plate and is overhung by the sphenoid bone.

The convex cranial surface of the frontal bone separates the brain from the orbit and bears impressions of cerebral gyri and small grooves for meningeal vessels. Posteriorly, it joins the anterior border of the lesser wing of the sphenoid bone, which forms the posterior boundary of the anterior cranial fossa. The medial end of the lesser wing constitutes the anterior clinoid process. The lesser wing joins the body of the sphenoid body by two roots that are separated by the optic canal. The anterior root, broad and flat, is continuous with the jugum sphenoidale; the smaller and thicker posterior root joins the body of the sphenoid bone near the posterior bank of the sulcus chiasmatis. The frontosphenoid and sphenoethmoidal sutures divide the sphenoid from the adjacent bones.

The posterior border of each lesser wing fits the stem of the lateral cerebral sulcus and may be grooved by the sphenoparietal sinus. Above is the inferior surface of the frontal lobe of the cerebral hemisphere, and medial is the anterior perforated substance. Inferiorly, the lesser wing bounds the superior orbital fissure and completes the orbital roof. Each anterior clinoid process gives attachment to the free margin of the tentorium cerebelli and is grooved medially by the internal carotid artery as it leaves the cavernous sinus. It may be connected to the middle clinoid process by a thin osseous bar, completing a caroticoclinoid foramen around the artery.

CASE 1   FOSTER KENNEDY SYNDROME

A 49-year-old woman undergoes surgery for a subfrontal tumour, which is found to be a meningioma arising in the olfactory groove. Her clinical abnormalities include a mild contralateral hemiparesis, behavioural change, ipsilateral optic atrophy with contralateral papilloedema and ipsilateral anosmia. Similar symptoms may also appear with other tumours, such as meningioma involving the sphenoid wing.

Discussion: Owing to the subfrontal site of this woman's tumour, she developed anosmia due to primary involvement of the olfactory nerve in the olfactory groove by the tumour, along with mild frontal signs such as behavioural change. Reduced visual acuity with optic atrophy is due to direct compression of the ipsilateral optic nerve or optic chiasma, whereas papilloedema involving the contralateral optic nerve clearly indicates the presence of increased intracranial pressure, a combination that is uncommon today in light of early diagnostic studies. See Figure 9.4.

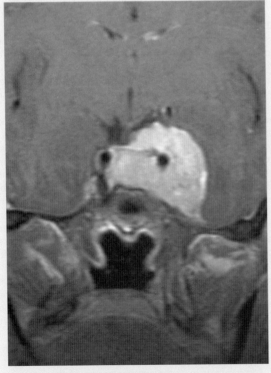

Fig. 9.4

Middle Cranial Fossa

The middle cranial fossa is deeper and more extensive than the anterior cranial fossa, particularly laterally. It is bounded in front by the lesser wings and part of the body of the sphenoid, behind by the superior borders of the petrous part of the temporal bone and the dorsum sellae of the sphenoid and laterally by the squamous parts of the temporal bone, parietal bone and greater wings of the sphenoid. This region corresponds with the middle part of the cranial base.

Centrally, the floor is narrower and formed by the body of the sphenoid bone. The hollowed-out area is the site of the hypophysial (pituitary) gland and is therefore termed the hypophysial (pituitary) fossa. The area has the shape of a Turkish saddle and is also known as the sella turcica. The anterior edge of the hypophysial fossa is completed laterally by a middle clinoid process. The floor forms the roof of the sphenoidal air sinuses, and the posterior boundary presents a vertical pillar of bone, the dorsum sellae. The superolateral angles of the dorsum sellae are expanded as the posterior clinoid processes. A fold of dura, the diaphragma sella, is attached to the anterior and posterior clinoid processes and roofs the hypophysial fossa. The smooth upper part of the anterior wall of the fossa is the jugum sphenoidale, which is bounded behind by the anterior border of the grooved sulcus chiasmatis, leading laterally to the optic canals. The optic nerve and ophthalmic artery pass through the optic canal, and the optic chiasma usually lies posterosuperior to the sulcus chiasmatis. Below the sulcus chiasmatis is the tuberculum sellae. The cavernous sinus lies lateral to the hypophysial fossa, and the lateral wall of the body of the sphenoid contains a shallow carotid groove related to the internal carotid artery as it ascends from the carotid canal and runs through the cavernous sinus. Posterolaterally, the groove may be deepened by a small projecting lingula.

Laterally, the middle cranial fossa is deep and supports the temporal lobes of the cerebral hemispheres. Anteriorly are the orbits, laterally the temporal fossae and inferiorly the infratemporal fossae. The middle cranial fossa communicates with the orbits by the superior orbital fissures, each bounded above by a lesser wing, below by a greater wing and medially by the body of the sphenoid bone. Each fissure is wider medially and has a long axis sloping inferomedially and forward. Many nerves and vessels pass through it: the oculomotor, trochlear and abducens nerves and the lacrimal, frontal and nasociliary branches of the ophthalmic division of the trigeminal nerve, together with filaments from the internal carotid plexus (sympathetic), the ophthalmic veins, the orbital branch of the middle meningeal artery and the recurrent branch of the lacrimal artery.

Three foramina can be identified in the greater wing of the sphenoid bone. The foramen rotundum is situated just below and behind the medial end of the superior orbital fissure and leads forward into the pterygopalatine fossa, to which it conducts the maxillary nerve. Behind the foramen rotundum is the foramen ovale, which transmits the mandibular nerve. The foramen spinosum is posterolateral to the foramen ovale and transmits the middle meningeal artery. The latter, with companion veins, ascends lateral to the squamous part of the temporal bone and turns anterolaterally across the sphenosquamosal suture to the greater wing of the sphenoid bone, where it divides into frontal and parietal branches. The frontal branch ascends across the pterion to the anterior part of the parietal bone; at or near the pterion it is often in a bony canal. The parietal branch runs back and up onto the squamous part of the temporal bone, crossing the squamosal suture to gain the parietal bone. These arteries and veins groove the floor and lateral wall of the middle cranial fossa. The foramen ovale and foramen spinosum connect with the underlying infratemporal fossa.

The foramen lacerum is situated at the posterior end of the carotid groove, posteromedial to the foramen ovale. Its boundaries and contents were already described in the section on the intermediate part of the cranial base. A small foramen may occur at the root of the greater wing of the sphenoid medial to the foramen lacerum; when present, this emissary sphenoidal foramen transmits a vein from the cavernous sinus.

A shallow trigeminal impression, adapted to the trigeminal ganglion, is situated posterior to the foramen lacerum on the anterior surface of the petrous part of the temporal bone, near its apex. Posterolateral to this impression is a shallow pit, limited posteriorly by a rounded arcuate eminence produced by the anterior semicircular canal. Lateral to the trigeminal impression, a narrow groove passes posterolaterally into the hiatus for the greater petrosal nerve, and even farther laterally is the hiatus for the lesser petrosal nerve. The anterior surface of the petrous part of the temporal bone is formed by the tegmen tympani, a thin osseous lamina in the roof of the tympanic cavity, which extends anteromedially above the auditory tube, anterolateral to the arcuate eminence. The posterior part of the tegmen tympani roofs the mastoid antrum, lateral to the eminence. The superior border of the petrous part of the temporal bone separates the middle and posterior cranial fossae and is grooved by the superior petrosal sinus. In young skulls, a petrosquamous suture may be visible at the lateral limit of the tegmen tympani, but it is obliterated in adults. The tegmen tympani then turns down as the lateral wall of the osseous auditory tube, and its lower border may appear in the squamotympanic fissure. Lateral to the anterior part of the tegmen tympani, the squamous part of the temporal bone is thin over a small area that coincides with the deepest part of the mandibular fossa.

A smooth trigeminal notch leads into the trigeminal impression and lies on the upper border of the petrous temporal bone, anteromedial to the groove for the superior petrosal sinus. At this point, the trigeminal nerve separates the sinus from bone. The petrosphenoidal ligament is attached to a tiny bony spicule, directed anteromedially at the anterior end of the trigeminal notch. The abducens nerve bends sharply across the upper petrous border, passing between the ligament and the dorsum sellae anterior to the petrosphenoidal ligament.

CASE 2 PITUITARY TUMOUR WITH BITEMPORAL VISUAL FIELD DEFECT

A 56-year-old woman presents with a 6-month history of worsening bifrontal headache and difficulty reading. She can read single words but has difficulty tracking a sentence across the page. Evaluation was prompted when she struck her husband's car on the right side as she drove into the garage; she stated she did not see his parked car.

Neuro-ophthalmological examination shows 20/25 vision bilaterally, bitemporal visual field defects, normal-appearing optic discs, intact pupillary function and normal extraocular motility. Magnetic resonance imaging demonstrates a large intrasellar and suprasellar mass. There are no endocrine abnormalities.

Discussion: Bitemporal hemianopsia localizes the lesion to the optic chiasma, with involvement primarily of the decussating fibres originating in the nasal portion of the retina. Tumours in this area can compress both the optic nerves and optic chiasma, sometimes producing a mixed defect consisting of bitemporal visual field disturbances (as in this woman) and a superimposed monocular visual field disturbance—a so-called junctional defect. Such a combination of monocular and bitemporal visual field defects can be diagnostically challenging. See lesion 3, Figure 12.11. As this case demonstrates, patients with bitemporal visual field defects may be unaware of the vision loss.

Posterior Cranial Fossa

The posterior cranial fossa is the largest and deepest of the cranial fossae. It is bounded in front by the dorsum sellae, posterior aspects of the sphenoidal body and basilar part of occipital bone; behind by the squamous part of the occipital bone; laterally by the petrous and mastoid parts of the temporal bone and by the lateral parts of the occipital bone; and above and behind by the mastoid angles of the parietal bones. The posterior cranial fossa contains the cerebellum, pons and medulla oblongata. The region corresponds extracranially with the posterior part of the cranial base.

The most prominent feature in the floor of the posterior cranial fossa is the foramen magnum in the occipital bone. A sloping surface called the clivus—formed successively by the basilar part of the occipital bone, the posterior part of the body and the dorsum sellae of the sphenoid bone—lies anterior to the foramen magnum. The clivus is gently concave from side to side. On each side it is separated from the petrous part of the temporal bone by a petro-occipital fissure, filled by a thin plate of cartilage and limited behind by the jugular foramen. Its margins are grooved by the inferior petrosal sinus. The spheno-occipital synchondrosis is evident on the clivus of a growing child.

A large jugular foramen, sited at the posterior end of the petro-occipital fissure, lies above and lateral to the foramen magnum. Its upper border is

sharp and irregular and contains a notch for the glossopharyngeal nerve. The cochlear canaliculus, which contains the perilymphatic 'duct,' is sited in the deepest part of the notch. The lower border of the jugular foramen is smooth. Posteriorly, it is grooved by the sigmoid sinus, which continues into the foramen as the internal jugular vein. The accessory, vagus and glossopharyngeal nerves pass forward through the anterior part of the jugular foramen from behind, and they may groove the jugular tubercle as they enter the foramen. The hypoglossal (anterior condylar) canal lies medial to and below the lower border of the jugular foramen at the junction of the basilar and lateral parts of the occipital bone. This canal transmits the hypoglossal nerve (and its recurrent branch), the meningeal branch of the ascending pharyngeal artery and an emissary vein linking the basilar plexus intracranially with the internal jugular vein extracranially. If a posterior condylar canal is present behind the occipital condyle, its internal orifice is posterolateral to that of the hypoglossal canal and contains a sigmoid emissary vein (associated with the occipital veins) and a meningeal branch of the occipital artery. The occipital condyles lie within the anterior aspect of the foramen magnum; their medial aspects are roughened for the attachments of the alar ligaments associated with the atlanto-axial joints.

The posterior surface of the petrous part of the temporal bone forms much of the anterolateral wall of the posterior cranial fossa. It contains the internal acoustic meatus, which lies anterosuperior to the jugular foramen, and transmits the facial and vestibulocochlear nerves, nervus intermedius and labyrinthine vessels.

The mastoid part of the temporal bone lies behind the petrous part of the temporal bone in the lateral wall of the posterior cranial fossa. Anteriorly, it is grooved by a wide sigmoid sulcus (groove) running forward and downward, then downward and medially and finally forward to the jugular foramen. It contains the sigmoid sinus. Superiorly, where the groove touches the mastoid angle of the parietal bone, it is continuous with a groove transmitting the transverse sinus; it next crosses the parietomastoid suture and then descends behind the mastoid antrum. A mastoid foramen for an emissary vein from the sigmoid sinus and a meningeal branch of the occipital artery, sometimes large enough to groove the squamous part of the occipital bone, may be sited there. The lowest part of the sigmoid sulcus crosses the occipitomastoid suture and grooves the jugular process of the occipital bone. The right sigmoid sulcus is usually larger than the left.

A thin plate with an irregularly curved margin projects back behind the internal acoustic meatus and bounds a slit containing the opening of the vestibular aqueduct (which contains the saccus and ductus endolymphaticus and a small artery and vein). A small subarcuate fossa lies between the internal acoustic meatus and the aqueductal opening. It contains dura mater. Near the superior border of the petrous part of the temporal bone, it is pierced by a small vein. In infants, the fossa is a relatively large blind tunnel under the anterior semicircular canal.

The squamous part of the occipital bone displays a median internal occipital crest, which runs posteriorly from the foramen magnum to an internal occipital protuberance and gives attachment to the falx cerebelli. The internal occipital crest may be grooved by the occipital sinus. The internal occipital protuberance is close to the confluence of the sinuses and is grooved bilaterally by the transverse sinuses. The latter curve laterally, with an upward convexity, to the mastoid angles of the parietal bones. The groove for the transverse sinus is usually deeper on the right, where it is generally a continuation of the superior sagittal sinus; on the left, it is frequently a continuation of the straight sinus. On both sides, the transverse sulcus is continuous with the sigmoid sulcus. Below the transverse sulcus, the internal occipital crest separates two shallow fossae, adapted to the cerebellar hemispheres. The margins of the grooves for the transverse sinus and superior petrosal sinus, together with the posterior clinoid process, all provide anchorage for the attached margin of the tentorium cerebelli.

References

Berkovitz, B.K.B., Moxham, B.J., 1994. Color Atlas of the Skull. Mosby-Wolfe, London.

Howells, W.W., 1973. Cranial Variation in Man, vol. 67. Papers of the Peabody Museum of Archaeology and Ethnography, Cambridge, MA.

Lieberman, D.E., McCarthy, R.C., 1999. The ontogeny of cranial base angulation in humans and chimpanzees and its implications for reconstructing pharyngeal dimensions. J. Hum. E. 36, 487–517.

Lieberman, D.E., Pearson, O.M., Mowbray, K.M., 2000. Basicranial influence on overall cranial shape. J. Hum. E. 38 (2), 291–315.

Moos, K.F., Baker, A.W., 1998. Craniofacial surgery: Assessment and techniques. In: Langdon, J.D., Patel, M.F., (Eds.), Operative Maxillofacial Surgery. Chapman & Hall, London, pp. 407–436. *A detailed description of the various craniosynostoses.*

Relethford, J.H., 1994. Craniometric variation among modern human populations. Am. J. Phys. Anthropol. 95, 53–62.

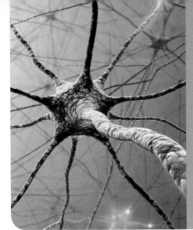

Brain Stem

The brain stem consists of the medulla oblongata, pons and midbrain. It is sited in the posterior cranial fossa, and its ventral surface lies on the clivus. It contains numerous intrinsic neurone cell bodies and their processes, some of which are the brain stem homologues of spinal neuronal groups. These include the sites of termination and cells of origin of axons that enter or leave the brain stem through the cranial nerves. They provide the sensory, motor and autonomic innervation of structures that are mostly in the head and neck. Autonomic fibres, which arise from the brain stem, are distributed more widely. Additional groups of neurones receive input related to the special senses of hearing, vestibular function and taste (Ch. 12). The reticular formation is an extensive and often ill-defined network of neurones that extends throughout the length of the brain stem and is continuous caudally with its spinal counterpart. Some of its nuclei are concerned with cardiac, respiratory and alimentary control; some are involved in aspects of many neural activities, and others provide or receive massive afferent and efferent cerebellar projections.

The brain stem is the site of termination of numerous ascending and descending fibres and is traversed by many others. The spinothalamic (spinal lemniscal), medial lemniscal and trigeminal systems ascend through the brain stem to reach the thalamus (see Figs 8.32, 10.22). Prominent corticospinal projections descend through the brain stem, and corticobulbar projections end within it (see Fig. 8.41).

Clinically, damage to the brain stem is often devastating and life threatening. This is because it is a structurally and functionally compact region, where even small lesions can destroy vital cardiac and respiratory centres, disconnect forebrain motor areas from brain stem and spinal motor neurones and sever incoming sensory fibres from higher centres of consciousness, perception and cognition. Irreversible cardiac and respiratory arrest follows complete destruction of the neural respiratory and cardiac centres in the medulla.

This chapter starts with a brief systematic overview of the cranial nerves that attach to the brain stem, their central origins and their connections within the cranial nerve nuclei. The major subdivisions of the brain stem are then described. Many structures, including nuclei and tracts, extend longitudinally across their boundaries. The structure and function of the most notable of these are discussed in detail at the most appropriate point in the text. As is customary, transverse sections of the brain stem are included to illustrate the relationships between structures and the regional variation that occurs at different levels.

OVERVIEW OF CRANIAL NERVES AND CRANIAL NERVE NUCLEI

The cranial nerves are the conduits by which the brain receives information directly from, and controls the functions of, structures that are mainly, but not exclusively, within the head and neck. All but 2 of the 12 pairs of cranial nerves attach to the brain stem; this chapter is therefore an appropriate place to describe their structure and function.

The cranial nerves are individually named and numbered (using roman numerals) in a rostrocaudal sequence (see Table 1.1). Cranial nerve I (olfactory) terminates directly in cortical and subcortical areas of the frontal and temporal lobes. It is closely associated functionally with the limbic system and is described in that context (Ch. 16). The fibres of cranial nerve II (optic) pass into the optic chiasma and emerge as the optic tract, which terminates in the lateral geniculate nucleus of the thalamus. Cranial nerves III (oculomotor) and IV (trochlear) attach to the midbrain. Cranial nerve V (trigeminal) attaches to the pons, medial to the middle cerebellar peduncle. Cranial nerves VI (abducens), VII (facial) and VIII (vestibulocochlear) attach to the brain stem at or close to the junction of the pons and the medulla. Cranial nerves IX (glossopharyngeal) and X (vagus), the cranial part of cranial nerve XI (accessory) and cranial nerve XII (hypoglossal) all attach to the medulla.

Cranial nerves III to XII, which attach to the brain stem, are associated with a number of cell groupings of varying size, referred to collectively as the cranial nerve nuclei (Fig. 10.1). The nuclei are either the origin of efferent cranial nerve fibres or the site of termination of cranial nerve afferents. For convenience, they are considered to be organized into six discontinuous, longitudinal cell columns that correspond to the columns that can be identified in the embryo (see Fig. 1.4). Three columns are 'sensory' and three are 'motor' in function.

The trigeminal sensory nucleus, which extends throughout the length of the brain stem and into the cervical spinal cord, represents a general somatic afferent cell column. Its principal afferents are carried in the trigeminal nerve. General visceral afferents carried by the facial, glossopharyngeal and vagus nerves end in the nucleus solitarius of the medulla. The special visceral afferent column corresponds to the vestibular and cochlear nuclei, which are located beneath the vestibular area of the floor of the fourth ventricle.

The general somatic efferent cell column consists of four nuclei that lie near the midline and give rise to motor fibres that run in nerves of the same name. From rostral to caudal, these are the oculomotor, trochlear and abducens nuclei, which innervate the extraocular muscles, and the hypoglossal nucleus, which innervates all but one of the muscles of the tongue. The general visceral efferent, or parasympathetic, cell column is made up of the Edinger–Westphal nucleus of the midbrain, salivary nuclei of the pons and vagal nucleus of the medulla. Cells in the special visceral efferent column innervate muscles derived from the branchial arches and lie in the trigeminal motor nucleus, facial nucleus and nucleus ambiguus.

MEDULLA OBLONGATA

External Features and Relations

The medulla oblongata extends from the lower pontine margin to a transverse plane that is above the first pair of cervical spinal nerves and intersects the upper border of the atlas dorsally and the centre of the dens ventrally (Fig. 10.2). It is approximately 3 cm long and 2 cm in diameter at its widest. The ventral surface of the medulla is separated from the basilar part of the occipital bone and apex of the dens by the meninges and occipito-axial ligaments. Caudally, the dorsal surface of the medulla occupies the midline notch between the cerebellar hemispheres.

The ventral and dorsal surfaces of the medulla (Fig. 10.3; see also Fig. 5.11) possess a longitudinal median fissure and sulcus, respectively, which are continuous with their spinal counterparts. Caudally, the ventral median fissure is interrupted by the obliquely crossing fascicles of the pyramidal decussation. Rostrally, it ends at the pontine border in a diminutive depression, the foramen caecum. Immediately lateral to the ventral median fissure is a prominent elongated ridge called the pyramid, which contains descending pyramidal, or corticospinal, axons (see Fig. 10.3). The lateral margin of the pyramid is indicated by a shallow ventrolateral sulcus. From this emerges, in line with the ventral spinal nerve roots, a linear series of rootlets that constitute the hypoglossal nerve. The abducens nerve emerges at the slightly narrowed rostral end of the pyramid, where it adjoins the pons. Caudally, the pyramid tapers into the spinal ventral funiculus. Lateral to the pyramid and the ventrolateral sulcus is an oval prominence, the olive (Figs 10.3, 10.4), which contains the inferior olivary nucleus. Lateral to the olive is the posterolateral sulcus. The glossopharyngeal, vagus and accessory nerves join the brain stem along the line of this sulcus, in line with the dorsal spinal nerve roots.

The spinal central canal extends into the caudal half of the medulla, migrating progressively more dorsally until it opens out into the lumen of the fourth ventricle. This divides the medulla into a closed part, which contains the central canal, and an open part, which contains the caudal half of the fourth ventricle (see Figs 10.2, 5.11).

In the closed part of the medulla, a shallow posterointermediate sulcus on either side of the dorsal median sulcus, continuous with its cervical spinal counterpart, indicates the location of the ascending dorsal columns

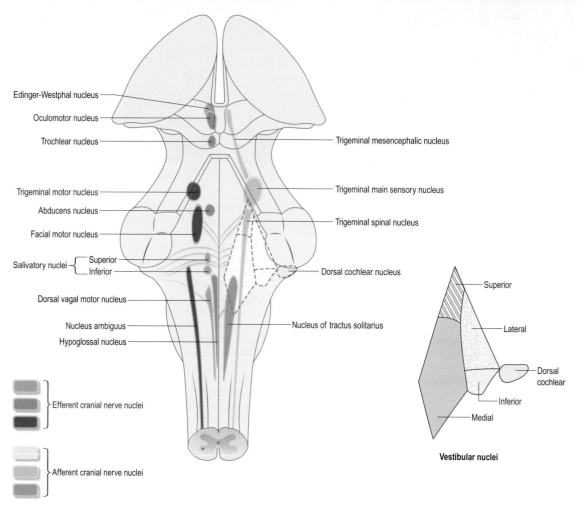

Fig. 10.1 *Cranial nerve nuclei.*

(fasciculus gracilis and fasciculus cuneatus). The ascending fasciculi are at first parallel to each other, but at the caudal end of the fourth ventricle they diverge, and each develops an elongated swelling, the gracile and cuneate tubercles, produced by the subjacent nuclei gracilis and cuneatus, respectively (Figs 10.5, 10.6). Most fibres in the fasciculi synapse with neurones in their respective nuclei, and these project to the contralateral thalamus, which in turn projects to the primary somaesthetic cortex (see Fig. 8.32). The inferior cerebellar peduncle forms a rounded ridge between the caudal part of the fourth ventricle and the glossopharyngeal and vagal rootlets. The two peduncles diverge and incline to enter the cerebellar hemispheres, where they are crossed by the striae medullares, which run to the median ventricular sulcus (see Fig. 5.11). Here also the peduncles form the anterior and rostral boundaries of the lateral recess of the fourth ventricle. This becomes continuous with the subarachnoid space through the lateral apertures of the fourth ventricle, the foramina of Luschka. A tuft of choroid plexus, continuous with that of the fourth ventricle, protrudes from the foramina on either side. The fibre composition of the inferior cerebellar peduncle is described in Chapter 13.

Internal Structure
Transverse Section of the Medulla at the Level of the Pyramidal Decussation
A transverse section across the lower medulla oblongata (see Fig. 10.5) intersects the dorsal, lateral and ventral funiculi, which are continuous with their counterparts in the spinal cord. The ventral funiculi are separated from the central grey matter by corticospinal fibres, which cross in the pyramidal decussation to reach the contralateral lateral funiculi (see Fig. 10.11). The decussation displaces the ventral intersegmental tract, the central grey matter and the central canal dorsally. Continuity between the ventral grey column and central grey matter, which is maintained throughout the spinal cord, is lost. The column subdivides into the supraspinal nucleus (continuous above with that of the hypoglossal nerve), which is the efferent source of the first cervical nerve, and the spinal nucleus of the accessory nerve, which provides some spinal accessory fibres and merges rostrally with the nucleus ambiguus.

The dorsal grey column is also modified at this level where the nucleus gracilis appears as a grey lamina in the ventral part of the fasciculus gracilis. The nucleus begins caudal to the nucleus cuneatus, which invades the fasciculus cuneatus from its ventral aspect in similar fashion.

The spinal nucleus and spinal tract of the trigeminal nerve are visible ventrolateral to the dorsal columns. They are continuous with the substantia gelatinosa and tract of Lissauer of the spinal cord.

Transverse Section of the Medulla at the Level of the Decussation of the Medial Lemniscus
The medullary white matter is rearranged above the level of the pyramidal decussation (see Fig. 10.6). The pyramids contain ipsilateral corticospinal and corticonuclear fibres, the latter distributed to nuclei of cranial nerves and other medullary nuclei. At this level, they form two large ventral bundles flanking the ventral median fissure. The accessory olivary nuclei and lemniscal decussation are dorsal.

The nucleus gracilis is broader at this level, and the fibres of its fasciculus are located on its dorsal, medial and lateral surfaces. The nucleus cuneatus is well developed. Both nuclei retain continuity with the central grey matter at this level, but this is subsequently lost. First-order gracile and cuneate fascicular fibres, which have ascended ipsilaterally and uninterrupted from their origin in the spinal cord, synapse on neurones in their respective nuclei. Second-order axons emerge from the nuclei as internal arcuate fibres, at first curving ventrolaterally around the central grey matter and then ventromedially between the trigeminal spinal tract and the central grey matter. They decussate to form an ascending contralateral tract, the medial lemniscus. The lemniscal decussation is located dorsal to the pyramids and ventral to the central grey matter. The latter is therefore more dorsally displaced than in the previous section.

The medial lemniscus ascends from the lemniscal decussation on each side as a flattened tract near the median raphe. As the tracts ascend, they increase in size because fibres join from upper levels of the decussation. Corticospinal fibres are ventral, and the medial longitudinal fasciculus and tectospinal tract are dorsal. Fibres are rearranged in the decussation, so that those from the nucleus gracilis come to lie ventral to those from the nucleus cuneatus. Above

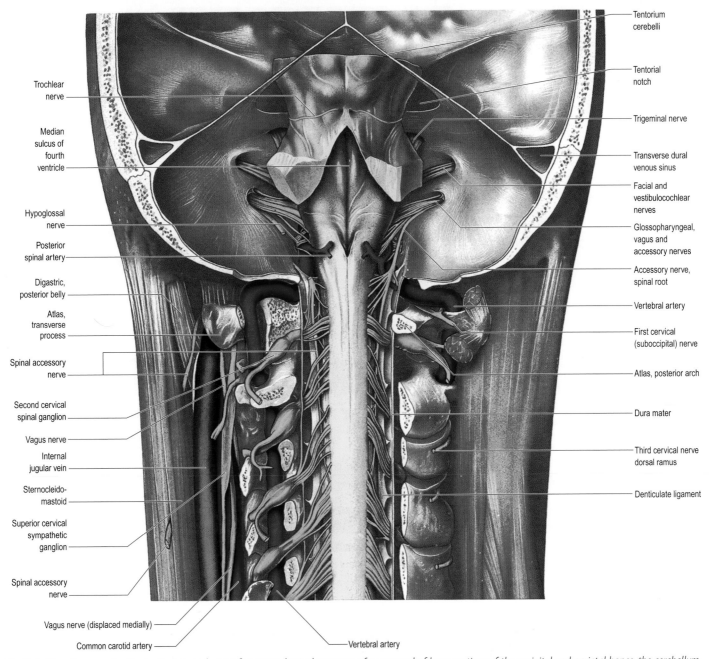

Fig. 10.2 *Dissection exposing the brain stem and upper five cervical spinal segments after removal of large portions of the occipital and parietal bones, the cerebellum and the roof of the fourth ventricle. On the left, the foramina transversaria of the atlas and the third, fourth and fifth cervical vertebrae have been opened to expose the vertebral artery. On the right, the posterior arch of the atlas and the laminae of the succeeding cervical vertebrae have been removed.*

this, the medial lemniscus is also rearranged, with ventral (gracile) fibres becoming lateral and dorsal (cuneate) fibres medial. At this level, medial lemniscal fibres show a laminar somatotopy on a segmental basis, in that fibres from C1 to S4 spinal segments are segregated sequentially from medial to lateral.

The nucleus of the spinal tract of the trigeminal nerve (see Fig. 10.22) is separated from the central grey matter by internal arcuate fibres; it is separated from the lateral medullary surface by the trigeminal spinal tract, which ends in it, and by some dorsal spinocerebellar tract fibres. The latter progressively incline dorsally and enter the inferior cerebellar peduncle at a higher level.

Two other nuclei occur at this level. One is dorsolateral to the pyramid, and the other is medial to it and near the median plane. These are parts of the precerebellar medial accessory olivary nucleus, described with the inferior olivary nuclear complex. Precerebellar nuclei of the vestibular, pontine and reticular system are described in Chapter 13.

Transverse Section of the Medulla at the Caudal End of the Fourth Ventricle

A transverse section level with the lower end of the fourth ventricle shows some new features, along with most of those already described (Fig. 10.8). The

total area of grey matter is increased by the presence of the large olivary nuclear complex and nuclei of the vestibulocochlear, glossopharyngeal, vagus and accessory nerves.

A smooth, oval elevation—the olive—lies between the ventrolateral and dorsolateral sulci of the medulla. It is formed by the underlying inferior olivary complex of nuclei and lies lateral to the pyramid, separated from it by the ventrolateral sulcus and emerging hypoglossal nerve fibres. The roots of the facial nerve emerge between its rostral end and the lower pontine border, in the cerebellopontine angle. The arcuate nuclei are curved, interrupted bands, ventral to the pyramids, and are said to be displaced pontine nuclei. Anterior external arcuate fibres and those of the striae medullares are derived from them. They project mainly to the contralateral cerebellum through the inferior cerebellar peduncle (Fig. 10.9).

The inferior olivary nucleus is a hollow, irregularly crenated grey mass. It has a longitudinal medial hilum and is surrounded by myelinated fibres that form the olivary amiculum. Dorsolateral to the pyramid, it underlies the olive but ascends within the pons.

The central grey matter at this level constitutes the ventricular floor. It contains (sequentially from medial to lateral) the hypoglossal nucleus, dorsal vagal nucleus, nucleus solitarius and caudal ends of the inferior and medial vestibular nuclei.

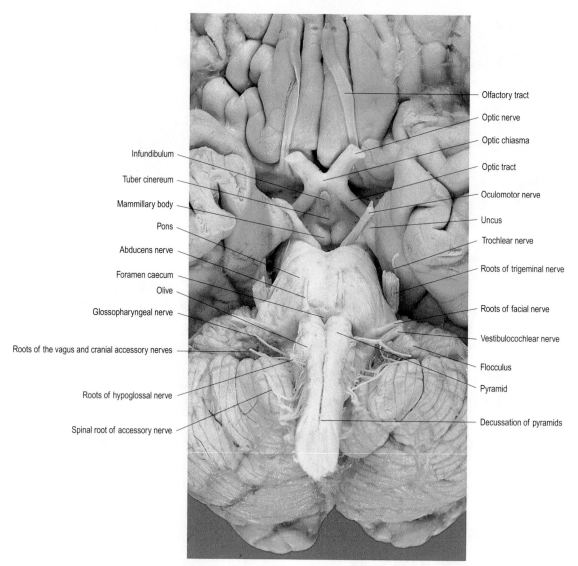

Infundibulum
Tuber cinereum
Mammillary body
Pons
Abducens nerve
Foramen caecum
Olive
Glossopharyngeal nerve
Roots of the vagus and cranial accessory nerves
Roots of hypoglossal nerve
Spinal root of accessory nerve

Olfactory tract
Optic nerve
Optic chiasma
Optic tract
Oculomotor nerve
Uncus
Trochlear nerve
Roots of trigeminal nerve
Roots of facial nerve
Vestibulocochlear nerve
Flocculus
Pyramid
Decussation of pyramids

Fig. 10.3 *Ventral aspect of the brain stem.*

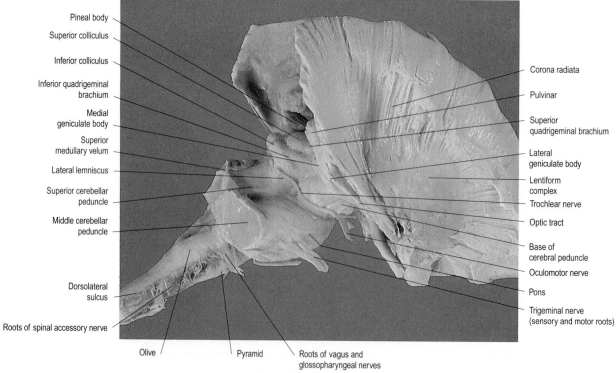

Pineal body
Superior colliculus
Inferior colliculus
Inferior quadrigeminal brachium
Medial geniculate body
Superior medullary velum
Lateral lemniscus
Superior cerebellar peduncle
Middle cerebellar peduncle
Dorsolateral sulcus
Roots of spinal accessory nerve

Olive
Pyramid
Roots of vagus and glossopharyngeal nerves

Corona radiata
Pulvinar
Superior quadrigeminal brachium
Lateral geniculate body
Lentiform complex
Trochlear nerve
Optic tract
Base of cerebral peduncle
Oculomotor nerve
Pons
Trigeminal nerve (sensory and motor roots)

Fig. 10.4 *Lateral aspect of the brain stem.*

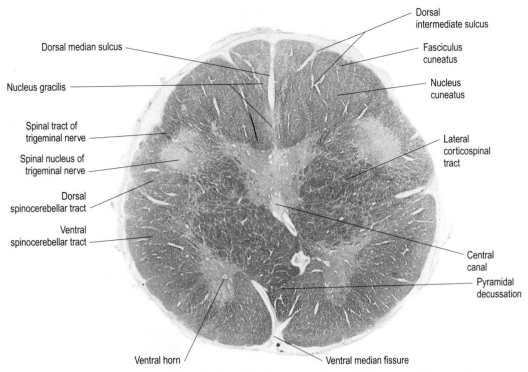

Dorsal median sulcus

Nucleus gracilis

Spinal tract of trigeminal nerve

Spinal nucleus of trigeminal nerve

Dorsal spinocerebellar tract

Ventral spinocerebellar tract

Ventral horn

Dorsal intermediate sulcus

Fasciculus cuneatus

Nucleus cuneatus

Lateral corticospinal tract

Central canal

Pyramidal decussation

Ventral median fissure

Fig. 10.5 *Transverse section through the medulla oblongata at the level of the pyramidal decussation.*

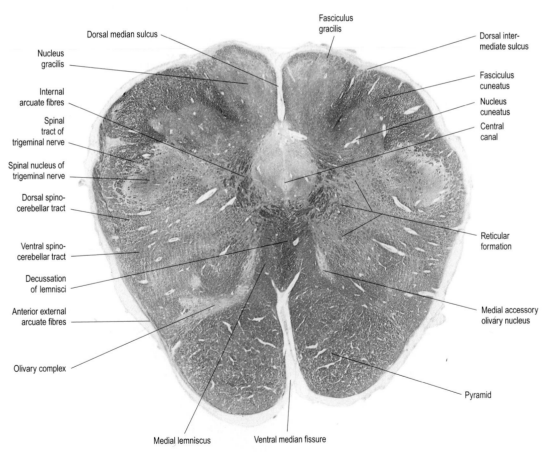

Dorsal median sulcus

Nucleus gracilis

Internal arcuate fibres

Spinal tract of trigeminal nerve

Spinal nucleus of trigeminal nerve

Dorsal spino-cerebellar tract

Ventral spino-cerebellar tract

Decussation of lemnisci

Anterior external arcuate fibres

Olivary complex

Medial lemniscus

Fasciculus gracilis

Dorsal inter-mediate sulcus

Fasciculus cuneatus

Nucleus cuneatus

Central canal

Reticular formation

Medial accessory olivary nucleus

Pyramid

Ventral median fissure

Fig. 10.6 *Transverse section through the medulla oblongata at the level of the decussation of the medial lemniscus.*

The tractus solitarius and its associated circumferential nucleus solitarius extend throughout the length of the medulla. The tract is composed of general visceral afferents from the vagus and glossopharyngeal nerves. The nucleus and its central connections with the reticular formation subserve the reflex control of cardiovascular, respiratory and cardiac functions. The rostral fibres of the tract consist of gustatory fibres from the facial, glossopharyngeal and vagal nerves that project to the rostral pole of the nucleus solitarius, which is sometimes referred to as the gustatory nucleus.

The medial longitudinal fasciculus, a small, compact tract near the midline and ventral to the hypoglossal nucleus, is continuous with the ventral vestibulospinal tract. At this medullary level it is displaced dorsally by the pyramidal and lemniscal decussations. It ascends in the pons and midbrain, maintaining its relationship to the central grey matter and midline, so it is

CASE 1   DOWNBEAT NYSTAGMUS AND ARNOLD–CHIARI MALFORMATION

A 24-year-old woman presents with a long history of increasing headache, blurred vision when attempting to read and an increasingly unsteady gait with intermittent falls. Neurological examination reveals downbeat nystagmus with the eyes in the primary position, amplified by down-gaze; dysmetria of the lower extremities with heel-to-shin testing; and hyperreflexia in both lower extremities.

Magnetic resonance imaging (MRI) shows 'beaking' of the dorsal midbrain and enlargement of the lateral and third ventricles, with herniation of the cerebellar tonsils through the foramen magnum. See Figure 10.7.

A ventriculoperitoneal shunt is placed, with marked symptomatic improvement.

Discussion: Downbeat nystagmus consists of a rapid downbeat motion of the eyes followed by a slower upward movement. This is usually present with the eyes in the primary position, but at times it is so subtle that it can be seen only with ophthalmoscopy. The amplitude of the movements is usually increased by down-gaze and sometimes by horizontal gaze to either side. It is characteristically associated with conditions involving the medulla oblongata, particularly at the level of the craniocervical junction. These conditions include Arnold–Chiari malformation, as is the case in this woman. It has also been reported with drug toxicity involving lithium and phenytoin.

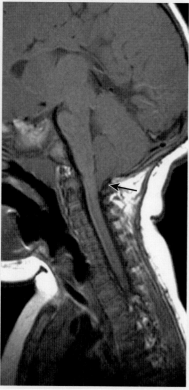

Fig. 10.7 *Arnold–Chiari malformation. MRI demonstrates downward displacement of the cerebellar tonsil (arrow) below the plane of the foramen magnum. (© 2010 Thomas Jefferson University. All rights reserved. Reproduced with the permission of Thomas Jefferson University.)*

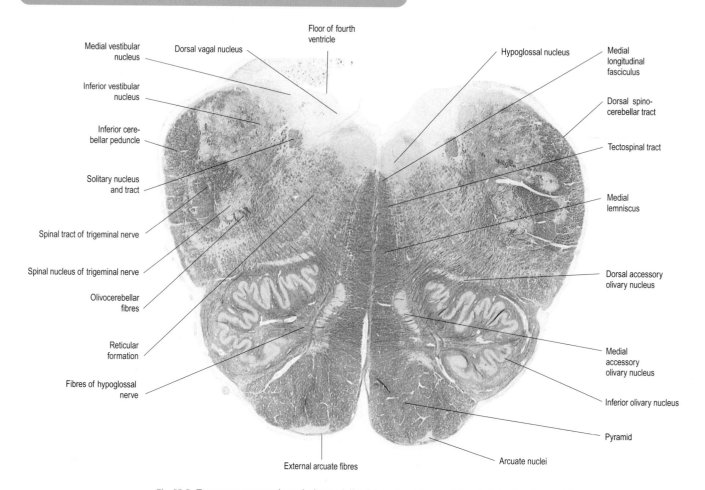

Fig. 10.8 *Transverse section through the medulla oblongata at the caudal end of the fourth ventricle.*

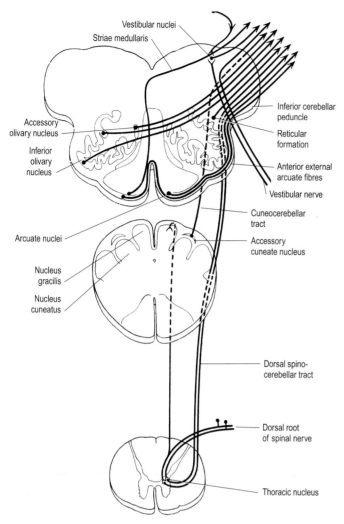

Fig. 10.9 *Some of the afferent components of the inferior cerebellar peduncles. The efferent components have been omitted.*

Labels (top to bottom, left and right):
Vestibular nuclei
Striae medullaris
Accessory olivary nucleus
Inferior olivary nucleus
Arcuate nuclei
Nucleus gracilis
Nucleus cuneatus
Inferior cerebellar peduncle
Reticular formation
Anterior external arcuate fibres
Vestibular nerve
Cuneocerebellar tract
Accessory cuneate nucleus
Dorsal spino-cerebellar tract
Dorsal root of spinal nerve
Thoracic nucleus

near the somatic efferent nuclear column. Fibres from a variety of sources course for short distances in the tract.

The spinocerebellar, spinotectal, vestibulospinal, rubrospinal and lateral spinothalamic (spinal lemniscal) tracts all lie in the ventrolateral area of the medulla at this level. The tracts are limited dorsally by the spinal trigeminal nucleus and ventrally by the pyramid.

Numerous islets of grey matter are scattered centrally in the ventrolateral medulla, an area intersected by nerve fibres that run in all directions. This is the reticular formation, which exists throughout the medulla and extends into the pontine tegmentum and midbrain.

Pyramidal Tract

Each pyramid contains descending corticospinal fibres, derived from the ipsilateral cerebral cortex, which have traversed the internal capsule, midbrain and pons (Fig. 10.11). Approximately 70% to 90% of the axons leave the pyramids in successive bundles, crossing in and deep to the ventral median fissure as the pyramidal decussation. In the rostral medulla, fibres cross by inclining ventromedially, whereas more caudally, they pass dorsally, decussating ventral to the central grey matter. The decussation is orderly, with fibres destined to end in the cervical segments crossing first. They continue to pass dorsally as they descend, reaching the contralateral spinal lateral funiculus as the crossed lateral corticospinal tract. Most uncrossed corticospinal fibres descend ventromedially in the ipsilateral ventral funiculus, as the ventral corticospinal tract. A minority run dorsolaterally to join the lateral corticospinal tracts as a small uncrossed component. The corticospinal tracts display somatotopy at almost all levels. In the pyramids the arrangement is like that at higher levels, in that the most lateral fibres subserve the most medial arm and neck movements. Similar somatotopy is ascribed to the lateral corticospinal tracts within the spinal cord.

Dorsal Column Nuclei

The nuclei gracilis and cuneatus are part of the pathway that is considered the major route for discriminative aspects of tactile and locomotor

CASE 2   AVELLIS' SYNDROME

A 47 year old man, previously well, suddenly developed numbness of the left hand. Within 2 days, the sensory loss spread to involve the entire left arm, then the left leg; at that point he developed an increasingly severe left hemiparesis. Speech was described as occasionally slurred. Examination demonstrated a flaccid left hemiparesis with exaggerated reflex activity bilaterally. Plantar response on the left arm was extensor. There was reduction in vibratory sense on the left side; sensation was otherwise normal. There was mild wasting on the left side of the tongue, with fasciculation and the left sternomastoid muscle was slightly atrophic.

MRI demonstrated an acute infarction in the right medial lowermost medulla involving the pyramid, the medial lemniscus, and the hypoglossal nerve in its course through the medulla.

COMMENT: The patient demonstrated the classic features of Avellis syndrome due to a lesion (infarction) in the medial aspect of the lower medulla involving to variable extents. The neuro-anatomic structures involved include the corticospinal tracts causing contralateral hemiparesis, the medial lemniscus leading to impaired posterior column sensibility, the accessory nerve causing mild atrophy of the sternomastoid muscle, and the hypoglossal nerve producing atrophy of the tongue with fasciculations. This syndrome is rare, and variably described; in a number of cases, palatal weakness has been observed. See Figure 10.10.

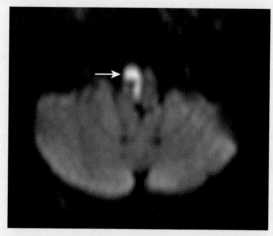

Fig. 10.10 *Diffusion-weighted MRI showing acute infarction of the medulla (arrow).*

(proprioceptive) sensation. The upper regions of both nuclei are reticular and contain small and large multipolar neurones with long dendrites. The lower regions contain clusters of large, round neurones with short and profusely branching dendrites. Upper and lower zones differ in their connections, but both receive terminals from the dorsal spinal roots at all levels. Dorsal funicular fibres from neurones in the spinal grey matter terminate only in the superior, reticular zone. Variable ordering and overlap of terminals, on the basis of spinal root levels, occur in both zones. The lower extremity is represented medially, the trunk ventrally and the digits dorsally. There is modal specificity; that is, lower levels respond to low-threshold cutaneous stimuli, and upper reticular levels respond to inputs from fibres serving receptors in the skin, joints and muscles. The cuneate nucleus is divided into several parts. Its middle zone contains a large pars rotunda, in which rostrocaudally elongated, medium-sized neurones are clustered between bundles of densely myelinated fibres. The reticular poles of its rostral and caudal zones contain scattered but evenly distributed neurones of various sizes. The pars triangularis is smaller

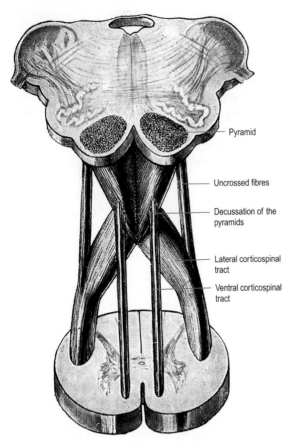

Pyramid

Uncrossed fibres

Decussation of the
pyramids

Lateral corticospinal
tract

Ventral corticospinal
tract

Fig. 10.11 *Schematic dissection to show the decussation of the pyramids.*

and laterally placed. There is a somatotopic pattern of termination of cutaneous inputs from the upper limb on the cell clusters of the pars rotunda. Terminations are diffuse in the reticular poles.

The gracile and cuneate nuclei serve as relays between the spinal cord and higher levels. Primary spinal afferents synapse with multipolar neurones in the nuclei to form the major nuclear efferent projection. The nuclei also contain interneurones, many of which are inhibitory. Descending afferents from the somatosensory cortex reach the nuclei through the corticobulbar tracts and appear to be restricted to the upper, reticular zones. Because these afferents both inhibit and enhance activity, the nuclear region is clearly one of sensory modulation. The reticular zones also receive connections from the reticular formation. Feedback from the gracile and cuneate nuclei to the spinal cord probably occurs.

Neurones of dorsal column nuclei receive terminals of long, uncrossed, primary afferent fibres of the fasciculi gracilis and cuneatus, which carry information concerning deformation of the skin, movement of hairs, joint movement and vibration. Unit recording of the neurones in dorsal column nuclei shows that their tactile receptive fields (i.e. the skin area in which a response can be elicited) vary in size, although they are mostly small and are smallest for the digits. Some fields have excitatory centres and inhibitory surrounds, which means that stimulation just outside its excitatory field inhibits the neurone. Neurones in the nuclei are spatially organized into a somatotopic map of the periphery (in accord with the similar localization in the dorsal columns). In general, specificity is high. Many cells receive input from one or a few specific receptor types (e.g. hair, type I and II slowly adapting receptors and Pacinian corpuscles), and some cells respond to Ia muscle spindle input. However, some neurones receive convergent input from tactile pressure and hair follicle receptors.

A variety of control mechanisms can modulate the transmission of impulses through the dorsal column–medial lemniscus pathway. Concomitant activity in adjacent dorsal column fibres may result in presynaptic inhibition by depolarization of the presynaptic terminals of one of them. Stimulation of the sensorimotor cortex also modulates the transmission of impulses by both pre- and postsynaptic inhibitory mechanisms, and sometimes by facilitation. These descending influences are mediated by the corticospinal tract. Modulation of transmission by inhibition also results from stimulation of the reticular formation, raphe nuclei and other sites.

The accessory cuneate nucleus, dorsolateral to the cuneate, is part of the spinocerebellar system of precerebellar nuclei (see Fig. 10.9); it contains large neurones like those in the spinal thoracic nucleus. These form the posterior

external arcuate fibres, which enter the cerebellum by the ipsilateral inferior peduncle. The nucleus receives the lateral fibres of the fasciculus cuneatus, carrying proprioceptive impulses from the upper limb (which enter the cervical spinal cord rostral to the thoracic nucleus). Its efferent fibres form the cuneocerebellar tract. A group of neurones, called nucleus Z, has been identified in animals between the upper pole of the nucleus gracilis and the inferior vestibular nucleus and is said to be present in the human medulla. Its input is probably from the dorsal spinocerebellar tract, which carries proprioceptive information from the ipsilateral lower limb, and it projects through internal arcuate fibres to the contralateral medial lemniscus.

Trigeminal Sensory Nucleus

The trigeminal sensory nucleus receives the primary afferents of the trigeminal nerve. It is a large nucleus and extends caudally into the cervical spinal cord and rostrally into the midbrain. The principal and largest division of the nucleus is located in the pontine tegmentum.

On entering the pons, the fibres of the sensory root of the trigeminal nerve run dorsomedially toward the principal sensory nucleus, which is situated at this level (Fig. 10.12). Before reaching the nucleus, approximately 50% of the fibres divide into ascending and descending branches; the others ascend or descend without division. The descending fibres, 90% of which are less than 4 μm in diameter, form the spinal tract of the trigeminal nerve, which reaches the upper cervical spinal cord. The tract embraces the spinal trigeminal nucleus (Figs 10.5, 10.6, 10.8, 10.13, 10.14). There is a precise somatotopic organization in the tract. Fibres from the ophthalmic root lie ventrolaterally, those from the mandibular root lie dorsomedially and the maxillary fibres lie between them. The tract is completed on its dorsal rim by fibres from the sensory roots of the facial, glossopharyngeal and vagus nerves. All these fibres synapse in the nucleus caudalis.

The detailed anatomy of the trigeminospinal tract excited early clinical interest because it was recognized that dissociated sensory loss could occur in the trigeminal area. For example, in Wallenberg's syndrome (see Case 3), occlusion of the posterior inferior cerebellar branch of the vertebral artery leads to loss of pain and temperature sensation in the ipsilateral half of the face, with retention of common sensation.

There are conflicting opinions about the termination pattern of fibres in the spinal nucleus. It has long been held that fibres are organized rostrocaudally within the tract. According to this view, ophthalmic fibres are ventral and descend to the lower limit of the first cervical spinal segment, maxillary fibres are central and do not extend below the medulla oblongata and mandibular fibres are dorsal and do not extend much below the mid-medullary level. The results of section of the spinal tract in cases of severe trigeminal neuralgia support this distribution. It was found that sectioning 4 mm below the obex produced analgesia in the ophthalmic and maxillary areas, but tactile sensibility, apart from the abolition of 'tickle,' was much less affected. To include the mandibular area, it was necessary to section at the level of the obex. More recently, it has been proposed that fibres are arranged dorsoventrally within the spinal tract. There appear to be sound anatomical, physiological and clinical reasons for believing that all divisions terminate throughout the whole nucleus, although the ophthalmic division may not project fibres as far caudally as the maxillary and mandibular divisions do. Fibres from the posterior face (adjacent to C2) terminate in the lower (caudal) part, whereas those from the upper lip, mouth and nasal tip terminate at a higher level. This can give rise to a segmental (cross-divisional) sensory loss in syringobulbia. Tractotomy of the spinal tract, if carried out at a lower level, can spare the perioral region, a finding that would accord with the 'onionskin' pattern of loss of pain sensation. However, in clinical practice, the progression of anaesthesia on the face is most commonly 'divisional' rather than 'onionskin' in distribution.

Fibres of the glossopharyngeal, vagus and facial nerves subserving common sensation (general visceral afferent) form a column dorsally within the spinal tract of the trigeminal nerve and synapse with cells in the lowest part of the spinal trigeminal nucleus. Consequently, operative section of the dorsal part of the spinal tract results in analgesia that extends to the mucosa of the tonsillar sinus, the posterior third of the tongue and adjoining parts of the pharyngeal wall (glossopharyngeal nerve) and the cutaneous area supplied by the auricular branch of the vagus.

Other afferents that reach the spinal nucleus are from the dorsal roots of the upper cervical nerves and from the sensorimotor cortex.

The spinal nucleus is considered to consist of three parts: the subnucleus oralis (which is most rostral and adjoins the principal sensory nucleus), the subnucleus interpolaris and the subnucleus caudalis (which is the most caudal part and is continuous below with the dorsal grey column of the spinal cord). The structure of the subnucleus caudalis is different from that of the other trigeminal sensory nuclei. It has a structure analogous to that of the dorsal horn of the spinal cord, with a similar arrangement of cell laminae, and it is

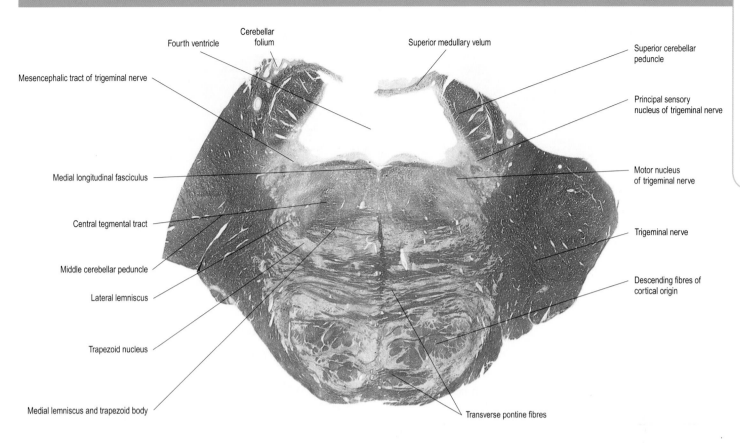

Fourth ventricle

Cerebellar folium

Superior medullary velum

Superior cerebellar peduncle

Mesencephalic tract of trigeminal nerve

Principal sensory nucleus of trigeminal nerve

Medial longitudinal fasciculus

Motor nucleus of trigeminal nerve

Central tegmental tract

Trigeminal nerve

Middle cerebellar peduncle

Descending fibres of cortical origin

Lateral lemniscus

Trapezoid nucleus

Medial lemniscus and trapezoid body

Transverse pontine fibres

Fig. 10.12 *Transverse section of the pons at the level of the trigeminal nerve.*

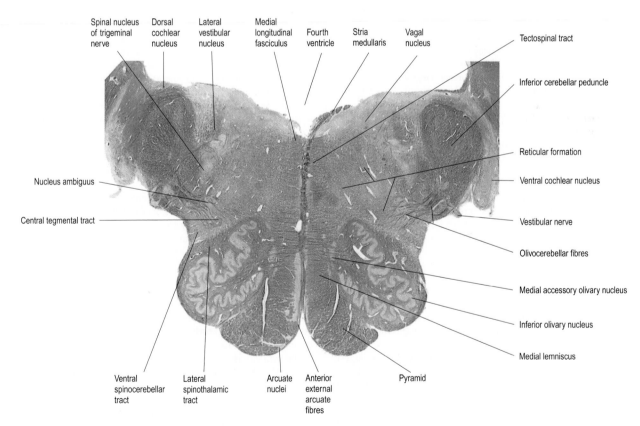

Spinal nucleus of trigeminal nerve

Dorsal cochlear nucleus

Lateral vestibular nucleus

Medial longitudinal fasciculus

Fourth ventricle

Stria medullaris

Vagal nucleus

Tectospinal tract

Inferior cerebellar peduncle

Nucleus ambiguus

Reticular formation

Ventral cochlear nucleus

Central tegmental tract

Vestibular nerve

Olivocerebellar fibres

Medial accessory olivary nucleus

Inferior olivary nucleus

Medial lemniscus

Ventral spinocerebellar tract

Lateral spinothalamic tract

Arcuate nuclei

Anterior external arcuate fibres

Pyramid

Fig. 10.13 *Transverse section through the superior half of the medulla oblongata at the level of the inferior olivary nucleus.*

involved in trigeminal pain perception. Cutaneous nociceptive afferents and small-diameter muscle afferents terminate in layers I, II, V and VI of the sub-nucleus caudalis. Low-threshold mechanosensitive afferents of Aβ neurones terminate in layers III and IV of the subnucleus caudalis and rostral (interpo-laris, oralis and main sensory) nuclei.

Many of the neurones in the subnucleus caudalis that respond to cutaneous or tooth pulp stimulation are also excited by noxious electrical, mechanical or chemical stimuli derived from the jaw or tongue muscles. This indicates

that convergence of superficial and deep afferent inputs via wide dynamic range or nociceptive-specific neurones occurs in the nucleus. Similar conver-gence of superficial and deep inputs occurs in the rostral nuclei and may account for the poor localization of trigeminal pain and for the spread of pain, which often makes diagnosis difficult.

There are distinct subtypes of cells in lamina II. Afferents from 'higher centres' arborize within it, as do axons from nociceptive and low-threshold afferents. Descending influences from these higher centres include fibres from

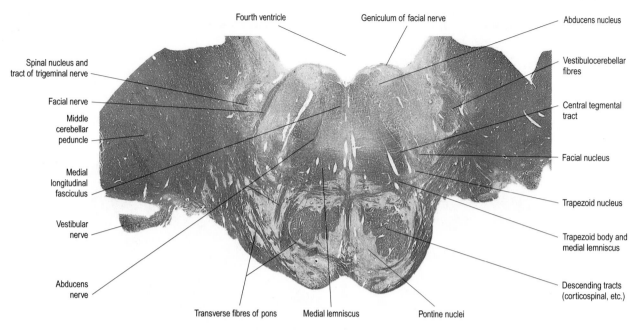

Fourth ventricle
Geniculum of facial nerve
Abducens nucleus
Spinal nucleus and tract of trigeminal nerve
Vestibulocerebellar fibres
Facial nerve
Central tegmental tract
Middle cerebellar peduncle
Facial nucleus
Medial longitudinal fasciculus
Trapezoid nucleus
Vestibular nerve
Trapezoid body and medial lemniscus
Descending tracts (corticospinal, etc.)
Abducens nerve
Transverse fibres of pons
Medial lemniscus
Pontine nuclei

Fig. 10.14 *Transverse section through the pons at the level of the facial colliculus.*

the periaqueductal grey matter and from the nucleus raphe magnus and associated reticular formation.

The nucleus raphe magnus projects directly to the subnucleus caudalis, probably via enkephalin-, noradrenaline- and 5-HT–containing terminals. These fibres directly or indirectly (through local interneurones) influence pain perception. Stimulation of the periaqueductal grey matter or nucleus raphe magnus inhibits the jaw opening reflex to nociception and may induce primary afferent depolarization in tooth pulp afferents and other nociceptive facial afferents. Neurones in the subnucleus caudalis can be suppressed by stimuli applied outside their receptive field, particularly by noxious stimuli. The subnucleus caudalis is an important site for relay of nociceptive input and functions as part of the pain 'gate control.' However, rostral nuclei also have a nociceptive role. Tooth pulp afferents via wide dynamic range and nociceptive-specific neurones may terminate in rostral nuclei, which all project to the subnucleus caudalis.

Most fibres arising in the trigeminal sensory nuclei cross the midline and ascend in the trigeminal lemniscus. They end in the contralateral thalamic nucleus ventralis posterior medialis, from which third-order neurones project to the cortical postcentral gyrus (areas 1, 2 and 3). However, some trigeminal nucleus efferents ascend to the nucleus ventralis posterior medialis of the ipsilateral thalamus.

Fibres from the subnucleus caudalis, especially from laminae I, V and VI, also project to the rostral trigeminal nuclei, cerebellum, periaqueductal grey of the midbrain, parabrachial area of the pons, brain stem reticular formation and spinal cord. Fibres from lamina I project to the subnucleus medius of the medial thalamus.

Vagal Nucleus

The vagal nucleus (also known as the dorsal motor nucleus of the vagus) lies dorsolateral to the hypoglossal nucleus, from which it is separated by the nucleus intercalatus. It extends caudally to the first cervical spinal segment and rostrally to the open part of the medulla under the vagal triangle (see Fig. 10.1).

The vagal nucleus is a general visceral efferent nucleus and is the largest parasympathetic nucleus in the brain stem. Most of its neurones (80%) give rise to the preganglionic parasympathetic fibres of the vagus nerve. The remainder are interneurones or project centrally. Its fibres control the nonstriated muscle of the viscera of the thorax (heart, bronchi, lungs and oesophagus) and abdomen (stomach, liver, pancreas, spleen, small intestine and proximal part of the colon). Neurones within the nucleus are heterogeneous and can be classified into nine subnuclei, which are regionally grouped into rostral, intermediate and caudal divisions. Topographical maps of visceral representation in animals suggest that the heart and lungs are represented in the caudal and lateral part of the nucleus, the stomach and pancreas in intermediate regions and the remaining abdominal organs in the rostral and medial part of the nucleus.

There may be a sparse sensory afferent supply that arises in the nodose ganglion and projects directly to the nucleus and possibly beyond into the nucleus tractus solitarius.

Hypoglossal Nucleus

The prominent hypoglossal nucleus lies near the midline in the dorsal medullary grey matter. It is approximately 2 cm long. Its rostral part lies beneath the hypoglossal triangle in the floor of the fourth ventricle, and its caudal part extends into the closed part of the medulla (see Figs 10.2, 10.6, 5.11).

The hypoglossal nucleus consists of large motor neurones interspersed with myelinated fibres. It is organized into dorsal and ventral nuclear tiers, each divisible into medial and lateral subnuclei. There is a musculotopic organization of motor neurones within the nuclei that corresponds to the structural and functional divisions of tongue musculature. Thus, motor neurones innervating tongue retrusor muscles are located in dorsal and dorsolateral nuclei, whereas motor neurones innervating the main tongue protrusor muscle are located in ventral and ventromedial regions of the nucleus. Although relatively little is known about the organization of motor neurones innervating the intrinsic muscles of the tongue, experimental evidence suggests that motor neurones of the medial division of the hypoglossal nucleus innervate tongue muscles that are oriented in planes transverse to the long axis of the tongue (transverse and vertical intrinsics and genioglossus), whereas motor neurones of the lateral division innervate tongue muscles that are oriented parallel to this axis (styloglossus, hyoglossus, superior and inferior longitudinal).

Several smaller groups of cells lie near the hypoglossal nucleus. They are perhaps misnamed the 'perihypoglossal complex' or 'perihypoglossal grey,' for none is known with certainty to be connected to the hypoglossal nerve or nucleus. They include the nucleus intercalatus, sublingual nucleus, nucleus prepositus hypoglossi and nucleus paramedianus dorsalis (reticularis). Gustatory and visceral connections are attributed to the nucleus intercalatus.

Hypoglossal fibres emerge ventrally from their nucleus, traverse the reticular formation lateral to the medial lemniscus, pass medial to (or sometimes through) the inferior olivary nucleus and curve laterally to emerge superficially as a linear series of 10 to 15 rootlets in the ventrolateral sulcus between the pyramid and olive (see Fig. 10.3).

The hypoglossal nucleus receives corticonuclear fibres from the precentral gyrus and adjacent areas of mainly the contralateral hemisphere. They synapse either directly on motor neurones of the nucleus or on interneurones. Evidence indicates that the most medial hypoglossal subnuclei receive projections from both hemispheres. The nucleus may connect with the cerebellum via adjacent perihypoglossal nuclei and perhaps with the medullary reticular formation, trigeminal sensory nuclei and solitary nucleus.

Inferior Olivary Nucleus

The olivary nuclear complex consists of the large inferior olivary nucleus and the much smaller medial and dorsal accessory olivary nuclei. They are the so-called precerebellar nuclei, a group that also includes the pontine, arcuate, vestibular, reticulocerebellar and spinocerebellar nuclei, all of which receive afferents from specific sources and project to the cerebellum. The inferior olivary nucleus contains small neurones, most of which form the olivocerebellar tract, which emerges either from the hilum or through the adjacent wall to run medially and intersect the medial lemniscus (see Fig. 10.9). Its fibres cross the midline and sweep either dorsal to or through the opposite olivary nucleus. They intersect the lateral spinothalamic and rubrospinal tracts and the spinal trigeminal nucleus and enter the contralateral inferior cerebellar peduncle, where they constitute its major component. Fibres from the contralateral inferior olivary complex terminate on Purkinje cells in the cerebellum as climbing fibres; there is a one-to-one relationship between Purkinje cells and neurones in the complex. Afferent connections to the inferior olivary nucleus are both ascending and descending. Ascending fibres, mainly crossed, arrive from all spinal levels in the spino-olivary tracts and via the dorsal columns. Descending ipsilateral fibres come from the cerebral cortex, thalamus, red nucleus and central grey of the midbrain. In part, the two latter projections make up the central tegmental tract (fasciculus) that forms the olivary amiculum.

The medial accessory olivary nucleus is a curved grey lamina that is concave laterally and located between the medial lemniscus and pyramid and the ventromedial aspect of the inferior olivary nucleus. The dorsal accessory olivary nucleus is a similar lamina dorsomedial to the inferior olivary nucleus. Both nuclei are connected to the cerebellum. The accessory nuclei are phylogenetically older than the inferior and are connected with the palaeocerebellum. In all connections—cerebral, spinal and cerebellar—the olivary nuclei sometimes display very specific somatotopy, particularly in their cerebellar connections, which are described in detail in Chapter 13.

Nucleus Solitarius

The nucleus solitarius (solitary nucleus, nucleus of the solitary tract) lies ventrolateral to the vagal nucleus and is almost coextensive with it. A neuronal group ventrolateral to the nucleus solitarius has been termed the nucleus parasolitarius. The nucleus solitarius is intimately related to, and receives fibres from, the tractus solitarius, which carries afferent fibres from the facial, glossopharyngeal and vagus nerves. These fibres enter the tract in descending order and convey gustatory information from the lingual and palatal mucosa. They may also convey visceral impulses from the pharynx (glossopharyngeal and vagus) and from the oesophagus and abdominal alimentary canal (vagus). There is some overlap in this vertical representation.

Termination of special visceral gustatory afferents within the nucleus shows a viscerotopic pattern, predominantly in the rostral region. Experimental evidence suggests that fibres from the anterior two-thirds of the tongue and the roof of the oral cavity (which travel via the chorda tympani and greater petrosal branches of the facial nerve) terminate in the extreme rostral part of the solitary complex. Those from the circumvallate and foliate papillae of the posterior third of the tongue, tonsils, palate and pharynx (which travel via the lingual branch of the glossopharyngeal nerve) are distributed throughout the rostrocaudal extent of the nucleus, predominantly rostral to the obex. Gustatory afferents from the larynx and epiglottis (which travel via the superior laryngeal branch of the vagus) have a more caudal and lateral distribution. The nucleus solitarius may also receive fibres from the spinal cord, cerebral cortex and cerebellum.

Medial and commissural subnuclei in the caudal part of the nucleus appear to be the primary site of termination for gastrointestinal afferents. Ventral and interstitial subnuclei probably receive tracheal, laryngeal and pulmonary afferents and play an important role in respiratory control and possibly rhythm generation. The carotid sinus and aortic body nerves terminate in the dorsal and dorsolateral region of the nucleus solitarius, which may be involved in cardiovascular regulation.

The nucleus solitarius is thought to project to the sensory thalamus with a relay to the cerebral cortex. It may also project to the upper levels of the spinal cord through a solitariospinal tract. Secondary gustatory axons cross the midline. Many subsequently ascend the brain stem in the dorsomedial part of the medial lemniscus and synapse on the most medial neurones of the thalamic nucleus ventralis posterior medialis (in a region sometimes termed the accessory arcuate nucleus). Axons from the nucleus ventralis posterior medialis radiate through the internal capsule to the anteroinferior area of the sensorimotor cortex and the insula. It is thought that other ascending paths end in a number of hypothalamic nuclei and thus mediate the route by which gustatory information reaches the limbic system, allowing appropriate autonomic reactions.

Swallowing and Gag Reflexes — During the normal processes of eating and drinking, passage of material to the rear of the mouth stimulates branches of the glossopharyngeal nerve in the oropharynx (Fig. 10.15). This information is relayed via the nucleus solitarius to the nucleus ambiguus, which contains the motor neurones innervating the muscles of the palate, pharynx and larynx. The nasopharynx is closed off from the oropharynx by elevation of the soft palate. The larynx is raised, its entrance narrows and the glottis is closed. Peristaltic activity down the oesophagus to the stomach is mediated through the pharyngeal plexus.

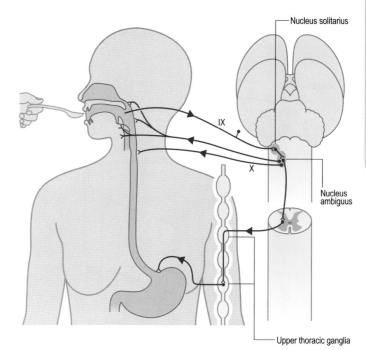

Fig. 10.15 *Swallowing and gag reflexes. (Redrawn from MacKinnon, P., Morris, J. (Eds.), 1990. Oxford Textbook of Functional Anatomy, vol 3, Head and Neck. Oxford University Press, Oxford. By permission of Oxford University Press.)*

If stimulation of the oropharynx occurs other than during swallowing, the gag reflex may be initiated. There is a reflex contraction of the muscles of the pharynx, soft palate and fauces that, if extreme, may result in retching and vomiting.

Nucleus Ambiguus

The nucleus ambiguus is a group of large motor neurones situated deep in the medullary reticular formation. It extends rostrally as far as the upper end of the vagal nucleus; caudally, it is continuous with the nucleus of the spinal accessory nerve. Fibres emerging from it pass dorsomedially, then curve laterally. Rostral fibres join the glossopharyngeal nerve. Caudal fibres join the vagus and cranial accessory nerves and are distributed to the pharyngeal constrictors, intrinsic laryngeal muscles and striated muscles of the palate and upper oesophagus.

The nucleus ambiguus contains several cellular subgroups, and some topographical representation of the muscles innervated has been established. Individual laryngeal muscles are innervated by relatively discrete groups of cells in more caudal zones. Neurones that innervate the pharynx lie in the intermediate area, and neurones that innervate the oesophagus and soft palate are rostral.

The nucleus ambiguus is connected to corticonuclear tracts bilaterally and to many brain stem centres. At its upper end, a small retrofacial nucleus intervenes between it and the facial nucleus. Although the nucleus ambiguus lies in line with the special visceral efferent nuclei, it is a reputed source of general visceral efferent vagal fibres.

Cough and Sneeze Reflexes — Irritation of the larynx or trachea is conveyed via laryngeal branches of the vagus nerve to the trigeminal sensory nucleus of the brain stem. Impulses are relayed to medullary respiratory centres and to the nucleus ambiguus. More or less energetic exhalation (coughing) occurs, caused by the contraction of intercostal and abdominal wall muscles after a buildup of pressure against a closed glottis.

A similar mechanism underlies sneezing (Fig. 10.16), except that the stimulus arises from the nasal mucosa, and afferent impulses are conveyed by the ophthalmic or maxillary divisions of the trigeminal nerve to the trigeminal sensory nucleus. After sharp inhalation, explosive exhalation occurs, with closure of the oropharyngeal isthmus by action of the palatoglossus, which diverts air through the nasal cavity and expels the irritant.

PONS

External Features and Relations

The pons lies rostral to the medulla and caudal to the midbrain. Ventrally, the site of transition with the medulla is demarcated superficially by a transverse sulcus. Laterally, in a region known as the cerebellopontine angle (see Figs 10.2, 10.3), the facial, vestibulocochlear and glossopharyngeal roots and the nervus intermedius all lie on the choroid plexus of the fourth ventricle (which

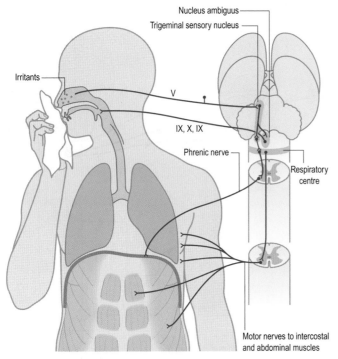

Fig. 10.16 *Sneeze and cough reflexes. (Redrawn from MacKinnon, P., Morris, J. (Eds.), 1990. Oxford Textbook of Functional Anatomy, vol 3, Head and Neck. Oxford University Press, Oxford. By permission of Oxford University Press.)*

protrudes from the foramen of Luschka into the subarachnoid space). The ventral surface of the pons (see Fig. 10.3) is separated from the clivus (basisphenoid and dorsum sellae) by the cisterna pontis. It is markedly convex transversely and less so vertically; it grooves the petrous part of the temporal bone laterally up to the internal acoustic meatus. The surface has a shallow vertical median sulcus in which the basilar artery runs, bounded bilaterally by prominences that are formed partly by underlying corticospinal fibres as they descend through the pons. Bundles of transverse fibres, bridging the midline and originating from nuclei in the basal pons (nuclei pontis), converge on each side into the large middle cerebellar peduncle and project to the cerebellum. The trigeminal nerve emerges near the mid-pontine level. It has a small superomedial motor root and a large inferolateral sensory root.

The dorsal surface of the pons is hidden by the cerebellum, which covers the rostral half of the rhomboid fossa, into which the aqueduct of the midbrain empties. The roof of the fossa is formed by a thin sheet of tissue, the superior medullary velum, and is overlain by the lingula of the vermis of the cerebellum. The velum is attached on each side to the superior cerebellar peduncles and is enclosed by pia mater above and ependyma below (see Fig. 5.11). The abducens nerves decussate in the velum.

Internal Structure
Transverse Sections of the Pons
Transverse sections (see Figs 10.12, 10.14) reveal that the pons consists of a dorsal tegmentum, which is a continuation of the medulla (excluding the pyramids), and a ventral (basilar) part. The latter contains bundles of longitudinal descending fibres, some of which continue into the pyramids; others end in the many pontine or medullary nuclei. It also contains numerous transverse fibres and scattered pontine nuclei.

Ventral Pons
The ventral pons is similar in structure at all levels. The longitudinal fibres of the corticopontine, corticonuclear and corticospinal tracts descend from the crus cerebri of the midbrain and enter the pons compactly. They rapidly disperse into fascicles, which are separated by the pontine nuclei and transverse pontine fibres. Corticospinal fibres run through the pons to the medullary pyramids, where they again converge into compact tracts. They are accompanied by corticonuclear fibres, some of which diverge to contralateral (and some ipsilateral) nuclei of cranial nerves and other nuclei in the pontine tegmentum, while others reach the pyramids. Clinical evidence supports the view that the facial and other nuclei receive ipsilateral corticonuclear fibres.

Corticopontine fibres from the frontal, temporal, parietal and occipital cortices end in the pontine nuclei (see Fig. 10.14). Axons from the latter constitute the transverse pontine (pontocerebellar) fibres, which, after

decussation, continue as the contralateral middle cerebellar peduncle. Frontopontine axons end in the pontine nuclei above the level of the emerging trigeminal roots and are relayed to the contralateral cerebellum in the upper transverse pontine fibres. All pontocerebellar fibres end as mossy fibres in the cerebellar cortex, and a degree of somatotopy is maintained in these connections.

The precerebellar pontine nuclei include all the neurones scattered in the ventral pons. In humans, there are some 20 million pontine neurones. They are probably all glutamatergic, and most project to the cerebellar cortex, with some input to the deep cerebellar nuclei. Corticopontine fibres arise mainly from neurones in layer V of the premotor, somatosensory, posterior parietal, extrastriate visual and cingulate neocortices. Projections from prefrontal, temporal and striate cortices are sparse. The terminal fields, although divergent, form topographically segmented patterns resembling overlapping columns, slabs or lamellae within the pons. Subcortical projections to the pontine nuclei include those from the superior colliculus to the dorsolateral pons, and from the medial mammillary nucleus to the rostromedial pons and pretectal nuclei. The lateral geniculate nucleus, dorsal column nuclei, trigeminal nuclei, hypothalamus and intracerebellar nuclei also project to restricted neurones of the pons. Functionally related subcortical and cerebrocortical afferents converge, for example, those from the somatosensory cortex, dorsal column nuclei and medial mammillary nucleus. There is also non-specific input from the reticular formation, raphe nuclei, locus coeruleus and paraqueductal grey matter.

Pontine Tegmentum
The pontine tegmentum varies in cytoarchitecture at different levels. A transverse section through the lower pontine tegmentum transects the facial colliculi (Figs 10.14, 10.20). Each colliculus contains the motor nucleus of the abducens nerve and the geniculum of the facial nerve. More deeply placed are the facial nuclei, the nearby vestibular and cochlear nuclei and other isolated neuronal groups. The medial vestibular nucleus continues from the medulla slightly into the pontine tegmentum and is separated from the inferior cerebellar peduncle by the lateral vestibular nucleus.

The vestibular nuclei are laterally placed in the rhomboid fossa of the fourth ventricle, subjacent to the vestibular area, which spans the rostral medulla and caudal pons (see Fig. 10.1). They consist of medial, lateral (Deiters' nucleus), superior and inferior vestibular groups. They all receive fibres from the vestibulocochlear nerve and send axons to the cerebellum, medial longitudinal fasciculus, spinal cord and lateral lemniscus. Evidence suggests that the vestibular apparatus is spatially represented in the nuclei. The medial vestibular nucleus broadens, then narrows, as it ascends from the upper olivary level into the lower pons, where it separates the vagal nucleus from the floor of the fourth ventricle. It is crossed by the striae medullares nearer the floor. Below, it is continuous with the nucleus intercalatus. The inferior vestibular nucleus (which is the smallest) lies between the medial vestibular nucleus and inferior cerebellar peduncle from the level of the upper end of the nucleus gracilis to the pontomedullary junction. It is crossed by descending fibres of the vestibulocochlear nerve and the vestibulospinal tract. The lateral vestibular nucleus lies just above the inferior nucleus and ascends almost to the level of the abducens nucleus. It is composed of large multipolar neurones, which are the main source of the vestibulospinal tract. The superior vestibular nucleus is small and lies above the medial and lateral nuclei.

Vestibular fibres of the vestibulocochlear nerve enter the medulla between the inferior cerebellar peduncle and the trigeminal spinal tract and approach the vestibular area, where they bifurcate into descending and ascending branches. The former descend medial to the inferior cerebellar peduncle and end in medial, lateral and inferior vestibular nuclei, and the latter enter the superior and medial nuclei. A few vestibular fibres enter the cerebellum directly through the inferior peduncle (superficially in the juxtarestiform body) and end in the fastigial nucleus, flocculonodular lobe and uvula. Vestibular nuclei project extensively to the cerebellum and also receive axons from the cerebellar cortex and the fastigial nuclei. Their uncrossed spinal projections run in the vestibulospinal tracts. Vestibular axons also reach the spinal cord in the medial longitudinal fasciculus (see Figs 8.42, 10.26). Some reach cerebral levels, possibly for bilateral cortical representation. The vestibular nuclear complex projects to the pontine reticular nuclei and to motor nuclei of the ocular muscles in the medial longitudinal fasciculus.

Fibres of the cochlear division of the vestibulocochlear nerve partially encircle the inferior cerebellar peduncle laterally and end in the dorsal and ventral cochlear nuclei. The dorsal cochlear nucleus forms a bulge, the auditory tubercle, on the posterior surface of the peduncle and is continuous medially with the vestibular area in the rhomboid fossa. The ventral cochlear nucleus is ventrolateral to the dorsal cochlear nucleus and lies between the cochlear and vestibular fibres of the vestibulocochlear nerve.

CASE 3   WALLENBERG'S SYNDROME

A 60-year-old retired teacher with known hypertension and diabetes presents with the acute onset of difficulty walking, along with incoordination of his left arm and leg. He has noticed that a soda can does not feel cold in his left hand, and the beverage does not feel cold in the right side of his mouth. He also complains of nausea and hiccups and of a change in his speech.

On examination, he has a mild left eyelid ptosis and impaired elevation of the soft palate on the left. His speech is nasal, and the left pupil fails to dilate in the dark. Cranial nerve functions are otherwise intact. Motor power is normal throughout, as is reflex activity; the plantar responses are flexor. Sensory testing shows reduced pain and temperature sensations on his left face and throughout his right arm and leg; proprioception is normal. He has incoordination and ataxia with finger–nose–finger and heel–shin testing on the left.

MRI shows an infarct in the left lateral medullary tegmentum (Fig. 10.17).

Discussion: Lateral medullary (or Wallenberg's) syndrome is due to infarction in the distribution of the posterior inferior cerebellar artery. This vessel arises from the vertebral artery and supplies the tegmentum of the lateral medulla (the so-called lateral medullary plate) and the inferior cerebellum. Symptoms of lateral medullary syndrome include ipsilateral facial sensory loss due to involvement of the descending spinal trigeminal nucleus and tract; ispsilateral ataxia, reflecting the lesion in the inferior cerebellar peduncle (restiform body); contralateral pain and temperature loss due to involvement of the lateral spinothalamic tract; and Horner's syndrome due to involvement of the descending sympathetic tracts in the tegmentum. Patients may also have vertigo and nystagmus, indicating that the vestibular complex is affected, and hoarseness due to involvement of the vagal nerve nucleus. There is no motor involvement because the descending corticospinal tracts lie medial and inferior to this vascular supply.

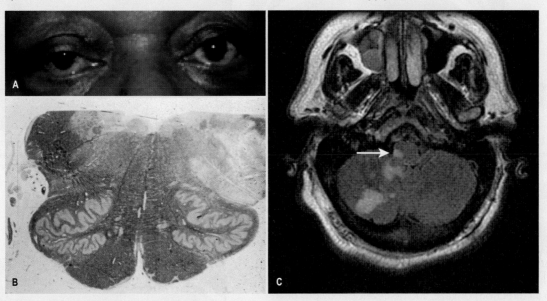

Fig. 10.17 *Wallenberg's syndrome.* **A,** *Typical changes in Horner's syndrome (ptosis, miosis) as part of Wallenberg's syndrome.* **B,** *Section through medulla shows an infarction of the lateral medullary plate.* **C,** *MRI demonstrates infarction in the lateral medullary plate (arrow) in the distribution of the posterior inferior cerebellar artery. Infarction is also noted in the ipsilateral cerebellum. (© 2010 Thomas Jefferson University. All rights reserved. Reproduced with the permission of Thomas Jefferson University.)*

The striae medullares of the fourth ventricle (see Figs 5.11, 10.13) are an aberrant cerebropontocerebellar connection in which the arcuate nuclei and external arcuate fibres are involved. Axons from arcuate nuclei spread around the medulla, above and below the inferior olive, where they are superficially visible as the circumolivary fasciculus. All these fibres, which are known collectively as the external arcuate fibres, enter the inferior cerebellar peduncle (see Fig. 10.8). Some fibres from arcuate nuclei pass dorsally through the medulla near its midline, decussate near the floor of the fourth ventricle, then turn laterally under the ependyma and enter the cerebellum through the inferior peduncle.

In addition to the tracts already noted at lower levels, the lower pontine tegmentum contains the trapezoid body, lateral lemniscus and emerging fibres of the abducens and facial nerves. The medial lemniscus is ventral, its transverse outline now a flat oval. It extends laterally from the median raphe (see Figs 10.12, 10.14) and is laterally related to the lateral spinothalamic tract and trigeminal lemniscus. The fibres of the latter originate from neurones of the contralateral spinal nucleus, serving pain and thermal sensibility in facial skin and mucosa of the conjunctiva, tongue, mouth, and nose. Here the lemnisci form a transverse band composed of, in lateral order from the midline, the medial and trigeminal lemnisci, the lateral spinothalamic tract and the lateral lemniscus.

The trapezoid body contains cochlear fibres, mainly from the ventral cochlear and trapezoid nuclei. They ascend transversely in the ventral

tegmentum, pass either through or ventral to the vertical medial lemniscal fibres and decussate with the contralateral fibres in the median raphe. Below the emerging facial axons, the trapezoid fibres turn up into the lateral lemniscus. As the lateral lemniscus ascends, it lies near the dorsolateral surface of the brain stem. Above, its fibres enter the inferior colliculus and medial geniculate body. The ascending auditory pathway is described in detail in Chapter 12.

The medial longitudinal fasciculus is paramedian, ventral to the fourth ventricle and near the abducens nucleus, from which it is separated by facial nerve fibres. It is the main intersegmental tract in the brain stem, particularly for interactions between nuclei of cranial nerves innervating the extraocular muscles and the vestibular system (see Fig. 10.26). In the lower pons it receives fibres from vestibular and perhaps dorsal trapezoid nuclei. Its greater part is formed by vestibulocochlear contributions.

A transverse section at an upper pontine tegmental level contains trigeminal elements (see Fig. 10.12) but otherwise shows little notable alteration from a section through a lower pontine tegmental level. Its dorsolateral parts are invaded by the superior cerebellar peduncles. The small lateral lemniscal nucleus is medial to its tract in the upper pons and receives some lemniscal terminals. Some of its efferent fibres enter the medial longitudinal fasciculus; others return to the lemniscus. The lateral lemniscal nucleus is a relay station in the auditory pathway associated with the trapezoid nucleus.

CASE 4 CENTRAL PONTINE MYELINOLYSIS

A 58-year-old poorly nourished chronic alcoholic is found to have severe hyponatremia when brought to the emergency room. The sodium deficit is corrected vigorously, but within a day or two of admission, he experiences a rapidly progressive motor deficit, with flaccid paralysis of all limbs and inability to speak or swallow, along with a facial diplegia. Ocular motility is preserved, and although he is unable to speak, he can communicate by eye-blinking responses.

Discussion: This patient exhibits a so-called locked-in syndrome, reflecting the development of central pontine myelinolysis (also called osmotic demyelination syndrome), with extensive demyelination of the mid and upper basis pontis. Paralysis of the limbs with bulbar palsy is due to an extensive symmetrically placed lesion in the basis pontis, with involvement of the descending corticobulbar and corticospinal fibres. The pontine tegmentum is usually preserved; there is little if any significant impairment of consciousness. Rapid shifts in serum osmolarity due to overvigorous correction of hyponatremia is generally believed to be the cause of this disorder. In some patients, extrapontine lesions may appear. See Figure 10.18.

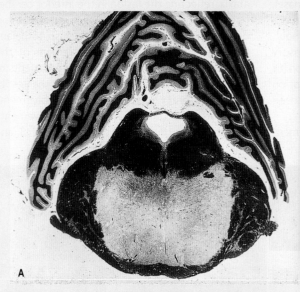 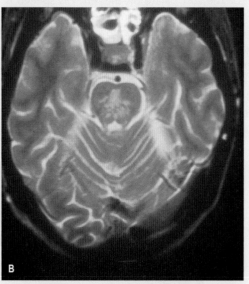

Fig. 10.18 *Central pontine myelinolysis.* **A,** *Myelin sheath stain demonstrates marked symmetric demyelination in the basis pontis.* **B,** *MRI demonstrates demyelination in the basis pontis. (A, From Adams, R.D., Victor, M., Mancall, E.L., 1959. Central pontine myelinolysis: a hitherto undescribed disease occurring in alcoholic and malnourished patients. AMA Arch. Neurol. Psychiatry. 1959; 81(2): 154–172. Copyright © 1959 American Medical Association. All rights reserved.)*

CASE 5 BRAIN STEM GLIOMA

A 12-year-old boy complains to his parents of seeing double, especially when looking to the side. Diplopia is subsequently noted in all directions of gaze, and he develops obvious bilateral but somewhat asymmetric abducens palsies. Drooling with facial weakness, numbness over the right side of the face and incoordination of his limbs are noted, and he becomes increasingly unsteady on his feet. At times he experiences frontal headaches. Examination demonstrates multiple cranial nerve palsies, along with ataxia of gait and of the arms; later in the clinical course, bilateral hyperreflexia and spasticity appear in the legs.

Discussion: This subacutely evolving syndrome is most suggestive of a brain stem (pontine) glioma, a slow-growing brain stem tumor that, by virtue of its infiltrating growth characteristics, presents initially with segmental brain stem signs such as ocular palsies. Long tract signs and increased intracranial pressure due to hydrocephalus appear late in the course. See Figure 10.19.

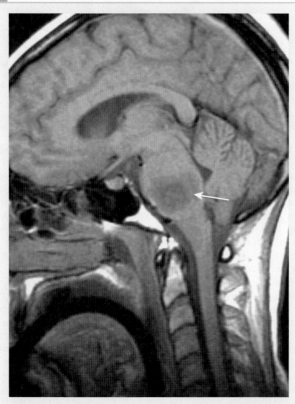

Fig. 10.19 *Pontine glioma. Swollen appearance of the pons is evident on MRI (arrow). (© 2010 Thomas Jefferson University. All rights reserved. Reproduced with the permission of Thomas Jefferson University.)*

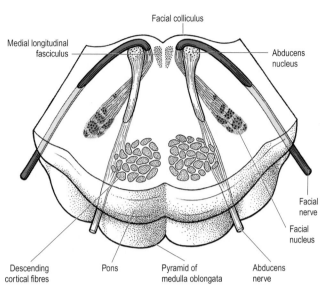

Fig. 10.20 *Central course of fibres of the facial nerve in a transverse section of the pons, viewed from the rostral aspect.*

Labels: Facial colliculus; Medial longitudinal fasciculus; Abducens nucleus; Facial nerve; Facial nucleus; Abducens nerve; Descending cortical fibres; Pons; Pyramid of medulla oblongata

The medial lemniscus (see Figs 10.12, 8.32) retains its paramedian position in the ventral pontine tegmentum, where it lies a little lateral to the median raphe and is joined medially by fibres from the principal trigeminal sensory nucleus. The trigeminal lemniscus, lateral spinothalamic tract and lateral lemniscus and its nucleus all lie dorsolaterally.

CASE 6 MILLARD–GUBLER AND FOVILLE'S SYNDROMES

A 49-year-old woman with a long history of cigarette smoking develops acute left-sided neck pain. One day later she notes double vision when looking to the left and suddenly becomes paralysed on the right side. On examination, she has a left abducens palsy, left peripheral facial paralysis and right hemiparesis. MRI demonstrates an infarct in the ventral paramedian pons.

Discussion: Millard–Gubler syndrome is a result of a paramedian pontine lesion affecting the facial nerve (cranial nerve VII) and abducens nerve (cranial nerve VI) in the mid-pontine tegmentum. This results in complete ipsilateral facial paralysis involving the forehead and lower face and loss of abduction of the eye. There is an associated contralateral hemiparesis due to involvement of the ipsilateral corticospinal tract.

Similar to Millard–Gubler syndrome is Foville's syndrome, caused by a lesion in the caudal pons affecting the pontine tegmentum. In addition to the contralateral hemiparesis and ipsilateral cranial nerve palsies of Millard–Gubler syndrome, there is inability of the contralateral eye to cross the midline medially due to injury to the paramedian pontine reticular formation. This results in complete loss of lateral (horizontal) gaze toward the side of the lesion—a key feature distinguishing the two clinical syndromes.

Cochlear Nuclei — Cochlear nerve fibres, which are derived from neuronal somata in the spiral ganglion, bifurcate on entering the brain stem and terminate in both dorsal and ventral cochlear nuclei.

The ventral cochlear nucleus has a complex cytoarchitecture. It contains many neuronal types with distinct dendritic field characteristics. Marked topographical order has been demonstrated in cochlear nerve terminals

within the nucleus. Different parts of the spiral ganglion and different stimulation frequencies are related to neurones that are serially arrayed anteroinferiorly in the ventral nucleus. All cochlear nerve fibres enter the nucleus. There are approximately 25,000 axons in the human cochlear nerve, and they project onto a much larger number of neurones in the cochlear nucleus. The number of cochlear fibres in the lateral lemniscus greatly exceeds that in the cochlear nerve. A minor fraction of the cochlear neurones receive terminals from the nerve, although each fibre may connect with several neurones. Terminals are limited to the anteroinferior region of the ventral nucleus, where the neurones are probably mostly local interneurones.

The dorsal cochlear nucleus is almost continuous with the ventral nucleus, from which it is separated only by a thin stratum of nerve fibres. Giant cells predominate, and their dendritic fields are aligned with the incoming auditory fibres.

Although the cellular origins are not precisely known, axons of most neuronal types in the cochlear nuclei leave to end at pontine levels in the superior olivary, trapezoid and lateral lemniscal nuclei (see Fig. 10.12). They leave the cochlear nuclei by three routes. The largest group of axons lies ventrally and decussates as the trapezoid body, level with the pontomedullary junction (see Figs 10.12, 10.14). Most of these axons ascend slightly, decussate and relay in the contralateral nuclei. A few do not cross and synapse in the ipsilateral superior olivary nuclei. From both nuclei, the next-order axons ascend in the corresponding lateral lemniscus. Occasional decussating fibres traverse the contralateral superior olive and enter the lateral lemniscus to relay in lemniscal nuclei.

Some axons from ventral cochlear neurones pass dorsally, superficial to descending trigeminal spinal fibres, cerebellar fibres in the inferior peduncle and axons of the dorsal cochlear nucleus. This bundle of ventral cochlear fibres is smaller than that of the trapezoid decussation. It swerves ventromedially across the midline, ventral to the medial longitudinal fasciculus, as the intermediate acoustic striae. Its further path is uncertain, but it probably ascends in the contralateral lateral lemniscus.

The most dorsally placed axons issue from the dorsal cochlear nucleus. They curve dorsomedially around the inferior cerebellar peduncle toward the midline as the dorsal acoustic striae, ventral to the striae medullares. They incline ventromedially and cross the midline to ascend in the contralateral lateral lemniscus, probably relaying in its nuclei.

The superior olivary complex is sited in the tegmentum of the caudal pons, lateral in the reticular formation at the level of the pontomedullary junction. The superior complex includes several named nuclei and nameless smaller groups. In humans, the lateral superior olivary nucleus is made up of some six small cellular clusters. The medial (accessory) superior olivary nucleus is large and compact. The trapezoid nucleus is medial. A retro-olivary group, the reputed origin of some efferent cochlear fibres, is dorsal. Some internuclear connections have been described. The medial superior olivary nucleus receives impulses from both spiral organs and may be involved in auditory sound source localization. The superior olivary complexes and the trapezoid nuclei are relay stations in the ascending auditory projection. These intricate connections have not been well established in humans.

The medial nucleus of the trapezoid body is small in humans. It has a ventral component, which consists of large neurones scattered among the trapezoid fascicles, and a more compact dorsal nucleus, medial to the superior olivary complex. The nucleus lies at the level of the exiting abducens nerve roots, anterior to the central tegmental tract. It is not known whether the human trapezoid nuclei function in the auditory relay. Some trapezoid axons may enter the medial longitudinal fasciculus and ascend to end in trigeminal, facial, oculomotor, trochlear and abducens nuclei, where they mediate reflexes involving tensor tympani, stapedius and oculogyric muscles, respectively.

The nucleus of the lateral lemniscus consists of small groups of neurones that lie among the fibres of the lateral lemniscus. Dorsal, ventral and intermediate groups probably receive afferent axons from both cochlear nuclei. Their efferents enter the midbrain along the lateral lemniscus and terminate in the inferior colliculi (see Fig. 10.4). Total neuronal counts of 18,000 to 24,000 have been recorded in human lemniscal nuclei.

Efferent cochlear axons travel in the cochlear nerves to the spiral organ. Although few in number, they may be involved in hearing, perhaps by modulating sensory transduction through reflexes via cochlear nuclei. The neurones of origin are located at the hilus and along the lateral border of the lateral superior olivary nucleus and lateral edge of the ventral trapezoid nucleus. Fibres from both sides proceed to both cochleae.

Vestibular Nuclei — The vestibular nuclear complex contains medial, lateral, inferior and superior nuclei. The medial vestibular nucleus is the largest subdivision and extends up from the medulla oblongata into the pons. It lies under the vestibular area of the floor of the fourth ventricle and is crossed dorsally by the striae medullares. The inferior vestibular nucleus is lateral to the medial nucleus and extends to a lower medullary level. It lies between the medial nucleus and the inferior cerebellar peduncle. Descending branches of afferent vestibular fibres end among its cells. The lateral nucleus is ventro-lateral to the upper part of the medial nucleus and is characterized by its large neurones. Its rostral end is continuous with the caudal end of the superior nucleus, which extends higher into the pons than other subdivisions and occupies the upper part of the vestibular area.

All vestibular nuclei receive fibres from the vestibulocochlear nerve and also from the spinal cord and the reticular formation. Vestibulocerebellar fibres from the nuclei travel via the inferior cerebellar peduncle mainly to the flocculus and nodule. Some afferent fibres bypass the nuclei and reach the flocculus and nodule directly via the inferior cerebellar peduncle. Cerebellovestibular fibres pass to the nuclei in the inferior cerebellar peduncle. They arise mainly in the flocculus and nodule (posterior lobe), but some fibres are derived from the anterior lobe and fastigial nucleus (see Case 3).

In summary, the vestibular nuclear complex is a relay station on an afferent cerebellar path and a distributing station for vestibulocerebellar fibres. Fibres from vestibular nuclei also enter the medial longitudinal fasciculus (see Fig. 10.26) and ascend or descend to motor nuclei of the oculogyric and nuchal muscles. It is suggested that excitatory and inhibitory projections exist, mediating complex and subtle integration between vestibular signals and eye movements. From the vestibular nuclei, and from the lateral nucleus in particular, fibres descend in the ventral funiculus of the spinal cord as the vestibulospinal tracts. Information from the vestibular nuclei also reaches the cerebral cortex by way of the thalamus (probably via posterior parts of the ventroposterior complex and the medial pulvinar). The primary vestibular cortical area is located in the parietal lobe at the junction between the intraparietal and postcentral sulci, which is adjacent to that portion of the postcentral gyrus where the head is represented. This makes sense functionally, because this region of the somatosensory cortex is concerned with conscious appreciation of body position. There may be an additional representation of the vestibular system in the superior temporal gyrus near the auditory cortex. Through its connections, the vestibular system influences movements of the eyes, head and muscles of the trunk and limbs to maintain equilibrium.

Abducens Nucleus — The abducens nucleus occupies a paramedian position in the central grey matter, in line with the trochlear, oculomotor and hypoglossal nuclei, with which it forms a somatic motor column (see Fig. 10.1). It lies ventromedial to the medial longitudinal fasciculus, which is the means by which vestibular, cochlear and other cranial nerve nuclei, especially the oculomotor, connect with the abducens. The abducens nucleus contains large motor neurones and small multipolar interneurones, which are intermixed, although the latter are most heavily concentrated in its lateral and ventral aspects. Axons from the motor neurones cross the midline at the level of the nucleus and ascend in the medial longitudinal fasciculus to all three medial rectus subnuclei of the oculomotor nucleus. The total number of neurones in the nucleus is approximately 6500.

Efferent abducens axons pass ventrally; descend through the reticular formation, trapezoid body and medial lemniscus; and traverse the ventral pons to emerge at its inferior border (see Fig. 10.20 and Case 6).

The abducens nucleus receives afferent connections from corticonuclear fibres, which are principally contralateral (some of the fibres being aberrant corticospinal fibres that descend from the midbrain to this level in the medial lemniscus); the medial longitudinal fasciculus, by which it is connected to oculomotor, trochlear and vestibular nuclei; the tectobulbar tract from the deep layers of the superior colliculus; the paramedian pontine reticular formation, which lies rostral and caudal to the nucleus; the nucleus prepositus hypoglossi; and the contralateral medullary reticular formation.

Facial nucleus — The facial (motor) nucleus lies in the caudal pontine reticular formation, posterior to the dorsal trapezoid nucleus and ventromedial to the trigeminal spinal tract and nucleus. Groups of facial neurones form columns that innervate individual muscles or correspond to branches of the facial nerve. Neurones innervating muscles in the scalp and upper face are dorsal, and those supplying the lower facial musculature are ventral.

Efferent fibres of the large motor neurones of the facial nucleus form the motor root of the facial nerve. The motor nucleus represents the branchial efferent column, but it lies much more deeply in the pons than might be expected, and its axons have an unusual course (see Fig. 10.20). At first they incline dorsomedially toward the fourth ventricle, below the abducens nucleus, and ascend medial to it, near the medial longitudinal fasciculus. They then curve around the upper pole of the abducens nucleus and descend ventrolaterally through the reticular formation. Finally, they pass between their own nucleus medially and the spinal trigeminal nucleus. They emerge between the olive and the inferior cerebellar peduncle at the cerebellopontine angle (see Fig. 10.3).

The facial nucleus receives corticobulbar fibres for volitional control. Neurones that innervate muscles in the scalp and upper face are believed to receive bilateral corticobulbar fibres, whereas those supplying lower facial

musculature receive only a contralateral innervation. Clinically, upper and lower motor neurone lesions of the facial nerve can be differentiated: the former results in paralysis confined to the contralateral lower face, and the latter results in complete ipsilateral paralysis (Bell's palsy; see Ch. 11, Case 9).

The facial nucleus also receives ipsilateral rubroreticular tract fibres and afferents from its own sensory root (via the nucleus solitarius) and from the spinal trigeminal nucleus. These infracortical afferents complete local reflex loops.

Some efferent fibres of the facial nerve originate from neurones in the superior salivatory nucleus, which is thought to be in the reticular formation dorsolateral to the caudal end of the motor nucleus. These preganglionic parasympathetic neurones belong to the general visceral efferent column. They send fibres into the sensory root of the facial nerve. These travel via the chorda tympani to the submandibular ganglion and via the greater petrosal nerve and the nerve of the pterygoid canal to the pterygopalatine ganglion.

Corneal Reflex — Touching the cornea or shining a bright light into the eye elicits reflex closure of the eye. The former action stimulates nasociliary branches of the ophthalmic nerve, and the latter stimulates the retina and optic pathway. In both cases, afferent impulses enter the central nervous system and spread via interneurones to activate neurones in the facial motor nucleus in the pons (Fig. 10.21). The efferent impulses pass along the facial nerve to activate the palpebral component of orbicularis oculi, which contracts, producing a 'blink.' The sweep of the eyelids carries lacrimal secretions across the eye, which helps remove any irritating particles.

Trigeminal Sensory Nucleus — On entering the pons, the fibres of the sensory root of the trigeminal nerve run dorsomedially toward the principal sensory nucleus (see Fig. 10.12). About 50% of the fibres divide into ascending and descending branches; the others ascend or descend without division. The descending fibres form the spinal tract of the trigeminal, which terminates in the subjacent spinal nucleus of the trigeminal nerve. The spinal nucleus was described in detail earlier.

Some ascending trigeminal fibres, many of them heavily myelinated, synapse around the small neurones in the principal sensory nucleus (Fig. 10.22), which lies lateral to the motor nucleus and medial to the middle cerebellar peduncle and is continuous inferiorly with the spinal nucleus. The principal nucleus is thought to be concerned mainly with tactile stimuli.

Other ascending fibres enter the mesencephalic nucleus, a column of unipolar cells whose peripheral branches may convey proprioceptive impulses from the masticatory muscles and possibly from the teeth and the facial and oculogyric muscles. Its neurones are unique, in that they are the only primary sensory neurones with somata in the central nervous system. It is the relay for the jaw-jerk reflex, which is the only supraspinal monosynaptic reflex. Nerve fibres that ascend to the mesencephalic nucleus may give collaterals to the motor nucleus of the trigeminal nerve and to the cerebellum.

Most fibres that arise in the trigeminal sensory nuclei cross the midline and ascend in the trigeminal lemniscus. They end in the contralateral thalamic nucleus ventralis posterior medialis, from which third-order neurones project to the cortical postcentral gyrus (areas 1, 2 and 3). Some trigeminal nucleus efferents ascend to the nucleus ventralis posterior medialis of the ipsilateral thalamus.

Jaw-Jerk Reflex — Rapid stretching of the muscles that close the jaw (masseter, temporalis, medial pterygoid) activates muscle spindle afferents, which travel via the mandibular division of the trigeminal nerve to the brain stem (Fig. 10.23). The cell bodies of these primary afferent neurones are located in the mesencephalic nucleus of the trigeminal. Collaterals project monosynaptically to the motor nucleus of the trigeminal nerve in the pons. From there, motor axons of the mandibular nerve innervate the muscles that close the

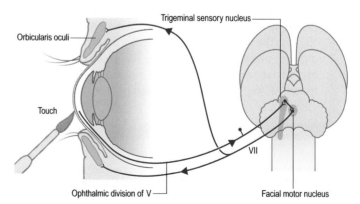

Fig. 10.21 *Corneal reflex. (Redrawn from MacKinnon, P., Morris, J. (Eds.), 1990. Oxford Textbook of Functional Anatomy, vol 3, Head and Neck. Oxford University Press, Oxford. By permission of Oxford University Press.)*

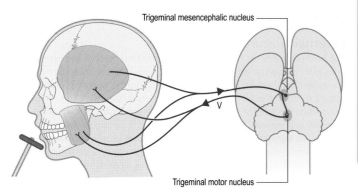

Fig. 10.23 *Jaw-jerk reflex. (Redrawn from MacKinnon, P., Morris, J. (Eds.), 1990. Oxford Textbook of Functional Anatomy, vol 3, Head and Neck. Oxford University Press, Oxford. By permission of Oxford University Press.)*

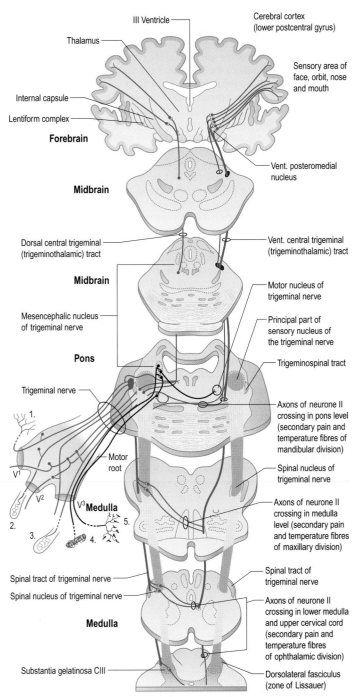

Fig. 10.22 *Trigeminal nerve and its central connections.*

jaw. Clinically, an exaggerated jaw jerk is noted with bilateral lesions in the upper brain stem.

Trigeminal Motor Nucleus — The trigeminal motor nucleus is ovoid in outline and lies in the upper pontine tegmentum, under the lateral part of the floor of the fourth ventricle (see Fig. 10.1). It lies medial to the principal sensory nucleus and is separated from it by fibres of the trigeminal nerve. It occupies the position of the branchial (special visceral) efferent column.

The motor nucleus contains characteristic large multipolar neurones interspersed with smaller multipolar cells. The neurones are organized into a number of relatively discrete subnuclei, the axons from which innervate individual muscles. It receives fibres from both corticobulbar tracts. These fibres leave the tracts at the nuclear level or higher in the pons (aberrant corticospinal fibres) and descend in the medial lemniscus. They may end on motor neurones or interneurones. The motor nucleus receives afferents from the sensory nuclei of the trigeminal nerve, possibly including some from the mesencephalic nucleus; these form monosynaptic reflex arcs for proprioceptive control of the masticatory muscles. It also receives afferents from the reticular formation, red nucleus, tectum and medial longitudinal fasciculus, and possibly from the locus coeruleus. Collectively, these represent pathways by which salivary secretion and mastication may be coordinated.

Tensor Tympani and Stapedius Reflex — Loud sound elicits reflex contraction of tensor tympani and stapedius, which attenuates movement of the tympanic membrane and middle ear ossicles. Afferent impulses travel in the cochlear nerve to the cochlear nuclei in the brain stem. Efferent fibres to tensor tympani arise in the trigeminal motor nucleus and travel in the mandibular division of the trigeminal nerve. Efferent fibres to stapedius originate in the facial nucleus and travel in the facial nerve.

Salivary Nucleus — The salivary (salivatory) nucleus is near the upper pole of the vagal nucleus, just above the pontomedullary junction and near the inferior pole of the facial nucleus. It is customarily divided into superior and inferior salivary nuclei, which send preganglionic parasympathetic fibres into the facial and glossopharyngeal nerves for control of the salivary and lacrimal glands.

CASE 7   OCULAR BOBBING

A 78-year-old man falls to the floor while in the bathroom and is unresponsive to his wife's attempts to arouse him. He has a history of hypertension for 15 years and a myocardial infarction followed by coronary artery bypass surgery 4 years ago.

On arrival in the emergency room he is comatose. The pupils are 1 mm and reactive to light under magnification. Oculocephalic ('doll's eye') and vestibulo-ocular ('cold water caloric') reflexes are absent. There are intermittent spontaneous, conjugate, rapid downward movements of the eyes, followed by a slow return to mid position. There are no spontaneous movements of the extremities. Tendon reflexes are reduced throughout; there are bilateral extensor plantar responses. Computed tomography demonstrates a large intrapontine haematoma.

Discussion: This combination of neurological and neuro-ophthalmologic findings points to a pontine lesion. The spontaneous eye movement is referred to as ocular bobbing. Various spontaneous eye movements can be noted in comatose patients, including ocular dipping, reverse ocular bobbing and reverse ocular dipping. Of all these movements, ocular bobbing is the most reliable for localization. It is a classic sign of intrinsic pontine lesions, most commonly haemorrhage, as in this man. However, it has been reported in other settings, such as expanding cerebellar lesions compressing the pons.

Ocular bobbing is a reflection of the fact that pathways that mediate upward and downward eye movements differ anatomically. Large pontine lesions affect the paramedian pontine reticular formation and related structures responsible for horizontal gaze but ordinarily spare pathways responsible for vertical eye movements, which are largely localized to the rostral midbrain.

MIDBRAIN

External Features and Relations

The midbrain traverses the hiatus in the tentorium cerebelli and connects the pons and cerebellum with the forebrain. It is the shortest brain stem segment, no more than 2 cm long, and most of it lies in the posterior cranial fossa. Lateral to it are the parahippocampal gyri, which hide the sides of the midbrain when the inferior surface of the brain is examined. Its long axis inclines ventrally as it ascends. For descriptive purposes, it can be divided into a dorsal tectum and right and left cerebral peduncles, each of which is further divided into a ventral crus cerebri and a dorsal tegmentum by a pigmented lamina, the substantia nigra. The two crura are separate, whereas the tegmental parts are united and traversed by the cerebral aqueduct that connects the third and fourth ventricles. The tectum lies dorsal to an oblique coronal plane that includes the aqueduct and consists of the pretectal area and the corpora quadrigemina (the paired superior and inferior colliculi).

The crura cerebri are superficially corrugated and emerge from the cerebral hemispheres. They converge as they descend and meet as they enter the pons, where they form the caudolateral boundaries of the interpeduncular fossa (Figs 10.24, 10.25). At the level of the tentorial incisure, the basilar artery divides in the interpeduncular fossa into the right and left posterior cerebral arteries. The superior cerebellar arteries branch from the basilar artery immediately distal to this bifurcation. The posterior cerebral and superior cerebellar arteries both run laterally around the ventral (basilar) crural surfaces. The former passes above the tentorium cerebelli, the latter below it. The oculomotor and trochlear nerves lie between the two arteries. The roots of the oculomotor nerve emerge from a medial sulcus on each crus (see Figs 10.3, 10.24, 10.25). The posterior communicating artery joins the posterior cerebral artery on the medial surface of the peduncle in the interpeduncular fossa. The median caudal part of the interpeduncular fossa is a greyish area called the posterior perforated substance, which is pierced by central branches of the posterior cerebral arteries. The optic tract winds dorsolaterally around the crus near the crural entry into the hemispheres. Its lateral surface adjoins the parahippocampal gyrus and is crossed by the trochlear nerve (see Figs 5.11, 10.4). It bears a longitudinal lateral sulcus in which fibres of the lateral lemniscus reach and form a surface elevation. The latter inclines rostrodorsally; part joins the inferior colliculus, while the rest continues into the inferior quadrigeminal brachium.

The colliculi or corpora quadrigemina are two paired eminences (see Figs 5.11, 10.4). They lie rostral to the superior medullary velum, inferior to the pineal gland and caudal to the posterior commissure, the whole sloping ventrally as it ascends. Below the splenium of the corpus callosum, they are partly overlapped on each side by the pulvinar of the dorsal thalamus. The superior and inferior colliculi are separated by a cruciform sulcus. The upper limit of the sulcus expands into a depression for the pineal gland, and a median frenulum veli is prolonged from its caudal end down over the superior medullary velum. The trochlear nerves emerge lateral to the frenulum. They pass ventrally over the lateral aspects of the cerebral peduncles and traverse the interpeduncular cistern to the petrosal end of the cavernous sinus. The superior colliculi, larger and darker than the inferior, are stations for visual responses. The inferior colliculi, smaller but more prominent, are associated with auditory paths. The difference in colour is attributed to the presence of superficial layers of neurones in the superior colliculi.

A brachium ascends ventrolaterally from the lateral aspect of each colliculus (see Figs 5.11, 10.4). The brachium of the superior colliculus (superior quadrigeminal brachium) passes below the pulvinar, partly overlapping the medial geniculate body, and continues partly into the lateral geniculate body and partly into the optic tract. It conveys fibres from the retina and optic radiation to the superior colliculus. The brachium of the inferior colliculus (inferior quadrigeminal brachium) ascends ventrally. It conveys fibres from the lateral lemniscus and inferior colliculus to the medial geniculate body.

Internal Structure
Transverse Sections of the Midbrain

In transverse section, the cerebral peduncles are composed of dorsal and ventral regions separated by the substantia nigra (see Figs 10.24, 10.25). On each side, the dorsal region is the tegmentum and the ventral part is the crus cerebri. The tegmenti are continuous across the midline, but the crura are separated.

Crus Cerebri

Each crus cerebri is semilunar in section. It contains corticospinal, corticonuclear and corticopontine fibres. Corticonuclear and corticospinal fibres occupy the middle two-thirds of the crura and descend via the pons and medulla. Corticonuclear fibres end in the nuclei of the cranial nerves and other

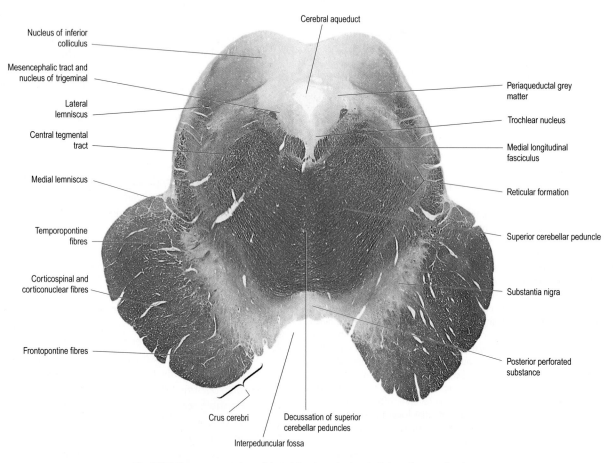

Fig. 10.24 *Transverse section of the midbrain at the level of the inferior colliculi.*

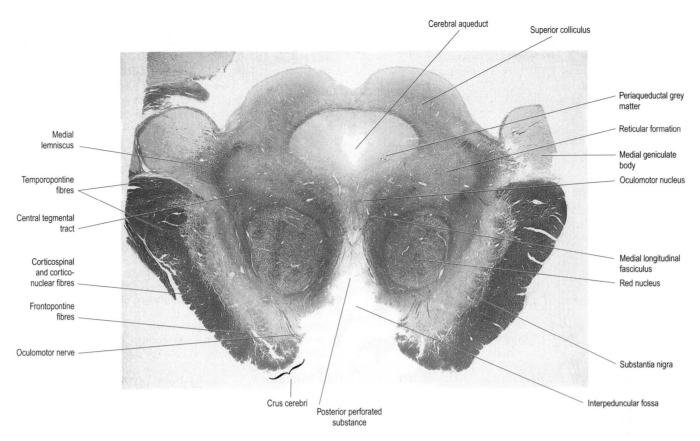

Fig. 10.25 *Transverse section of the midbrain at the level of the superior colliculi.*

brain stem nuclei, whereas corticospinal fibres continue into the medullary pyramid (see Fig. 8.41). Corticopontine fibres arise in the cerebral cortex and form two groups, both of which end in the pontine nuclei. The frontopontine fibres from the frontal lobe, principally areas 6 and 4, traverse the internal capsule and then occupy the medial sixth of the ipsilateral crus cerebri. The temporopontine fibres, which are largely from the posterior region of the temporal lobe, traverse the internal capsule but occupy the lateral sixth of the ipsilateral crus. Parietopontine and occipitopontine fibres are also described in the crus, lying medial to the temporopontine fibres. There are few fibres from the primary sensory cortex in corticopontine projections.

Mesencephalic Tegmentum

The mesencephalic tegmentum is directly continuous with the pontine tegmentum and contains the same tracts. At inferior collicular levels, grey matter is restricted to scattered collections of neurones in the reticular formation and the tectum near the cerebral aqueduct. The trochlear nucleus is in the ventral grey matter near the midline, in a position corresponding to the abducens and hypoglossal nuclei at other levels. It extends through the lower half of the midbrain, just caudal to the oculomotor nucleus and immediately dorsal to the medial longitudinal fasciculus.

The trigeminal mesencephalic nucleus occupies a lateral position in the central grey matter. It ascends from the upper pole of the main trigeminal sensory nucleus in the pons to the level of the superior colliculus in the midbrain and is accompanied by a tract of both peripheral and central branches from its axons. Its large ovoid neurones are unipolar, like those in peripheral sensory ganglia. They are arranged in many small groups that extend as curved laminae on the lateral margins of the periaqueductal grey matter. Neurones are most numerous in its lower level.

Apart from these nuclei, the mesencephalic tegmentum contains many other scattered neurones, most of which are included in the reticular formation.

The white matter contains all the tracts mentioned in the pontine tegmentum. The decussation of the superior cerebellar peduncles is particularly prominent. Fibres enter the tegmentum and pass ventromedially around the central grey matter to the median raphe, where most cross in the decussation of the superior cerebellar peduncles and then separate into ascending and descending fascicles. Some ascending fibres either end in or give collaterals to the red nucleus, which they encapsulate and penetrate. Many other fibres ascend to the nucleus ventralis lateralis of the thalamus. Some uncrossed fibres are believed to end in the periaqueductal grey matter and reticular formation, interstitial nucleus and posterior commissural nucleus (nucleus of

Darkshevich). The latter nucleus may send efferent fibres to the medial longitudinal fasciculus and posterior commissure. Descending fascicles end in the pontine and medullary reticular formation, the olivary complex and, possibly, cranial motor nuclei.

The medial longitudinal fasciculus adjoins the somatic efferent column, dorsal to the decussating superior cerebellar peduncles (Fig. 10.26). The medial, trigeminal, lateral and spinal lemnisci form a curved band dorsolateral to the substantia nigra. Fibres in the medial, spinal and trigeminal lemnisci continue a rostral course to synapse with neurones in the lateral and medial ventral posterior nuclei of the thalamus, respectively (see Figs 8.33, 10.22). Some fibres of the lateral lemniscus end in the nucleus of the inferior colliculus, encapsulating it and synapsing with its neurones. The remaining fibres (direct lemniscal) join inferior colliculus–derived fibres and enter the inferior quadrigeminal brachium, which starts at this level and carries the fibres to the medial geniculate body. Some fibres to the inferior colliculus are collaterals of direct lemniscal fibres.

Superiorly, level with the superior colliculus, the tegmentum contains the red nucleus, which extends into the subthalamic region. The ventromedial central grey matter around the aqueduct contains the oculomotor nucleus, which is elongated and is related ventrolaterally to the medial longitudinal fasciculus and caudally reaches the trochlear nucleus. The oculomotor nucleus is divisible into neuronal groups that are partially correlated with the motor distribution of the oculomotor nerve. A group of preganglionic parasympathetic neurones, the accessory oculomotor (Edinger–Westphal) nucleus, which controls the activity of smooth muscle within the eyeball (for pupillary constriction), lies dorsal to the oculomotor nucleus (Ch. 12).

Substantia Nigra

The substantia nigra is a lamina of many multipolar neurones that extends through the whole midbrain, from the medial to the lateral crural sulcus and from the pons to the subthalamic region. It is connected massively with the basal ganglia but has other projections.

The substantia nigra is semilunar in transverse section, concave dorsally and thicker medially, where it is traversed by oculomotor axons as they stream ventrally to their point of exit in the interpeduncular fossa. Extensions from its convex ventral surface pass between fibres of the crus cerebri. The substantia nigra is subdivided into a dorsal pars compacta and a ventral pars reticulata (reticularis), and the cells of these two parts have different connections. The pars compacta consists of many darkly pigmented neurones that contain neuromelanin granules. Their arrangement is irregular, and they partially penetrate the subjacent pars reticulata. The pigmentation is easily

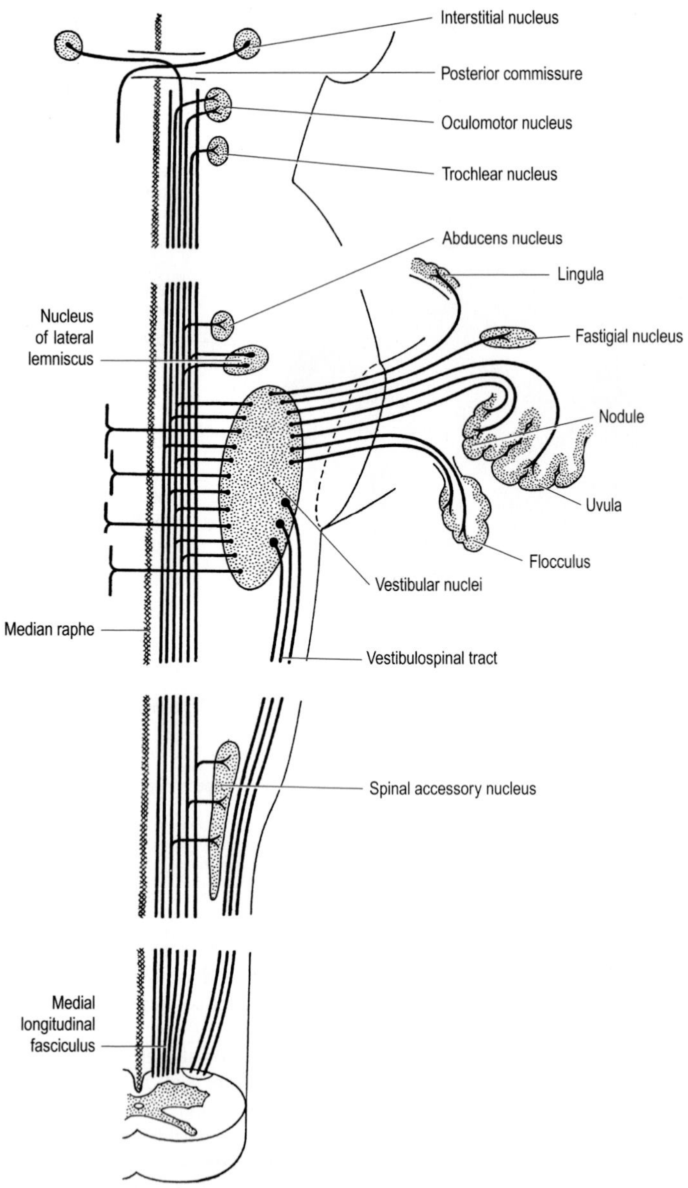
Interstitial nucleus
Posterior commissure
Oculomotor nucleus
Trochlear nucleus
Abducens nucleus
Lingula
Nucleus of lateral lemniscus
Fastigial nucleus
Nodule
Uvula
Flocculus
Vestibular nuclei
Median raphe
Vestibulospinal tract
Spinal accessory nucleus
Medial longitudinal fasciculus

Fig. 10.26 *Some of the fibre components of the medial longitudinal fasciculus.*

visible in transverse or coronal sections and is related to the aminergic status of the neurones (see Figs 10.24, 10.25). Pigmentation increases with age; it is most abundant in primates, maximal in humans, and is present even in albinos. The pigmented pars compacta neurones synthesize dopamine as their neurotransmitter and project to the corpus striatum of the basal ganglia and other sites.

The pars compacta of the substantia nigra corresponds to the dopaminergic cell group A9 (see Fig. 14.10). Two other dopaminergic cell groups are found in the ventral tegmentum: cell group A10 in the rostromedial region, which constitutes the ventral tegmental area (of Tsai), and cell group A8 in the dorsolateral reticular area, which forms the nucleus parabrachialis pigmentosus. The whole ventral tegmental system of dopaminergic neurones appears to act as an integrative centre for adaptive behaviour. It projects via a number of pathways, mainly through ipsilateral fibres in the medial forebrain bundle. These pathways are a mesodiencephalic system, which terminates in thalamic and hypothalamic nuclei; a mesostriatal projection; a mesolimbic (mesorhombic) pathway to the nucleus accumbens, olfactory tubercle, lateral septum, interstitial nucleus of the stria terminalis, amygdala and entorhinal cortex; and mesocortical fibres to most cortical areas, particularly the prefrontal, orbitofrontal and cingulate cortex.

The pars compacta projects heavily to the caudate nucleus and putamen in a topographically organized fashion (nigrostriatal fibres). Lesser projections end in the globus pallidus and subthalamic nucleus. In Parkinson's disease, the levels of dopamine in the substantia nigra and striatum decrease dramatically as a result of the degeneration of pars compacta neurones (see Ch. 14, Case 5).

The ventral pars reticulata of the substantia nigra contains clusters of neurones, most of which are GABAergic, that intermingle with fibres of the crus cerebri. The pars reticulata extends rostrally as far as the subthalamic region and is considered to be homologous with the medial segment of the globus pallidus, which it resembles structurally. The neurones in both contain high levels of iron.

There are reciprocal connections between the substantia nigra and the basal ganglia. Efferent fibres from the basal ganglia end largely, but by no means exclusively, in the pars reticulata. Topographically organized striatonigral fibres originate from the caudate nucleus and putamen and project to the pars reticulata. The head of the caudate nucleus projects to the rostral third of the substantia nigra, while the putamen projects to all parts. The fibres end in axodendritic synapses. A small number of GABAergic pallidonigral fibres from the lateral segment of the globus pallidus end mostly in the pars reticulata. The subthalamic nucleus sends an important glutamatergic projection to the pars reticulata and to the globus pallidus. Subthalamonigral and subthalamopallidal projections are important in the pathophysiology of movement disorders such as Parkinson's disease and dyskinesias.

GABAergic neurones in the pars reticulata project through a nigrothalamic tract to the ventral anterior and dorsomedial thalamic nuclei, and through a nigrotegmental tract to the pedunculopontine nucleus and reticular formation, where impulses are relayed to spinal ventral column neurones. A pars lateralis of the substantia nigra is small but recognizable in humans. It projects to the ipsilateral superior colliculus, which may control saccadic eye movements.

Corticonigral fibres arise from precentral and probably postcentral gyri. A few terminate on neurones in the pars reticulata, but many more are fibres of passage to the red nucleus and reticular formation.

Red Nucleus

The red nucleus is an ovoid mass approximately 5 mm in diameter, with a pink tinge, dorsomedial to the substantia nigra (see Fig. 10.25). The tint appears only in fresh material and is caused by a ferric iron pigment in its multipolar neurones. The latter are of varying size. Their proportions and arrangements vary among species; for example, in primates, the magnocellular element is decreased, and there is a reciprocal increase in the size of the parvocellular component. Small multipolar neurones occur in all parts of the nucleus. In humans, the larger neurones are restricted to the caudal part of the nucleus and have been estimated to be as few as 200 in number. The magnocellular element is considered phylogenetically old, which accords with the parvocellular predominance in primates. Rostrally, the red nucleus is poorly demarcated, and it blends into the reticular formation and caudal pole of the interstitial nucleus. It is traversed and surrounded by fascicles of nerve fibres, including many from the oculomotor nucleus.

Principal afferent connections of the red nucleus travel via corticorubral and cerebellorubral fibres. Uncrossed corticorubral fibres originate from primary somatomotor and somatosensory areas. In animals, the red nucleus receives fibres from the contralateral nucleus interpositus (which corresponds to the human globose and emboliform nuclei) and dentate nucleus, via the superior cerebellar peduncle. It has bilateral, probably reciprocal connections with the superior colliculi. In humans, the rubrospinal tract is small and originates from the caudal magnocellular part of the red nucleus. Few fibres reach the cervical cord. The fibres decussate and then run obliquely laterally in the ventral tegmental decussation, ventral to the tectospinal decussation and dorsal to the medial lemniscus. On reaching the grey matter ventral to the inferior cerebellar peduncle, the tract turns caudally to enter the lateral part of the lateral lemniscus. It continues descending ventral to the tract and nucleus of the trigeminal nerve throughout the medulla and enters the upper part of the cervical cord, intermingled with fibres of the lateral corticospinal tract (Ch. 8). Some efferent axons form a rubrobulbar tract to motor nuclei of the trigeminal, facial, oculomotor, trochlear and abducens nerves.

The largest group of efferents from the red nucleus in humans is found in the massive uncrossed central tegmental tract (fasciculus), which lies in the ventral part of the midbrain. Initially it lies lateral to the medial longitudinal fasciculus and dorsolateral to both the red nucleus and the decussation of the superior cerebellar peduncles (see Figs 10.12–10.14, 10.24). Most fibres arise from the parvocellular part of the red nucleus and join the tract as it traverses the nucleus on its way to the ipsilateral inferior olivary nucleus in the medulla. Some tract fibres terminate in the brain stem reticular nuclei. Ascending and descending axons from the brain stem reticular formation run in the central tegmental tract. Their collaterals and terminals innervate other 'reticular' or adjacent 'specific' nuclei. These axons include dorsal and ventral ascending noradrenergic bundles, a ventral ascending serotoninergic bundle and some fibres of dorsal and ventral ascending cholinergic bundles.

Lesions of the corticospinal system in humans result in permanent paresis. In monkeys, although the paralysis is initially complete, it eventually disappears, and a good recovery ensues. The explanation for this interprimate variability in recovery from corticospinal lesions could lie in the differential capacity of the rubrospinal system to compensate for the loss of corticospinal drive. Monkeys never fully recover from combined lesions of both the corticospinal and rubrospinal tracts, which suggests that the two systems are functionally interrelated in the control of movement. Both encode force, velocity and direction parameters, but the rubrospinal system primarily directs activity both during the terminal phase of a movement and preceding a movement. There is thus overlap of activity in the two systems for all parameters during the movements of limbs and even of individual digits. The corticospinal system is most active during the learning of new movements, whereas the rubrospinal system is most active during the execution of learned automated movements.

The rubro-olivary projection, which travels in the central tegmental tract, connects the red nucleus directly to the contralateral cerebellar cortex and indirectly to the ipsilateral motor cortex, which is where both the corticospinal and central tegmental tracts originate. The cerebellum is thought to play a role in motor learning, so the rubro-olivary system could switch the control of movements from the corticospinal to the rubrospinal system for programmed automation. The relative absence of a rubrospinal system in humans could explain the poor recovery of motor function after stroke.

Oculomotor Nucleus

The nuclear complex from which the efferent fibres of the oculomotor nerve arise consists of several groups of large motor neurones and smaller preganglionic parasympathetic neurones. On each side, the large-celled motor neurone groups innervate, in dorsoventral order, the ipsilateral inferior rectus, inferior oblique and medial rectus. There is also a medially placed column, almost in the long axis of the midbrain, that innervates the contralateral superior rectus. The axons from this nucleus decussate in its caudal part. The medial rectus subnucleus consists of three anatomically distinct subpopulations. The ventral portion, which contains the largest number of motor neurones, occupies the rostral two-thirds. A subpopulation of smaller-diameter motor neurones lies dorsally throughout the rostral two-thirds of the nucleus and innervates the small orbital fibres of the medial rectus. They are thought to be involved in vergence movements. Another subpopulation lies dorsolaterally in the caudal two-thirds of the nucleus.

A median nucleus of large neurones, the caudal central nucleus, lies at the caudal pole of the oculomotor nucleus adjacent to the superior rectus and medial rectus subnuclei. In experimental primates, approximately 30% of the motor neurones in this subnucleus innervate levator palpebrae superioris bilaterally, which is a unique condition among all paired skeletal muscles.

The Edinger–Westphal nucleus lies dorsal to the main oculomotor nucleus. It is composed of small multipolar, preganglionic parasympathetic neurones, which give rise to axons that travel in the oculomotor nerve and relay in the ciliary ganglion.

Separate fascicles from these subnuclei course forward in the midbrain and emerge on the surface of the brain stem in the interpeduncular fossa. The fascicles are probably arranged from medial to lateral, subserving the pupil, inferior rectus, medial rectus, levator palpebrae superioris, superior rectus and inferior oblique. The human oculomotor nerve contains approximately 15,000 axons.

Afferent inputs to the oculomotor nuclear complex include fibres from the rostral interstitial nucleus of the medial longitudinal fasciculus and the interstitial nucleus of Cajal, both of which are involved in the control of vertical and torsional gaze; the nuclei of the posterior commissure, both directly and via the interstitial nucleus of Cajal, and, via these nuclei, the frontal eye fields, superior colliculus, dentate nucleus and other cortical areas; the medial longitudinal fasciculus (including fibres from the trochlear, abducens and vestibular nuclei); the medial and lateral vestibular nuclei to the medial rectus subnucleus; the superior colliculus; and the nucleus prepositus hypoglossi, primarily to the medial rectus subnucleus.

Afferent inputs to the Edinger–Westphal nucleus come from the pretectal nuclei (primarily the pretectal olivary nucleus) bilaterally and mediate the pupillary light reflex. Afferents also come from the visual cortex, mediating accommodation. Efferent fibres relay through the ciliary ganglion in the orbit.

The oculomotor nucleus also contains neurones connected with other nuclei concerned with ocular motor function. In particular, reciprocal connections exist between the oculomotor and abducens nuclei, both ipsilateral and contralateral. These internuclear connections are predictable, based on the results of experimental stimulation of or damage to the medial longitudinal fasciculus and clinicopathological data derived from cases of internuclear ophthalmoplegia.

Trochlear Nucleus

The trochlear nucleus lies in the grey matter in the floor of the cerebral aqueduct, level with the upper part of the inferior colliculus (see Figs 10.1, 10.24). It is in line with the ventromedial part of the oculomotor nucleus, in

CASE 8   NUCLEAR THIRD NERVE PALSY

A 68-year-old man experiences the sudden onset of double vision and unsteadiness. He is found to have atrial fibrillation, with no prior history of cardiac arrhythmia, and is admitted to the hospital and started on intravenous heparin.

Evaluation demonstrates that the right eye is slightly exodeviated and immobile, with the exception of intact abduction. The right pupil is midriatic, and there is right lid ptosis. The left eye is normal, with the exception of paralysis of up-gaze and ptosis.

MRI of the brain with diffusion images demonstrates an acute infarct in the right paramedian midbrain tegmentum and in both cerebellar hemispheres.

Discussion: Isolated lesions of the oculomotor nerve nucleus are rare. In this patient, localization of the lesion to the right oculomotor nerve nucleus is supported by the findings in the left eye; innervation of each superior rectus muscle, unlike all other oculomotor nerve–innervated muscles, is crossed, with axons to the superior rectus passing through the contralateral superior rectus subnucleus. Hence a lesion affecting the right ipsilateral subnucleus results in bilateral up-gaze paresis. Bilateral ptosis is explained by involvement of the caudal central subnucleus that supplies axons to both levator palpebrae muscles.

the position of the somatic efferent column. The medial longitudinal fasciculus is ventral and lateral to it. The oculomotor and trochlear nuclei often overlap slightly but can be distinguished by the smaller size of the trochlear neurones.

The afferent inputs to the trochlear nucleus are similar to those described for the oculomotor nucleus.

Trochlear efferent fibres pass laterodorsally around the central grey matter, then descend medial to the trigeminal mesencephalic nucleus to reach the upper end of the superior medullary velum, where they decussate and emerge lateral to the frenulum. A few fibres remain ipsilateral.

Medial Longitudinal Fasciculus

The medial longitudinal fasciculus (see Fig. 10.26) is a heavily myelinated composite tract lying near the midline, ventral to the periaqueductal grey matter. It ascends to the interstitial nucleus (of Cajal), which lies in the lateral wall of the third ventricle, just above the cerebral aqueduct. The fasciculus retains its position relative to the central grey matter through the midbrain, pons and upper medulla, but it is displaced ventrally by successive decussations of the medial lemnisci and lateral corticospinal tracts. At spinal levels, it is synonymous with the medial vestibulospinal tract.

The medial longitudinal fasciculus interconnects the oculomotor, trochlear, abducens, Edinger–Westphal, vestibular, reticular and spinal accessory nuclei, coordinating conjugate eye movements and associated movements of the head and neck. Lesions cause internuclear ophthalmoplegia. All four vestibular nuclei contribute ascending fibres. Those from the superior nucleus remain uncrossed, while the others are partly crossed. Some fibres reach the interstitial and posterior commissural nuclei, and some decussate to the contralateral nuclei. Descending axons, from the medial vestibular nuclei and perhaps the lateral and inferior nuclei, partially decussate and descend in the fasciculus as the medial vestibulospinal tract (see Fig. 8.42). Fibres join from the dorsal trapezoid, lateral lemniscal and posterior commissural nuclei, which means that both the cochlear and vestibular components of the vestibulocochlear nerve may influence movements of the eyes and head via the medial longitudinal fasciculus. Some vestibular fibres may ascend in the medial longitudinal fasciculus as far as the thalamus (see Ch. 12, Case 6).

Tectum

Inferior Colliculus — The inferior colliculus (see Fig. 10.24) has a central, ovoid main nucleus that is continuous with the periaqueductal grey matter. It is surrounded by a lamina of nerve fibres, many from the lateral lemniscus, which terminate in it. The central nucleus has dorsomedial and ventrolateral zones, which are covered by a dorsal cortex. In humans, the cortex has four cytoarchitectonic layers: layer I contains small neurones with flattened radial dendritic fields; layer II, medium-sized neurones with ovoid dendritic fields aligned parallel with the collicular surface; layer III, medium-sized neurones with spherical dendritic fields; and layer IV, large neurones with variably shaped dendritic fields. The central nucleus is laminated. Bands of cells with disc-shaped or stellate dendritic fields orthogonally span the fibre layers in which the terminals of lateral lemniscal fibres ramify. The neurones are sharply tuned to frequency, and the laminae may represent the structural basis of tonal discrimination. Experimental studies have found cells driven by low frequencies in the dorsal laminae, and others driven by high frequencies in the ventral laminae. Neurones are broadly frequency tuned in the dorsal cortex and lateral nucleus.

Most efferent fibres travel via the inferior brachium to the ipsilateral medial geniculate body. Lemniscal fibres relay only in the central nucleus, and some pass without relay to the medial geniculate body. In humans, the ventral division of the medial geniculate body receives a topographical projection from the central nucleus, and the dorsal division receives a similar projection from the dorsal cortex. Some colliculogeniculate fibres do not relay in the geniculate body but continue, with those that do, via the auditory radiation to the auditory cortex area. A descending projection from the auditory cortex reaches the inferior colliculus via the medial geniculate body. Some fibres may traverse this projection without relay. This descending path may produce effects at levels from the medial geniculate body downward, and it probably links with efferent cochlear fibres through the superior olivary and cochlear nuclei.

Inferior collicular projections to the brain stem and spinal cord appear to traverse the superior colliculi before they descend. In this way they connect with the origins of the tectospinal and tectotegmental tracts. These projections are relatively small and probably mediate reflex turning of the head and eyes in response to sounds.

In experimental animals, lesions of either the inferior colliculus or its brachium produce defects in tonal discrimination, sound localization and auditory reflexes. The effects of such lesions are poorly documented in humans.

The inferior colliculus is part of the ascending auditory pathway, which is described in more detail later.

Superior Colliculus — The superior colliculi are laminated structures. At successive depths from the external surface, each superior colliculus can be divided into a stratum zonale, cinereum, opticum and lemnisci. The stratum lemnisci can be subdivided into the stratum griseum medium, album medium, griseum profundum and album profundum. These seven layers have also been termed zonal, superficial grey, optic, intermediate grey, deep grey, deep white and periventricular strata. The two schemes are not in complete accord, but in general, layers can be considered to be composed alternately of neuronal somata or their processes. The zonal layer consists chiefly of myelinated and non-myelinated fibres from the occipital cortex (areas 17, 18 and 19), which arrive as the external corticotectal tract. It also contains a few small neurones that are horizontally arrayed. The superficial grey layer (stratum cinereum) forms a crescentic lamina over the deeper layers and contains many small multipolar interneurones, on which cortical fibres synapse. The optic layer consists partly of fibres from the optic tract. As they terminate, they permeate the entire anterior–posterior extent of the superficial layers with numerous collateral branches. This arrangement provides a retinotopic map of the contralateral visual field, in which the fovea is represented anterolaterally. Retinal axons terminate in clusters from specific retinotectal neurones and as collaterals of retinogeniculate fibres. The layer also contains some large multipolar neurones. Efferent fibres to the retina are said to start in this layer.

The intermediate grey and white layers collectively constitute the main reception zone. The main afferent input is the medial corticotectal path from layer V neurones of the ipsilateral occipital cortex (area 18) and from other neocortical areas concerned with ocular following movements. Afferent fibres are also received from the contralateral spinal cord (via spinotectal and spinothalamic routes), inferior colliculus, locus coeruleus and raphe nuclei (from noradrenergic and serotoninergic neurones). The deep grey and deep white layers adjacent to the periaqueductal grey matter are collectively called the parabigeminal nucleus. They contain neurones whose dendrites extend into the optic layer, and their axons form many of the collicular efferents.

The superior colliculus receives afferents from many sources, including the retina, spinal cord, inferior colliculus and occipital and temporal cortices. The first three of these pathways convey visual, tactile and probably thermal, pain and auditory impulses. Collicular efferents pass to the retina; lateral geniculate nucleus; pretectum; parabigeminal nucleus; inferior, medial and lateral pulvinar; and numerous sites in the brain stem and spinal cord. Fibres passing from the pulvinar are relayed to primary and secondary visual cortices and

form an extrageniculate retinocortical pathway for visual orientation and attention.

The tectospinal and tectobulbar tracts start from neurones in the superior colliculi. They sweep ventrally around the central grey matter to decussate ventral to the oculomotor nuclei and medial longitudinal fasciculi as part of the dorsal tegmental decussations. The tectospinal tract descends ventral to the medial longitudinal fasciculus as far as the medial lemniscal decussation in the medulla, where it diverges ventrolaterally to reach the spinal ventral white column near the ventral lip of the vental median fissure. Tectospinal fibres descend to cervical segments. The tectobulbar tract, mainly crossed, descends near the tectospinal tract and ends in the pontine nuclei and motor nuclei of the cranial nerves, particularly those innervating the oculogyric muscles. It subserves reflex ocular movements. Other tectotegmental fibres reach various tegmental reticular nuclei in the ipsilateral mesencephalic and contralateral pontomedullary reticular formation (gigantocellular reticular, caudal pontine reticular, oral pontine reticular nuclei), substantia nigra and red nucleus. Tectopontine fibres, which probably descend with the tectospinal tract, terminate in dorsolateral pontine nuclei, with a relay to the cerebellum. A tecto-olivary projection, from deeper collicular laminae to the upper third of the medial accessory olivary nucleus, exists in primates; it is crossed and links with the posterior vermis.

In animals, central collicular stimulation produces contralateral head movement as well as movements involving the eyes, trunk and limbs, which implicates the superior colliculus in complex integrations between vision and widespread body activity.

Pretectal Nucleus — The pretectal nucleus is a poorly defined mass of neurones at the junction of the mesencephalon and diencephalon. It extends from a position dorsolateral to the posterior commissure, caudally toward the superior colliculus, with which it is partly continuous. It receives fibres from the visual cortex via the superior quadrigeminal brachium, the lateral root of the optic tract from the retina and the superior colliculus. Its efferent fibres reach both parasympathetic Edinger–Westphal nuclei. Those that decussate pass ventral to the aqueduct or through the posterior commissure. In this way, sphincter pupillae contract in both eyes in response to impulses from either eye. This bilateral light reflex may not be the sole activity of the pretectal nucleus. Some of its efferents project to the pulvinar and deep laminae of the superior colliculus and provide another extrageniculate path to the cerebral cortex.

BRAIN STEM RETICULAR FORMATION

The brain stem contains extensive fields of intermingled neurones and nerve fibres, which are collectively termed the reticular formation. The reticular regions are often regarded as phylogenetically ancient, representing a primitive nerve network on which more anatomically organized, functionally selective connections have developed during evolution. However, the most primitive nervous systems show both diffuse and highly organized regions, which cooperate in response to different demands.

The general characteristics of reticular regions can be summarized as follows. They tend to be ill-defined collections of neurones and fibres with diffuse connections. Their conduction paths are difficult to define, complex and often polysynaptic, and they have ascending and descending components that are partly crossed and partly uncrossed. Their components subserve somatic and visceral functions. They include distinct chemoarchitectonic nuclear groups, including clusters of serotoninergic neurones (group B cells), which synthesize the indolamine 5-hydroxytryptamine (serotonin); cholinergic neurones (group Ch cells), which contain acetyltransferase, the enzyme that catalyses the synthesis of acetylcholine; and three catecholaminergic groups composed of noradrenergic (group A), adrenergic (group C) and dopaminergic (group A) neurones, which synthesize noradrenaline (norepinephrine), adrenaline (epinephrine) and dopamine, respectively, as neurotransmitters.

Studies with the Golgi technique show that few brain stem reticular neurones are classic Golgi type II neurones (i.e. with short axons that branch locally). In contrast, they have long dendrites that spread across the long axis of the brain stem in transverse sheets. These radiating dendrites may spread into 50% of the cross-sectional area of their half of the brain stem, and they are intersected by, and may synapse with, a complex of ascending and descending fibres. Many axons of the reticular neurones ascend or descend, or bifurcate to do both. They travel far, perhaps through the whole brain stem and often beyond. As an example, a bifurcating axon from a cell in the magnocellular medullary nucleus may project rostrally into the upper medulla, pons, midbrain tegmentum, subthalamus, hypothalamus, dorsal thalamus, septum, limbic system and neocortex, while its descending branch innervates the reticular core of the lower medulla and may reach the cervical spinal intermediate grey matter (laminae V and VI). Many reticular neurones have unidirectional, shorter axons that synapse with the radiating dendrites of

CASE 9   PARINAUD'S SYNDROME

A 13-year-old boy has complained of headaches for several months. On examination, he is found to have bilateral disc edema (papilloedema) with paresis of up-gaze. His pupils fail to constrict in bright light but constrict normally with accommodation. He also has convergence retraction nystagmus. MRI reveals a tumor involving the dorsal midbrain (collicular plate) that is also responsible for obstructive hydrocephalus.

Discussion: This boy has classic Parinaud's (dorsal midbrain) syndrome, with prominent light–near dissociation, paresis of up-gaze convergence, retraction nystagmus and eyelid retraction. It is caused by lesions affecting the dorsal midbrain (tectum) in the region of the superior colliculi and involving the pretectal nuclei. Supranuclear fibres destined for the oculomotor nerve complex are spared. Pupils are midsize or enlarged. Light–near dissociation (characterized by a poor pupillary response (reflex) to light, but preservation of pupillary constriction to a near target) usually results from bilateral midbrain lesions, but not necessarily. Responsible lesions include tumour (e.g. pinealoma), hydrocephalus and infarction. It is of interest that Argyll Robertson pupils, seen, for example, in cases of neurosyphilis, may also exhibit light–near dissociation; however, in this case, the pupil is typically very small and irregular, with reduced dilatation in the dark. Again, the supranuclear connection between the protector and the midbrain Edinger–Westphal nucleus is spared, so the pupillary near reflex is preserved. The so-called tonic pupil of Adie's syndrome, with a lesion involving primarily the ciliary ganglia, similarly exhibits light–near dissociation.

CASE 10   SEE-SAW NYSTAGMUS

A 36-year-old woman develops increasing headaches with intermittent nausea and vomiting. Neurological examination shows bilateral papilloedema, bitemporal visual field defects and see-saw nystagmus.

Skull X-rays show suprasellar calcifications, and MRI demonstrates a suprasellar cystic-appearing mass with extension posteriorly, compressing the diencephalon and rostral ventral mesencephalon. At surgery, this is found to be a craniopharyngioma. Following a course of radiation therapy, all clinical symptoms resolve except for a persistent bitemporal visual field defect.

Discussion: See-saw nystagmus is an uncommon form of pendular nystagmus characterized by synchronous alternating elevation and intorsion of one eye, with simultaneous depression and extorsion of the other eye, followed in the next half cycle by reversal of the vertical and torsional movements. It has been reported in association with a number of conditions, most commonly parasellar masses. Underlying disorders appear to affect multiple structures; as a result, the exact pathophysiological basis for this form of nystagmus remains uncertain. Several cases of brain stem stroke with discrete lesions in the region of the interstitial nucleus of Cajal have been associated with see-saw nystagmus, suggesting that this may be a significant anatomical substrate.

innumerable other neurones en route and give off collaterals, which synapse with cells in 'specific' brain stem nuclei or cortical formations, such as the cerebellum. Multitudes of afferent fibres converging on individual neurones and their myriad synapses and destinations provide the structural basis for the polymodal responses elicited by experiments, and also for such terms as 'diffuse, non-specific polysynaptic systems.'

A contrasting dendritic form is also found, in which the dendrites are short, sinuous or curved, branch profusely and pursue reentrant courses at the perimeter of a nuclear group, defining a boundary between it and its environs. Neurones with an intermediate dendritic complexity occur in and near such nuclei and vary in density in much of the remaining reticular formation. In different zones, the proportion of different sizes of neuronal somata varies. Some regions contain only small to intermediate multipolar cells ('parvocellular' regions). However, there are a few areas where these mingle with large multipolar neurones in 'gigantocellular' or 'magnocellular' nuclei.

In general terms, the reticular formation is a continuous core that traverses the whole brain stem and is continuous below with the reticular intermediate spinal grey laminae. It is divisible, on the basis of cytoarchitectonic, chemoarchitectonic and functional criteria, into three bilateral longitudinal columns: median; medial, containing mostly large reticular neurones; and lateral, containing mostly small to intermediate neurones (Fig. 10.27).

Median Column of Reticular Nuclei

The median column of reticular nuclei extends throughout the medulla, pons and midbrain and contains neurones that are largely aggregated in bilateral, vertical sheets, blended in the midline and occupying the paramedian zones. Collectively, they are called the nuclei of the raphe, or raphe nuclei (see Fig. 10.27). Many neurones in raphe nuclei are serotoninergic and are grouped into nine clusters, B1 to B9. The raphe pallidus nucleus and associated raphe obscurus nucleus lie in the upper two-thirds of the medulla and cross the pontomedullary junction. The raphe magnus nucleus, corresponding to many B3 neurones, partly overlaps them and ascends into the pons. Above it is the pontine raphe nucleus, which is formed by the cell group B5. Also located in the pons is the central superior raphe nucleus, which contains parts of cell groups B6 and B8. The dorsal (rostral) raphe nucleus, approximating cell group B7, ascends—expanding, then narrowing—through much of the midbrain.

The serotoninergic raphe system ramifies extensively throughout the entire central nervous system. Although many of these fibres may be diffusely distributed, recent work has revealed substantial preferential innervation by discrete parts of the system. For example, whereas the central superior raphe nucleus projects divergently to all areas of the cortex, different neurones in the dorsal raphe nucleus project not only to circumscribed regions of the frontal, parietal and occipital cortices but also to functionally related regions of the cerebellar cortex. Similarly, the caudate nucleus and putamen receive a preferential input from the dorsal raphe nucleus, whereas the hippocampus, septum and hypothalamus are innervated mainly by cells in the central superior mesencephalic raphe nucleus.

All raphe nuclei provide mainly serotoninergic descending projections, which terminate in the brain stem and spinal cord. Brain stem connections are multiple and complex. For example, the dorsal raphe nucleus, in addition to sending a large number of fibres to the locus coeruleus, projects to the dorsal tegmental nucleus and most of the rhombencephalic reticular formation, together with the central superior, pontine raphe and raphe magnus nuclei.

Raphe spinal serotoninergic axons originate mainly from neurones in the raphe magnus, pallidus and obscurus nuclei. They project as ventral, dorsal and intermediate spinal tracts in the ventral and lateral funiculi and terminate, respectively, in the ventral horns and laminae I, II and V of the dorsal horns of all segments and in the thoracolumbar intermediolateral sympathetic and sacral parasympathetic preganglionic cell columns. The dorsal raphe spinal projections function as a pain-control pathway that descends from the mesencephalic pain-control centre, which is located in the periaqueductal grey matter, dorsal raphe and cuneiform nuclei. The intermediate raphe spinal projection is inhibitory and, in part, modulates central sympathetic control of cardiovascular function. The ventral raphe spinal system excites ventral horn cells and could function to enhance motor responses to nociceptive stimuli and promote the fight-or-flight response.

Principally, the mesencephalic serotoninergic raphe system is reciprocally interconnected rostrally with the limbic system, septum, prefrontal cortex and hypothalamus. Efferents ascend and form a large ventral pathway and a diminutive dorsal pathway. Both originate from neurones in the dorsal and central superior raphe nuclei. The raphe magnus nucleus also contributes to the dorsal ascending serotoninergic pathway, which is at first incorporated into the dorsal longitudinal fasciculus (of Schütz). A few fibres terminate in the central mesencephalic grey matter and posterior hypothalamus, but most continue into the medial forebrain bundle and merge with the axons of the

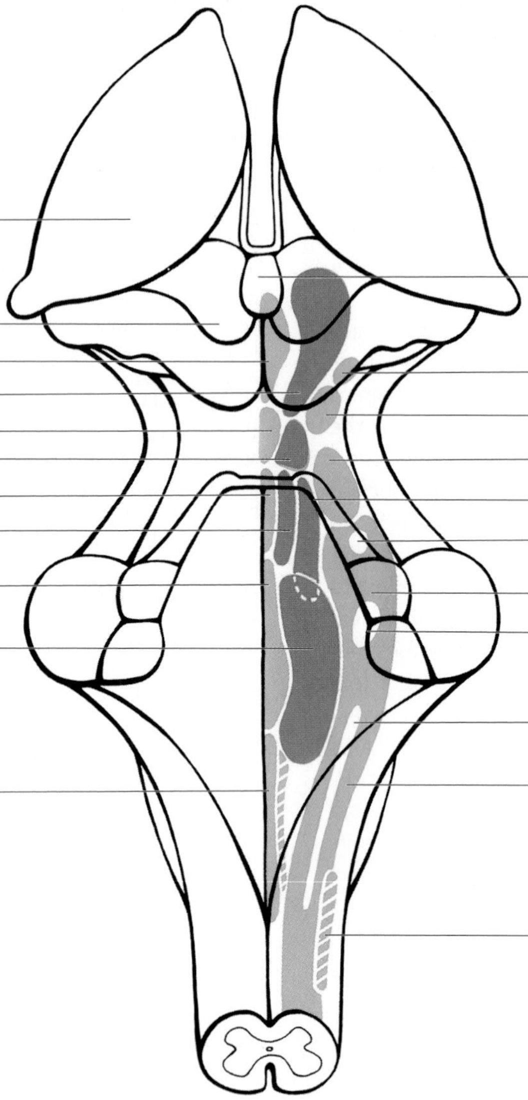

Dorsal thalamus
Pineal gland
Superior colliculus
Dorsal raphe nucleus
Cuneiform and subcuneiform nuclei
Pedunculopontine tegmental nucleus pars compacta
Lateral parabrachial nucleus
Superior central nucleus
Oral pontine reticular nucleus
Medial parabrachial nucleus
Pontine raphe nucleus
Caudal pontine reticular nucleus
Pontine tegmental reticular nucleus
Motor nucleus of trigeminal nerve
Nucleus raphe magnus
Central pontine nucleus
Motor nucleus of facial nerve
Gigantocellular nucleus (magnocellularis)
Nucleus ambiguus
Nucleus raphe obscuris and pallidus
Central nucleus of the medulla oblongata
Lateral funicular nucleus
(nucleus reticularis lateralis of medulla
oblongata)

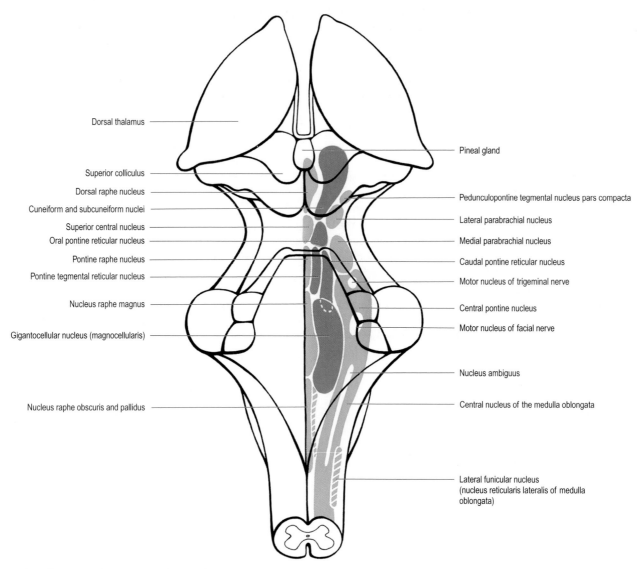

Fig. 10.27 *Outline of the human brain stem* (black) *extending from the caudal end of the medulla to the dorsal thalami. Note the margins of the rhomboid fossa, the lateral angles of which indicate the pontomedullary junction. Note also the profiles of the transected surfaces of the cerebellar penducles, colliculi and pineal gland. The principal nuclear derivatives of the brain stem reticular formation are indicated in approximate outline. Those from the median and paramedian nuclear column are in* magenta, *medial column derivatives are* purple *and lateral column derivatives are* blue. *In reality, considerable overlap of the nuclear profiles would be present when the third dimension is considered. A number of 'non-reticular' nuclei are also included.*

ventral pathway, which are distributed to the same targets. The fibres of the ventral ascending serotoninergic pathway exit the ventral aspect of the mesencephalic raphe nuclei and then course rostrally through the ventral tegmentum, where fibres pass to the ventral tegmental area, substantia nigra and interpeduncular nucleus. A large number of fibres then enter the habenulo-interpeduncular tract and run rostrally to innervate the habenular nucleus; intralaminar, midline, anterior, ventral and lateral dorsal thalamic nuclei; and lateral geniculate body. The ventral ascending serotoninergic pathway enters the median forebrain bundle in the lateral hypothalamic area and splits to pass medially and laterally. The fibres in the medial tract terminate in the mammillary body; dorsomedial, ventromedial, infundibular, anterior and lateral hypothalamic nuclei; medial and lateral preoptic nuclei; and suprachiasmatic nuclei. Those in the lateral tract take the ansa peduncularis–ventral amygdalofugal path to the amygdala, striatum and caudal neocortex. The medial forebrain bundle carries the remaining ventral ascending serotoninergic axons into the medullary stria, stria terminalis, fornix, diagonal band, external capsule, cingulate fasciculus and medial olfactory stria, to terminate in all the structures that these systems interconnect.

Major afferents into the mesencephalic raphe nuclei include those from the interpeduncular nucleus linking the limbic and serotoninergic systems; the lateral habenular nucleus linking the septum, preoptic hypothalamus and prefrontal cortex via the habenulo-interpeduncular tract and the medial forebrain bundle; and the pontine central grey matter.

The ascending raphe system probably functions to moderate forebrain activities, particularly limbic, septal and hypothalamic activities. Recent demonstrations of specific connectivity suggest that it exerts precise as well as tonal control.

Medial Column of Reticular Nuclei

The medial column of reticular nuclei is composed predominantly of neurones of medium size, although very large neurones are found in some regions, and most have processes oriented in the transverse plane (see Fig. 10.27). In the lower medulla, the column is indistinct and is perhaps represented by a thin lamina lateral to the raphe nuclei. However, in the upper medulla, it expands into the medullary gigantocellular (magnocellular) nucleus, which lies ventrolateral to the hypoglossal nucleus, ventral to the vagal nuclei and dorsal to the inferior olivary complex. Ascending farther, the column continues as the pontine gigantocellular (magnocellular) nucleus, which lies medially in the tegmentum. Its neurones suddenly diminish in size to form, in rostral order, the almost coextensive caudal and oral pontine tegmental reticular nuclei. It then expands into the cuneiform nucleus and subcuneiform nucleus before fading away in the midbrain tegmentum.

Axons of medial reticular column neurones form a multisynaptic ascending and descending system within the column and ultimately enter the spinal cord and diencephalon. Descending fibres form the pontospinal (lateral reticulospinal) and bulbospinal (medial reticulospinal) tracts. Pontospinal axons arise from neurones in the caudal and oral parts of the pontine reticular nucleus, descend uncrossed in the ventral spinal funiculus and terminate in spinal cord laminae VII, VIII and IX. Bulbospinal axons descend bilaterally to end in laminae VII, VIII, IX and X and ipsilaterally to end in laminae IV, V and VI. The system modulates spinal motor function and segmental nociceptive input.

Afferent components to the medial reticular nuclear column include the spinoreticular projection and collaterals of centrally projecting spinal trigeminal, vestibular and cochlear fibres. Spinoreticular fibres arise from neurones in the intermediate grey matter of the spinal cord. They decussate in the ventral white commissure; ascend in the ventrolateral funiculus, usually via several neurones; and terminate not only at all levels of the medial column of reticular nuclei but also in the intralaminar nuclei of the thalamus. Three areas of the medial reticular zone receive particularly high densities of terminations: the combined caudal and rostral ends of the gigantocellular and central nuclei, respectively; the caudal pontine reticular nucleus; and the pontine tegmentum. Retinotectal and tectoreticular fibres relay visual information, and the medial forebrain bundle transmits olfactory impulses.

Efferents from the medial column of reticular nuclei project through a multisynaptic pathway within the column to the thalamus. Areas of maximal termination of spinoreticular fibres also project directly to the intralaminar thalamic nuclei. The multisynaptic pathway is integrated into the lateral column of reticular nuclei with cholinergic neurones in the lateral pontine tegmentum. The intralaminar thalamic nuclei project directly to the striatum and neocortex.

Lateral Column of Reticular Nuclei

The lateral column of reticular nuclei contains six nuclear groups, which include the parvocellular reticular area; superficial ventrolateral reticular area; lateral pontine tegmental noradrenergic cell groups A1, A2 and A4 to A7 (A3 is absent in primates); adrenergic cell groups C1 and C2; and cholinergic cell groups Ch5 and Ch6. The column descends through the lower two-thirds of the lateral pontine tegmentum and upper medulla, where it lies between the gigantocellular nucleus medially and the sensory trigeminal nuclei laterally. It continues caudally and expands to form most of the reticular formation lateral to the raphe nuclei. It abuts the superficial ventrolateral reticular area, nucleus solitarius, nucleus ambiguus and vagal nucleus, where it contains the adrenergic cell group C2 and the noradrenergic group A2.

The lateral paragigantocellular nucleus lies at the rostral pole of the diffuse superficial ventrolateral reticular area (at the level of the facial nucleus). The zone extends caudally as the nucleus retroambiguus and descends into the spinal cord. It contains noradrenergic cell groups A1, A2, A4 and A5 and the adrenergic cell group C1. The ventrolateral reticular area is involved in cardiovascular, respiratory, vasoreceptor and chemoreceptor reflexes and in the modulation of nociception. The A2 or noradrenergic dorsal medullary cell group lies in the nucleus of the tractus solitarius, vagal nucleus and adjoining parvocellular reticular area. Adrenergic group C1 lies rostral to the A2 cell group. Noradrenergic cell group A4 extends into the lateral pontine tegmentum, along the subependymal surface of the superior cerebellar peduncle. Noradrenergic group A5 forms part of the paragigantocellular nucleus in the caudolateral pontine tegmentum. Noradrenergic cell group A5 and adrenergic cell group C1 probably function as centres of vasomotor control. The entire region is subdivided into functional areas on the basis of stimulation experiments in animals, in which vasoconstrictor, cardioaccelerator, depressor, inspiratory, expiratory and sudomotor effects have been elicited.

The lateral pontine tegmental reticular grey matter is related to the superior cerebellar peduncle and forms the medial and lateral parabrachial nuclei and the ventral Kölliker-Fuse nucleus, a pneumotaxic centre. The locus coeruleus (noradrenergic cell group A6), area subcoeruleus, noradrenergic cell group A7 and cholinergic group Ch5 in the pedunculopontine tegmental nucleus are all located in the lateral pontine and mesencephalic tegmental reticular zones. The mesencephalic group Ch5 is continuous caudally with cell group Ch6 in the pontine central grey matter.

Cell group A6 contains all the noradrenergic cells in the central region of the locus coeruleus. Group A6 has ventral (nucleus subcoeruleus), rostral and caudolateral extensions; the last merges with the A4 group. The locus coeruleus probably functions as an attention centre, focusing neural functions on prevailing needs. The noradrenergic A7 group occupies the rostroventral part of the pontine tegmentum and is continuous with groups A5 and A1 through the lateral rhombencephalic tegmentum. The A7, A5, A1 complex is also connected by noradrenergic cell clusters with group A2 caudally and with group A6 rostrally. The A5 and A7 groups lie mainly within the medial parabrachial and Kölliker-Fuse nuclei. Reticular neurones in the lateral pontine tegmental reticular area, like those of the ventrolateral zone, function to regulate respiratory, cardiovascular and gastrointestinal activity. Two micturition centres are located in the dorsomedial and ventrolateral parts of the lateral pontine tegmentum.

The connections of the lateral column reticular nuclei are complex. The short ascending and descending axons of the parvocellular reticular area constitute bulbar reflex pathways, which connect all branchiomotor nuclei and the hypoglossal nucleus with central afferent cranial nerve complexes through a propriobulbar system. The area also receives descending afferents from the contralateral motor cortex via the corticotegmental tract and from the contralateral red nucleus via the rubrospinal tract. The longitudinal catecholamine bundle passes through the parvocellular reticular formation.

The superficial ventrolateral reticular area receives some input from the spinal cord, insular cortex and amygdala, but the principal projection is from the nucleus solitarius and subserves cardiovascular, baroreceptor, chemoreceptor and respiratory reflexes. Reticulospinal afferents from the region terminate bilaterally on sympathetic preganglionic neurones in the thoracic spinal cord. Afferents from the pneumotaxic centre project to an inspiratory centre in the ventrolateral part of the nucleus solitarius and to a mixed expiratory–inspiratory centre in the superficial ventrolateral reticular area. Inspiratory neurones in both centres monosynaptically project to the phrenic and intercostal motor neurones. Axons of expiratory neurones terminate on lower motor neurones that innervate intercostal and abdominal musculature.

The superficial ventrolateral area is also the seat of the visceral alerting response. Fibres from the hypothalamus, periaqueductal grey matter and midbrain tegmentum mediate increased respiratory activity, raised blood pressure, tachycardia, vasodilatation in skeletal muscle and renal and gastrointestinal vasoconstriction. Ascending efferents from the superficial ventrolateral area synapse on neurones of the supraoptic and paraventricular hypothalamic nuclei. Excitation of these neurones causes release of vasopressin from the neurohypophysis. Medullary noradrenergic cell groups A1 and A2 also innervate (directly and indirectly) the median eminence and control the release of growth hormone, luteinizing hormone and adrenocorticotropic hormone (ACTH).

The lateral pontine tegmentum, particularly the parabrachial region, is reciprocally connected to the insular cortex. It shares reciprocal projections with the amygdala through the ventral amygdalofugal pathway, medial forebrain bundle and central tegmental tract, and with the hypothalamic, median preoptic and paraventricular nuclei, which preferentially project to the lateral parabrachial nucleus and the micturition centres. It also shares reciprocal bulbar projections, many from the pneumotaxic centre, with the nucleus solitarius and superficial ventrolateral reticular area.

Reticulospinal fibres descend from the lateral pontine tegmentum. A mainly ipsilateral subcoeruleospinal pathway is distributed to all spinal segments of the cord through the lateral spinal funiculus. Crossed pontospinal fibres descend from the ventrolateral pontine tegmentum, decussate in the rostral pons and occupy the contralateral dorsolateral spinal funiculus. They terminate in laminae I, II, V and VI of all spinal segments of the cord. Fibres from the pneumotaxic centre innervate the phrenic nucleus and T1–3 sympathetic preganglionic neurones bilaterally through this projection system.

Bilateral projections from the micturition centres travel in the lateral spinal funiculus. They terminate on preganglionic parasympathetic neurones in the sacral cord (which innervate the detrusor muscle in the urinary bladder) and on neurones in the nucleus of Onuf (which innervate the musculature of the pelvic floor and the anal and urethral sphincters).

Descending fibres of the A6 noradrenergic neurones of the locus coeruleus project into the longitudinal dorsal fasciculus (as the caudal limb of the dorsal periventricular pathway) and into the caudal limb of the dorsal noradrenergic bundle (as part of the longitudinal catecholamine bundle). In this way, they innervate, mainly ipsilaterally, all other rhombencephalic reticular areas, principal and spinal trigeminal nuclei, pontine nuclei, cochlear nuclei, nuclei of the lateral lemniscus and, bilaterally, all spinal preganglionic autonomic neurones and the ventral region of the dorsal horn in all segments of the spinal cord. Other axons that contribute to the longitudinal catecholamine bundle originate from cell groups C1, A1, A2, A5 and A7. The main projection is a descending one from cell groups C1 and A5, which are sudomotor neural control centres and innervate preganglionic sympathetic neurones.

Most ascending fibres from the locus coeruleus pass in the dorsal noradrenergic (or tegmental) bundle; others run in either the rostral limb of the dorsal periventricular pathway or the superior cerebellar peduncle. The latter fibres terminate on the deep cerebellar nuclei. The dorsal noradrenergic bundle is large and runs through the ventrolateral periaqueductal grey matter to join the medial forebrain bundle in the hypothalamus, where fibres continue forward to innervate all rostral areas of the brain. The pathway contains efferent and afferent axons that reciprocally connect the locus coeruleus with adjacent structures along its course, including the central mesencephalic grey matter, dorsal raphe nucleus, superior and inferior colliculi, interpeduncular nucleus, epithalamus, dorsal thalamus, habenular nuclei, amygdala, septum, olfactory bulb, anterior olfactory nucleus, entire hippocampal formation and neocortex. Fibres from the locus coeruleus travel in the rostral limb of the dorsal periventricular pathway, ascend in the ventromedial periaqueductal grey matter adjacent to the longitudinal dorsal fasciculus and terminate in the parvocellular part of the paraventricular nucleus in the hypothalamus.

The functions of the locus coeruleus and related tegmental noradrenergic cell groups are poorly understood, largely because the afferent neurones that drive them have yet to be identified. The diversity of their rostral and caudal projections suggests a holistic role in central processing. In animals, firing rates

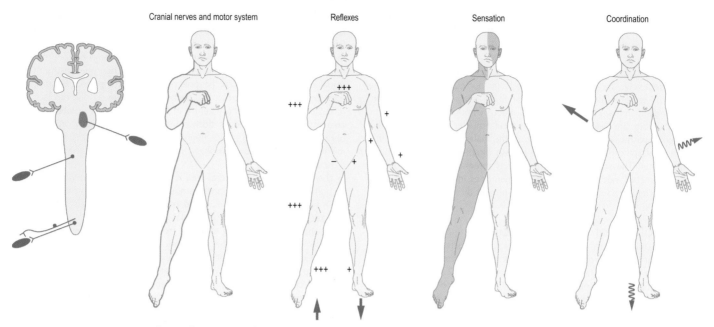

Cranial nerves and motor system   Reflexes   Sensation   Coordination

Fig. 10.28 *Brain stem lesions. (By permission from Crossman, A.R., Neary, D., 2000. Neuroanatomy, 2nd ed. Churchill Livingstone, Edinburgh.)*

of locus coeruleus neurones peak during wakefulness and decrease during sleep—they cease almost completely during rapid eye movement (REM) sleep. During wakefulness, firing rates are augmented when novel stimuli are presented. The locus coeruleus may therefore function to control the level of attentiveness. Other functions that have been ascribed to the locus coeruleus include control of the wake–sleep cycle, regulation of blood flow and maintenance of synaptic plasticity.

The A1, A2, A5 and A7 noradrenergic cell groups project rostrally, mainly through the central tegmental tract. Their axons constitute a major longitudinal catecholamine pathway that continues through the medial forebrain bundle and ends in the amygdala, lateral septal nucleus, bed nucleus of the stria terminalis, nucleus of the diagonal band and hypothalamus. The ascending dorsal periventricular pathway contains a few non-coerulean noradrenergic fibres, which terminate in the periventricular region of the thalamus.

Propriobulbar projections receive a contribution from the diffusely organized dorsal medullary and lateral tegmental noradrenergic cell groups. These interconnect cranial nerve nuclei and other reticular cell groups, particularly those of the vagus, facial and trigeminal nerves, and the rhombencephalic raphe and parabrachial nuclei.

Three precerebellar nuclei—the lateral and paramedian reticular nuclei and the nucleus of the pontine tegmentum—are involved in the relay of spinal information into the vermis and paravermal regions of the ipsilateral cerebellar hemisphere. They receive inputs from the contralateral primary motor and sensory neocortices and the ipsilateral cerebellar and vestibular nuclei and spinal cord (the latter through the ascending spinoreticular pathway). This system augments the dorsal and ventral spinocerebellar, cuneocerebellar, accessory cuneocerebellar and trigeminocerebellar tracts.

BRAIN STEM LESIONS

Unilateral brain stem lesions may arise as a result of extrinsic compression of the brain stem by space-occupying tumours (e.g. meningioma, acoustic neuroma, metastatic carcinoma) or may be caused by intrinsic disease (e.g. glioma, demyelination, stroke) (Figs 10.28, 10.29). The clinical syndrome is determined by the neuroanatomical site of the lesion. At the segmental level, an ipsilateral cranial nerve palsy occurs. Below the level of the lesion, there is a contralateral loss of power and sensation in the limbs (corresponding to dysfunction of the decussating corticospinal and ascending sensory pathways) and ipsilateral incoordination of the limbs (as a result of the interruption of efferent and afferent cerebellar connections).

The ipsilateral cranial nerve dysfunction reflects the segmental level of the lesion in the midbrain, pons and medulla. Midbrain lesions cause ophthalmoplegia, pupillary dilatation and ptosis (oculomotor nerve palsy) and impaired upward gaze (e.g. due to pinealoma). Pontine lesions (e.g. acoustic neuroma in the cerebellopontine angle) lead to ophthalmoplegia (abducens nerve lesion), loss of facial sensation and weakness of masticatory muscles (trigeminal nerve lesion), weakness of facial muscles (facial nerve lesion) or deafness and vertigo (vestibulocochlear nerve lesion). Medullary lesions cause a 'bulbar palsy' consisting of dysarthria, dysphagia and dysphonia, with wasting of the hemitongue and palate (glossopharyngeal, vagal and hypoglossal nerve

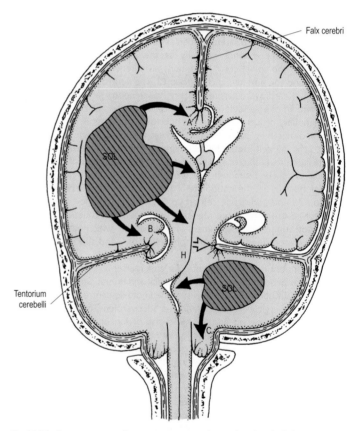

Fig. 10.29 *Consequences of a space-occupying lesion (SOL) include herniation of the cingulate gyrus under the falx (A), tentorial herniation of the parahippocampal gyrus (B) and herniation of cerebellar tonsils through the foramen magnum (C). The open arrow points out compression of the cerebral peduncle against the free edge of the tentorium cerebelli. H, haemorrhage into the midbrain.*

lesions) and weakness and wasting of sternocleidomastoid and trapezius (accessory nerve lesion).

In addition to this focal brain stem syndrome, blockage of the outflow of cerebrospinal fluid from the fourth ventricle via the foramina of Magendie and Luschka (e.g. by extrinsic tumours) produces hydrocephalus, which is characterized by headache, papilloedema and progressive stupor and coma.

Bilateral destructive lesions of the brain stem are fatal if untreated because of damage to centres in the medulla that control respiration, heart rate and blood pressure. Impairment of the reticular activating system in the core of the brain stem leads to progressive impairment of consciousness, followed

CASE 11   BRAIN STEM VASCULAR SYNDROMES

Patient 1: A 59-year-old woman with diabetes and hypertension awakens with right-sided weakness and complains of double vision. On examination, she has a dense right hemiparesis. The left eye cannot move medially, she has ptosis, and the left pupil is dilated. MRI shows an infarct in the right ventral midbrain.

Discussion: The findings are those of Weber's syndrome, caused by a ventral midbrain lesion, usually infarction, and characterized by ipsilateral oculomotor paralysis and ptosis with contralateral hemiparesis, reflecting injury to the third cranial nerve and crus cerebri (corticospinal and corticobulbar tracts). If the Edinger–Westphal nucleus is implicated in the lesion, a fixed, dilated pupil is observed, reflecting loss of parasympathetic function; in some cases with more caudal lesions, the pupil may still react (pupil sparing).

Patient 2: A 61-year-old man with coronary artery disease develops double vision (diplopia) and difficulty walking. He exhibits right oculomotor palsy and left-sided ataxia. On finger–nose–finger testing, he has a prominent tremor that worsens as he approaches the target (rubral tremor) and dysmetria. He cannot perform rapid alternating movements with the left hand (dysdiadochokinesia). MRI demonstrates a lesion in the medial midbrain.

Discussion: This patient has Claude's syndrome, caused by a midbrain lesion, usually ischaemic, that affects the third cranial nerve and the red nucleus, resulting in ipsilateral oculomotor palsy and contralateral hemiataxia. The red nucleus is involved in motor coordination, with connections to the superior cerebellar peduncle, thalamus and spinal cord.

Patient 3: A 60-year-old woman develops a right third nerve palsy with left-sided hemiparesis, along with a left-sided tremor. MRI demonstrates a large ventral midbrain infarction.

Discussion: This constellation of findings, known as Benedikt's syndrome, can be considered a combination of Weber's and Claude's syndromes.

Focal lesions in the brain stem, most commonly vascular in nature, result in syndromes that, as a group, are characterized by 'crossed' findings, with ipsilateral cranial nerve involvement and contralateral (hemibody) abnormalities (motor, sensory or cerebellar). The level of the brain stem lesion (midbrain, pons, medulla) and its dorsal or ventral extent determine precisely which structures or tracts are involved. Although the majority of such focal brain stem syndromes are caused by vascular lesions (stroke, haemorrhage), as in the preceding three cases, they may result from tumours or inflammatory lesions. In contrast, metabolic lesions involving the brain stem, such as Wernicke's encephalopathy or central pontine myelinolysis (osmotic dysequilibrium syndrome), tend to produce bilateral alterations both clinically and anatomically.

CASE 12   OPSOCLONUS

A 68-year-old man, an insulin-dependent diabetic, is found unconscious by his wife after returning home from an overnight trip. He has been non-compliant with glucose monitoring and insulin injections.

In the emergency room, he is found to be comatose. Cranial nerve examination shows spontaneous continuous, rapid, conjugate eye movements in all directions. The pupils are 2 mm in diameter and minimally reactive to light. The extremities are flaccid, with reduced patellar, biceps and triceps reflexes. There are bilateral extensor plantar responses (Babinski's sign). His blood glucose level is 630 mg/dl. There are no ketones in the urine.

He is treated aggressively with intravenous insulin and fluids. A computed tomography scan is normal; electroencephalography demonstrates diffuse slowing without epileptiform activity. After several hours, the patient begins to regain consciousness. By the next morning, his eye movements are normal, and he is fully awake.

Discussion: Opsoclonus (saccadomania) is characterized by continuous, involuntary, conjugate, multidirectional saccades. This uncommon but well-described eye movement disorder is associated with a number of systemic disorders in adults (metabolic, toxic, infectious, paraneoplastic). In children it is a classic manifestation of neuroblastoma. The mechanism of action, though variable, is most likely the result of interference with brain stem oculomotor control systems.

by stupor and coma. In this state of 'brain stem death,' life can only be supported artificially. This is the fate of all untreated expanding space-occupying lesions in the cranium (e.g. haematoma, abscess or tumour, whether extrinsic or intrinsic to the brain; cerebral oedema). A space-occupying lesion within the unyielding skull raises the intracranial pressure directly as well as indirectly by obstruction of cerebrospinal fluid flow, which causes headache and papilloedema. The brain is distorted and displaced downward (rostrocaudally) within the skull and meningeal framework. The brain stem is vulnerable to compression at two critical sites, which are determined by the neuroanatomical relationship of the meningeal tentorium and foramen magnum to the cerebral hemisphere (supratentorial) and brain stem (infratentorial). Downward displacement of the cerebral hemisphere leads to herniation of the ipsilateral medial temporal lobe (uncus) through the tentorial notch. There may be direct ipsilateral compression of the midbrain and emergent oculomotor and trochlear cranial nerves or contralateral compression of the upper brain stem by the abutting sharp edge of the tentorium. The ipsilateral posterior cerebral artery is vulnerable to compression at this site. Unilateral herniation is heralded by a progressive oculomotor nerve palsy (ophthalmoplegia, pupillary dilatation and ptosis), contralateral limb weakness, falling level of consciousness and, if treatment is long delayed, contralateral homonymous hemianopia. Compression of the contralateral brain stem by the tentorium leads to ipsilateral 'false localizing' signs (Kernohan's syndrome).

Further progressive rostrocaudal displacement of the brain ultimately leads to herniation of the medulla through the foramen magnum and into the spinal canal. This is accompanied by bilateral cranial nerve dysfunction, quadriplegia, deepening coma and finally apnoea—brain stem death. These neuroanatomical and functional processes underlie the diagnosis and management of traumatically brain-injured patients and the complications of intracranial haematoma (extradural, subdural and intracerebral) and cerebral oedema.

References

Adams, R.D., Victor, M., Mancall, E.L., 1959. Central pontine myelinolysis. A hitherto undescribed disease occurring in alcoholic and malnourished patients. Arch. Neurol. Psychiatry 81, 154.

Brodal, P., Bjaalie, J.G., 1992. Organization of the pontine nuclei. Neurosci. Res. 13, 83–118.

Ciriello, J., 1983. Brainstem projections of aortic baroreceptor afferent fibres in the rat. Neurosci. Lett. 36, 37–42.

Dahlström, A., Fuxe, K., 1964. Evidence for the existence of monamine-containing neurones in the central nervous system. Acta. Physiol. Scand. Suppl. 232, 1–55.

Dahlström, A., Fuxe, K., 1965. Evidence for the existence of monoamine neurones in the central nervous system. II. Experimentally induced changes in the intraneuronal amine levels of bulbospinal neurone systems. Acta. Physiol. Scand. Suppl. 247, 1–36.

Hamilton, R.B., Norgren, R., 1984. Central projections of gustatory nerves in the rat. J. Comp. Neurol. 222, 560–577.

Johnston, J.B., 1909. The morphology of the forebrain vesicle in vertebrates. J. Comp. Neurol. 19, 458–539.

Kleinschmidt-DeMasters, B.K., Rojiani, A.M., Filley, C.M., 2006. Central and extrapontine myelinolysis: then and now. J. Neuropathol. Exp. Neurol. 65, 1–11.

Leigh, R.J., 1991. Zee DS the Neurology of Eye Movements, second ed. FA Davis, Philadelphia, p. 462.

Millar, J., Basbaum, A.I., 1975. Topography of the projection of the body surface of the cat to cuneate and gracile nuclei. Exp. Neurol. 49, 281–290.

Nathan, P.W., Smith, M.C., 1982. The rubrospinal and central tegmental tracts in man. Brain 105, 223–269.

Nieuwenhuys, R., Voogd, J., van Huijzen, C., 1988. The human central nervous system. A synopsis and atlas, third ed. Springer Verlag, Berlin.

Olszewski, J., 1950. On the anatomical and functional organization of the spinal trigeminal nucleus. J. Comp. Neurol. 92, 401–409.

Schmeichel, A.M., Buchhalter, L.C., Low, P.A., et al, 2008. Mesopontine cholingeric neuron involvement in Lewy body dementia and multiple system atrophy. Neurology 70, 368–373.

Wolf, J.K., 1971. The classical brain stem syndromes. Charles C. Thomas, Springfield.

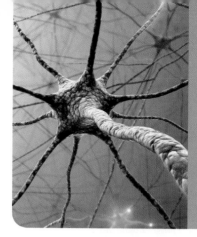

Cranial Nerves

Cranial nerves are the means by which the brain receives information from, and controls the activities of, the head and neck and, to a lesser extent, the thoracic and abdominal viscera. Briefly, there are 12 pairs of cranial nerves that are individually named and numbered (using roman numerals) in a rostrocaudal sequence (see Table 1.1). Unlike spinal nerves, only some are mixed in function and thus carry both sensory and motor fibres. Others are purely sensory or purely motor. The first cranial nerve (I; olfactory) has an ancient lineage and is derived from the forerunner of the cerebral hemisphere. It retains this unique position through the connections of the olfactory bulb and is the only sensory cranial nerve that projects directly to the cerebral cortex rather than via the thalamus, as do all other sensory modalities. The areas of cerebral cortex involved have a primitive cellular organization and are an integral part of the limbic system, which is concerned with the emotional aspects of behaviour. The second cranial nerve (II; optic) consists of the axons of second-order visual neurones and terminates in the thalamus. The other 10 pairs of cranial nerves attach to the brain stem. Most of the component fibres originate from, or terminate in, named cranial nerve nuclei (Ch. 10).

The sensory fibres in individual spinal and cranial nerves have characteristic, but often overlapping, peripheral distributions. As far as the innervation of the body surface is concerned, the area supplied by a particular spinal or cranial nerve is referred to as a dermatome. Detailed dermatome maps are described on a regional basis. The motor axons of individual spinal and cranial nerves tend to innervate anatomically and functionally related groups of skeletal muscles, which are referred to as myotomes.

OLFACTORY NERVE (I)

The cell of origin of the olfactory nerves serving the sense of smell is in the olfactory mucosa covering the superior nasal concha, the upper part of the vertical portion of the middle concha and the opposite part of the nasal septum. The axons, which are unmyelinated, originate as the central or deep processes of the olfactory neurones and collect in bundles that cross in various directions, forming a plexiform network in the mucosa. The bundles finally form approximately 20 branches that traverse the cribriform plate in lateral and medial groups and end in the glomeruli of the olfactory bulb. Each branch has a sheath consisting of dura mater and pia-arachnoid; the former continues into the nasal periosteum, and the latter into the connective tissue sheaths surrounding the nerve bundles (Figs 11.1, 11.2).

Olfactory pathways subserving the sense of smell are described in Chapter 12.

OPTIC NERVE (II)

The optic nerve is the second cranial nerve (Figs 11.3, 11.4). It arises from the optic chiasma on the floor of the diencephalon and enters the orbit through the optic canal, accompanied by the ophthalmic artery. It changes shape, starting out flat at the chiasma and becoming rounded as it passes through the optic canal. In the orbit it passes forward, laterally and downward and pierces the sclera at the lamina cribrosa, slightly medial to the posterior pole. It has a somewhat tortuous course within the orbit to allow for movements of the eyeball. It is surrounded by extensions of the three layers of meninges.

The optic nerve has important relationships with other orbital structures. As it leaves the optic canal, it lies superomedial to the ophthalmic artery and is separated from the lateral rectus by the oculomotor, nasociliary and abducens nerves and sometimes by the ophthalmic veins. The optic nerve is closely related to the origins of the four recti muscles, whereas more anteriorly, where the muscles diverge, it is separated from them by a substantial amount of orbital fat. Just beyond the optic canal, the ophthalmic artery and the nasociliary nerve cross the optic nerve to reach the medial wall of the orbit. The central artery of the retina enters the substance of the optic nerve about halfway along its length. Near the back of the eye, it becomes surrounded by long and short ciliary nerves and vessels.

CASE 1   ANOSMIA

A 52-year-old man falls approximately 10 feet from a ladder, striking his head on the pavement below. He loses consciousness for a short time. He is found to have a left frontal skull fracture involving the base of the anterior fossa, responsible for a right hemiparesis and mild language dysfunction. He also experiences a leak of spinal fluid through his nose for several months thereafter. Although he recovers normal neurological function with the passage of time, it becomes clear that he has lost the sense of smell on the side of the skull fracture.

Discussion: This man has suffered a basal skull fracture involving the floor of the anterior fossa. The fracture line crosses the olfactory groove, resulting in laceration of the olfactory nerve and thus anosmia. Tumours and other mass lesions on the floor of the anterior fossa may similarly result in ipsilateral loss of the sense of smell; bilateral anosmia, with or without impairment of taste, may be due to the use of a variety of drugs, such as calcium channel blockers, some antibiotics, anticonvulsants and opiates, among others. (See also Ch. 9, Case 1.)

Retina

The retina is described in Chapter 12.

OCULOMOTOR NERVE (III)

The oculomotor nerve is the third cranial nerve (Figs 11.3, 11.4, 11.8). It is the main source of innervation to the extraocular muscles and also contains parasympathetic fibres that relay in the ciliary ganglion.

The oculomotor nerve emerges at the midbrain, on the medial side of the crus of the cerebral peduncle. It passes along the lateral dural wall of the cavernous sinus, where it divides into superior and inferior divisions that run beneath the trochlear and ophthalmic nerves. The two divisions of the oculomotor nerve enter the orbit through the superior orbital fissure, within the common tendinous ring of the recti muscles, separated by the nasociliary branch of the ophthalmic nerve.

The superior division of the oculomotor nerve passes above the optic nerve to enter the inferior (ocular) surface of superior rectus. It supplies this muscle and gives off a branch that runs to supply levator palpebrae superioris. The inferior division of the oculomotor nerve divides into three branches: medial, central and lateral. The medial branch passes beneath the optic nerve to enter the lateral (ocular) surface of the medial rectus. The central branch runs downward and forward to enter the superior (ocular) surface of the inferior rectus. The lateral branch travels forward on the lateral side of inferior rectus to enter the orbital surface of the inferior oblique. The lateral branch also communicates with the ciliary ganglion to distribute parasympathetic fibres to sphincter pupillae and ciliaris.

Ciliary Ganglion

The ciliary ganglion is a parasympathetic ganglion concerned functionally with the motor innervation of certain intraocular muscles (Figs 11.5, 11.6). It is a small, flat, reddish grey swelling, 1 to 2 mm in diameter, connected to the nasociliary nerve and located near the apex of the orbit in loose fat approximately 1 cm

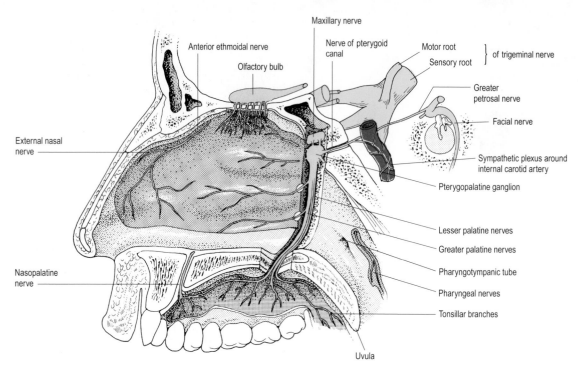

Fig. 11.1 *Sensory innervation of the lateral wall of the nasal cavity, hard and soft palates and nasopharynx. Secretomotor fibres to mucous glands are distributed in branches from the pterygopalatine ganglion.*

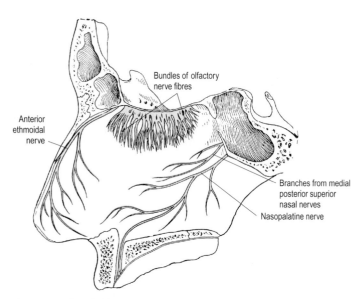

Fig. 11.2 *Bundles of olfactory nerve fibres and nerves associated with the septum (left side).*

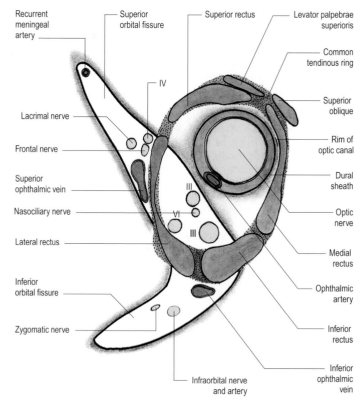

Fig. 11.3 *The common tendinous ring with its muscle origins superimposed, and the relative positions of the nerves entering the orbital cavity through the superior orbital fissure and optic canal. Note that the attachments of levator palpebrae superioris and superior oblique lie external to the common tendinous ring but are attached to it. The ophthalmic veins frequently pass through the ring. The recurrent meningeal artery, a branch of the ophthalmic artery, is often conducted from the orbit to the cranial cavity through its own foramen. (Based mainly on the data of Whitnall, S.E., 1932. Anatomy of the Human Orbit, 2nd ed. Oxford University Press, London; and Koornneef, I., 1977. Spatial Aspects of Orbital Musculo-fibrous Tissue in Man. Swestsa Zeitlinger, Amsterdam. Provided by the late Gordon L. Ruskell, Department of Optometry and Visual Science, The City University, London.)*

in front of the medial end of the superior orbital fissure. It lies between the optic nerve and lateral rectus, usually lateral to the ophthalmic artery. Its neurones, which are multipolar, are larger than in typical autonomic ganglia; a very small number of more typical neurones are also present.

Its connections or roots enter or leave it posteriorly. Eight to 10 delicate filaments, termed the short ciliary nerves, emerge anteriorly from the ganglion arranged in two or three bundles, the lower being larger. They run forward sinuously with the ciliary arteries, above and below the optic nerve, and divide into 15 to 20 branches that pierce the sclera around the optic nerve and run in small grooves on the internal scleral surface. They convey parasympathetic, sympathetic and sensory fibres between the eyeball and the ciliary ganglion; only the parasympathetic fibres synapse in the ganglion.

The parasympathetic root, derived from the branch of the oculomotor nerve to the inferior oblique, consists of preganglionic fibres from the Edinger–Westphal nucleus, which relay in the ganglion. Postganglionic fibres travel in the short ciliary nerves to the sphincter pupillae and ciliaris. More than 95% of these fibres supply the ciliaris, which is a much larger muscle in volume.

The sympathetic root contains fibres from the plexus around the internal carotid artery within the cavernous sinus. These postganglionic fibres, derived from the superior cervical ganglion, form a fine branch that enters the orbit through the superior orbital fissure inside the common tendinous ring of recti muscles. The fibres either pass directly to the ganglion or join the nasociliary nerve and travel to the ganglion in its sensory root. Either way, they traverse the ganglion without synapsing to emerge into the short ciliary nerves. They are distributed to the blood vessels of the eyeball. Sympathetic fibres innervating dilator pupillae may sometimes travel via the short ciliary nerves (rather than the more usual route via the ophthalmic, nasociliary and long ciliary nerves).

The sensory fibres that pass through the ciliary ganglion are derived from the nasociliary nerve. They enter the short ciliary nerves and carry sensation from the cornea, the ciliary body and the iris.

TROCHLEAR NERVE (IV)

The trochlear nerve is the fourth cranial nerve and is the only one that emerges from the dorsal surface of the brainstem (see Fig. 11.35). It passes from

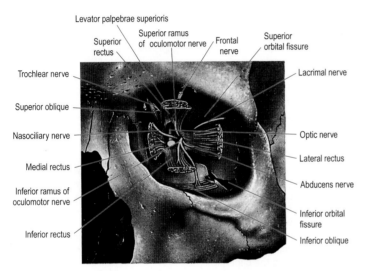

Fig. 11.4 *Dissection of the left orbit, viewed from the front, to show the origins of the orbital muscles and the relative positions of the nerves of the orbit.*

the midbrain onto the lateral surface of the crus of the cerebral peduncle and runs through the lateral dural wall of the cavernous sinus. It then crosses the oculomotor nerve and enters the orbit through the superior orbital fissure, above the common tendinous ring of the recti muscles and levator palpebrae superioris and medial to the frontal and lacrimal nerves. The trochlear nerve travels only a short distance to enter the superior (orbital) surface of superior oblique, which is its sole target (see Fig. 11.8).

TRIGEMINAL NERVE (V)
Innervation of the Face and Scalp

The sensory innervation of the face and scalp is primarily from the three divisions of the mandibular nerve, with smaller contributions from the cervical spinal nerves. The two muscles of mastication that relate to the face are innervated by the mandibular division of the trigeminal nerve.

Three large areas of the face can be mapped to indicate the peripheral nerve fields associated with the three divisions of the trigeminal nerve. The fields are not horizontal but curve upward (Fig. 11.11A), apparently because the facial skin moves upward with growth of the brain and skull. Embryologically, each division of the trigeminal nerve is associated with a developing facial process that gives rise to a specific area of the face in the adult. Thus the ophthalmic nerve is associated with the frontonasal process, the maxillary nerve with the maxillary process and the mandibular nerve with the mandibular process.

Ophthalmic Nerve

The ophthalmic nerve (Fig. 11.11B), a division of the trigeminal nerve, travels through the orbit to supply targets primarily in the upper part of the face. It arises from the trigeminal ganglion in the middle cranial fossa and passes forward along the lateral dural wall of the cavernous sinus. It gives off three main branches—the lacrimal, frontal and nasociliary nerves—just before it reaches the superior orbital fissure. The cutaneous branches of the ophthalmic nerve supply the conjunctiva, skin over the forehead, upper eyelids and much of the external surface of the nose.

Lacrimal Nerve

The lacrimal nerve enters the orbit through the superior orbital fissure, above the common tendinous ring of the recti muscles and lateral to the frontal and trochlear nerves (see Figs 11.4, 11.5, 11.8). It passes forward along the lateral wall of the orbit on the superior border of the lateral rectus and travels through the lacrimal gland and the orbital septum to supply conjunctiva and skin covering the lateral part of the upper eyelid. The lacrimal nerve communicates with the zygomatic branch of the maxillary nerve, so parasympathetic

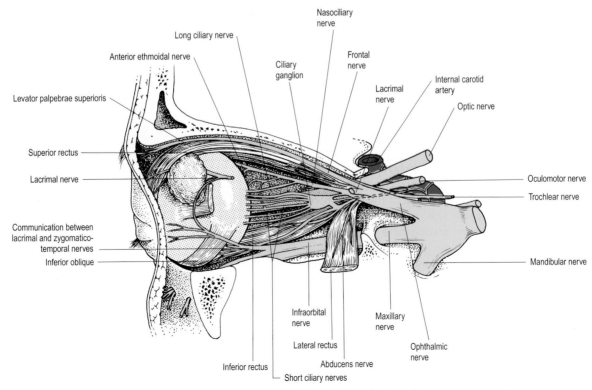

Fig. 11.5 *Nerves of the left orbit and the ciliary ganglion: lateral aspect.*

fibres associated with the pterygopalatine ganglion might be conveyed to the lacrimal gland.

Frontal Nerve

The frontal nerve is the largest branch of the ophthalmic nerve (see Figs 11.4, 11.5, 11.8). It enters the orbit through the superior orbital fissure, above the common tendinous ring of the recti muscles, and lies between the lacrimal nerve laterally and the trochlear nerve medially. It passes forward on the levator palpebrae superioris, toward the rim of the orbit; about halfway along this course it divides into the supraorbital and supratrochlear nerves.

The supraorbital nerve is the larger of the terminal branches of the frontal nerve. It continues forward along levator palpebrae superioris and leaves the orbit through the supraorbital notch or foramen to emerge onto the forehead. It ascends on the forehead with the supraorbital artery and divides into medial and lateral branches, which supply the skin of the scalp nearly as far back as the lambdoid suture. The supraorbital nerve supplies the mucous membrane that lines the frontal sinus, the skin and conjunctiva covering the upper eyelid and the skin over the forehead and scalp. The postganglionic sympathetic fibres that innervate the sweat glands of the supraorbital area probably travel in the supraorbital nerve, having entered the ophthalmic nerve through its communication with the abducens nerve within the cavernous sinus.

The supratrochlear nerve runs medially above the superior oblique pulley. It gives a descending branch to the infratrochlear nerve and ascends onto the forehead through the frontal notch to supply the skin and conjunctiva covering the upper eyelid and the skin over the forehead.

Nasociliary Nerve

The nasociliary nerve is intermediate in size between the frontal and lacrimal nerves and is more deeply placed in the orbit, which it enters through the

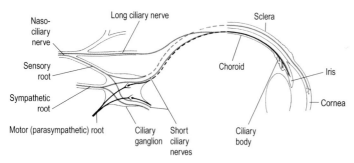

Fig. 11.6 *Ciliary ganglion, with its roots and branches of distribution.* Red, *sympathetic fibres;* heavy black, *parasympathetic fibres;* blue, *sensory (cerebrospinal) fibres. Alternative pathways are given for the sympathetic fibres.*

common tendinous ring, lying between the two rami of the oculomotor nerve (see Figs 11.4, 11.5, 11.8). It crosses the optic nerve with the ophthalmic artery and runs obliquely below superior rectus and superior oblique to reach the medial orbital wall. Here, as the anterior ethmoidal nerve, it passes through the anterior ethmoidal foramen and canal and enters the cranial cavity. It runs forward in a groove on the upper surface of the cribriform plate beneath the dura mater and descends through a slit lateral to the crista galli into the nasal cavity, where it occupies a groove on the internal surface of the nasal bone and gives off two internal nasal branches. The medial internal nasal nerve supplies the anterior septal mucosa, and the lateral internal nasal nerve supplies the anterior part of the lateral nasal wall. The anterior ethmoidal nerve emerges, as the external nasal nerve, at the lower border of the nasal bone and descends under the transverse part of the nasalis to supply the skin of the nasal alae, apex and vestibule.

The nasociliary nerve has connections with the ciliary ganglion and has long ciliary, infratrochlear and posterior ethmoidal branches.

The ramus communicans to the ciliary ganglion usually branches from the nerve as it enters the orbit lateral to the optic nerve. It is sometimes joined by a filament from the internal carotid sympathetic plexus or from the superior ramus of the oculomotor nerve as it enters the posterosuperior angle of the ganglion.

Two or three long ciliary nerves branch from the nasociliary nerve as it crosses the optic nerve (see Fig. 11.5). They accompany the short ciliary nerves and pierce the sclera near the attachment of the optic nerve. Running forward between the sclera and choroid, they supply the ciliary body, iris and cornea and are thought to contain postganglionic sympathetic fibres for the dilator pupillae from neurones in the superior cervical ganglion. An alternative pathway for the supply of the dilator pupillae is via the sympathetic root associated with the ciliary ganglion.

The posterior ethmoidal nerve leaves the orbit by the posterior ethmoidal foramen and supplies the ethmoidal and sphenoidal sinuses.

Maxillary Nerve

The maxillary nerve is a sensory division of the trigeminal nerve. Most of the branches from the maxillary nerve arise in the pterygopalatine fossa. It gives rise to the zygomatic and infraorbital nerves that pass into the orbit through the inferior orbital fissure and two others that pass through the pterygopalatine ganglion without synapsing and are distributed to the nose, palate and pharynx. The maxillary nerve passes through the orbit to supply the skin of the lower eyelid, the prominence of the cheek, the alar part of the nose, part of the temple and the upper lip.

Zygomatic Nerve

The zygomatic nerve is located close to the base of the lateral wall of the orbit. It soon divides into two branches—the zygomaticotemporal and zygomaticofacial nerves—which run for only a short distance in the orbit before

---

CASE 2   NUTRITIONAL AMBLYOPIA

A 58-year-old malnourished chronic alcoholic notes subacute loss of vision bilaterally. Examination demonstrates markedly reduced visual acuity in both eyes, with impairment of color vision and bilateral central scotomata on testing of the visual fields. His pupils respond sluggishly to direct light. The fundi do not appear unusual. There is no other neurological deficit.

Discussion: This man has nutritional amblyopia, sometimes referred to as tobacco-alcohol amblyopia. The clinical manifestations are due to bilateral involvement of the neural fibres constituting the macular projection system, resulting in a macular syndrome. The lesions predominate in the central portion of the optic nerves bilaterally, where the macular fibres are found, thus making it a disorder of the anterior conducting system (Fig. 11.7). Although tobacco use is sometimes implicated as a cause, this is in all likelihood a nutritional disorder due to deficiency of one or more B vitamins. It responds quickly to vitamin supplementation.

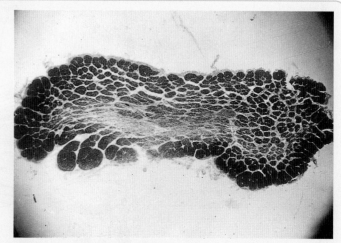

Fig. 11.7 *Deficiency amblyopia. Myelin sheath stain of a cross-section through an optic nerve in a case of deficiency (nutritional, tobacco-alcohol) amblyopia demonstrates degeneration in the fibres derived from the macula (papillomacular bundle). (From Victor, M., Mancall E.L., Dreyfus, P.M. Deficiency amblyopia in the alcoholic patient. Arch. Ophthalmol. 1960; 64, (1): 1–33. Copyright © 1960 American Medical Association. All rights reserved.)*

passing onto the face through the lateral wall of the orbit. Either these two branches enter separate canals within the zygomatic bone or the zygomatic nerve itself enters the bone before dividing.

The zygomaticotemporal nerve exits the zygomatic bone on its medial surface and pierces the temporal fascia to supply the skin over the temple. It

also gives a branch to the lacrimal nerve, which may carry parasympathetic fibres to the lacrimal gland (Figs 11.5, 11.13).

The zygomaticofacial nerve leaves the zygomatic bone on its lateral surface to supply skin overlying the prominence of the cheek.

Infraorbital Nerve

The infraorbital nerve emerges onto the face at the infraorbital foramen (see Fig. 11.5), where it lies between the levator labii superioris and levator anguli oris. It divides into three additional groups of branches. The palpebral branches ascend deep to orbicularis oculi and pierce the muscle to supply the skin of the lower eyelid and join with the facial and zygomaticofacial nerves near the lateral canthus. Nasal branches supply the skin of the side of the nose and movable part of the nasal septum and join the external nasal branch of the anterior ethmoidal nerve. Superior labial branches, large and numerous, descend behind levator labii superioris to supply the skin of the anterior part of the cheek and upper lip. They are joined by branches from the facial nerve to form the infraorbital plexus.

Orbital Branches of Pterygopalatine Ganglion

Several rami orbitales arise dorsally from the pterygopalatine ganglion and enter the orbit through the inferior orbital fissure. Branches leave the orbit through the posterior ethmoidal air sinus. There is strong experimental evidence from studies in animals, including monkeys, that postganglionic parasympathetic branches pass directly to the lacrimal gland, ophthalmic artery and choroid.

Mandibular Nerve

The mandibular nerve is the largest trigeminal division and is a mixed nerve (Figs 11.11, 11.13, 11.14). Its sensory branches supply the teeth and gums of the mandible; the skin in the temporal region; part of the auricle, including the external meatus and tympanic membrane, and the lower lip; the lower part of the face (see Fig. 11.11); and the mucosa of the anterior two-thirds (presulcal

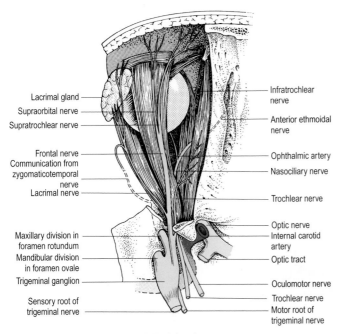

Lacrimal gland
Supraorbital nerve
Supratrochlear nerve

Frontal nerve
Communication from zygomaticotemporal nerve
Lacrimal nerve

Maxillary division in foramen rotundum
Mandibular division in foramen ovale
Trigeminal ganglion

Sensory root of trigeminal nerve

Infratrochlear nerve

Anterior ethmoidal nerve

Ophthalmic artery
Nasociliary nerve

Trochlear nerve

Optic nerve
Internal carotid artery

Optic tract

Oculomotor nerve

Trochlear nerve
Motor root of trigeminal nerve

Fig. 11.8 *Nerves of the left orbit: superior aspect.*

CASE 3   THYROID-ASSOCIATED OPHTHALMOPATHY (GRAVES' DISEASE)

A 45-year-old woman is referred for evaluation of a mild action tremor. She has a history of a mixed seizure disorder in the first two decades of her life, completely controlled by sodium divalproate. She subsequently complains of double vision, and neuro-ophthalmological a examination shows impaired up-gaze of the right eye with resultant vertical diplopia. There is slight lid retraction. Thyroid function testing reveals an elevated thyroxine (T_4) level and reduced thyroid-stimulating hormone (TSH). Orbital magnetic resonance imaging (MRI) documents thickening of the extraocular muscles, particularly involving the medial and inferior recti of the right eye (Fig. 11.9).

A diagnosis of thyroid-associated ophthalmopathy (Graves' disease) is made on the basis of the clinical presentation,

abnormalities on thyroid testing and MRI findings. Treatment of the hyperthyroidism with radioactive iodine and of the ophthalmopathy with prednisone results in resolution of the tremor and less lid retraction, although the patient continues to have slight limitation of up-gaze in the right eye.

Discussion: Thyroid-associated ophthalmopathy (Graves' disease) is a complicated and multifaceted disorder thought to be of autoimmune origin, usually occurring in association with demonstrable hyperthyroidism. Plasma cells, lymphocytes and mast cells migrate into the orbital tissues and extraocular muscles, with deposition of hydrophilic glycosaminoglycans and collagen. In some cases, the neuro-ophthalmological features may precede the clinical and laboratory manifestations of hyperthyroidism.

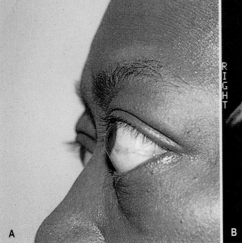
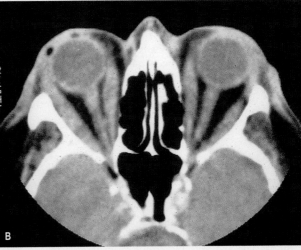

Fig. 11.9 *Thyrotoxicosis (Graves' disease).* **A,** *Exophthalmos is evident clinically.* **B,** *MRI demonstrates thickening of the extraocular muscles in the orbits.*

CASE 4   DIABETIC THIRD NERVE PALSY

A 48-year-old obese, hypertensive woman with a 7-year history of type 2 diabetes mellitus treated with an oral hypoglycemic agent suddenly develops left orbital pain and double vision. The double vision is sometimes vertical, sometimes horizontal. Upon awakening the next morning, she is unable to open her left eye. Evaluation later that same day shows nearly complete ptosis of the left lid; slight exodeviation of the left eye when attempting to look straight ahead, with complete ophthalmoplegia except for intact abduction, and slight anisocoria, the left pupil being 1 mm larger than the right in ambient room light with normal pupillary constriction to light and accommodation.

MRI of the brain demonstrates small, scattered areas of increased signal intensity on the T2-weighted and FLAIR images. Her fasting blood glucose level is 190 mg/dl. Magnetic resonance angiography of the intracranial vessels demonstrates mild irregularities in the distal carotid and middle cerebral arteries bilaterally, consistent with atherosclerotic disease.

Two months later the patient is entirely normal except for persistent mild left ptosis.

Discussion: Vasculopathic third nerve palsies are most commonly associated with diabetes mellitus and usually come under the rubric of diabetic ophthalmoplegia. Other conditions associated with microvascular disease, such as hypertension and dyslipidemia, may also be responsible. Most cases are thought to be the result of ischaemia affecting the central portion of the oculomotor nerve, sparing the peripherally located pupillary fibre bundle; nonetheless, a small proportion of patients exhibits minor pupillary involvement. In contrast, compressive third nerve palsies, such as those associated with an intracranial aneurysm, almost always have marked pupillary involvement and usually present with more pain. See Figure 11.10.

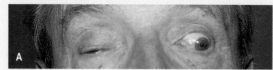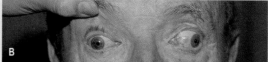

Fig. 11.10 *Third cranial nerve palsy (diabetic ophthalmoplegia) evidenced by eyelid ptosis (**A**) and inability to direct the involved eye medially on request (**B**).*

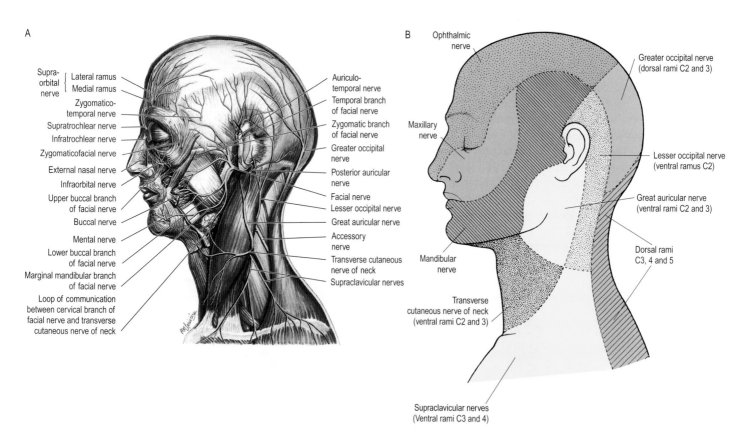

Fig. 11.11 *A, Sensory nerves of the left side of the scalp, face and neck, and the branches of the facial nerve, which are distributed to the muscles of 'facial expression.' The pinna has been reflected forward. **B**, Cutaneous innervation of the face and neck, showing dermatomes.*

part) of the tongue and floor of the oral cavity. The motor branches innervate the muscles of mastication. The large sensory root emerges from the lateral part of the trigeminal ganglion and exits the cranial cavity through the foramen ovale. The small motor root passes under the ganglion and through the foramen ovale to unite with the sensory root just outside the skull. As it descends from the foramen ovale, the nerve is approximately 4 cm from the surface and a little anterior to the neck of the mandible. The mandibular nerve immediately passes between tensor veli palatini, which is medial, and lateral pterygoid, which is lateral, and gives off a meningeal branch and nerve to the medial pterygoid from its medial side. The nerve then divides into small anterior and large posterior trunks. The anterior division gives off branches to the four main muscles of mastication and a buccal branch that

CASE 5   HERPES ZOSTER OPHTHALMICUS

A 32-year-old woman is referred for pain in the right side of the forehead. Pain in the right supraorbital region spreading into the right superior frontal region began several days before the initial evaluation and was unremitting. She has a prior history of migraine and is being treated for non-Hodgkin's lymphoma, with good response to chemotherapy. Her only other complaint is mild photophobia in the right eye.

The initial neurological examination demonstrates slightly decreased pin appreciation in the territory of the ophthalmic division of the right trigeminal nerve but is otherwise normal. There is slight conjunctival injection. One day later she reports a rash, and evaluation shows several vesicles in the right supraorbital region, with intense right conjunctival injection. Visual acuity is decreased in the right eye. Ocular motility is normal.

She is diagnosed with herpes zoster ophthalmicus. Within several days, vesicles appear in the territory of the ophthalmic division of the right trigeminal nerve, along with keratitis, conjunctivitis and iritis of the right eye (Fig. 11.12).

Treatment with acyclovir is instituted. Pain largely subsides after a week, and after several more weeks the vesicles begin to heal. Her vision returns to near normal.

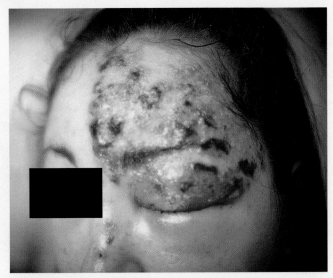

Fig. 11.12 Herpes zoster ophthalmicus. The distribution of the ophthalmic division of the trigeminal nerve (VI) is sharply demarcated by the crusting herpetic lesions.

CASE 6   TRIGEMINAL NEURALGIA

A 63-year-old woman, previously well, complains of severe intermittent, paroxysmal, lancinating right facial pain of 8 months' duration. The pain generally begins just anterior to the ear, radiating in lightning-like fashion to the lower jaw and occasionally to the upper jaw as well. Attacks of pain may be precipitated by speaking, chewing or swallowing or by minor cutaneous stimulation. These attacks last up to 15 minutes and recur at unpredictable intervals. Facial grimacing or tearing may accompany these episodes, but no other neurological changes have been observed, and the neurological examination is normal.

Discussion: This woman describes typical trigeminal neuralgia (tic douloureux). The cause is generally unknown; in younger patients, multiple sclerosis may be implicated. Degenerative changes in the Gasserian ganglion, compression of the ganglion by tumour and vascular compression of the trigeminal nerve have been described in individual patients. Pain classically radiates along the peripheral distribution of the branches of the trigeminal nerve, most commonly the mandibular and maxillary divisions. Typically, examination demonstrates no abnormality. Management, whether pharmacological or surgical, is often unsatisfactory.

Nerve to medial pterygoid — The nerve to the medial pterygoid is a slender ramus that enters the deep aspect of the muscle. It supplies one or two filaments that pass through the otic ganglion without interruption to supply tensor tympani and tensor veli palatini (see Fig. 11.14).

Anterior Trunk

The anterior trunk of the mandibular nerve gives rise to the buccal nerve, which is sensory, and the masseteric, deep temporal and lateral pterygoid nerves, which are motor.

Buccal nerve — The buccal nerve (Fig. 11.15) passes between the two heads of the lateral pterygoid. It descends deep to the temporalis tendon, passes laterally in front of the masseter, and anastomoses with the buccal branches of the facial nerve. It carries the motor fibres to the lateral pterygoid, and these are given off as the buccal nerve passes through the muscle. It may also give off the anterior deep temporal nerve. The buccal nerve supplies sensation to the skin over the anterior part of the buccinator and buccal mucous membrane, together with the posterior part of the buccal gingivae adjacent to the second and third molar teeth.

Nerve to masseter — The nerve to the masseter (see Fig. 11.15) passes laterally above the lateral pterygoid and on to the skull base, anterior to the temporomandibular joint and posterior to the temporalis tendon. It crosses the posterior part of the mandibular notch with the masseteric artery and ramifies on and enters the deep surface of the masseter. It also provides articular branches that supply the temporomandibular joint.

Deep temporal nerves — The deep temporal nerves usually consist of two branches, anterior and posterior, although there may be a middle branch. They pass above the lateral pterygoid to enter the deep surface of the temporalis. The anterior nerve frequently arises as a branch of the buccal nerve. The small posterior nerve sometimes arises in common with the nerve to the masseter.

Nerve to lateral pterygoid — The nerve to the lateral pterygoid enters the deep surface of the muscle. It may arise separately from the anterior division of the mandibular nerve or from the buccal nerve.

Posterior Trunk

The posterior trunk of the mandibular nerve is larger than the anterior and is mainly sensory, although it receives fibres from the motor root for the nerve to the mylohyoid. It divides into auriculotemporal, lingual and inferior alveolar (dental) nerves.

Auriculotemporal nerve — The auriculotemporal nerve usually has two roots that encircle the middle meningeal artery (see Figs 11.13, 11.14). It runs back under the lateral pterygoid on the surface of tensor veli palatini, passes between the sphenomandibular ligament and neck of the mandible and then runs laterally behind the temporomandibular joint related to the upper part

is sensory to the cheek. The posterior division gives off three main sensory branches—the auriculotemporal, lingual and inferior alveolar nerves—and motor fibres to supply the mylohyoid and anterior belly of the digastric (see Figs 11.13, 11.14).

Meningeal branch — The meningeal branch (nervus spinosus) reenters the cranium through the foramen spinosum with the middle meningeal artery. It divides into anterior and posterior branches that accompany the main divisions of the middle meningeal artery and supply the dura mater in the middle cranial fossa and, to a lesser extent, in the anterior fossa and calvaria.

A

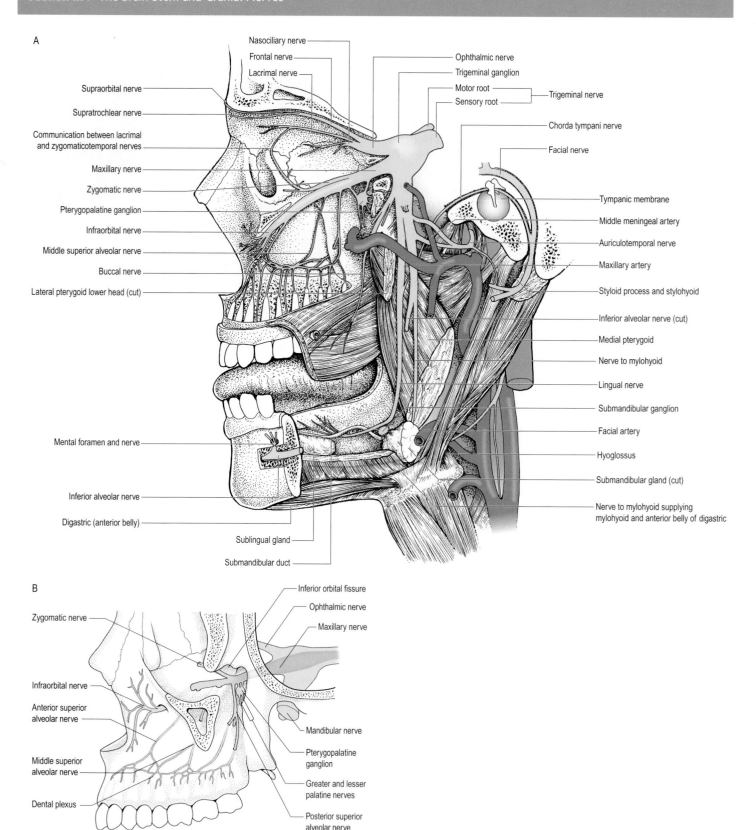

Nasociliary nerve
Frontal nerve
Lacrimal nerve
Ophthalmic nerve
Trigeminal ganglion
Motor root
Sensory root
Trigeminal nerve
Supraorbital nerve
Supratrochlear nerve
Communication between lacrimal and zygomaticotemporal nerves
Chorda tympani nerve
Facial nerve
Maxillary nerve
Zygomatic nerve
Pterygopalatine ganglion
Tympanic membrane
Infraorbital nerve
Middle meningeal artery
Middle superior alveolar nerve
Auriculotemporal nerve
Buccal nerve
Maxillary artery
Lateral pterygoid lower head (cut)
Styloid process and stylohyoid
Inferior alveolar nerve (cut)
Medial pterygoid
Nerve to mylohyoid
Lingual nerve
Submandibular ganglion
Facial artery
Mental foramen and nerve
Hyoglossus
Submandibular gland (cut)
Inferior alveolar nerve
Digastric (anterior belly)
Nerve to mylohyoid supplying mylohyoid and anterior belly of digastric
Sublingual gland
Submandibular duct

B

Zygomatic nerve
Inferior orbital fissure
Ophthalmic nerve
Maxillary nerve
Infraorbital nerve
Anterior superior alveolar nerve
Mandibular nerve
Pterygopalatine ganglion
Middle superior alveolar nerve
Greater and lesser palatine nerves
Dental plexus
Posterior superior alveolar nerve

Fig. 11.13 *A and B, Left ophthalmic, maxillary and mandibular nerves and the submandibular and pterygopalatine ganglia.*

of the parotid gland. Emerging from behind the joint, it ascends over the posterior root of the zygoma, posterior to the superficial temporal vessels, and divides into superficial temporal branches. It communicates with the facial nerve and otic ganglion. The rami to the facial nerve, usually two, pass anterolaterally behind the neck of the mandible to join the facial nerve at the posterior border of the masseter. Filaments from the otic ganglion join the roots of the auriculotemporal nerve close to their origin (Figs 11.14, 11.16). The cutaneous branches of the auriculotemporal nerve supply the tragus and part of the adjoining auricle of the ear and posterior part of the temple.

Lingual nerve — The lingual nerve (see Figs 11.13–11.15) is sensory to the mucosa of the anterior two-thirds of the tongue, the floor of the mouth and the mandibular lingual gingivae. It arises from the posterior trunk of the man-dibular nerve and at first runs beneath the lateral pterygoid and superficial to

tensor veli palatini, where it is joined by the chorda tympani branch of the facial nerve and often by a branch of the inferior alveolar nerve. Emerging from under cover of the lateral pterygoid, the lingual nerve then runs down-ward and forward on the surface of the medial pterygoid and is thus carried progressively closer to the medial surface of the mandibular ramus. It becomes intimately related to the bone a few millimetres below and behind the junc-tion of the vertical ramus and horizontal body of the mandible. Here it lies anterior to, and slightly deeper than, the inferior alveolar (dental) nerve. It next passes below the mandibular attachment of the superior pharyngeal constrictor and pterygomandibular raphe, closely applied to the periosteum of the medial surface of the mandible, until it lies opposite the posterior root of the third molar tooth, where it is covered only by the gingival mucoperi-osteum. At this point it usually lies 2 to 3 mm below the alveolar crest and

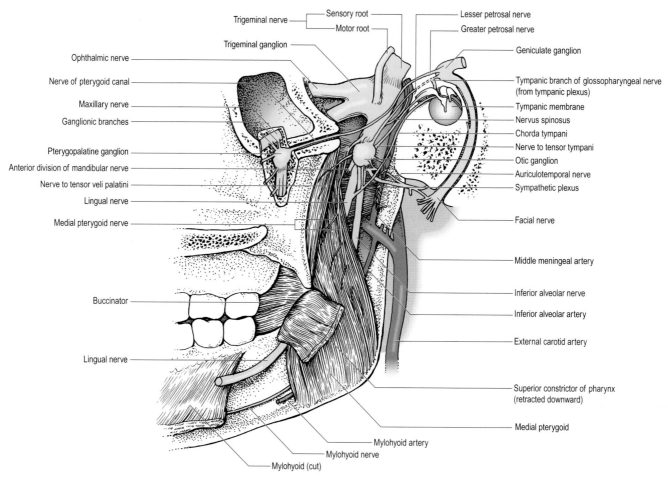

Fig. 11.14 *Right otic and pterygopalatine ganglia and their branches displayed from the medial side.*

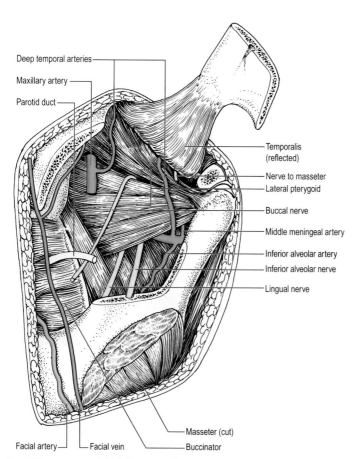

Fig. 11.15 *Dissection of the left pterygoid region, showing some of the branches of the mandibular nerve and maxillary artery. The temporalis and the coronoid process of the mandible have been reflected upward. The masseter has been removed (with the exception of a small inferior portion). The zygomatic arch has also been removed.*

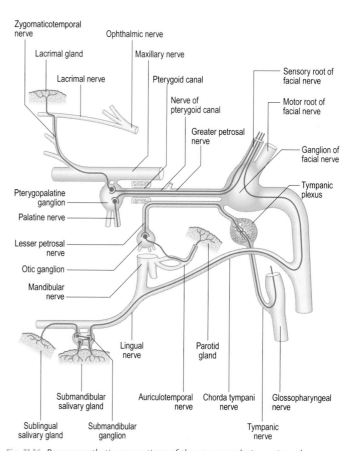

Fig. 11.16 *Parasympathetic connections of the pterygopalatine, otic and submandibular ganglia. The parasympathetic fibres, both pre- and postganglionic, are shown as blue lines. The parasympathetic fibres in the palatine nerves are secretomotor to the nasal, palatine and pharyngeal glands.*

0.6 mm from the bone; however, in approximately 5% of cases, it lies above the alveolar crest. It next passes medial to the mandibular origin of mylohyoid, and this carries it progressively away from the mandible and separates it from the alveolar bone covering the mesial root of the third molar tooth.

Inferior alveolar nerve — The inferior alveolar (dental) nerve descends behind the lateral pterygoid. At the lower border of the muscle the nerve passes between the sphenomandibular ligament and the mandibular ramus and enters the mandibular canal via the mandibular foramen. Below the lateral pterygoid it is accompanied by the inferior alveolar artery, a branch of the first part of the maxillary artery, which also enters the canal with associated veins. The mental nerve is the terminal branch of the inferior alveolar nerve. It enters the face through the mental foramen, where it is directed backward. It supplies the skin of the lower lip.

CASE 7   MENTAL NEUROPATHY

A 64-year-old woman with no recognized prior illness develops pain and numbness in a very restricted pattern in the left lower jaw. She has no known dental problems. On examination, pain appreciation is found to be decreased in a sharply limited zone involving the skin over the left mandible, below the lower lip and extending to but not beyond the midline. The examination is otherwise normal.

Neuroimaging demonstrates a lytic lesion in the left mandible, involving the mental foramen. The patient is found to have a mass in her left breast, which is proved on biopsy to be carcinomatous. No lesions are found elsewhere.

Discussion: This woman has a very focal neuropathy involving the left mental nerve, a branch of the inferior alveolar nerve, as it exits the left mental foramen. As in this patient, the majority of cases of so-called mental neuropathy are due to metastatic disease.

ABDUCENS NERVE (VI)

The abducens nerve is the sixth cranial nerve, and it emerges from the brainstem between the pons and the medulla oblongata (see Figs 11.5, 11.35). It is related to the cavernous sinus, but unlike the oculomotor, trochlear, ophthalmic and maxillary nerves, which merely invaginate the lateral dural wall, it passes through the sinus itself, lying lateral to the internal carotid artery (see Fig. 4.6). The abducens nerve enters the orbit through the superior orbital fissure, within the common tendinous ring of the recti muscles (see Fig. 11.3), at first below and then between the two divisions of the oculomotor nerve and lateral to the nasociliary nerve. It passes forward to enter the medial (ocular) surface of the lateral rectus, which is its sole target.

FACIAL NERVE (VII)

The facial nerve enters the temporal bone through the internal acoustic meatus accompanied by the vestibulocochlear nerve (Fig. 11.18; see also Fig. 10.20). At this point, the motor root, which supplies the muscles of the face, and the nervus intermedius, which contains sensory fibres concerned with the perception of taste and parasympathetic (secretomotor) fibres to various glands, are separate components. They merge within the meatus. At the end of the meatus, the facial nerve enters its own canal, the facial canal, which runs across the medial wall and down the posterior wall of the tympanic cavity to the stylomastoid foramen (Fig. 11.19). As the nerve enters the facial canal, there is a bend that contains the geniculate ganglion (Figs 11.18, 11.20). The branches that arise from the facial nerve within the temporal bone can be divided into those that come from the geniculate ganglion and those that arise within the facial canal.

The main branch from the geniculate ganglion is the greater (superficial) petrosal nerve. It is a branch of the nervus intermedius. The greater petrosal nerve passes anteriorly, receives a branch from the tympanic plexus and traverses a hiatus on the anterior surface of the petrous part of the temporal bone. It enters the middle cranial fossa and runs forward in a groove on the bone above the lesser petrosal nerve. It passes beneath the trigeminal ganglion to reach the foramen lacerum. There it is joined by the deep petrosal nerve from the internal carotid sympathetic plexus to become the nerve of the pterygoid canal (Vidian's nerve). The greater petrosal nerve contains parasympathetic fibres destined for the pterygopalatine ganglion and taste fibres from the palate.

The nerve to the stapedius arises from the facial nerve in the facial nerve canal behind the pyramidal eminence of the posterior wall of the tympanic cavity. It passes forward through a small canal to reach the muscle.

The chorda tympani (Figs 11.14, 11.21) leaves the facial nerve approximately 6 mm above the stylomastoid foramen and runs anterosuperiorly in a canal to enter the tympanic cavity via the posterior canaliculus. It then curves anteriorly in the substance of the tympanic membrane between its mucous and fibrous layers (Fig. 11.22) and crosses medial to the upper part of the handle of the malleus to the anterior wall, where it enters the anterior canaliculus (Fig. 11.23). It exits the skull at the petrotympanic fissure. It contains parasympathetic fibres that supply the submandibular and sublingual salivary glands via the submandibular ganglion (see Fig. 11.16) and taste fibres from the anterior two-thirds of the tongue.

The geniculate ganglion also communicates with the lesser petrosal nerve.

The facial nerve emerges from the base of the skull at the stylomastoid foramen. At this point, the facial nerve lies approximately 9 mm from the posterior belly of the digastric muscle and 11 mm from the bony external acoustic meatus. It gains access to the face by passing through the substance of the parotid gland. Although mainly motor, there are some cutaneous fibres

CASE 8   SIXTH CRANIAL NERVE PALSY

A 61-year-old woman with diabetes and hypertension complains of double vision while looking to the left. On examination, she has incomplete paralysis of gaze past the midline bilaterally, worse in the left eye (Fig. 11.17). Upward gaze is also slightly impaired. She complains of headache and difficulty walking. Neuroimaging reveals a posterior fossa ependymoma with hydrocephalus. She undergoes a suboccipital craniectomy for resection of the ependymoma; after several months, her vision returns to normal.

Discussion: Sixth cranial nerve (abducens) palsies may occur as a complication of hydrocephalus and may be present bilaterally or unilaterally. The precise pathophysiology is unknown but is thought to be related to the long intracranial course of the nerve. Other causes of isolated abducens nerve palsies include nerve infarction (microvascular abducens palsy), skull base tumour, otitis media, trauma or post viral infection. Myasthenia gravis may mimic an abducens palsy.

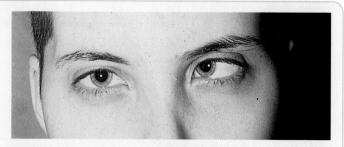

Fig. 11.17 *Abducens palsy in a case of obstructive hydrocephalus due to an ependymoma.*

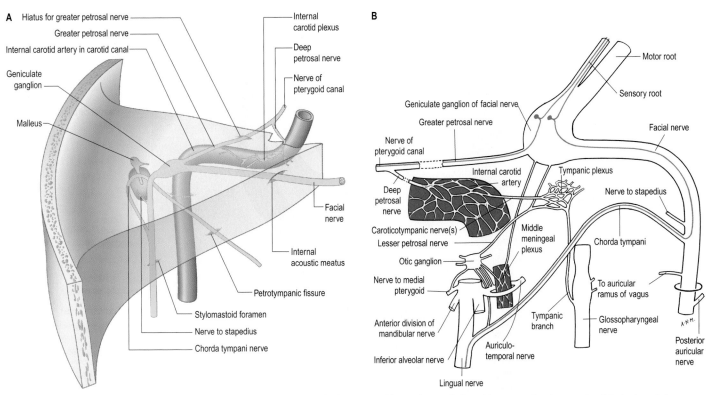

Fig. 11.18 *Facial nerve.* **A**, *Course of the facial nerve and its branches through the temporal bone; the vestibulocochlear nerve has been omitted.* **B**, *A plan of the intrapetrous section of the facial nerve, its branches and communications. The course of the taste fibres from the mucous membrane of the palate and from the anterior presulcal part of the tongue is represented by blue lines.* (**A**, *Reprinted by permission from Hall-Craggs, E.C.B., 1986. Anatomy as a Basis for Clinical Medicine, 2nd ed. Baltimore, Urban and Schwarzenberg.*)

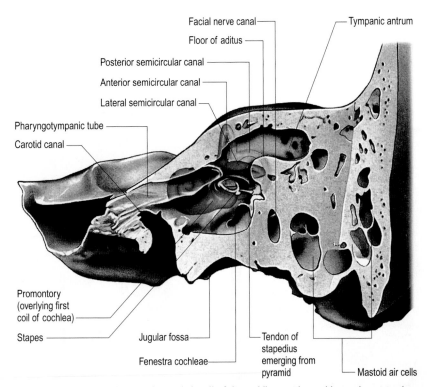

Fig. 11.19 *Oblique section through the left temporal bone, showing the medial wall of the middle ear. The cochlea and semicircular canals are in blue. Note the relationship of the first coil of the cochlea to the promontory and the closeness of the facial nerve canal and the lateral semicircular canal to the medial wall of the aditus.*

from the facial nerve that accompany the auricular branch of the vagus and probably innervate the skin on both auricular aspects, in the conchal depression and over its eminence.

Close to the stylomastoid foramen the facial nerve gives off the posterior auricular nerve, which supplies the occipital belly of occipitofrontalis and some of the auricular muscles, and the nerves to the posterior belly of the digastric and stylohyoid. The nerve then enters the parotid gland high up on the posteromedial surface and passes forward and downward behind the mandibular ramus. Within the substance of the gland, the facial nerve branches

into the temporofacial and cervicofacial trunks, just behind (within about 5 mm of) the retromandibular vein. In approximately 90% of cases, the two trunks lie superficial to the vein, in intimate contact with it. Occasionally (temporofacial trunk, about 9% of cases; cervicofacial trunk, about 2%), the trunks pass beneath the retromandibular vein. The trunks branch farther to form a parotid plexus (pes anserinus), which exhibits variations in its branching pattern. Five main terminal branches arise from the plexus and diverge within the gland. They leave the parotid gland by its anteromedial surface, medial to its anterior margin, and supply the muscles of facial expression.

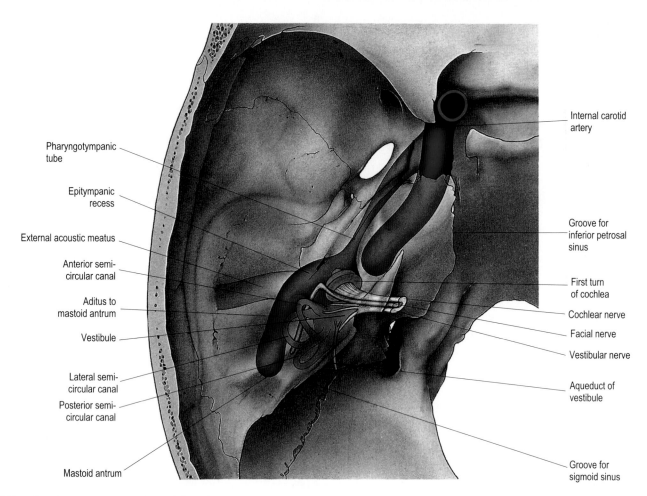

Pharyngotympanic tube

Epitympanic recess

External acoustic meatus

Anterior semi-circular canal

Aditus to mastoid antrum

Vestibule

Lateral semi-circular canal

Posterior semi-circular canal

Mastoid antrum

Internal carotid artery

Groove for inferior petrosal sinus

First turn of cochlea

Cochlear nerve

Facial nerve

Vestibular nerve

Aqueduct of vestibule

Groove for sigmoid sinus

Fig. 11.20 *Left auditory apparatus, as if viewed through a semitransparent temporal bone. Compare with Figure 11.19. Note the bend (genu) in the facial nerve at the site of the geniculate ganglion.*

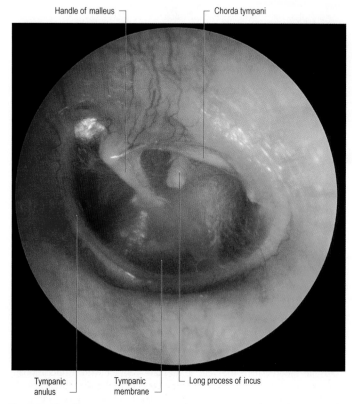

Handle of malleus

Chorda tympani

Tympanic anulus

Tympanic membrane

Long process of incus

Fig. 11.21 *Chorda tympani nerve crossing the tympanic membrane. (Courtesy of Mr. Simon A. Hickey.)*

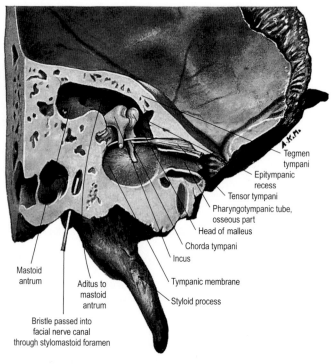

Tegmen tympani

Epitympanic recess

Tensor tympani

Pharyngotympanic tube, osseous part

Head of malleus

Chorda tympani

Incus

Tympanic membrane

Styloid process

Mastoid antrum

Aditus to mastoid antrum

Bristle passed into facial nerve canal through stylomastoid foramen

Fig. 11.22 *Oblique vertical section through the left temporal bone, showing the roof and lateral wall of the middle ear and the mastoid antrum.*

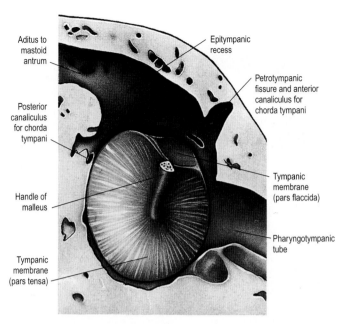

Fig. 11.23 *Lateral wall of the left tympanic cavity.*

The temporal branches are generally multiple and pass across the zygomatic arch to the temple to supply intrinsic muscles on the lateral surface of the auricle and the anterior and superior auricular muscles. They join with the zygomaticotemporal branch of the maxillary nerve and the auriculotemporal branch of the mandibular nerve. The more anterior branches supply the frontal belly of occipitofrontalis, orbicularis oculi and corrugator and join the supraorbital and lacrimal branches of the ophthalmic nerve.

Zygomatic branches are generally multiple and cross the zygomatic bone to the lateral canthus of the eye, supplying orbicularis oculi, and join filaments of the lacrimal nerve and zygomaticofacial branch of the maxillary nerve. The branches may also help supply muscles associated with the buccal branch of the facial nerve.

The buccal branch has a variable origin and passes horizontally to a distribution below the orbit and around the mouth. It is usually single, but two branches occur in 15% of cases. The buccal branch has a close relationship to the parotid duct and usually lies below it. Superficial branches run deep to subcutaneous fat and the superficial musculo-aponeurotic system. Some branches pass deep to procerus and join the infratrochlear and external nasal nerves. Upper deep branches pass under the zygomaticus major and levator labii superioris, supply them and form an infraorbital plexus with the superior labial branches of the infraorbital nerve. They also supply levator anguli oris, zygomaticus minor, levator labii superioris alaequae nasi and the small nasal muscles. These branches are sometimes described as lower zygomatic branches. Lower deep branches supply the buccinator and orbicularis oris and join filaments of the buccal branch of the mandibular nerve.

The marginal mandibular branches, of which there are usually two, run forward toward the angle of the mandible under platysma, at first superficial to the upper part of the digastric triangle, then turning up and running forward across the body of the mandible to pass under depressor anguli oris. The branches supply risorius and the muscles of the lower lip and chin and join the mental nerve. The marginal mandibular branch has an important surgical relationship with the lower border of the mandible and may pass below the lower border with a reported incidence of 20% to 50%, the farthest distance being 1.2 cm.

The cervical branch issues from the lower part of the parotid gland and runs anteroinferiorly under platysma to the front of the neck, to supply platysma and communicate with the transverse cutaneous cervical nerve. In 20% of cases there are two branches.

The peripheral branches of the facial nerve just described are joined by anastomotic arcades between adjacent branches to form the parotid plexus of nerves, which shows considerable variation. In surgical terms, these anastomoses are important and presumably explain why accidental or essential division of a small branch often fails to result in the expected facial nerve weakness. Six distinctive anastomotic patterns were originally classified by Davis and colleagues (1956) and are illustrated in Figure 11.24. These observations have been confirmed by others, although some variation in the frequency has been reported.

Facial Nerve Lesions

Facial nerve paralysis may be due to an upper motor neurone lesion (when frontalis is partially spared due to bilateral innervation of the muscle of the

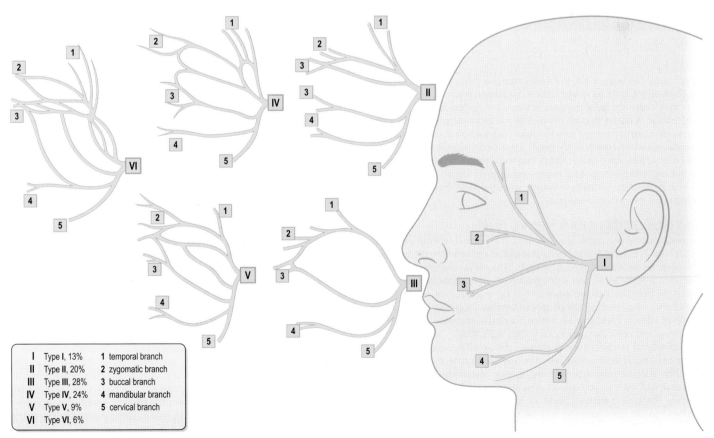

I	Type I, 13%	1	temporal branch
II	Type II, 20%	2	zygomatic branch
III	Type III, 28%	3	buccal branch
IV	Type IV, 24%	4	mandibular branch
V	Type V, 9%	5	cervical branch
VI	Type VI, 6%		

Fig. 11.24 *Patterns of branching of the facial nerve. (Modified with permission from Berkovitz, B.K.B., Moxham, B.J., Head and Neck Anatomy. 2002. © 2002 Informa Healthcare and from Davis, R.A., Anson, B.J., Budinger, J.M., Kurth, I.E., 1956. Surgical anatomy of the facial nerve and parotid gland based upon a study of 350 cervicofacial halves. Surg. Gynecol. Obstet. 102, 385–412, with permission from the American College of Surgeons.)*

CASE 9   BELL'S PALSY

A 36-year-old previously healthy woman presents with a 2-day history of drooling from the left corner of her mouth. Later in the day that the drooling began, she noted a tendency for food to become lodged between her left cheek and left lower gum while eating. She could not whistle or purse her lips. The next morning she awoke with left retro-auricular pain. When she attempted to brush her teeth, she noticed that the left side of her mouth did not move; when she blinked, her left eyelid did not fully close. When applying makeup, she observed that the left eyebrow was lower than the right. During breakfast she noted a disturbed sense of taste and mildly slurred speech.

Neurological evaluation the next day documents near complete paralysis of the left facial muscles, including frontalis, orbicularis oculi, orbicularis oris, platysma and buccinator. A Schirmer test reveals decreased left eye tearing. There is decreased perception of taste on the anterior two-thirds of the tongue on the involved side. Inspection of the left ear and external auditory canal demonstrates no vesicles suggestive of herpes zoster, and results of routine laboratory tests are normal. Serum Lyme titres are negative.

Discussion: This woman has typical Bell's palsy, or idiopathic peripheral facial palsy (Fig. 11.25). The seventh cranial (facial) nerve has a complex anatomy and subserves multiple functions. Idiopathic facial palsy is most often the result of a lesion (probably inflammatory) within the confines of the fallopian canal. This often impacts the greater superficial petrosal nerve (decreased tearing), nerve to the stapedius (hyperacusis) and chorda tympani (dysgeusia, with impaired taste on the ipsilateral anterior two-thirds of the tongue), in addition to the main branch of the facial nerve (ipsilateral facial paralysis and subtle sensory disturbance in the region of the ipsilateral ear).

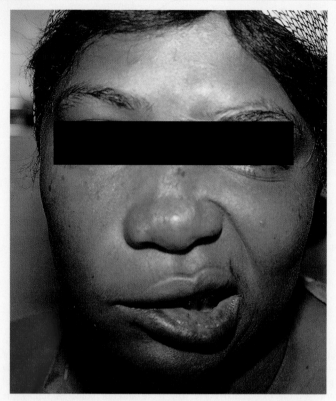

Fig. 11.25 Bell's palsy. Weakness reflecting involvement of both the upper and lower divisions of the facial nerve is evident when the patient attempts to smile or elevate the eyebrow.

upper part of the face) or a lower motor neurone lesion (when all branches may be involved). Bell's palsy and acoustic neuromas can produce a complete lower motor neurone facial paralysis as a result of compression of the facial nerve trunk as it passes through the middle ear. More commonly, cheek lacerations or malignant parotid tumours result in weakness in part of the face, depending on which branch of the nerve is involved. Unfortunately, the presence of facial paralysis is not a reliable diagnostic sign of a malignant tumour. It is not uncommon for a facial nerve infiltrated by a malignant tumour to continue to function normally. However, when paralysis does accompany a parotid mass, it is certainly malignant.

VESTIBULOCOCHLEAR NERVE (VIII)

The vestibulocochlear nerve emerges from the pontocerebellar angle (Fig. 11.35). It courses through the posterior cranial fossa to enter the petrous temporal bone via the internal acoustic meatus, where it divides into an anterior trunk, the cochlear nerve, and a posterior trunk, the vestibular nerve. Both contain the centrally directed axons of bipolar neurones, the cell bodies of which are situated close to their peripheral terminals, together with a smaller number of efferent fibres that arise from brain stem neurones and terminate on cochlear and vestibular sensory cells (Figs. 11.20, 11.29).

In audiological practice, it is important to distinguish between intratemporal and intracranial lesions. However, it is relevant to note that this surgical distinction does not correlate with the precise anatomical descriptions of peripheral and central portions of the auditory and vestibular systems. Clinically, the term 'peripheral auditory lesion' is used to describe lesions peripheral to the spiral ganglion, and the term 'peripheral vestibular disturbance' includes lesions of the vestibular ganglion and the entire vestibular nerve. Furthermore, the intratemporal portion of the vestibulocochlear nerve in humans consists of two histologically distinct portions: a central glial zone adjacent to the brain stem, and a peripheral or non-glial zone. In the glial zone,

the axons are supported by central neuroglia, whereas in the non-glial zone, they are ensheathed by Schwann cells. The non-glial zone extends into the cerebellopontine angle medial to the internal acoustic meatus in more than 50% of human vestibulocochlear nerves.

Intratemporal Vestibular Nerve

The maculae and crests are innervated by dendrites of bipolar neurones in the vestibular (Scarpa's) ganglion situated in the trunk of the nerve within the lateral end of the internal auditory meatus (Fig. 11.27).

The peripheral processes of the ganglion cells are aggregated into definable nerves, each with a specific distribution (Fig. 11.28). The main nerve divides at and within the ganglion into superior and inferior divisions, which are connected by an isthmus. The superior division, the larger of the two, passes through the small holes in the superior vestibular area to supply the ampullary crests of the lateral and anterior semicircular canals via the lateral and anterior ampullary nerves, respectively. A secondary branch of the lateral ampullary nerve supplies the macula of the utricle; however, the greater part of the utricular macula is innervated by the utricular nerve, which is a separate branch of the superior division. Another branch of the superior division, Voit's nerve, supplies part of the saccule.

The inferior division of the vestibular nerve passes through small holes in the inferior vestibular area to supply the remainder of the saccule and the posterior ampullary crest via saccular and singular branches, respectively; the latter passes through the foramen singulare. Occasionally, a very small supplementary or accessory branch supplies the posterior crest; it is probably a vestigial remnant of the crista neglecta, an additional area of sensory epithelium found in some other mammals but seldom in humans.

Afferent and efferent cochlear fibres are also present in the inferior division of the vestibular nerve, but they leave at the anastomosis of Oort to join the main cochlear nerve (see review by Warr 1992). Another anastomosis, the

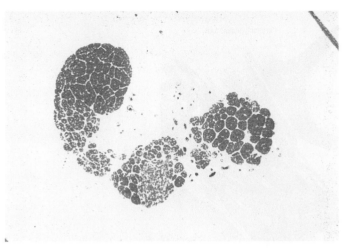

Fig. 11.26 *Human vestibulocochlear nerve, in transverse section. On the left, the cochlear nerve (seen as a comma-shaped profile) abuts the inferior division of the vestibular nerve* (right). *The singular nerve is a separate fascicle between the superior and inferior divisions of the vestibular nerve. (Courtesy of H. Felix, M. Gleeson and L.-G. Johnsson, ENT Department, University of Zurich and GKT School of Medicine, London.)*

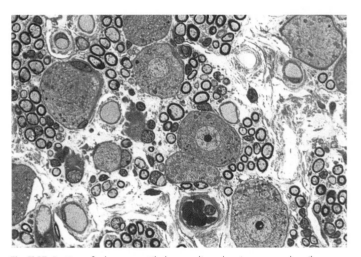

Fig. 11.27 *Portion of a human vestibular ganglion, showing neuronal perikarya, myelinated axons and small blood vessels* (toluidine blue stained resin section). *(Courtesy of H. Felix, M. Gleeson and L.-G. Johnsson, ENT Department, University of Zurich and GKT School of Medicine, London.)*

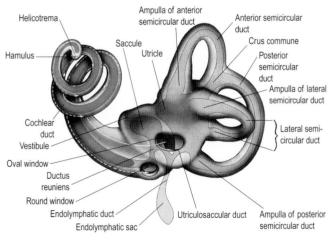

Fig. 11.28 *The membranous labyrinth* (blue) *projected onto the bony labyrinth. The* arrows indicate the direction of pressure waves in the cochlea.

vestibulofacial anastomosis, is situated more centrally between the facial and vestibular nerves and is the point at which fibres originating in the intermediate nerve pass from the vestibular nerve to the main trunk of the facial nerve.

There are approximately 20,000 fibres in the vestibular nerve, of which 12,000 travel in the superior division and 8000 in the inferior division. The distribution of fibre diameters is bimodal, with peaks at 4 and 6.5 μm. The smaller fibres go mainly to the Type II hair cells, and the larger fibres tend to supply the Type I hair cells. In addition to the afferents, efferent and

autonomic fibres have been identified. Efferent fibres synapse exclusively with the afferent calyceal terminals around Type I cells and usually with the afferent boutons on Type II cells, although a few are in direct contact with the cell bodies of Type II cells. The autonomic fibres do not contact vestibular sensory cells but terminate beneath the sensory epithelia. Two distinct sympathetic components have been identified in the vestibular ganglion: a perivascular adrenergic system derived from the stellate ganglion, and a blood vessel–independent system derived from the superior cervical ganglion.

The cell bodies of the bipolar neurones that contribute to the vestibular nerve vary considerably in size: their circumferences range from 45 to 160 μm (Felix et al 1987). No topographically ordered distribution relating to size has been found. The cell bodies are notable for their abundant granular endoplasmic reticulum, which forms Nissl bodies in places, and their prominent Golgi complexes (see Fig. 11.27). They are covered by a thin layer of satellite cells and are often arranged in pairs, closely abutting each other so that only a thin layer of endoneurium separates the adjacent coverings of satellite cells. This arrangement has led to speculation that ganglion cells may affect one another directly by electrotonic spread (ephaptic transmission).

Intratemporal Cochlear Nerve

The cochlear nerve connects the organ of Corti to the cochlear and related nuclei of the brain stem. The cochlear nerve lies inferior to the facial nerve throughout the internal acoustic meatus. It becomes intimately associated with the superior and inferior divisions of the vestibular nerve, which are situated in the posterior compartment of the canal, and leaves the internal acoustic meatus in a common fascicle (Fig. 11.29).

There are approximately 30,000 to 40,000 nerve fibres in the human cochlear nerve (for review, see Nadol 1988). Their fibre diameter distribution is unimodal and ranges from 1 to 11 μm, with a peak at 4 to 5 μm. Functionally, the nerve contains both afferent and efferent somatic fibres, together with adrenergic postganglionic sympathetic fibres from the cervical sympathetic system.

Afferent Cochlear Innervation

The afferent fibres are myelinated axons with bipolar cell bodies that lie in the spiral ganglion in the modiolus (Fig. 11.30). There are two types of ganglion cell: most (90% to 95%) are large Type I cells, and the remainder are smaller Type II cells (see reviews by Nadol 1988, Eybalin 1993). Type I cells contain a prominent spherical nucleus, abundant ribosomes and many mitochondria; in many mammals (although possibly not in humans) they are surrounded by myelin sheaths. In contrast, Type II cells are smaller, are always unmyelinated and have a lobulated nucleus. The cytoplasm of Type II cells is enriched with neurofilaments but has fewer mitochondria and ribosomes than Type I cells.

Each inner hair cell is in synaptic contact with the unbranched peripheral processes of approximately ten Type I ganglion cells. The processes of Type II ganglion cells diverge within the organ of Corti and innervate more than ten outer hair cells. The peripheral and central processes of Type I ganglion cells are relatively large in diameter and are myelinated, whereas those of Type II are smaller and unmyelinated. The peripheral processes of both types of cell radiate from the modiolus into the osseous spiral lamina, where the Type I axons lose their myelin sheaths before entering the organ of Corti through the habenula perforata.

Three distinct groupings of afferent fibres have been identified: inner radial, basilar and outer spiral fibres (Fig. 11.31).

Inner radial fibres — The inner radial fibre group consists of the majority of afferent fibres. They run directly in a radial direction to the inner hair cells, each of which receives endings from several of these fibres.

Basilar fibres — Basilar fibres are afferent to the outer hair cells and take an independent spiral course, turning toward the cochlear apex near the bases of the inner hair cells. They run for a distance of about five pillar cells before turning radially again and crossing the floor of the tunnel of Corti, often diagonally, to form part of the outer spiral bundle.

Outer spiral bundles — The afferent fibres of the bundles of the outer spiral group course toward the basal part of the cochlea, continually branching off en route to supply several outer hair cells. The outer spiral bundles also contain efferent fibres.

Efferent Cochlear Fibres

The efferent nerve fibres in the cochlear nerve are derived from the olivocochlear system (see reviews by Warr 1992, Guinan 1996). Within the modiolus, the efferent fibres form the intraganglionic spiral bundle, which may be one or more discrete groups of fibres situated at the periphery of the spiral ganglion (see Fig. 11.31). There are two main groups of olivocochlear efferents: lateral and medial. The lateral efferents come from small neurones in and near the lateral superior olivary nucleus and arise mainly, but not exclusively, ipsilaterally. They are organized into inner spiral fibres that run in the inner

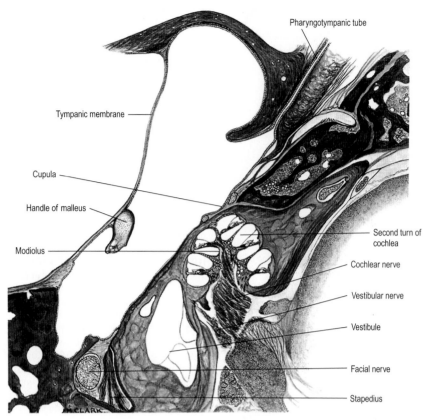

Pharyngotympanic tube

Tympanic membrane

Cupula

Handle of malleus

Modiolus

Second turn of cochlea

Cochlear nerve

Vestibular nerve

Vestibule

Facial nerve

Stapedius

Fig. 11.29 *Horizontal section through the left temporal bone. (Drawn from a section prepared at the Ferens Institute and lent by the late J. Kirk.)*

spiral bundle before terminating on the afferent axons that supply the inner hair cells. The medial efferents originate from larger neurones in the vicinity of the medial superior olivary nucleus, and the majority arise contralaterally. They are myelinated and cross the tunnel of Corti to synapse with the outer hair cells mainly by direct contact with their bases, although a few synapse with the afferent terminals. The efferent innervation of the outer hair cells decreases along the organ of Corti from cochlear base to apex, and from the first (inner) row to the third. The efferents use acetylcholine, γ-aminobutyric acid (GABA) or both as their neurotransmitter. They may also contain other neurotransmitters and neuromodulators.

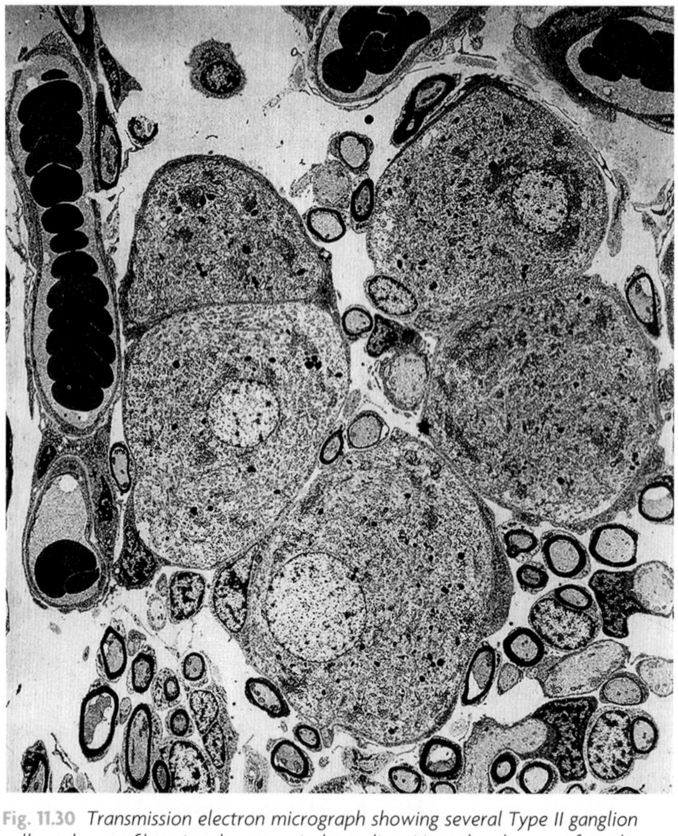

Activity of the medial efferents inhibits cochlear responses to sound; the strength of the activity grows slowly with increasing sound levels. They are believed to modulate the micromechanics of the cochlea by altering the mechanical responses of the outer hair cells, thus changing their contribution to frequency sensitivity and selectivity. The lateral efferents related to the inner hair cells also respond to sound. They appear to modify transmission through their postsynaptic action on inner hair cell afferents. The cholinergic fibres may excite the radial fibres, whereas those containing GABA may inhibit them, although their role is less well understood than that of the medial efferents (see review by Guinan 1996).

Autonomic Cochlear Innervation

Autonomic nerve endings appear to be entirely sympathetic. Two adrenergic systems have been described within the cochlea: a perivascular plexus derived from the stellate ganglion, and a blood vessel–independent system derived from the superior cervical ganglion. Both systems travel with the afferent and efferent cochlear fibres and seem to be restricted to regions away from the organ of Corti. The sympathetic nervous system may cause primary and secondary effects in the cochlea by remotely altering the metabolism of various cell types and by influencing the blood vessels and nerve fibres with which it makes contact.

GLOSSOPHARYNGEAL NERVE (IX)

The glossopharyngeal nerve (Figs 11.33–11.35) supplies motor fibres to stylopharyngeus; parasympathetic secretomotor fibres to the parotid gland (derived from the inferior salivatory nucleus); sensory fibres to the tympanic cavity, pharyngotympanic tube, fauces, tonsils, nasopharynx, uvula and posterior (postsulcal) third of the tongue; and gustatory fibres to the postsulcal part of the tongue.

The nerve leaves the skull through the anteromedial part of the jugular foramen, anterior to the vagus and accessory nerves, and in a separate dural sheath. In the foramen it is lodged in a deep groove leading from the cochlear aqueductal depression and is separated by the inferior petrosal sinus from the vagus and accessory nerves. The groove is bridged by fibrous tissue, which is calcified in approximately 25% of skulls. After leaving the foramen, the nerve passes forward between the internal jugular vein and internal carotid artery and then descends anterior to the latter, deep to the styloid process and its attached muscles, to reach the posterior border of stylopharyngeus. It curves

Fig. 11.30 *Transmission electron micrograph showing several Type II ganglion cells and nerve fibres in a human spiral ganglion. Note the absence of myelin from the surrounding sheaths of the ganglion cells. (Courtesy of H. Felix, M. Gleeson and L.-G. Johnsson, ENT Department, University of Zurich and GKT School of Medicine, London.)*

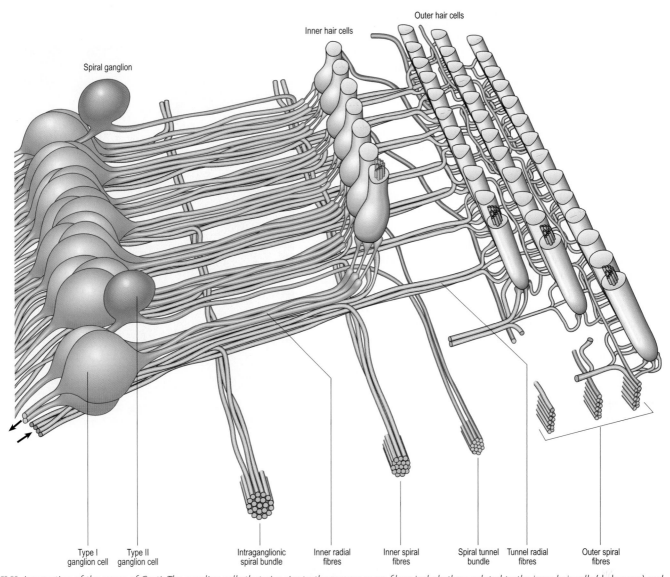

Inner hair cells

Outer hair cells

Spiral ganglion

| Type I ganglion cell | Type II ganglion cell | Intraganglionic spiral bundle | Inner radial fibres | Inner spiral fibres | Spiral tunnel bundle | Tunnel radial fibres | Outer spiral fibres |

Fig. 11.31 *Innervation of the organ of Corti. The ganglion cells that give rise to the sensory nerve fibres include those related to the inner hair cells* (dark green) *and others innervating the outer hair cells* (light green). *Efferent fibres are depicted in* purple. *There is a great contrast between the convergent afferent innervation of the inner hair cells (approximately 10 fibres to each cell) and the divergent supply of the outer hair cells (one afferent fibre to approximately 10 cells). This illustration is a simplified view of the complex innervation of the organ of Corti (see the text for further details).*

forward on the stylopharyngeus and either pierces the lower fibres of the superior pharyngeal constrictor or passes between it and the middle constrictor to be distributed to the tonsil, mucosa of the pharynx and postsulcal part of the tongue, vallate papillae and oral mucous glands.

Two ganglia, superior and inferior, are situated on the glossopharyngeal nerve as it traverses the jugular foramen (see Fig. 11.33). The superior ganglion is in the upper part of the groove occupied by the nerve in the jugular foramen. It is small, has no branches and is usually regarded as a detached part of the inferior ganglion. The inferior ganglion is larger and lies in a notch in the lower border of the petrous part of the temporal bone. Its cells are typical unipolar neurones, and their peripheral branches convey gustatory and tactile signals from the mucosa of the tongue (posterior third, including the sulcus terminalis and vallate papillae) and general sensation from the oropharynx, where it is responsible for initiating the gag reflex.

Communications

The glossopharyngeal nerve communicates with the sympathetic trunk, vagus and facial nerves. The inferior ganglion is connected with the superior cervical sympathetic ganglion. Two filaments from the inferior ganglion pass to the vagus—one to its auricular branch, and the other to its superior ganglion. A branch to the facial nerve arises from the glossopharyngeal nerve below the inferior ganglion and perforates the posterior belly of the digastric to join the facial nerve near the stylomastoid foramen.

Branches of Distribution

The branches of distribution are the tympanic, carotid, pharyngeal, muscular, tonsillar and lingual.

Tympanic nerve — The tympanic nerve leaves the inferior ganglion, ascends to the tympanic cavity through the inferior tympanic canaliculus and divides into branches that contribute to the tympanic plexus. The lesser petrosal nerve is derived from the tympanic plexus.

Carotid branch — The carotid branch is often double. It arises just below the jugular foramen and descends on the internal carotid artery to the wall of the carotid sinus and to the carotid body. The nerve contains primary afferent fibres from chemoreceptors in the carotid body and from the baroreceptors lying in the carotid sinus wall. It may communicate with the inferior ganglion of the vagus, or with one of its branches, and with a sympathetic branch from the superior cervical ganglion.

Pharyngeal branches — The pharyngeal branches are three or four filaments that unite with the pharyngeal branch of the vagus and the laryngopharyngeal branches of the sympathetic trunk to form the pharyngeal plexus near the middle pharyngeal constrictor. They constitute the route by which the glossopharyngeal nerve supplies sensory fibres to the mucosa of the pharynx.

Muscular branch — The muscular branch supplies stylopharyngeus.

Tonsillar branch — The palatine tonsil region receives its nerve supply through tonsillar branches of the maxillary nerve and the glossopharyngeal nerve. The maxillary nerve fibres pass through, but do not synapse in, the pterygopalatine ganglion and are distributed through the lesser palatine nerves. The latter, together with the tonsillar branches of the glossopharyngeal nerve, form a plexus around the tonsils. From this plexus (the circulus tonsillaris), nerve fibres are also distributed to the soft palate, and the pharyngeal nerve supplies the mucous membrane lining the tympanic cavity. Infection, malignancy and postoperative inflammation of the tonsils and tonsil fossa may therefore be accompanied by pain referred to the ear.

CASE 10 ACOUSTIC NEUROMA

A 45-year-old woman complains of right-sided tinnitus and reduced hearing, present for several years. With the passage of time, she has also experienced difficulty coordinating her right hand and, more recently, bifrontal headache. Examination demonstrates impaired hearing on the right; a reduced right corneal reflex, with variable impaired sensation on the right side of the face; and mild papilloedema. Somewhat later, right-sided facial weakness appears, but involvement of other cranial nerves is lacking until very late in the disease course.

Discussion: This patient exhibits an indolent clinical course typical of an acoustic neuroma, with early symptoms attributed to eighth nerve dysfunction reflecting the site of the tumour, which is virtually always within the internal auditory meatus (Fig. 11.32). Although the tumour is immediately adjacent to the facial nerve in this location, the first clinical manifestations beyond the eighth nerve itself are generally attributed to the trigeminal nerve. As in this patient, loss of the corneal reflex is a relatively early sign. As the tumour grows, other cranial nerves are affected. Eventually, the enlarging mass impinges, directly or indirectly, on the fourth ventricle, with resultant hydrocephalus; increased intracranial pressure is unusual under these circumstances, in light of contemporary diagnostic procedures.

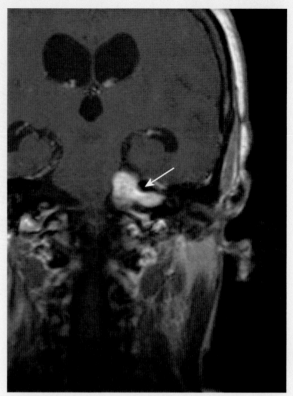

Fig. 11.32 *MRI demonstrates a large contrast-enhancing acoustic neuroma* (arrow) *with compression of the underlying brain stem and secondary ventriculomegaly.*

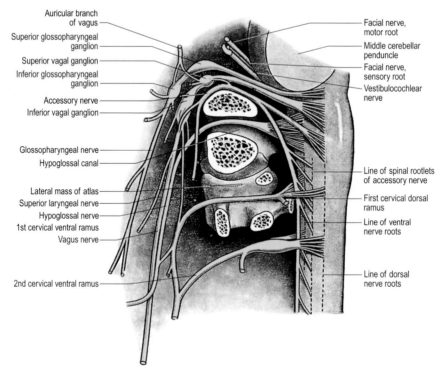

Fig. 11.33 *Communications between the last four cranial nerves of the left side viewed from the dorsolateral aspect. The hypoglossal canal has been split in its long axis, and the transverse process of the atlas has been divided close to the lateral mass. The descending branch of the hypoglossal nerve is not shown.*

Lingual branch — This branch supplies the mucous membranes at the base of the tongue and special visceral afferent innervation to the vallate papillae of the tongue.

Lesions of the Glossopharyngeal Nerve
Damage to the glossopharyngeal nerve rarely occurs without involvement of other lower cranial nerves. Transient or sustained hypertension may follow surgical section of the nerve, reflecting involvement of the carotid branch. Isolated lesions of the glossopharyngeal nerve lead to loss of sensation over the ipsilateral soft palate, fauces, pharynx and posterior third of the tongue, although this is difficult to assess clinically and requires galvanic stimulation. The palatal and pharyngeal (gag) reflexes are reduced or absent, and salivary secretion from the parotid gland may also be reduced. Stylopharyngeus weakness cannot be tested individually. Glossopharyngeal neuralgia consists of

CASE 11 Sudden Unilateral Hearing Loss

A 54-year-old man with a history of diabetes mellitus and a 40 pack-year smoking history awakens with loss of hearing in the left ear. He reports having had several episodes of vertigo in the previous month. He denies other neurological symptoms.

The neurological examination is remarkable primarily for profound sensorineural hearing loss on the left side. He has no nystagmus or ataxia, and with the exception of the hearing loss, cranial nerve functions are normal.

His hearing improves over the next several days, but he then develops severe hearing loss again, this time associated with tinnitus, vertigo and left-sided ataxia. MRI demonstrates an acute infarct involving the middle cerebellar peduncle.

Discussion: Sudden unilateral hearing loss may reflect ischaemic vascular disease involving the labyrinth or acoustic nerve, viral infection of the labyrinth, rupture of the cochlear membrane or immune-mediated injury to the inner ear. This man's symptoms are due to occlusive vascular disease (i.e. ischaemia) in the territory of the left anterior inferior cerebellar artery. It is especially noteworthy that stroke or transient ischaemic attacks involving the posterior circulation may present as acute hearing loss.

brief episodes of severe pain, often precipitated by swallowing, experienced in the throat, behind the angle of the jaw and within the ear. Superior jugular bulb thromboses (e.g. in otitis media) and jugular foramen syndrome (associated with nasopharyngeal carcinoma and glomus tumour) may cause lesions of the adjacent glossopharyngeal, vagus and accessory nerves, with associated weakness in the muscles supplied (in the pharynx and larynx).

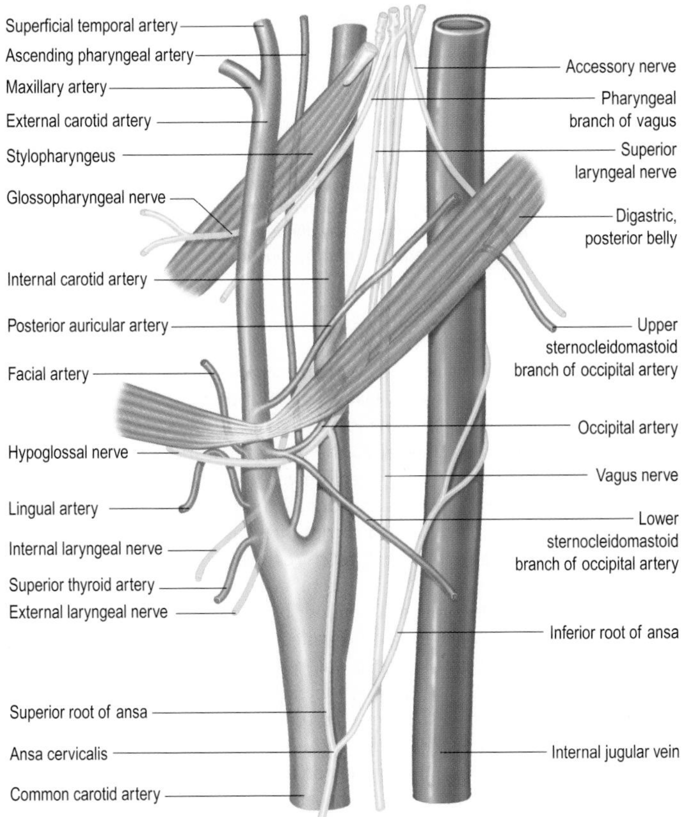
Superficial temporal artery
Ascending pharyngeal artery
Maxillary artery
External carotid artery
Stylopharyngeus
Glossopharyngeal nerve
Internal carotid artery
Posterior auricular artery
Facial artery
Hypoglossal nerve
Lingual artery
Internal laryngeal nerve
Superior thyroid artery
External laryngeal nerve
Superior root of ansa
Ansa cervicalis
Common carotid artery
Accessory nerve
Pharyngeal branch of vagus
Superior laryngeal nerve
Digastric, posterior belly
Upper sternocleidomastoid branch of occipital artery
Occipital artery
Vagus nerve
Lower sternocleidomastoid branch of occipital artery
Inferior root of ansa
Internal jugular vein

Fig. 11.34 *Structures crossing the internal jugular vein and carotid arteries and those intervening between the external and internal carotid arteries.*

VAGUS NERVE (X)

The vagus is a large mixed nerve. It has a more extensive course and distribution than any other cranial nerve and traverses the neck, thorax and abdomen (Figs 11.33, 11.34, 11.36; see also Figs 10.3, 10.8). Its central connections are described in Chapter 10.

The vagus exits the skull through the jugular foramen accompanied by the accessory nerve, with which it shares an arachnoid and a dural sheath. Both nerves lie anterior to a fibrous septum that separates them from the glossopharyngeal nerve. The vagus descends vertically in the neck in the carotid sheath, between the internal jugular vein and the internal carotid artery, to the upper border of the thyroid cartilage; it then passes between the vein and the common carotid artery to the root of the neck. Its relationships in this part of its course are therefore similar to those described for these structures. Its course then differs on the two sides. The right vagus descends posterior to the internal jugular vein to cross the first part of the subclavian artery and enter the thorax. The left vagus enters the thorax between the left common carotid and subclavian arteries and behind the left brachiocephalic vein.

After emerging from the jugular foramen, the vagus bears two marked enlargements: a small, round superior ganglion and a larger inferior ganglion (see Fig. 11.33).

Superior (Jugular) Ganglion

The superior ganglion is greyish, spherical and approximately 4 mm in diameter. It is connected to the cranial root of the accessory nerve, inferior glossopharyngeal ganglion and sympathetic trunk, the last by a filament from the superior cervical ganglion. The significance of these connections is not entirely clear, but the first probably contains aberrant motor fibres from the nucleus ambiguus that issue in the accessory nerve to be distributed to the palatal, pharyngeal, laryngeal and upper oesophageal musculature via the vagus.

Inferior (Nodose) Ganglion

The inferior or nodose ganglion is larger than the superior ganglion and is elongated and cylindrical in shape, with a length of approximately 25 mm and a maximum breadth of 5 mm. It is connected with the hypoglossal nerve, the loop between the first and second cervical spinal nerves, and with the superior cervical sympathetic ganglion. Just above the ganglion, the cranial accessory blends with the vagus nerve, its fibres being distributed mainly in pharyngeal and recurrent laryngeal vagal branches. Most visceral afferent fibres have their cell bodies in the nodose ganglion.

Both vagal ganglia are exclusively sensory and contain somatic, special visceral and general visceral afferent neurones. The superior ganglion is chiefly somatic, and most of its neurones enter the auricular nerve, whereas neurones in the inferior ganglion are concerned with visceral sensation from the heart, larynx, lungs and alimentary tract from the pharynx to the transverse colon. Some fibres transmit impulses from taste endings in the vallecula and epiglottis. Large afferent fibres are derived from muscle spindles in the laryngeal muscles. Vagal sensory neurones in the nodose ganglion may show some somatotopic organization. Both ganglia are traversed by parasympathetic and perhaps some sympathetic fibres, but there is no evidence that vagal parasympathetic components relay in the inferior ganglion. Preganglionic motor fibres from the dorsal vagal nucleus and the special visceral efferents from the nucleus ambiguus, which descend to the inferior vagal ganglion, commonly form a visible band skirting the ganglia in some mammals. These larger fibres probably provide motor innervation to the larynx in the recurrent laryngeal nerve, together with some contribution to the superior laryngeal nerve supplying the cricothyroid.

Branches in the Neck

The branches of the vagus in the neck are the meningeal, auricular, pharyngeal, carotid body, superior and recurrent laryngeal nerves and cardiac branches.

Meningeal Branches

Meningeal branches appear to start from the superior vagal ganglion and pass through the jugular foramen to be distributed to the dura mater in the posterior cranial fossa.

Auricular Branch

The auricular branch arises from the superior vagal ganglion and is joined by a branch from the inferior ganglion of the glossopharyngeal nerve. It passes behind the internal jugular vein and enters the mastoid canaliculus on the lateral wall of the jugular fossa. Traversing the temporal bone, it crosses the facial canal approximately 4 mm above the stylomastoid foramen and there supplies an ascending branch to the facial nerve. Fibres of the nervus intermedius may pass to the auricular branch at this point, which may explain the

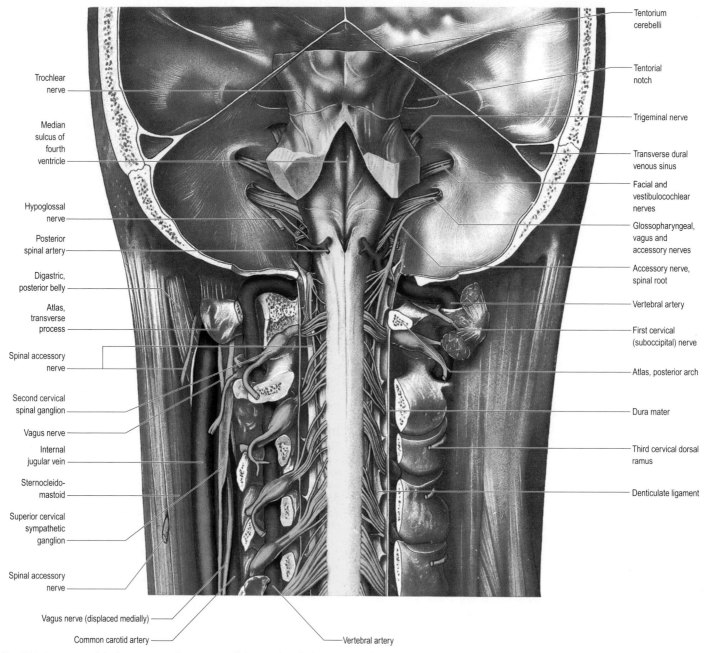

Trochlear nerve

Median sulcus of fourth ventricle

Hypoglossal nerve

Posterior spinal artery

Digastric, posterior belly

Atlas, transverse process

Spinal accessory nerve

Second cervical spinal ganglion

Vagus nerve

Internal jugular vein

Sternocleido-mastoid

Superior cervical sympathetic ganglion

Spinal accessory nerve

Vagus nerve (displaced medially)

Common carotid artery

Tentorium cerebelli

Tentorial notch

Trigeminal nerve

Transverse dural venous sinus

Facial and vestibulocochlear nerves

Glossopharyngeal, vagus and accessory nerves

Accessory nerve, spinal root

Vertebral artery

First cervical (suboccipital) nerve

Atlas, posterior arch

Dura mater

Third cervical dorsal ramus

Denticulate ligament

Vertebral artery

Fig. 11.35 *Dissection of the brain stem and upper part of the spinal cord after removal of large portions of the occipital and parietal bones, the cerebellum and the roof of the fourth ventricle. On the left side, the foramina transversaria of the atlas and the third, fourth and fifth cervical vertebrae have been opened to expose the vertebral artery. On the right side, the posterior arch of the atlas and the laminae of the succeeding cervical vertebrae have been divided and removed, together with the vertebral spines and the contralateral laminae. The tentorium cerebelli and the transverse sinuses have been divided and their posterior portions removed.*

cutaneous vesiculation in the auricle that sometimes accompanies geniculate herpes. The auricular branch then traverses the tympanomastoid fissure and divides into two rami. One ramus joins the posterior auricular nerve, and the other is distributed to the skin of part of the ear and to the external acoustic meatus.

Pharyngeal Branch

The pharyngeal branch of the vagus is the main motor nerve of the pharynx. It emerges from the upper part of the inferior vagal ganglion and consists chiefly of filaments from the cranial accessory nerve. It passes between the external and internal carotid arteries to the upper border of the middle pharyngeal constrictor and divides into numerous filaments that join rami of the sympathetic trunk and glossopharyngeal nerve to form a pharyngeal plexus. A minute filament, the ramus lingualis vagi, joins the hypoglossal nerve as it curves round the occipital artery.

Branches to the Carotid Body

Branches to the carotid body are variable in number. They may arise from the inferior ganglion or travel in the pharyngeal branch and sometimes in the superior laryngeal nerve. They form a plexus with the glossopharyngeal rami and branches of the cervical sympathetic trunk.

Superior Laryngeal Nerve

The superior laryngeal nerve is larger than the pharyngeal branch and issues from the middle of the inferior vagal ganglion. It receives a branch from the superior cervical sympathetic ganglion and descends alongside the pharynx, at first posterior and then medial to the internal carotid artery, and divides into the internal and external laryngeal nerves.

The internal laryngeal nerve is sensory to the laryngeal mucosa down to the level of the vocal folds. It also carries afferent fibres from the laryngeal neuromuscular spindles and other stretch receptors. It descends to the thyrohyoid membrane, pierces it above the superior laryngeal artery and divides into an upper and lower branch. The upper branch is horizontal and supplies the mucosa of the pharynx, epiglottis, vallecula and laryngeal vestibule. The lower branch descends in the medial wall of the piriform recess and supplies the aryepiglottic fold, the mucosa on the back of the arytenoid cartilage and one or two branches to the transverse arytenoid (which unite with twigs from the recurrent laryngeal nerve to supply the same muscle). The internal laryngeal nerve ends by piercing the inferior pharyngeal constrictor to unite with an ascending branch from the recurrent laryngeal nerve. As it ascends in the neck, it supplies branches, more numerous on the left, to the mucosa and tunica muscularis of the oesophagus and trachea and to the inferior constrictor.

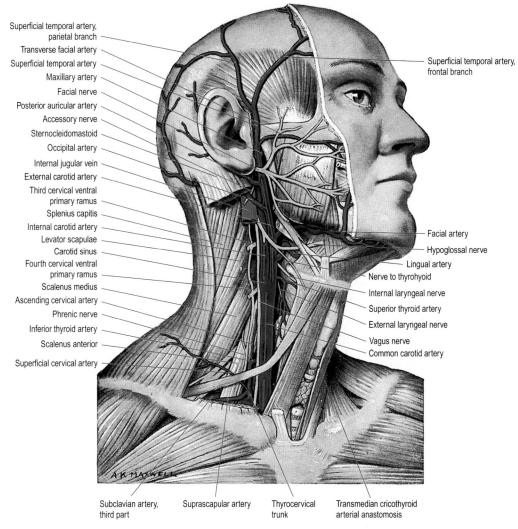

Superficial temporal artery, parietal branch
Transverse facial artery
Superficial temporal artery
Maxillary artery
Facial nerve
Posterior auricular artery
Accessory nerve
Sternocleidomastoid
Occipital artery
Internal jugular vein
External carotid artery
Third cervical ventral primary ramus
Splenius capitis
Internal carotid artery
Levator scapulae
Carotid sinus
Fourth cervical ventral primary ramus
Scalenus medius
Ascending cervical artery
Phrenic nerve
Inferior thyroid artery
Scalenus anterior
Superficial cervical artery

Superficial temporal artery, frontal branch

Facial artery
Hypoglossal nerve
Lingual artery
Nerve to thyrohyoid
Internal laryngeal nerve
Superior thyroid artery
External laryngeal nerve
Vagus nerve
Common carotid artery

Subclavian artery, third part
Suprascapular artery
Thyrocervical trunk
Transmedian cricothyroid arterial anastomosis

Fig. 11.36 *Dissection of the right side of the neck, showing the carotid and subclavian arteries and their branches. The parotid and submandibular glands have been removed, together with the lower part of the internal jugular vein, most of the sternocleidomastoid and the upper parts of the stylohyoid and posterior belly of the digastric.*

The external laryngeal nerve, smaller than the internal, descends behind the sternohyoid with the superior thyroid artery, but on a deeper plane. It lies first on the inferior pharyngeal constrictor, then pierces it to curve around the inferior thyroid tubercle and reach the cricothyroid, which it supplies. The nerve also gives branches to the pharyngeal plexus and inferior constrictor. Behind the common carotid artery, the external laryngeal nerve communicates with the superior cardiac nerve and superior cervical sympathetic ganglion.

Recurrent Laryngeal Nerve

The recurrent laryngeal nerve differs, in origin and course, on the two sides. On the right, it arises from the vagus anterior to the first part of the subclavian artery and curves backward, below and then behind it, to ascend obliquely to the side of the trachea behind the common carotid artery. Near the lower pole of the lateral lobe of the thyroid gland, it is closely related to the inferior thyroid artery and crosses in front of, behind or between its branches. On the left, the nerve arises from the vagus on the left of the aortic arch, curves below it immediately behind the attachment of the ligamentum arteriosum to the concavity of the aortic arch and ascends to the side of the trachea. As the recurrent laryngeal nerve curves around the subclavian artery or the aortic arch, it gives cardiac filaments to the deep cardiac plexus. On both sides, the recurrent laryngeal nerve ascends in or near a groove between the trachea and oesophagus. It is closely related to the medial surface of the thyroid gland before it passes under the lower border of the inferior constrictor, and it enters the larynx behind the articulation of the inferior thyroid cornu with the cricoid cartilage. The recurrent laryngeal nerve supplies all laryngeal muscles, except the cricothyroid, and it communicates with the internal laryngeal nerve, supplying sensory filaments to the laryngeal mucosa below the vocal folds. It also carries afferent fibres from laryngeal stretch receptors.

CASE 12   RECURRENT LARYNGEAL NERVE PALSY

A 36-year-old man complains of a weak voice and persistent hoarseness following thyroidectomy. His neurological examination is normal, but laryngoscopy demonstrates paralysis of the left vocal cord. A diagnosis of recurrent laryngeal nerve palsy secondary to operative trauma is made. He improves to a limited extent over several months.

Discussion: Although the relationship between surgery and vocal cord palsy appears clear in this case, recurrent laryngeal nerve palsy can be caused by a variety of mechanisms, including nerve compression by enlarged mediastinal lymph nodes, local invasion by metastatic carcinoma and compression by a large aortic aneurysm. The nerve can also be affected by systemic polyneuropathy or damaged during placement of an endotracheal tube. The left recurrent laryngeal nerve is more commonly involved than the right, presumably by virtue of its longer anatomical course.

ACCESSORY NERVE (XI)

The accessory nerve is conventionally described as a single entity (see Figs 11.33, 11.35, 11.37), even though its two components—the cranial root and spinal root, which join for a relatively short part of its course—are of separate origin.

Cranial Root

The cranial root of the accessory nerve is smaller than the spinal root. It exits the skull through the jugular foramen and unites for a short distance with the spinal root. It is also connected to the superior vagal ganglion. After traversing the foramen, the cranial root separates from the spinal part and immediately joins the vagus nerve superior to the inferior vagal ganglion. Those of its fibres that are distributed in the pharyngeal branches of the vagus are derived from the nucleus ambiguus and probably innervate the pharyngeal and palatal muscles, except tensor veli palatini. Other fibres enter the recurrent laryngeal nerve to supply the adductor muscles of the vocal cords, thyroarytenoid and lateral cricoarytenoid.

Spinal Root

The spinal root arises from an elongated nucleus of motor cells situated in the lateral aspect of the ventral horn that extends from the junction of the spinal cord and medulla to the sixth cervical segment (see Fig. 11.35). Some rootlets emerge directly; others turn cranially before exiting. Their line of exit is irregular rather than linear, and the spinal root usually passes through the first cervical dorsal root ganglion. The rootlets form a trunk that ascends between the ligamentum denticulatum and the dorsal roots of the spinal nerves and enters the skull via the foramen magnum, behind the vertebral artery. It then turns upward and passes laterally to reach the jugular foramen, which it traverses in a common dural sheath with the vagus, but separated from that nerve by a fold of arachnoid mater. As the spinal root exits the jugular foramen, it runs posterolaterally and passes either medial or lateral to the internal jugular vein. Occasionally, it passes through the vein. The nerve then crosses the transverse process of the atlas and is itself crossed by the occipital artery. It descends obliquely, medial to the styloid process, stylohyoid and posterior belly of the digastric. Running with the superior sternocleidomastoid branch of the occipital artery, it reaches the upper part of the sternocleidomastoid and enters its deep surface, to form an anastomosis with fibres from C2 alone, C3 alone, or C2 and C3, the ansa of Maubrac. The nerve occasionally terminates in the muscle. More commonly, it emerges a little above the midpoint of the posterior border of the sternocleidomastoid,

generally above the emergence of the great auricular nerve (usually within 2 cm of it) and between 4 and 6 cm from the tip of the mastoid process. However, the point of emergence is very variable. It crosses the posterior triangle on the levator scapulae (see Fig. 11.37), separated from it by the prevertebral layer of deep cervical fascia and adipose tissue. There the nerve is relatively superficial and related to the superficial cervical lymph nodes. About 3 to 5 cm above the clavicle, it passes behind the anterior border of the trapezius, often dividing to form a plexus on its deep surface that receives contributions from C3 and C4 or from C4 alone. It then enters the deep surface of the muscle.

The cervical course of the nerve follows a line from the lower anterior part of the tragus to the tip of the transverse process of the atlas and then across the sternocleidomastoid and the posterior triangle to a point on the anterior border of the trapezius 3 to 5 cm above the clavicle.

Conventionally, the spinal root is thought to provide the sole motor supply to the sternocleidomastoid, and the second and third cervical nerves are believed to carry proprioceptive fibres from it. The supranuclear pathway of fibres destined for the sternocleidomastoid is not simple: fibres may undergo a double decussation in the brain stem, or there may be a bilateral projection to the muscle from each hemisphere.

The motor supply to the upper and middle portions of the trapezius is primarily from the spinal accessory nerve. However, in approximately 75% of subjects, the lower two-thirds of the muscle receives an innervation from the cervical plexus. Based on the incomplete denervation of the muscle that sometimes occurs following sacrifice of both the accessory nerve and the cervical plexus, it has been suggested that the trapezius receives a partial motor supply from other sources, possibly via thoracic roots. In addition to their motor contribution, C3 and C4 carry proprioceptive fibres from the trapezius. In approximately 25% of subjects, the spinal accessory nerve receives no fibres from the cervical plexus.

Sensory ganglia have been described along the course of the spinal root.

Lesions Affecting the Accessory Nerve

Lesions of the accessory nerve may occur centrally, at its exit from the skull or in the neck. The supranuclear fibres that influence motor neurones innervating the sternocleidomastoid decussate twice; therefore, a lesion of the pyramidal system above the pons produces weakness of the ipsilateral sternocleidomastoid and contralateral trapezius. Episodic contraction of the sternocleidomastoid and trapezius, often accompanied by contraction of other muscle groups (e.g. splenius capitis), occurs in spasmodic torticollis, a focal dystonia. In jugular foramen syndrome, caused by disorders such as nasopharyngeal carcinoma or glomus tumour, lesions of the glossopharyngeal, vagus and accessory nerves coexist. The accessory nerve can be injured more distally in the neck by trauma or by surgical exploration in the posterior triangle. If the accessory nerve is sacrificed as part of a radical neck dissection and innervation of the trapezius is lost, the patient develops intractable neuralgia due to traction on the brachial plexus caused by the unsupported weight of the shoulder and arm.

HYPOGLOSSAL NERVE (XII)

The hypoglossal nerve is motor to all the muscles of the tongue, except the palatoglossus (see Figs 11.34, 11.36–11.38). The hypoglossal rootlets run laterally behind the vertebral artery, collected into two bundles that perforate the dura mater separately opposite the hypoglossal canal in the occipital bone and then unite after traversing it. The canal is sometimes divided by a spicule of bone. The nerve emerges from the canal in a plane medial to the internal jugular vein, internal carotid artery and ninth, tenth and eleventh cranial nerves and passes inferolaterally behind the internal carotid artery and glossopharyngeal and vagus nerves to the interval between the artery and the internal jugular vein. There it makes a half-spiral turn around the inferior vagal ganglion and is united with it by connective tissue. It then descends almost vertically between the vessels and anterior to the vagus to a point level with the angle of the mandible, becoming superficial below the posterior belly of the digastric and emerging between the internal jugular vein and internal carotid artery. It loops around the inferior sternocleidomastoid branch of the occipital artery and crosses lateral to both the internal and external carotid arteries and the loop of the lingual artery a little above the tip of the greater cornu of the hyoid; it is crossed itself by the facial vein.

Communications

The hypoglossal nerve communicates with the sympathetic trunk, vagus, first and second cervical nerves and lingual nerve. Near the atlas it is joined by branches from the superior cervical sympathetic ganglion and by a filament from the loop between the first and second cervical nerves, which leaves the hypoglossal as the upper root of the ansa cervicalis (see Fig. 11.38). The vagal connections occur close to the skull, and numerous filaments pass between

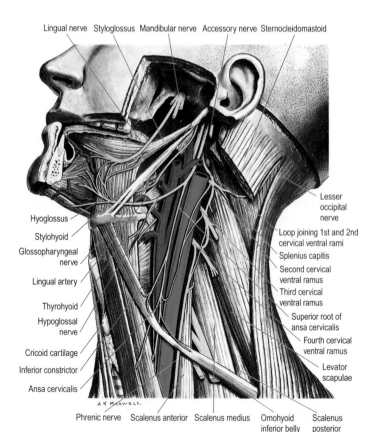

Lingual nerve Styloglossus Mandibular nerve Accessory nerve Sternocleidomastoid

Hyoglossus
Stylohyoid
Glossopharyngeal nerve
Lingual artery
Thyrohyoid
Hypoglossal nerve
Cricoid cartilage
Inferior constrictor
Ansa cervicalis

Lesser occipital nerve
Loop joining 1st and 2nd cervical ventral rami
Splenius capitis
Second cervical ventral ramus
Third cervical ventral ramus
Superior root of ansa cervicalis
Fourth cervical ventral ramus
Levator scapulae

A K MAXWELL

Phrenic nerve Scalenus anterior Scalenus medius Omohyoid inferior belly Scalenus posterior

Fig. 11.37 *Dissection showing the general distribution of the left hypoglossal and lingual nerves and the position and constitution of some parts of the cervical plexus of the left side.*

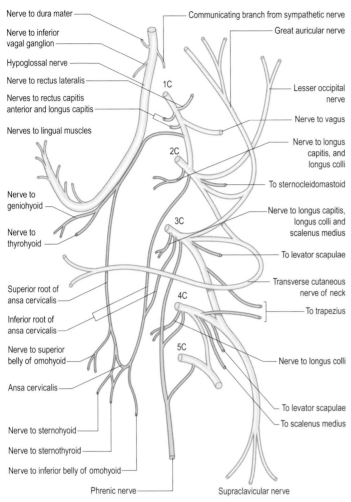

Fig. 11.38 *Plan of the cervical plexus.*

Labels (clockwise from top left):
Nerve to dura mater — Communicating branch from sympathetic nerve — Great auricular nerve — Nerve to inferior vagal ganglion — Hypoglossal nerve — Nerve to rectus lateralis — 1C — Lesser occipital nerve — Nerves to rectus capitis anterior and longus capitis — Nerve to vagus — Nerves to lingual muscles — 2C — Nerve to longus capitis, and longus colli — To sternocleidomastoid — Nerve to geniohyoid — Nerve to longus capitis, longus colli and scalenus medius — 3C — To levator scapulae — Nerve to thyrohyoid — Nerve to longus capitis, longus colli and scalenus medius — Superior root of ansa cervicalis — 4C — Transverse cutaneous nerve of neck — Inferior root of ansa cervicalis — To trapezius — Nerve to superior belly of omohyoid — 5C — Nerve to longus colli — Ansa cervicalis — To levator scapulae — Nerve to sternohyoid — To scalenus medius — Nerve to sternothyroid — Nerve to inferior belly of omohyoid — Phrenic nerve — Supraclavicular nerve

the hypoglossal nerve and the inferior vagal ganglion in the connective tissue uniting them. As the hypoglossal nerve curves around the occipital artery, it receives the ramus lingualis vagi from the pharyngeal plexus. Near the anterior border of the hyoglossus, it is connected with the lingual nerve by many filaments that ascend on the muscle.

Branches of Distribution

The branches of distribution of the hypoglossal nerve are meningeal, descending, thyrohyoid and muscular nerves.

Meningeal Branches

Meningeal branches leave the nerve in the hypoglossal canal and return through it to supply the diploë of the occipital bone, the dural walls of the occipital and inferior petrosal sinuses and much of the floor of the anterior wall of the posterior cranial fossa, probably through pathways other than those of the hypoglossal nerve (e.g. upper cervical spinal nerves).

Descending Branch

The descending branch (descendens hypoglossi) contains fibres from the first cervical spinal nerve. It leaves the hypoglossal nerve when it curves around the occipital artery and runs down on the carotid sheath. It provides a branch to the superior belly of the omohyoid before joining with the descendens cervicalis to form the ansa cervicalis (see Fig. 11.38).

Nerves to the Thyrohyoid and Geniohyoid

The nerves to the thyrohyoid and geniohyoid arise near the posterior border of the hyoglossus. They represent the remaining fibres from the first cervical spinal nerves.

Lesions of the Hypoglossal Nerve

The hypoglossal nerve may be damaged during neck dissection. Complete hypoglossal division causes unilateral lingual paralysis and eventual hemiatrophy. The protruded tongue deviates to the paralysed side; on retraction, the wasted and paralysed side rises higher than the unaffected side. The larynx may deviate toward the active side in swallowing, due to unilateral paralysis of the hyoid depressors associated with loss of the first cervical spinal nerve, which runs with the hypoglossal nerve. If paralysis is bilateral, the tongue is motionless. Taste and tactile sensibility are unaffected, but articulation is slow and swallowing is very difficult.

CASE 13   HYPOGLOSSAL NEUROPATHY

A 45-year-old man notes thinning of one side of his tongue. He denies any other symptoms. Examination demonstrates hemiatrophy of the tongue, with deviation to the wasted side when the tongue is protruded (Fig. 11.39). Otherwise, the examination is normal.

Discussion: This man has an isolated hypoglossal neuropathy. The lack of signs of other neurological dysfunction, in particular of the lower brain stem, indicates that the nerve is affected peripherally. Neuroimaging documents a focal lesion involving the hypoglossal foramen, in this case, a clivus meningioma. Other lesions of the skull base, such as chordoma or glomus jugulare tumour, must also be considered. The lack of other cranial nerve involvement argues against other potential diagnoses such as basal meningitis or meningeal carcinomatosis.

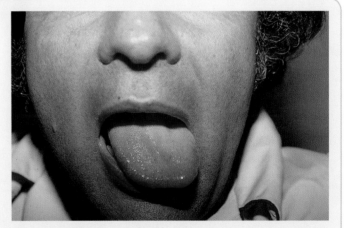

Fig. 11.39 *Hypoglossal palsy with deviation of the tongue to the side of the lesion.*

References

Brodal, A., 1981. Neurological Anatomy in Relation to Clinical Medicine, third ed. Oxford University Press, Oxford. *Unconventional but highly readable text of neuroanatomy with an emphasis on clinical relevance. Particularly good account of motor pathways.*

Crossman, A.R., Neary, D., 2000. Neuroanatomy: An Illustrated Colour Text, second ed. Churchill Livingstone, Edinburgh.

Davis, R.A., Anson, B.J., Budinger, J.M., Kurth, L.E., 1956. Surgical anatomy of the facial nerve and parotid gland based upon a study of 350 cervicofacial halves. Surg. Gynecol. Obstet. 102, 385–412.

England, M.A., Wakely, J., 1991. A Colour Atlas of the Brain and Spinal Cord. Wolfe Publishing, London.

Eybalin, M., 1993. Neurotransmitters and neuromodulators of the mammalian cochlea. Physiol. Rev. 73, 309–373.

Felix, H., Hoffman, V., Wright, A., Gleeson, M.J., 1987. Ultrastructural findings on human Scarpa's ganglion. Acta. Otolaryngol. Suppl. 436, 85–92.

Guinan, J., Jr., 1996. Physiology of olivocochlear efferents. In: Dallos, P., Popper, A.N., Fay, R.R., (Eds.), The Cochlea. Springer Verlag, New York, pp. 435–502. *Comprehensive description of the efferent innervation of the cochlea and its function.*

Haines, D.E., 2000. Neuroanatomy: An Atlas of Structures, Sections, and Systems, fifth ed. Lippincott Williams and Wilkins, Philadelphia.

Lee, H., et al., 2002. Sudden deafness and anterior inferior cerebellar artery infarction. Stroke 33, 2807.

Nadol, J.B., 1988. Comparative anatomy of the cochlea and auditory nerve in mammals. Hear Res. 34, 253–266.

Warr, W.B., 1992. Organization of olivocochlear efferent systems in mammals. In: Webster, D.B., Popper, A.N., Fay, R.R., (Eds.), Mammalian Auditory Pathway: Neuroanatomy. Springer Verlag, New York, pp. 410–448.

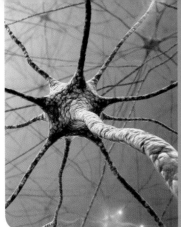

Special Senses

The special senses of olfaction, vision, taste, hearing and balance are conveyed to the brain in cranial nerves. In each case, highly specialized peripheral receptors respond to stimuli in the external environment or our relationship to it. The olfactory system has an ancient lineage, reflected by the fact that afferent olfactory pathways proceed directly to the cerebral cortex and bypass the thalamus. Its terminal fields are, likewise, primitive cortical areas in a phylogenetic sense and are considered to be parts of the limbic system. All other special senses have a thalamic representation that projects to specialized regions of the neocortex. The integrative functions related to the various special senses (e.g. control of ocular gaze) are also included here. Of particular importance is a detailed discussion of retinal functional anatomy.

OLFACTION

Olfactory pathways subserving the sense of smell are described in this section. Details of the relationship between the olfactory pathways and the limbic system are shown in Figure 16.7.

The olfactory nerves arise from olfactory receptor neurones in the olfactory mucosa. The axons collect into approximately 20 bundles and enter the anterior cranial fossa by passing through the foramina in the cribriform plate. They attach to the inferior surface of the olfactory bulb, which is situated at the anterior end of the olfactory sulcus on the orbital surface of the frontal lobe, and terminate in the bulb. Apparently unique in the nervous system, olfactory receptor neurones are continually replaced throughout life by differentiation of stem cells in the olfactory mucosa. The olfactory bulb is continuous posteriorly with the olfactory tract, through which the output of the bulb passes directly to the olfactory cortex.

There is a clear laminar structure in the olfactory bulb (Fig. 12.1). From the surface inward, the laminae are the olfactory nerve layer, glomerular layer, external plexiform layer, mitral cell layer, internal plexiform layer and granule cell layer.

The olfactory nerve layer consists of unmyelinated axons of the olfactory neurones. The continuous turnover of receptor cells means that axons in this layer are at different stages of growth, maturity or degeneration. The glomerular layer consists of a thin sheet of glomeruli, where the incoming olfactory axons divide and synapse on terminal dendrites of secondary olfactory neurones—that is, mitral, tufted and periglomerular cells. The external plexiform layer contains the principal and secondary dendrites of mitral and tufted cells. The mitral cell layer is a thin sheet composed of the cell bodies of mitral cells, each of which sends a single principal dendrite to a glomerulus, secondary dendrites to the external plexiform layer and a single axon to the olfactory tract. It also contains a few granule cell bodies. The internal plexiform layer contains axons, recurrent and deep collaterals of mitral and tufted cells and granule cell bodies. The granule cell layer contains the majority of the granule cells and their superficial and deep processes, together with numerous centripetal and centrifugal nerve fibres that pass through the layer.

The principal neurones in the olfactory bulb are the mitral and tufted cells; their axons form its output via the olfactory tract. These cells are morphologically similar, and most use an excitatory amino acid, probably glutamate or aspartate, as their neurotransmitter. The mitral cell spans the layers of the bulb and receives the sensory input superficially at its glomerular tuft. The axons of mitral and tufted cells appear to be parallel output pathways from the olfactory bulb. It is not known whether they receive inputs from different olfactory sensory neurones.

The main types of intrinsic neurones in the olfactory bulb are periglomerular cells and granule cells. The majority of periglomerular cells are dopaminergic (cell group A15); some are GABAergic. Their axons are distributed laterally and terminate within extraglomerular regions. Granule cells are similar in size to periglomerular cells. Their most characteristic feature is the absence of an axon, hence their resemblance to amacrine cells in the retina. Granule cells have two principal spine-bearing dendrites that pass radially in the bulb to ramify and terminate in the external plexiform layer. They appear to be GABAergic. The granule cell is likely to be a powerful inhibitory influence on the output neurones of the olfactory bulb.

Centrifugal inputs to the olfactory bulb arise from a variety of central sites. Neurones of the anterior olfactory nucleus and collaterals of pyramidal neurones in the olfactory cortex project to the granule cells of the olfactory bulb. Cholinergic neurones in the horizontal limb nucleus of the diagonal band of Broca, part of the basal forebrain cholinergic system, project to the granule cell layer and also to the glomerular layer. Other afferents to the granule cell layer and the glomeruli arise from the pontine locus coeruleus and the mesencephalic raphe nucleus.

The olfactory tract leaves the posterior pole of the olfactory bulb to run along the olfactory sulcus on the orbital surface of the frontal lobe (see Fig. 16.7). The granule cell layer of the bulb is extended into the olfactory tract as scattered medium-sized multipolar neurones that constitute the anterior olfactory nucleus. They continue into the olfactory striae and trigone to the grey matter of the prepiriform cortex, anterior perforated substance and precommissural septal areas. Many centripetal axons from mitral and tufted cells relay in, or give collaterals to, the anterior olfactory nucleus; the axons from the nucleus continue with the remaining direct fibres from the bulb into the olfactory striae.

As the olfactory tract approaches the anterior perforated substance, it flattens and splays as the olfactory trigone. Fibres of the tract continue from the caudal angles of the trigone as diverging medial and lateral olfactory striae, which border the anterior perforated substance. An intermediate stria sometimes passes from the centre of the trigone to end in a small olfactory tubercle. The lateral olfactory stria follows the anterolateral margin of the anterior perforated substance to the limen insulae, where it bends posteromedially to merge with an elevated region, the gyrus semilunaris, at the rostral margin of the uncus in the temporal lobe (see Fig. 16.7). The lateral olfactory gyrus forms a tenuous grey layer covering the lateral olfactory stria; it merges laterally with the gyrus ambiens, part of the limen insulae. The lateral olfactory gyrus and gyrus ambiens form the prepiriform region of the cortex, passing caudally into the entorhinal area of the parahippocampal gyrus. The prepiriform and periamygdaloid regions and the entorhinal area (area 28) together make up the piriform cortex. The medial olfactory stria, covered thinly by the grey matter of the medial olfactory gyrus, passes medially along the rostral boundary of the anterior perforated substance toward the medial continuation of the diagonal band of Broca. Together, they curve up on the medial aspect of the hemisphere, anterior to the attachment of the lamina terminalis. The diagonal band enters the paraterminal gyrus. The medial stria becomes indistinct as it approaches the boundary zone, which includes the paraterminal gyrus, parolfactory gyrus and, between them, prehippocampal rudiment (see Fig. 16.7).

The olfactory cortex receives a direct input from the olfactory bulb, which arrives via the olfactory tract without relay in the thalamus. The largest cortical olfactory area is the piriform cortex. The anterior olfactory nucleus, olfactory tubercle, regions of the entorhinal and insular cortex and amygdala also receive direct projections from the olfactory bulb.

The entorhinal cortex (Brodmann's area 28) is the most posterior part of the piriform cortex and is divided into medial and lateral areas (areas 28a and 28b). The lateral parts receive fibres mainly from the olfactory bulb and also from the piriform and periamygdaloid cortices.

Projections from the piriform olfactory cortex are widespread and include the neocortex (especially the orbitofrontal cortex), thalamus (especially the medial dorsal thalamic nucleus), hypothalamus, amygdala and hippocampal formation.

VISION

Eye

The eyeball, the peripheral organ of vision, is situated in the orbit, a skeletal cavity whose walls help protect the eye from injury (Fig. 12.2). The orbit also

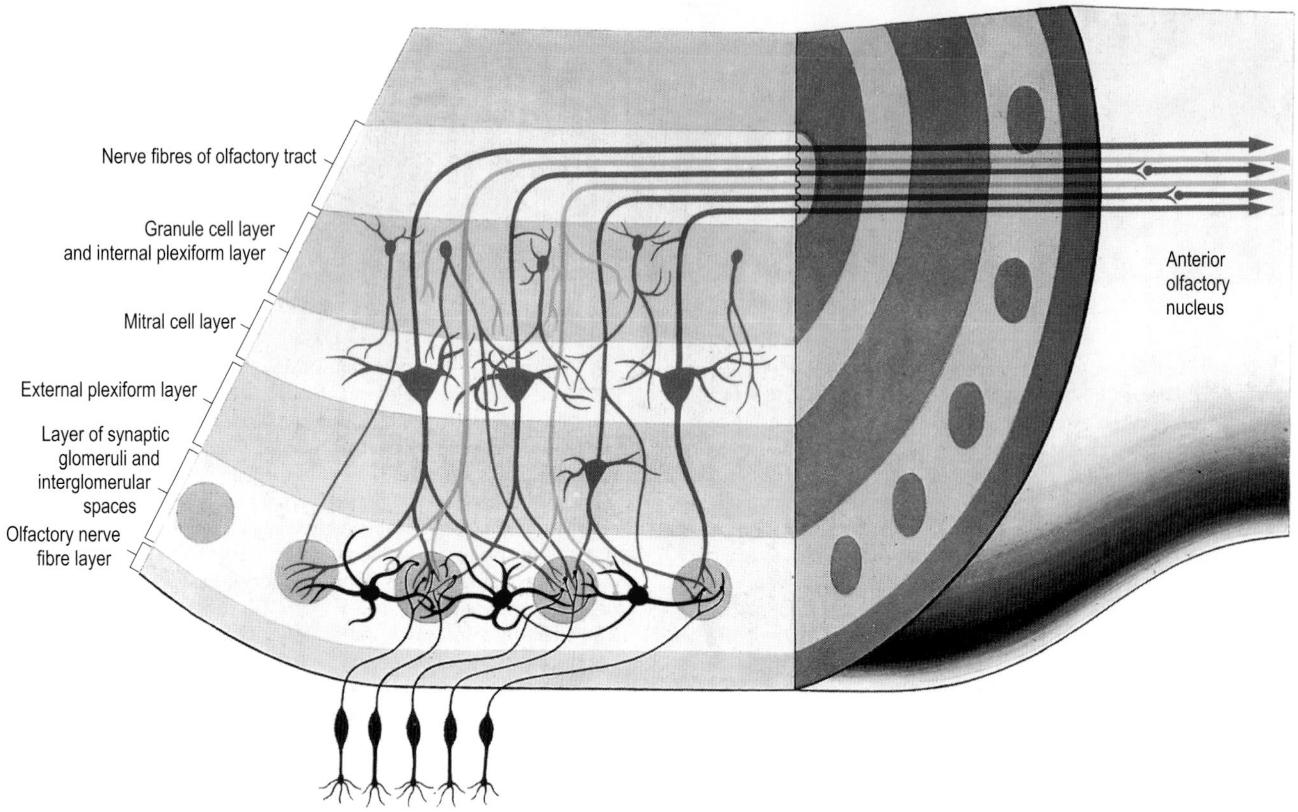
Nerve fibres of olfactory tract
Granule cell layer
and internal plexiform layer
Mitral cell layer
External plexiform layer
Layer of synaptic
glomeruli and
interglomerular
spaces
Olfactory nerve
fibre layer
Anterior
olfactory
nucleus

Fig. 12.1 *Organization of the olfactory bulb. The radial organization of the bulb into 'layers,' with their principal neurone types, and an indication of their main connections are shown.* Red, *mitral and tufted neurones and their processes;* light blue, *internal granule neurones;* dark blue, *dopaminergic periglomerular neurones;* black, *olfactory receptor neurones and their processes. The olfactory tract consists of (1) centripetal axons of mitral and tufted cells, some of which synapse with neurones in the anterior olfactory nucleus, and (2) centrifugal axons* (yellow), *which terminate in the different zones indicated.*

has a more fundamental role in the visual process itself: it provides rigid support and direction to the eye and forms the sites of attachment for its external muscles. This setting permits the accurate positioning of the visual axis under neuromuscular control and determines the spatial relationship between the two eyes—essential for binocular vision and conjugate eye movements.

The eyeball is embedded in orbital fat, separated from it by a thin fascial sheath. It is composed of the segments of two spheres of different radii. The anterior segment, part of the smaller sphere, is transparent and forms approximately 7% of the surface of the whole globe. It is more prominent than the posterior segment, which is part of the larger sphere and opaque and forms the remainder of the globe. The anterior segment is bounded by the cornea and the lens and is incompletely subdivided into anterior and posterior chambers by the iris. These chambers are continuous through the pupil. The anterior chamber is slightly overlapped by the sclera peripherally. The angle between the iris and cornea, therefore, forms an anulus of greater diameter than the limbus, the junction between the sclera and the cornea. The difference between these two varies from 1 to 2 mm, the angle being deeper above and below than at the sides of the eyeball. The posterior chamber lies between the posterior surface of the iris and the anterior aspect of the lens and its supporting ligament, the zonule, and is triangular in section. The apex of the triangle is the point where the iris touches the lens; the base, or zonular region, extends among the collagenous bundles of the zonule, sometimes even into a retrozonular space between the zonule and the vitreous humour in the posterior segment of the eyeball. The posterior segment consists of the parts of the eye posterior to the zonule and lens.

The anterior pole is the centre of the anterior (corneal) curvature, and the posterior pole is the centre of its posterior (scleral) curvature; a line joining these two points forms the optic axis. (By the same convention, the eye has an equator, equidistant between the poles: any circumferential line joining the poles is a meridian.) The optic axes of the two eyes, in their primary position, are parallel and do not correspond with the orbital axes, which diverge anterolaterally at a marked angle to each other. The optic nerves follow the orbital axes and are therefore not parallel; each enters its eye approximately 3 mm medial (nasal) to the posterior pole.

Visual Pathway

The visual pathway is illustrated in Figure 12.3. The first-order neurone of the visual system is a bipolar cell that is contained entirely within the retina. The second-order neurone is a ganglion cell whose axon enters the optic nerve.

The optic nerves pass posteromedially into the cranial cavity and meet in the midline, forming the optic chiasma, a flat mass of decussating fibres that lies at the junction of the anterior wall and floor of the third ventricle. The tuber cinereum and infundibulum lie posterior to the chiasma, and the third ventricle is dorsal to them. The termination of the internal carotid artery and the anterior perforated substance are lateral relations. The optic recess of the third ventricle passes over its superior surface to reach the lamina terminalis.

Optic nerve fibres arising from the nasal half of each retina, including half of the macula, cross in the chiasma to enter the contralateral optic tract. Fibres from the temporal hemiretinae continue into the ipsilateral optic tract. Decussating fibres loop a little backward into their ipsilateral optic nerve before crossing and then passing forward into the contralateral optic tract. Macular fibres, and those from an adjacent central area, occupy almost two-thirds of the central chiasma, dorsal to all peripheral decussating fibres. The most ventral axons are nasal fibres concerned with monocular fringes of the binocular field. They lie beneath fibres from the extramacular parts of both nasal hemiretinae, which occupy an intermediate position in the chiasma.

The optic chiasma is supplied with blood from a pial plexus that receives branches from the superior hypophysial, internal carotid, posterior communicating, anterior cerebral and anterior communicating arteries. The venous drainage of the chiasma is into the basal and anterior cerebral venous system.

Behind the optic chiasma, the optic tracts diverge dorsolaterally, each passing between the anterior perforated substance and tuber cinereum. The tract curves around the cerebral peduncle, to which it adheres. Optic tract fibres terminate primarily in the lateral geniculate nucleus of the thalamus, but also in the superior colliculus, pretectal area, suprachiasmatic nucleus of the hypothalamus and inferior pulvinar.

Axons from third-order visual neurones in the lateral geniculate nucleus run in the retrolenticular part of the internal capsule and form the optic radiation, which curves dorsomedially to the occipital cortex. Fibres representing the lower half of the visual field sweep superiorly to reach the visual cortex above

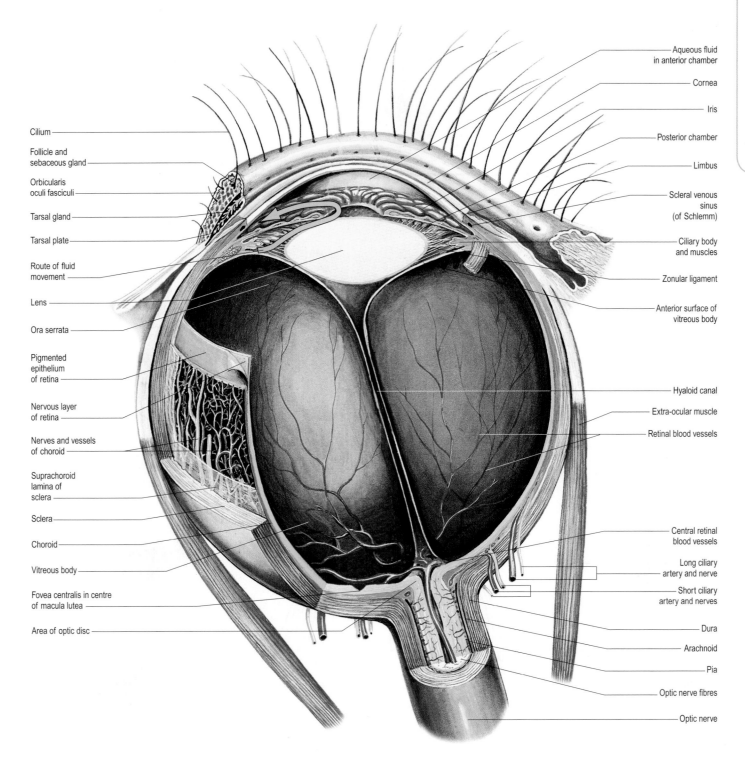

Cilium

Follicle and
sebaceous gland

Orbicularis
oculi fasciculi

Tarsal gland

Tarsal plate

Route of fluid
movement

Lens

Ora serrata

Pigmented
epithelium
of retina

Nervous layer
of retina

Nerves and vessels
of choroid

Suprachoroid
lamina of
sclera

Sclera

Choroid

Vitreous body

Fovea centralis in centre
of macula lutea

Area of optic disc

Aqueous fluid
in anterior chamber

Cornea

Iris

Posterior chamber

Limbus

Scleral venous
sinus
(of Schlemm)

Ciliary body
and muscles

Zonular ligament

Anterior surface of
vitreous body

Hyaloid canal

Extra-ocular muscle

Retinal blood vessels

Central retinal
blood vessels

Long ciliary
artery and nerve

Short ciliary
artery and nerves

Dura

Arachnoid

Pia

Optic nerve fibres

Optic nerve

Fig. 12.2 *The organization of the eye, viewed from above. In this illustration, the left eye and part of the lower eyelid are depicted in horizontal section and also cut away to show internal structure.*

the calcarine sulcus. Those representing the upper half of the visual field curve inferiorly into the temporal lobe (Meyer's loop) before reaching the visual cortex below the calcarine sulcus.

Some neurones in the occipital cortex send descending axons to the superior colliculus, which therefore receives cortical and retinal afferents. From there, fibres travel by tectobulbar tracts to motor nuclei of the third, fourth, sixth and eleventh cranial nerves and the ventral horn of the spinal cord.

Retina

The retina is the sensory neural layer of the eyeball (Figs 12.4–12.6). It is a very complex structure and should be considered a special area of the brain, from which it is derived by outgrowth from the diencephalon (Ch. 15). It is dedicated to the detection and early analysis of visual information and is an integrated part of the much larger apparatus of visual analysis present in the thalamus, cortex and other areas of the central nervous system.

The retina lies between the choroid externally and the vitreous body internally. It is thin, being thickest (0.56 mm) near the optic disc; it diminishes to 0.1 mm anterior to the equator and continues at this thickness to the ora serrata. It also thins locally at the fovea of the macula. The retina is continuous with the optic nerve at the optic disc. Anteriorly, at the ora serrata, a thin, non-neural prolongation of the retina extends forward over the ciliary processes and iris as the ciliary and iridial parts of the retina, respectively; they consist of pigmented and columnar epithelial layers only. The optic part of the retina extends from the optic disc to the ora serrata. It is soft, translucent and purple in the fresh, unbleached state because of the presence of rhodopsin (visual purple), but it soon becomes opaque and bleached when exposed to light.

Near the centre of the retina, there is a region 5 to 6 mm in diameter that contains the macula lutea (see Fig. 12.5C, D), an elliptical yellowish area measuring approximately 2 mm horizontally and 1 mm vertically. Its colour

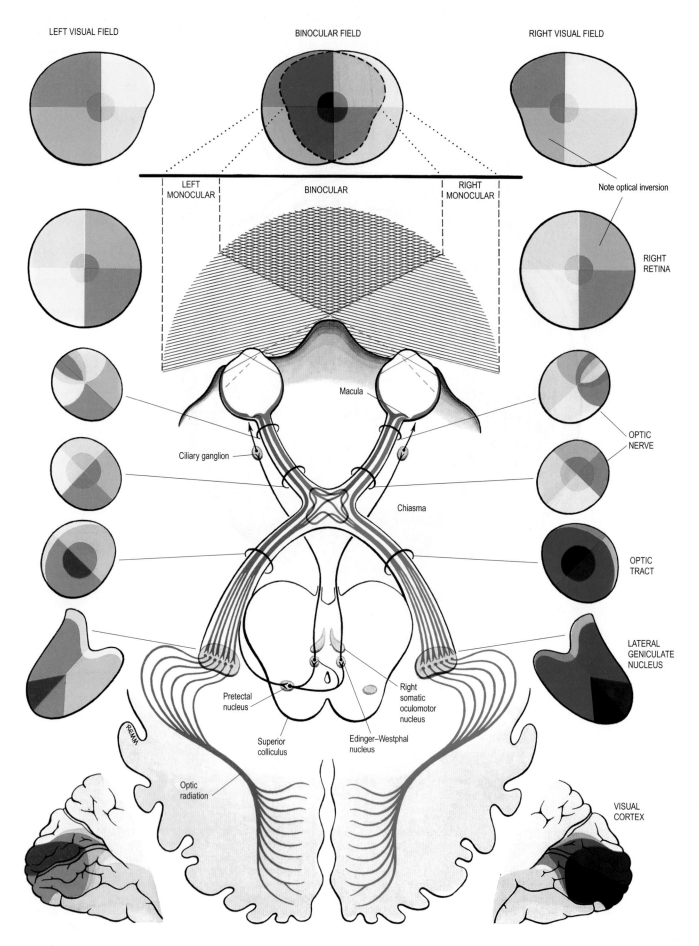

LEFT VISUAL FIELD

BINOCULAR FIELD

RIGHT VISUAL FIELD

LEFT
MONOCULAR

BINOCULAR

RIGHT
MONOCULAR

Note optical inversion

RIGHT
RETINA

Macula

Ciliary ganglion

OPTIC
NERVE

Chiasma

OPTIC
TRACT

LATERAL
GENICULATE
NUCLEUS

Pretectal
nucleus

Right
somatic
oculomotor
nucleus

Superior
colliculus

Edinger–Westphal
nucleus

Optic
radiation

VISUAL
CORTEX

Fig. 12.3 *The visual pathway, showing the spatial arrangement of neurones and their fibres in relation to the quadrants of the retinae and visual fields. The proportions at various levels are not exactly to scale; in particular, the macula is exaggerated in size in the visual fields and retinae. In each quadrant of the visual field and the parts of the visual pathway subserving it, two shades of the respective colour are used—paler for the peripheral fields, and darker for the macular part of the quadrant. From the optic tract onward, these two shades are both more saturated to denote the intermixture of neurones from both retinae, with the palest shade reserved for parts of the visual pathway concerned with monocular vision. The pathway subserving the pupillary light reflex is also indicated.*

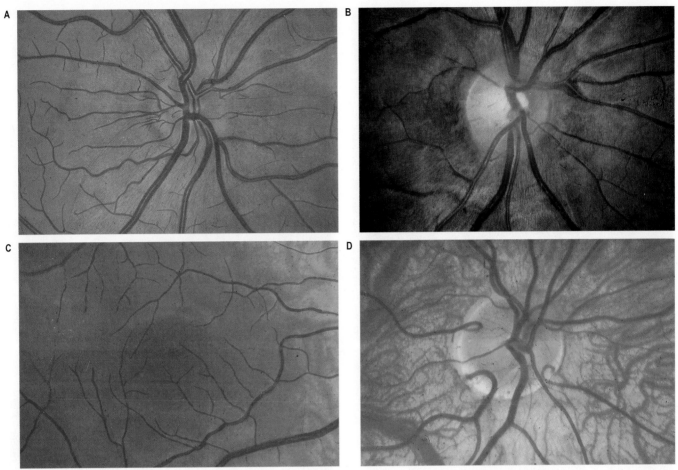

Fig. 12.4 *Ophthalmoscopic photographs of the right human retina.* **A,** *Note the dichotomous branching of vessels. Arteries are brighter red and show a more pronounced 'reflex' to light, as a pale stria along their length. The veins are also larger in calibre; more of them cross arteries superficially than is usual. The optic disc, around the entry of the vessels, is a light pink, with a surrounding zone of heavier pigmentation. Compare with Figure 12.5A from the same Caucasian adult.* **B,** *Appearances in a heavily pigmented individual (an adult of African origin), with a paler optic disc than in* **A.** *Note accentuation of the edge of the disc by retinal and choroidal pigmentation. The arteries cross the veins superficially in this retina.* **C,** *Normal macula of a young Caucasian subject. The vessels radiate from the centrally placed fovea. The macular branches of the central retinal artery are approaching from the right. The macula is largely free of vessels of macroscopic size, but the capillaries here form a particularly close network, except at the fovea.* **D,** *The region of the optic disc in an eye with poorly developed pigmentation. Three cilioretinal arteries are curving around the edge of the disc (two on the left, one on the right). Between the two cilioretinal arteries, a single macular artery is apparent. Due to the depressed pigmentation, choroidal vessels are also visible, especially veins; on the left of the photograph, two large vorticose venous tributaries can be seen.*

is due to the presence of xanthophyll derivatives. The macula lutea contains a central depression, the fovea centralis or foveola, with a diameter of approximately 0.4 mm, where visual resolution is highest (see Fig. 12.6.) Here, all elements except pigment epithelium cone photoreceptors are displaced laterally. The minute size of the foveola is the reason why the visual axes must be directed with great accuracy to achieve the most discriminative vision.

About 3 mm medial (nasal) and 1 mm superior to the foveola, the optic nerve becomes continuous with the retina at the optic disc ('blind spot'). It is approximately 1.5 mm in diameter. The name 'optic papilla,' which is often applied to the disc, is a misnomer because almost all of a normal disc is level with the retina. Centrally, it contains a shallow depression, where it is pierced by the central retinal vessels (see Figs 12.2, 12.4, 12.5A, B). The disc is devoid of photoreceptors and is therefore insensitive to light. By ophthalmoscopy, the disc is normally pink, but it is much paler than the retina and may be grey or almost white. In optic atrophy the capillary vessels disappear, and the disc is then white.

Microstructure

The retina is derived from the two layers of the invaginated optic vesicle; the outer layer becomes the layer of pigment cells, and the inner layer develops into a complex multilaminar structure of sensory and neural cells. Anteriorly, sensory and neural cells are absent from the retina as it approaches the ora serrata and merges into the ciliary body and iris.

The neural retina contains a variety of cell types, including photoreceptors (rod and cone cells), their first-order neurones (bipolar cells) and the somata and axons of the second-order neurones (ganglion cells); it also contains two major classes of interneurones, the horizontal and amacrine cells. In addition, the retina contains neuroglial elements and a rich vascular system, chiefly of capillaries. It is backed by specialized pigment epithelial cells.

Layers of the Retina

The retina is organized into layers or zones (Fig. 12.7), where distinctive components of its cells are clustered together or in register to form continuous strata. These layers extend uninterrupted throughout the photoreceptive retina except at the exit point of the optic nerve fibres at the optic disc, although certain layers are much reduced at the foveola where the photoreceptive elements predominate. The names given to the different layers reflect, in part, the components present within them, and also their position in the thickness of the retina. Conventionally, those structures farthest from the vitreous (i.e. toward the choroid) are designated as outer or external, and those toward the vitreous are inner or internal.

Customarily, 10 retinal layers are distinguished (Fig. 12.8), beginning at the choroidal edge and passing toward the vitreous. These are the retinal pigment epithelium, layer of rods and cones (outer and inner segments), external limiting membrane, outer nuclear layer, outer plexiform layer, inner nuclear layer, inner plexiform layer, ganglion cell layer, nerve fibre layer, and internal limiting membrane. Some of these are subdivided into substrata, and an innermost plexiform layer between layers 8 and 9 has also been demonstrated.

Rod and cone cells reach radially inward from the rod and cone lamina through the outer nuclear layer, where they have their nuclei, to the outer plexiform layer, where they synapse with bipolar and horizontal cells. Bipolar cells possess dendrites in the outer plexiform layer, cell bodies and nuclei in the inner nuclear layer, and axons in the inner plexiform layer, where they synapse with ganglion cell and amacrine cell dendrites. Horizontal cells have their dendrites and axons in the outer plexiform layer and their nuclei in the inner nuclear layer; ganglion cells have their dendrites in the inner plexiform layer, their cell bodies in the ganglion cell layer and their axons in the layer of nerve fibres (and within the optic nerve). Amacrine cell dendrites are mainly in the inner plexiform layer, although some (interplexiform cells) extend into the outer plexiform layer; amacrine cell dendrites are situated in either the

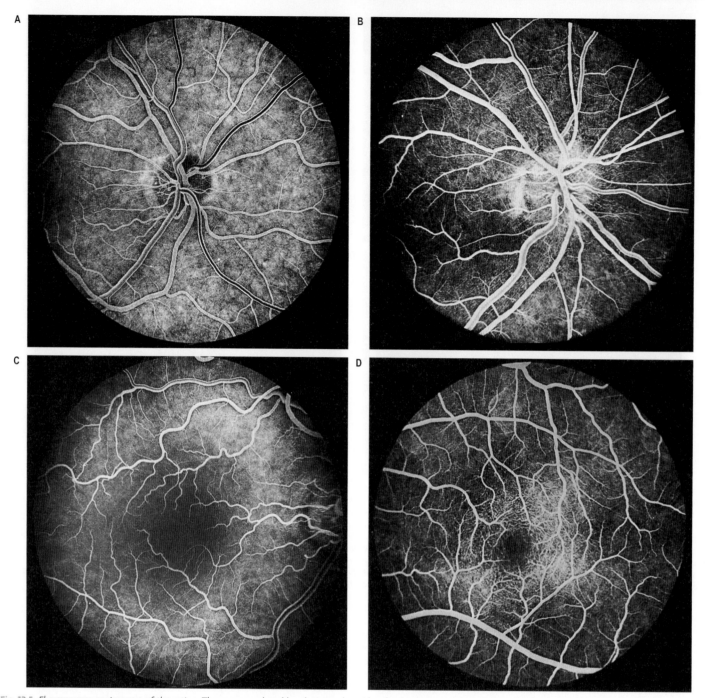

Fig. 12.5 *Fluorescence angiograms of the retina. These are produced by photography with a fundus camera at known periods of time following the introduction of fluorescein into the circulation. **A**, Angiogram of the same retina shown in Figure 12.4A, taken in 'mid-venous' phase. The arteries display an even fluorescence, but the veins appear striped, owing to laminar flow. This appearance is the reverse of the arterial 'reflex' shown in Figure 12.4A and should not be compared with it. The background mottling is due to fluorescence from the choroidal vessels. **B**, Angiogram of the left optic disc, showing the major arteries and veins and also their smaller branches. Note particularly the radial pattern in the retinal capillaries. The laminar flow in the veins is less obvious than in Figure 12.4A. **C**, Angiogram showing the macular region of a right eye. The main macular vessels are approaching from the right. The subject is an elderly person with considerable macular pigmentation, which masks fluorescence from the choroidal circulation. **D**, Angiogram of the macula of a young subject (left eye) showing the macular capillaries in detail. Note the central avascular fovea. Compare with **C**.*

inner nuclear layer or the outer part of the ganglionic layer (displaced amacrines). Pigment cells lie behind the retina, and several types of retinal glial cell are distributed in distinctive locations among its different layers.

The composition of the retinal layers is as follows:

Layer 1: Pigment Epithelium — This is a simple low cuboidal epithelium that forms the back of the retina and therefore forms the boundary with the choroid, from which it is separated by a thick composite basal lamina.

Layer 2: Rod and Cone Cell Processes — This contains the photoreceptive outer segments and the outer parts of the inner segments of rod and cone cells.

Layer 3: External Limiting Membrane — This layer appears as a distinct line by light microscopy. It consists of a zone of intercellular junctions of the zonula adherens type between the processes of radial glial cells and photoreceptor processes.

Layer 4: Outer Nuclear Layer — This consists of several tiers of rod and cone cell bodies and their nuclei, the cone nuclei lying outermost. Mingled

with these are the outer and inner fibres from the same cell bodies, directed outward to the bases of inner segments and inward toward the outer plexiform layer.

Layer 5: Outer Plexiform Layer — This is a region of complex synaptic arrangements between the processes of cells whose cell bodies lie in the adjacent layers. The outer plexiform layer contains the synaptic processes of rod and cone cells, bipolar cells, horizontal cells and some interplexiform cells (which, in this account, are grouped with the amacrines).

Layer 6: Inner Nuclear Layer — This is composed of three nuclear strata. Horizontal cell nuclei form the outermost zone; then, in sequence inward, are the nuclei and cell bodies of bipolar cells, radial glial cells and the outer set of amacrine cells, including the interplexiform cells whose dendrites cross this layer.

Layer 7: Inner Plexiform Layer — This is divisible into three layers, depending on the types of contact that occur. The outer or 'off' layer contains synapses between 'off' bipolar cells, ganglion cells and some amacrines; a middle

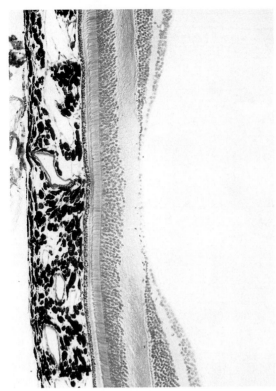

Fig. 12.6 *Section through the fovea centralis. (By permission from Young, B., Heath, J.W., 2000. Wheater's Functional Histology, Churchill Livingstone, Edinburgh.)*

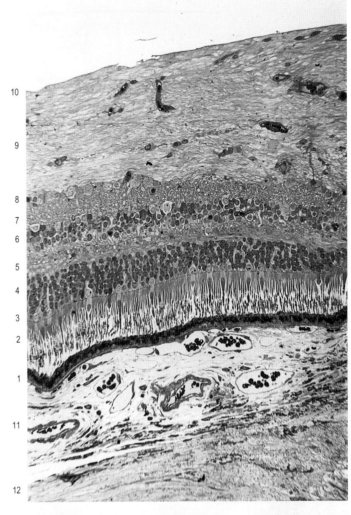

1. Pigment epithelial layer	5. Outer plexiform layer	9. Nerve fibre layer
2. Rod and cone layer	6. Inner nuclear layer	10. Internal limiting membrane
3. External limiting membrane	7. Inner plexiform layer	11. Choroid
4. Outer nuclear layer	8. Ganglion cell layer	12. Sclera

Fig. 12.7 *Retina of a 60-year-old man. The section was made close to the optic nerve head, explaining the thickened nerve fibre layer. 1, pigment epithelial layer; 2, rod and cone layer; 3, external limiting membrane; 4, outer nuclear layer; 5, outer plexiform layer; 6, inner nuclear layer; 7, inner plexiform layer; 8, ganglion cell layer; 9, nerve fibre layer; 10, internal limiting membrane; 11, choroid; 12, sclera. (Courtesy of the late Gordon L. Ruskell, Department of Optometry and Visual Science, The City University, London.)*

or 'on' layer contains synapses between the axons of 'on' bipolars and the dendrites of ganglion cells and displaced amacrines; and an inner 'rod' layer contains synapses between rod bipolars and displaced amacrines. (Refer to Wässle and Boycott 1991 for an explanation of the 'off' and 'on' cell designations.)

Layer 8: Ganglion Cell Layer — This layer contains the nuclei of the displaced amacrine cells. Its inner regions consist of the cell bodies, nuclei and initial segments of retinal ganglion cells of various classes.

Layer 9: Nerve Fibre Layer — This contains the unmyelinated axons of retinal ganglion cells. It forms a zone of variable thickness over the inner retinal surface and is the only component of the retina at the point where the fibres pass into the nerve at the optic disc. The inner aspect of this layer contains the nuclei and processes of astrocytes, which, together with radial glial cells, ensheathe the nerve fibres. Between the nerve fibre layer and the ganglion cells is another narrow innermost plexiform layer, where neuronal processes make synaptic contact with axon hillocks and initial segments of ganglion cells.

Layer 10: Internal Limiting Membrane — This is a glial boundary between the retina and the vitreous body. It is formed by the end-feet of radial glial cells and astrocytes and is separated from the vitreous body by a basal lamina.

Cells of the Retina

Retinal Pigment Epithelial Cells — The retinal pigment epithelial cells are low cuboidal cells that form a single continuous layer, extending from the periphery of the optic disc to the ora serrata and continue from there into the ciliary epithelium. They are flat in radial section and hexagonal or pentagonal in surface view. There are about 4 million to 6 million in the human retina. Their cytoplasm contains numerous melanin granules (Fig. 12.9). Apically (toward the rods and cones), the cells bear long (5 to 7 mm) microvilli that contact or project between the outer ends of rod and cone processes. The tips of rod outer segments are deeply inserted into invaginations in the apical membrane. The attachments are unsupported by junctional complexes and are broken in the clinical condition of retinal detachment arising from trauma or disease processes.

Pigment epithelial cells play a major role in the turnover of rod and cone photoreceptive components. Their cytoplasm contains the phagocytosed ends of rods and cones undergoing lysosomal destruction. The final products of this process are lipofuscin granules, which accumulate in these cells and add to their granular appearance. The failure of some part of this process may cause progressive loss of retinal function and eventual blindness, such as when enzyme deficiencies cause the buildup of shed but undegraded photoreceptor components within the retina.

The epithelium also acts as an antireflection device and prevents the light from bouncing back into the photoreceptive layer, with consequent loss of image sharpness. This process is complex, because the energy absorbed can be dissipated as heat or generate free radicals, both of which are potentially damaging. Indeed, very intense light may damage the pigment cells and cause epithelial breakdown.

The zone of tight junctions between the pigment cells allows the epithelium to function as an important blood–retinal barrier between the retina and the vascular system of the choroid. These junctions guard the special ionic environment of the retina and inhibit the entry of leukocytes into this immunologically sequestered compartment of the eye.

Cone and Rod Cells — The cone and rod cells are the retinal photoreceptor cells (Fig. 12.10). They are long, radially oriented structures with a cylindrical photoreceptive portion at the end nearest to the pigment epithelium and synaptic contacts at the other end, within the outer plexiform layer. Both types of cells have a similar organization, although their details differ. From the external (choroidal) end inward, the cells consist of outer and inner segments, a cell body containing the nucleus and either a cone pedicle or a rod spherule (depending on cell type); this is an area of synaptic contact with adjacent bipolar and horizontal cells and with other cone or rod cells. The outer and inner segments together form a cone process or a rod process (it should be noted that the terms *cone* and *rod* are often loosely applied to the whole cell); the cone process is wider but tapers (hence the name), whereas

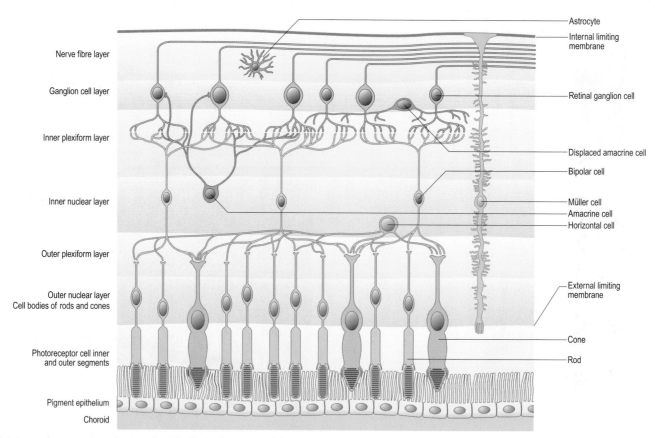

Fig. 12.8 *Layered arrangement of neuronal cell bodies in the retina and the interconnections of their processes in the intervening plexiform layers. Also shown are the two principal types of neuroglial cells in the retina; microglia are also present but are not shown.*

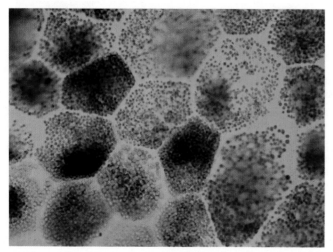

Fig. 12.9 *Unstained retinal pigment epithelium from a 40-year-old individual, seen in surface view. (Courtesy of John Marshall, Institute of Ophthalmology, London.)*

the rod processes are cylindrical. The outer and inner segments are connected by a short cilium.

Cone cells are chiefly responsible for high spatial resolution and colour vision in good lighting conditions (photopic vision). Rod cells provide high monochromatic sensitivity to a much wider range of illumination down to much lower intensities (scotopic vision), although with relatively low spatial discrimination because of their different neural connections. Cone cells are of three types—red, green and blue—according to their maximal spectral sensitivities. They are highly concentrated in the centre of the retina (the fovea), where visual acuity is greatest, but they populate the whole retina, intermingled with rods, as far as its neural edge. Rods are excluded from the fovea. The total number of rods in the human retina has been estimated at 110 million to 125 million, and cones at 63 million to 68 million (Osterberg 1935).

The outer segments of rods contain the photoreceptive protein rhodopsin (visual purple). Related photosensitive pigments with different absorption properties are present in cones. Photoreceptive pigments are incorporated

into flattened membranous discs that form as deep infoldings of the plasma membrane and stack together within the photoreceptor outer segments. They bud off as free discs within the outer segment of rods, where their turnover is rapid. New discs are generated at the proximal end closest to the soma and they are shed at the distal end embedded in the pigment epithelium, where they are phagocytosed. Turnover appears to be less rapid in cones, where the discs retain continuity with the plasma membrane, and a more random insertion of disc components may occur. Cones are much narrower at the fovea, where they closely resemble rods in size.

Bipolar Cells — Bipolar cells are radially oriented neurones, each with one or more dendrites that synapse with cones or rods and horizontal cells and interplexiform cells in the outer plexiform layer. Their somata are located in the inner nuclear layer, and axonal branches given off in the inner plexiform layer synapse with dendrites of ganglion cells or amacrine cells (see Fig. 12.8). Cone bipolars are of three major types—midget, blue cone or diffuse—according to their connectivity and size. As their name implies, midget cone bipolars are small cells, and each one is part of a single one-to-one channel from cone to ganglion cell; they are thought to mediate high spatial resolution. Blue cones have similar connectivity and selectively form part of a short wavelength-mediating channel. The larger diffuse cone bipolars are connected to up to 10 cones and are thought to signal luminosity rather than colour. Rod bipolars receive direct photoreceptive inputs from many rods and relate to ganglion cells indirectly via a synapse with amacrine cells.

Horizontal Cells — Horizontal cells (see Fig. 12.8) are inhibitory interneurones whose dendrites and axons extend within the outer plexiform layer, making synaptic contacts with the bases of cones and rods and, via gap junctions at the tips of their dendrites, with one another. Their cell bodies lie in the outer part of the inner nuclear layer. Because of their interactions with photoreceptor cells and bipolar cells, horizontal cells create inhibitory surrounds. When illumination of a photoreceptor cluster with a point of light causes depolarization of synaptically connected 'on' bipolars at its bright centre, horizontal cell dendrites cause inhibition at the edge of the illuminated area, thus sharpening contrast and maximizing spatial resolution.

Amacrine Cells — Amacrine cells (see Fig. 12.8) lack typical axons, but their dendrites function as axons and dendrites and make both incoming and outgoing synapses. Each neurone has a cell body in the inner nuclear layer; near its boundary with the inner plexiform layer; or on the outer aspect of the ganglion cell layer, where they are known as displaced amacrine cells. The processes of amacrine neurones make scattered chemical synaptic contacts

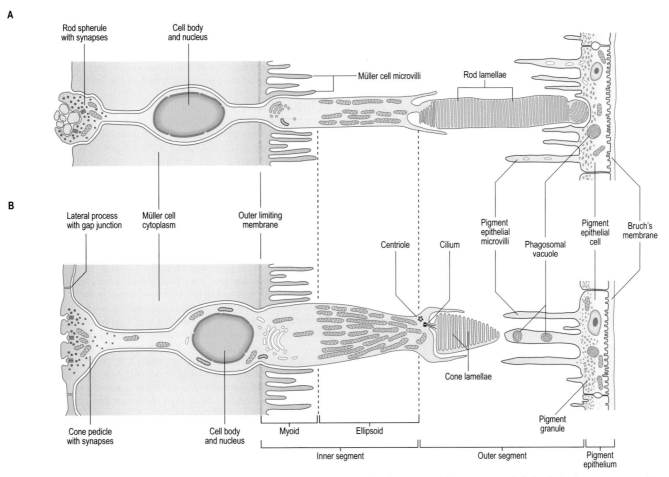

A

Rod spherule with synapses

Cell body and nucleus

Müller cell microvilli

Rod lamellae

B

Lateral process with gap junction

Müller cell cytoplasm

Outer limiting membrane

Centriole

Cilium

Pigment epithelial microvilli

Phagosomal vacuole

Pigment epithelial cell

Bruch's membrane

Cone pedicle with synapses

Cell body and nucleus

Myoid

Ellipsoid

Cone lamellae

Pigment granule

Inner segment

Outer segment

Pigment epithelium

Fig. 12.10 *Major features of a retinal rod cell (**A**) and a retinal cone cell (**B**). Note that the relative size of the pigment epithelial cells has been exaggerated for illustrative purposes.*

with the axons of bipolar cells, dendrites (and possibly axons) of ganglion cells and the processes of other amacrine cells. They also receive numerous synapses from bipolar cells. Some amacrine cells form electrical synapses with bipolar cells.

There are several classes of amacrine cells that variously serve a number of important functions in vision. One class (amacrine II cells) transmits signals from rod bipolars to ganglion cells and is therefore an essential element in the rod pathway. Others appear to be important modulators of photoreceptive signals and serve to adjust or maintain relative colour and luminosity inputs under changing light conditions, such as at different times of the day. They are probably responsible for some of the complex forms of image analysis known to occur within the retina (e.g. directional movement detection).

Ganglion Cells — Ganglion cells (see Fig. 12.8) are the final common pathway neurones of the retina. Their dendrites are synaptically connected with processes of bipolar and amacrine neurones in the inner plexiform layer, and their axons are likewise connected with neurones in the central nervous system. Their axons form the layer of nerve fibres on the inner surface of the retina. They turn tangentially to the optic disc, through which they leave the eye as fibres of the optic nerve. The axons are subsequently distributed to various parts of the brain, including the lateral geniculate nucleus, pretectal area and superior colliculus of the midbrain; the thalamic pulvinar; and the accessory optic system.

Ganglion cell bodies form a single stratum in most of the retina but become progressively more numerous near the macula. They are ranked in about 10 rows in the macular area, and their number diminishes again toward the fovea, from which they are almost totally excluded. Ganglion cells are multipolar neurones, varying from 10 to 30 mm or more in diameter. Their dendrites vary in number and branching pattern and usually emerge opposite the axon. Numbers of ganglion cells in the human macular area reach $38,000/mm^2$; they are more numerous in the nasal than the temporal retina and in the superior retina compared with the inferior, although numbers vary considerably in different eyes. In total, each human retina has approximately 106 ganglion cells, each of which receives signals from large numbers of photoreceptor cells.

In the nerve fibre layer, axons of ganglion cells converge on the optic disc from the whole retina. They converge in a simple radial pattern from the medial (nasal) half of the retina. However, the macular area, inferolateral to the optic disc, complicates the course of the lateral (temporal) axons. Axons from the macula form a papillomacular fasciculus that passes almost straight to the disc. The more temporal fibres, which are more peripheral, swerve circumferentially above and below the macula to reach the disc.

Axons of ganglion cells are almost always non-myelinated within the retina, which is an optical advantage because myelin is refractile. They are surrounded by the processes of radial glial cells and retinal astrocytes. A few small myelinated fibres may occur, but in general, myelin sheaths usually commence only as the axons enter the optic disc to become the optic nerve.

Retinal Glial Cells — Retinal glial cells are of three types: radial (Müller) cells, astrocytes and microglia. Radial glial cells are the predominant glial element in most of the retina. Retinal astrocytes are largely confined to the ganglion cell and nerve fibre layers. Microglial cells are scattered throughout the neural part of the retina in small numbers (see Fig. 12.8).

Radial glial cells span the entire thickness of the neural retina. They ensheathe and separate the various photoreceptive and neural cells, except at synaptic sites. They form the outer boundary of the retinal tissue at the level of the inner rod and cone segments and the inner boundary at the internal limiting membrane. Their nuclei lie within the inner nuclear layer, and from this region, a single thick fibre ascends radially, giving off complex lateral lamellae that branch among the processes of the outer plexiform layer. Apically, the central process terminates in a surface from which microvilli project into the space between the rod and cone processes. Just beneath this area, the radial glial cells form a line of dense zonulae adherentes with one another and with receptor inner segments, thus forming the external limiting membrane. On the inner aspect of the retina, the main radial glial cell process expands in a terminal footplate that contacts those of neighbouring radial glial cells and astrocytes and attaches to the internal limiting membrane. Like other neuroglia, radial glia also contact blood vessels, especially capillaries, and their basal laminae fuse with those of the vascular smooth muscle in the media of larger vessels or of the endothelia lining capillaries. These extensive neuroglial cells form much of the total retinal volume and almost totally fill the extracellular space between neural elements. Their functions appear to be similar to those of astrocytes—that is, maintenance of the stability of the retinal extracellular environment by ionic transport, uptake of neurotransmitter, removal of debris, storage of glycogen, electrical insulation of receptors and neurones and mechanical support of the neural retina.

The cell bodies of retinal astrocytes lie between the layer of nerve fibres and the internal limiting membrane, while their processes branch to form sheaths around ganglion cell axons. They are present only in regions of the retina that are vascularized and are therefore absent from the fovea. Astrocytes contribute substantially to the glia limitans, which surrounds the capillaries. Retinal microglia are scattered mainly within the inner plexiform layer. Their radiating branched processes spread mainly parallel to the retinal plane, and this gives them a star-like appearance when viewed microscopically from the surface of the retina. They can act as phagocytes, and their number increases in the injured retina.

The expanded end-feet of radial glial cells and astrocytes are separated from the vitreous body by a complex, rather thick (0.5 mm) internal limiting membrane that is continuous with the internal limiting membrane of the ciliary body. The delicate collagen fibrils of the vitreous body blend with the glial basal lamina. The internal limiting membrane is involved in fluid exchange between the vitreous and the retina and, perhaps through the latter, with the choroid. It has various other functions, including anchorage of retinal glial cells and inhibition of cell migration into the vitreous body.

Modifications in the Macular Area

All the retinal layers are modified in the macular area and, to a marked degree, in the fovea, which is largely devoid of rod cells or processes. Approximately 2500 close-packed, elongated, very narrow cone cells lie in the floor of the fovea (foveola), an arrangement that favours photopic vision and the high degree of spatial discrimination typical of foveal vision.

The general displacement of the outer nuclear layer to the foveal periphery means that the internal processes of the photoreceptors are stretched out tangentially in the external plexiform layer; consequently, there are no cone pedicles or rod spherules in the central fovea and foveola. The inner nuclear layer is also displaced to the edge of the foveal depression, and the internal plexiform, ganglionic and nerve fibre layers are almost absent from the whole fovea. Therefore, even on the foveal wall, the retina is thinner and more transparent than elsewhere. Capillaries reach the foveal margin, but they invade the ganglionic layer only at its circumference, so that the fovea is normally devoid of all blood vessels.

CASE 1 MACULAR DEGENERATION

An 81-year-old patient presents with a 6-month history of increasingly blurred vision initially involving the right eye and later the left. He has observed a decreased ability to read a newspaper, especially in dim light, and difficulty with dark adaptation. He has no other significant symptoms.

On examination, visual testing reveals best corrected vision of 20/100 in the right eye and 20/70 in the left. Visual fields are full with confrontation testing and perimetry. Funduscopic examination demonstrates macular oedema, and a small haemorrhage is present on the periphery of the macula in the right eye.

A fluorescein angiogram documents leakage in the region of the macula bilaterally, and the patient is diagnosed as having the neovascular subtype of age-related macular degeneration. He is treated with laser photocoagulation, but his vision gradually deteriorates over the next several years, with 20/400 acuity in the right eye and 20/200 in the left.

Discussion: Age-related macular degeneration is the leading cause of central visual loss in patients older than 65 years. The cause is unknown. Two forms of the disorder are recognized: non-neovascular (dry) and neovascular (wet). The non-neovascular form is more common, but the neovascular form is generally more severe, with a more rapid deterioration of vision.

Optic Disc and Retinal Blood Vessels

The retina is placed between two sets of arteries and veins—the ciliary vessels of the choroid, and the branches of the central retinal vessels. It depends on both circulations because neither is sufficient by itself to maintain full visual activity in the retina. The central retinal vessels enter and leave the retina at the optic disc, which is described first; then the vessels are considered.

Optic Disc

The optic disc is the region where retinal tissues meet the neural and glial elements of the optic nerve and the connective tissues of the sclera and meninges (see Figs 12.2, 12.4, 12.5). It is the exit point for the optic nerve fibres and a point of entry and exit for the retinal circulation. It is the only site where anastomoses occur with other arteries (the posterior ciliary arteries). It is visible, by ophthalmoscopy, and is a region of much clinical importance; it is here that the central vessels can be inspected directly—the only vessels so accessible in the whole body. Oedema of the disc (papilloedema) may be the first sign of raised intracranial pressure, which is transmitted into the subarachnoid space around the optic nerve and compresses the central retinal vein where it crosses the space.

The optic disc is superomedial to the posterior pole of the eye, so it lies away from the visual axis. It is round or oval, usually approximately 1.6 mm in transverse diameter and 1.8 mm in vertical diameter, and its appearance is very variable (for details, see Jonas, Gusek and Naumann 1988). In light-skinned subjects, the general retinal hue is a bright terra-cotta red, with which the pale pink of the disc contrasts sharply; its central part is usually even paler and may be light grey. These differences are due in part to the degree of vascularization of the two regions, which is much less at the optic disc; it is also due to the total absence of choroidal or retinal pigment cells, because the retina is represented in the disc by little more than the internal limiting membrane. In subjects with strongly melanized skin, both the retina and disc are darker (see Fig. 12.4B). The optic disc does not project at all in many eyes, and rarely does it project sufficiently to justify the term *papilla*. It is usually a little elevated on its lateral side, where the papillomacular nerve fibres turn into the optic nerve. There is usually a slight depression where the retinal vessels traverse its centre.

Retinal Vascular Supply

The central retinal artery enters the optic nerve as a branch of the ophthalmic artery, approximately 1.2 cm behind the eyeball. It travels in the optic nerve to its head, where its fascicles traverse the lamina cribrosa. At this level, which is usually not visible with ophthalmoscopy, the central artery divides into two equal branches, superior and inferior. After a few millimetres, these divide into superior and inferior nasal branches and superior and inferior temporal branches. Each of these four branches supplies its own 'quadrant' of the retina, although each territory is much more than a quadrant, because the branches ramify as far as the ora serrata. Corresponding retinal veins unite to form the central retinal vein. However, the courses of the venous and arterial vessels do not correspond exactly, and arteries often cross veins, usually lying superficial to them. In severe hypertension, the arteries may press on the veins and cause visible dilatation distal to these crossings. Arterial pulsation is not visible by routine ophthalmoscopy without higher magnification.

Visual Field Defects

Plotting visual field loss frequently reveals the approximate location of the causative lesion in the visual pathway and sometimes its nature (Fig. 12.11). Because retinal lesions can be visualized using an ophthalmoscope, these aids might appear to be redundant, but visual field measurement is still helpful in assessing the extent of the damage and may be the key factor in confirming a diagnosis. Glaucoma serves as an example. Field defects in glaucoma, occurring as a consequence of damage to the nerve fibre bundles at the optic nerve head, may be detectable ophthalmoscopically, but confirmation of the diagnosis frequently depends on field assessment. An initial constriction of the visual field is of little clinical significance, but later defects, characteristic of the disease, consist of a scotoma between 10 and 20 degrees of the fixation area, extending upward or, less commonly, downward from the blind spot. This later elongates circumferentially along the arcuate nerve fibres and subsequently extends farther. The field defect forms a linear limit or step along the horizontal meridian nasally; the loss continues, ultimately resulting in blindness.

With regard to the location of lesions central to the retina, deficits in the vision of one eye are usually attributable to optic nerve lesions. Lesions of the optic chiasma, involving crossing nerve fibres, produce a bilateral field loss, as exemplified by pituitary adenoma. The tumour expands upward from the pituitary fossa, compressing the inferior midline of the chiasma, and eventually produces bitemporal hemianopia, starting with an early loss in the upper temporal quadrants. Field defects in the rare cases of optic tract lesions

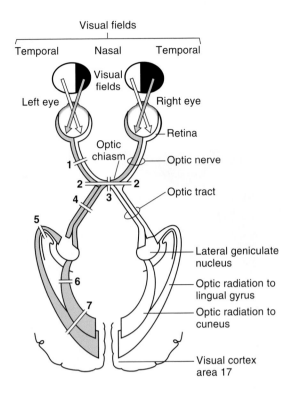

Lesion	Visual defect
1. Optic nerve	Ipsilateral blindness
Optic chiasm 2. Bilateral lateral compression	Binasal hemianopia
3. Midsagittal transection/pressure	Bitemporal hemianopia
4. Optic tract (left)	Right hemianopia
Optic radiation (left) 5. Lower division	Right upper quadrantanopia
6. Upper division	Right lower quadrantanopia
7. Both divisions	Right hemianopia with macular sparing

Fig. 12.11 *Schematic diagram of the visual system, demonstrating the visual field defects associated with various lesions along the visual pathways. From Brown, T.A., 2007. Rapid Review Physiology. Mosby, Philadelphia.*

CASE 2   RETINITIS PIGMENTOSA

A 25-year-old man presents with symptoms of approximately 5 years' duration. At age 18 he first noted difficulty running and unsteadiness; at that time, he demonstrated only mild gait ataxia. He has noted greater difficulty driving at might. There is no family history of secular symptoms.

Neurological examination shows gait ataxia with dysmetria and impaired limb dexterity throughout. Reflexes are generally hyperactive, but the Achilles reflexes are absent. Neuro-ophthalmological examination reveals constricted visual fields with normal visual acuity. Funduscopic examination demonstrates pigmentary changes in the retina with the appearance of bony spicules, along with narrowing of the retinal arterioles and slight pallor of the optic discs.

The electroretinogram is abnormal. An electromyogram and nerve conduction study document evidence of an axonal polyneuropathy. A diagnosis of retinitis pigmentosa (RP), associated with neuropathy and ataxia is made, subsequently supported by genetic testing. Over a period of years, the patient's neurological abnormalities increase, with marked impairment of night vision, gradual constriction of the visual fields and ultimately decreased visual acuity. RP is characterized by progressive visual loss, especially loss of night vision. It is a heterogenous group of genetic disorders leading to the death of rod photoreceptors, frequently associated with other neurological symptoms.

are distinctive. The tract contains contralateral nasal and ipsilateral temporal retinal projections, and damage causes a homonymous contralateral loss of field with substantial incongruity (dissimilar defects in the two fields). Incongruity probably results from a delay in achieving coincidence between retinal topographical projections of the two inputs of the visual pathway; as contiguous projections adjust their location, they gradually achieve coincidence. It also likely reflects the normal reorganization of fibres that occurs in the optic tracts, as some fibres leave the tract in the superior brachium and others progress to the lateral geniculate nucleus. The two defective fields may display incongruity as a result of lesions above the level of the chiasma. Incongruity is most marked in optic tract defects, less obvious in optic radiation defects and usually absent in cortically induced field defects, thus providing an additional clue to the location of the cause.

Lesions of the optic radiations are usually unilateral and commonly vascular in origin. Field defects therefore develop abruptly, in contrast to the slow progression of defects associated with tumours. Resulting hemifield loss follows the general rule that visual field defects central to the chiasma (i.e behind the chiasma) are on the side opposite the lesion. Little or no incongruity is seen in visual cortical lesions, but they commonly display the phenomenon of macular sparing, with the central 5 degrees to 10 degrees field retained in an otherwise hemianopic defect.

Neural Control of Gaze

Neural control systems are required to coordinate the movements of the eyes so that the image of the object of interest is simultaneously held on both foveae, despite movement of the object or the observer. A number of

CASE 3   OPTIC NEURITIS

A 26-year-old woman presents with a 2-day history of progressive loss of vision in her left eye, with accompanying left orbital pain, especially on eye movement. At the onset she noted blurring of vision. She performed a monocular cover test on herself and discovered that the blurring was confined to the left eye. She noted that when she looked at a computer screen with her left eye it became 'black and white.' Her visual loss stabilized after several days; she ultimately observed that she could see 'all around' a central visual loss in the left eye. It is noteworthy that 1 year before she had an episode of numbness and tingling sensations affecting her left arm and leg, lasting about 6 weeks. She did not seek medical attention at that time.

Examination shows a visual acuity of 20/20 on the right and 20/400 on the left. Impaired colour vision is noted on the left, and there is a central scotoma with visual field testing. There is a prominent left afferent pupillary defect (Marcus Gunn pupil). The fundi are normal, and extraocular motility is full, with the exception of occasional square wave jerks.

Magnetic resonance imaging (MRI) with and without gadolinium shows an area of increased signal intensity on T2 images in the left optic nerve, as well as scattered areas of increased signal intensity in the periventricular white matter. Lumbar puncture demonstrates a mild lymphocyte pleocytosis, with slight elevation of the protein content. Monoclonal antibodies are present.

Discussion: Progressive loss of central and colour vision over several days in association with orbital pain and normal fundi points to a left retro-orbital optic neuropathy, with clinical features of a Marcus Gunn pupil. Acutely there may be disc swelling and, with time, disc pallor may occur. These findings associated with aterial attenuation suggest acute ischemic optic neuropathy (Fig. 12.12). The observation of a central scotoma with intact peripheral visual fields emphasizes that about 90% of the axons in the optic nerve subserve macular vision.

Retrobulbar optic neuritis in a patient with a history of a hemisensory disturbance and an MRI demonstrating areas of increased signal intensity on T2 images in the periventricular white matter points strongly to a diagnosis of multiple sclerosis. Other disorders that can present with the same clinical and radiological features, such as systemic lupus erythematosus, must be excluded with appropriate testing.

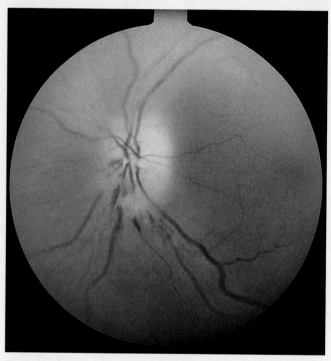

Fig. 12.12 *Ischaemic optic neuritis. The optic disc is pale and mildly swollen, and there is attenuation of some of the retinal vessels.*

CASE 4   SUPERIOR VISUAL FIELD DISTURBANCE

A 36-year-old woman with poorly controlled partial seizures, despite taking a variety of anticonvulsant medications, undergoes a right temporal lobectomy to remove an epileptogenic focus that was identified and localized by corticography. There is evidence of mesial temporal sclerosis on MRI. Following surgery, antiepileptic medication is resumed, and the woman's seizure disorder is completely controlled for the first time in 20 years.

Two months later, a routine ophthalmological examination demonstrates a left superior visual field defect to confrontation testing. Subsequent formal visual testing of the left eye reveals a wedge-shaped superior temporal field defect of about 20 degrees of arc and abutting the vertical meridian. In the right eye, a superior nasal field defect of about 40 degrees of arc is also present abutting the vertical meridian. The patient is unaware of the visual disturbance. The remainder of the neurological examination is normal.

Discussion: The 'pie in the sky' or wedge-shaped visual field defect noted in this patient is not uncommon following temporal lobectomy for epilepsy. Rostral geniculocalcarine pathway lesions produce incongruous visual field defects—that is, defects that are not exactly the same in both eyes—because geniculocalcarine fibres from corresponding retinal areas are not anatomically in close proximity until reaching the occipital lobe. Occipital lobe lesions, in contrast, produce congruous (i.e. identical) field defects that can be quadrantal. Because of the anatomical inversion of the visual pathways, inferiorly placed lesions in the optic tract or calcarine cortex tend to produce superior quadrantal defects, whereas inferior defects are consistent with lesions in the parietal lobe involving the tract from above. This case also demonstrates that visual field disturbances, particularly in the superior field, may go unnoticed by the patient. (See Fig. 12.11, optic radiation, lower division.)

CASE 5   HOMONYMOUS HEMIANOPIA

A 34-year-old, primarily healthy woman with a 2-week history of non-radiating neck pain has had three chiropractic treatments. On the drive home from the third treatment she notices that she cannot see well to the right; the next day her ophthalmologist notes a right visual field disturbance. There is no history of prior visual symptoms, migraine or smoking. She is not using oral contraceptives. With the exception of a dense right homonymous hemianopia, the neurological examination is completely normal. The visual acuity is 20/20 bilaterally.

An initial computed tomography (CT) scan is normal, but a repeat study several days later reveals an area of hypodensity in the left occipital lobe, most likely an ischaemic infarct. MRI of the brain (without diffusion images) shows a left occipital ischaemic infarct, and a magnetic resonance arteriogram of the cervical and cranial vessels demonstrates a right vertebral artery dissection at the C1 vertebral level and occlusion of the calcarine branch of the left posterior cerebral artery. Laboratory investigations are otherwise normal.

The patient is started on anticoagulation therapy. Follow-up assessment 4 months later documents a persistent right homonymous hemianopia, and repeat MRI of the brain reveals encephalomalacia in the left occipital lobe. Magnetic resonance angiography now demonstrates only slight irregularity of the lumen of the right vertebral artery.

Discussion: Cervical manipulation is a known risk factor for stroke. Vertebral artery dissection at the C1 level can be caused by rotation of the neck with an anatomically fixed vertebral artery.

It is noteworthy that the patient's visual field testing showed macular sparing. For many years, there has been debate whether such macular sparing has an underlying anatomical explanation, such as bilateral cortical representation of the macula or a dual blood supply, or whether this phenomenon is merely the result of slight horizontal movement of the eyes during field testing. The most commonly accepted explanation is the latter. (See Fig. 12.11, optic radiation, both divisions.)

separate neural systems are involved: first, to shift gaze to the object of interest using rapid movements, called saccades; and second, to stabilize the image on the fovea either during movement of the object of interest (smooth pursuit system) or during movement of the head or body (vestibulo-ocular and optokinetic systems). Although the detailed anatomical substrates for these systems differ, they share common circuitry that lies mainly in the pons and midbrain for horizontal and vertical gaze movements, respectively (Fig. 12.13).

The common element in all types of horizontal gaze movements is the abducens nucleus. This contains motor neurones that innervate the ipsilateral lateral rectus. It also contains interneurones that project via the

medial longitudinal fasciculus (MLF) to the contralateral oculomotor nucleus controlling the medial rectus. A lesion of the abducens nucleus leads to a total loss of ipsilateral horizontal conjugate gaze. A lesion of the MLF produces slowed or absent adduction of the ipsilateral eye, usually associated with jerky movements (nystagmus) of the abducting eye, a syndrome called internuclear ophthalmoplegia.

The gaze motor command involves specialized areas of the reticular formation of the brain stem that receive a variety of supranuclear inputs. The main region for horizontal gaze is the paramedian pontine reticular formation (PPRF), which is located on each side of the midline in the central paramedian part of the tegmentum and extends from the pontomedullary junction to the

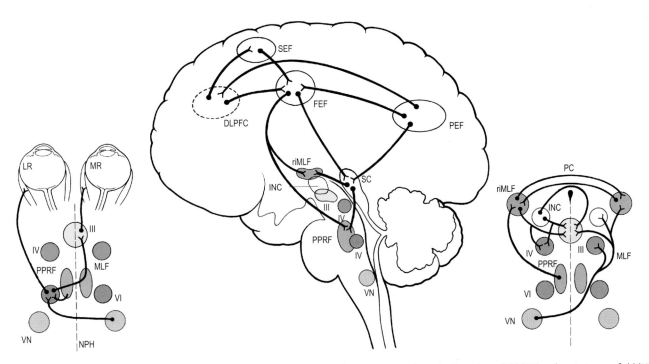

Fig. 12.13 *Summary of eye movement control. The central drawing shows the supranuclear connections from the frontal eye field (FEF) and posterior eye field (PEF) to the superior colliculus (SC), rostral interstitial nucleus of the medial longitudinal fasciculus (riMLF) and paramedian pontine reticular formation (PPRF). The FEF and SC are involved in the production of saccades, whereas the PEF is thought to be important in the production of pursuit. The drawing on the left shows the brain stem pathways for horizontal gaze. Axons from the PPRF travel to the ipsilateral abducens nucleus innervating the lateral rectus (LR). Abducens internuclear axons cross the midline and travel in the medial longitudinal fasciculus (MLF) to the portion of the oculomotor nucleus (III) innervating the medial rectus (MR) of the contralateral eye. The drawing on the right shows the brain stem pathways for vertical gaze. Important structures include the riMLF, PPRF, interstitial nucleus of Cajal (INC) and posterior commissure (PC). DLPFC, dorsolateral prefrontal cortex; IV, trochlear nucleus; NPH, nucleus prepositus hypoglossi; SEF, supplementary eye field; VI, abducens nucleus; VN, vestibular nucleus.*

pontopeduncular junction. Each PPRF contains excitatory neurones that discharge at high frequencies just before and during ipsilateral saccades. Pause neurones, which are located in a midline caudal pontine nucleus called the nucleus raphe interpositus, discharge tonically except just before and during saccades. They appear to exert an inhibitory influence on the burst neurones and thus prevent extraneous saccades occurring during fixation.

The vestibular nuclei and the perihypoglossal complex (especially the nucleus prepositus hypoglossi) project directly to the abducens nuclei. These projections probably carry both smooth pursuit signals, via the cerebellum, and vestibular signals. In addition, these nuclei, via reciprocal innervation with the PPRF, contain integrator neurones that control the step change in innervation required to maintain the eccentric position of the eye against the viscoelastic forces in the orbit. These forces tend to move the eyeball back to the position of looking straight ahead (i.e. the primary position) after a saccade.

The final common pathway of vertical gaze movements is formed by the oculomotor and trochlear nuclei. The rostral interstitial nucleus of the MLF (riMLF) contains neurones that discharge in relation to up-and-down vertical saccadic movements. The riMLF projects through the posterior commissure to its equivalent on the other side of the mesencephalon, as well as directly to the oculomotor nucleus. Therefore, lesions within the posterior commissure give rise to disturbance in vertical gaze, especially up-gaze (see Ch. 10, Case 9). Lesions located more ventrally in the region of the riMLF give rise to vertical gaze disorders that may be mixed up and down or mainly down-gaze. Slightly caudal to the riMLF, and directly connected to it, lies the interstitial nucleus of Cajal. It contains neurones that appear to be involved in vertical gaze by holding the vertical pursuit.

The cerebral hemispheres are extremely important for the programming and coordination of both saccadic and pursuit conjugate eye movements. There appear to be four main cortical areas in the cerebral hemispheres involved in the generation of saccades (see Fig. 12.13): the frontal eye field, which lies laterally at the caudal end of the second frontal gyrus in the premotor cortex (Brodmann's area 8); the supplementary eye field, which lies at the anterior region of the supplementary motor area in the first frontal gyrus (Brodmann's area 6); the dorsolateral prefrontal cortex, which lies anterior to the frontal eye field in the second frontal gyrus (Brodmann's area 46); and the posterior eye field, which lies in the parietal lobe, possibly in the superior part of the angular gyrus (Brodmann's area 39), and in the adjacent lateral intraparietal sulcus. These areas are apparently interconnected and send projections to the superior colliculus and the brain stem areas controlling saccades.

It seems that there are two parallel pathways involved in the cortical generation of saccades. An anterior pathway originates in the frontal eye field and projects both directly and via the superior colliculus to the brain stem saccadic generators. This pathway also passes indirectly via the basal ganglia to the superior colliculus. Projections from the frontal cortex influence cells in the pars reticulata of the substantia nigra, via a relay in the caudate nucleus. An inhibitory pathway from the pars reticulata projects directly to the superior colliculus. This appears to be a gating circuit related to volitional saccades, especially of the memory-guided type. A posterior pathway originates in the posterior eye field and passes to the brain stem saccadic generators via the superior colliculus.

To maintain foveation of a moving target, the smooth pursuit system has developed relatively independently of the saccadic oculomotor system, although there are inevitable interconnections between the two. The first task is to identify and code the velocity and direction of a moving target. This is carried out in the extrastriate visual area known as the middle temporal visual area (also called visual area V5), which contains neurones sensitive to visual target motion. In humans, this lies immediately posterior to the ascending limb of the inferior temporal sulcus at the occipitotemporal border. The middle temporal visual area sends this motion signal to the medial superior temporal visual area, which is thought to lie superior and a little anterior to area V5 within the inferior parietal lobe. Damage to this area results in impairment of smooth pursuit of targets moving toward the damaged hemisphere.

Both the medial superior temporal visual area and the frontal eye field send direct projections to a group of nuclei that lie in the basal part of the pons. In the monkey, the dorsolateral and lateral groups of pontine nuclei receive direct cortical inputs related to smooth pursuit. Lesions of similarly located nuclei in humans result in abnormal pursuit. These nuclei transfer the pursuit signal bilaterally to the posterior vermis, contralateral flocculus and fastigial nuclei of the cerebellum. The pursuit signal ultimately passes from the cerebellum to the brain stem, specifically to the medial vestibular nucleus and nucleus propositus hypoglossi, then to the PPRF and possibly directly to the ocular motor nuclei. This circuitry therefore involves a double decussation—first at the level of the mid-pons (pontocerebellar neurones), and second in the lower pons (vestibuloabducens neurones).

The vestibulo-ocular reflex maintains coordination of vision during movement of the head. It results in a compensatory conjugate eye movement that is equal but opposite to the movement of the head. This is essentially a three-neurone arc. It consists of primary vestibular neurones that project to the vestibular nuclei, secondary neurones that project from these nuclei directly to the abducens nucleus and tertiary neurones that are abducens motor neurones.

The optokinetic response is another visually mediated reflex that stabilizes retinal imagery during rotational movement. As the visual scene changes, the eyes follow, holding the retinal image steady until they shift rapidly in the opposite direction to another area of the visual scene. The full field of vision, rather than small objects within it, is the stimulus, and the alternating slow and fast phases of movement generated describes optokinetic nystagmus. The optokinetic reflex functions in collaboration with the rotational vestibulo-ocular reflex. Because of the mechanical arrangements of the semicircular canals, in the sustained rotations of the body described earlier, the vestibulo-ocular reflex fades. In darkness, the reflex, which is initially compensatory, loses velocity, and after approximately 45 seconds, the eyes become stationary.

CASE 6   INTERNUCLEAR OPHTHALMOPARESIS

A 69-year-old woman notes the sudden onset of side-by-side double vision when looking straight ahead and to the left. She performs a monocular cover test on herself and finds that her vision is normal in each eye when uncovered. Her past history is positive for hypertension, coronary artery angioplasty and dyslipidemia.

Examination shows failure of adduction of the right eye on left gaze, with monocular nystagmus involving the left eye on left gaze. Adduction with convergence is normal bilaterally.

Discussion: Selective involvement of the right medial rectus muscle on left gaze, in association with monocular nystagmus in the right abducting eye with intact convergence, indicates a right internuclear ophthalmoparesis due to a lesion in the right medial longitudinal fasciculus (MLF), the anatomical structure interconnecting the oculomotor nuclei and the abducens nucleus and associated PPRF in the pons. This is often due to multiple sclerosis in the young and to a vascular event in the elderly. The MLF is supplied by the paramedian branches of the basilar artery; internuclear ophthalmoparesis is a relatively common result of ischaemia due to small-vessel occlusive disease.

Pupillary Light Reflex

The pupillary light reflex is a dynamic system for controlling the amount of light reaching the retina (Fig. 12.14). Illumination of the retina causes reflex constriction of the pupil (miosis). The direct component of the light reflex mediates constriction of the pupil of the ipsilateral eye, and the consensual component elicits simultaneous constriction of the contralateral pupil.

A light stimulus acting on the retinal photoreceptors gives rise to activity in retinal ganglion cells, the axons of which form the optic nerve. Activity is conducted through the optic chiasma and along the optic tract, and the majority of fibres end in the lateral geniculate nucleus of the thalamus. However, a small number of fibres leave the optic tract before it reaches the thalamus and synapse in the pretectal nucleus. The information is relayed from the pretectal nucleus by short neurones that synapse bilaterally with preganglionic parasympathetic neurones in the Edinger–Westphal nucleus of the oculomotor nerve complex in the rostral midbrain. Efferent impulses pass along parasympathetic fibres of the oculomotor nerve to the orbit, where they synapse in the ciliary ganglion. Postganglionic fibres (short ciliary nerves) pass to the eyeball to supply the sphincter pupillae, which reduce the size of the pupil when it contracts.

There is also a connection to the spinal sympathetic centre controlling the dilator pupillae. The preganglionic fibres arise from neurones in the lateral column of the first and second thoracic segments and pass via the

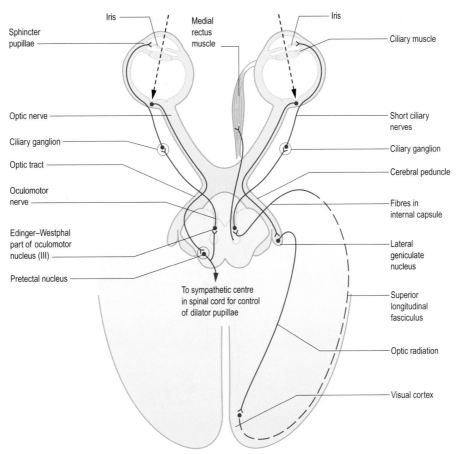

Fig. 12.14 *Pupillary light reflex and accommodation reflex. (From MacKinnon, P., Morris, J. [Eds.], 1990. Oxford Textbook of Functional Anatomy, vol 3, Head and Neck. Oxford University Press, Oxford. By permission of Oxford University Press.)*

sympathetic trunk to the superior cervical ganglion, where they synapse on postganglionic neurones. Postganglionic fibres arising from these neurones are distributed to the cavernous plexus; from there, they travel mainly through the long ciliary nerves to the anterior part of the eye, where they supply the dilator pupillae.

Because pupillary size results from the balanced action of these two innervations, the pupil dilates when the parasympathetic stimulus ceases. The pupil also dilates in response to painful stimulation of almost any part of the body. Presumably, fibres of sensory pathways connect with the sympathetic preganglionic neurones described earlier.

Accommodation Reflex

When focusing on a nearby object, the eyes converge, the lens becomes more convex and the pupils constrict (see Fig. 12.14).

Information from the retina passing to the visual cortex does not constitute the afferent limb of a simple reflex in the usual sense of the term, but it permits the visual areas to assess the clarity of objects in the visual field. Cortical efferent information passes to the pretectal area and then to the Edinger–Westphal nucleus, which contains preganglionic parasympathetic neurones whose axons travel in the oculomotor nerve. Efferent impulses pass in the oculomotor nerve to the orbit, where they synapse in the ciliary ganglion. Postganglionic fibres (short ciliary nerves) pass to the eyeball and stimulate contraction of the ciliary muscle, which slackens the ligament of the lens and increases the curvature of the lens for near vision. Contraction of the sphincter pupillae and relaxation of the dilator pupillae constrict the pupil. Simultaneously, contraction of the medial, superior and inferior recti (all innervated by the oculomotor nerve) converges the eyes on the near target. The pupillary changes may be secondary to convergence.

In certain central nervous system diseases (e.g. tabes dorsalis), the pupillary light reflex may be lost, but pupillary constriction as part of the accommodation reflex is retained (Argyll Robertson pupil). The site of a lesion producing such an effect is unclear, but it may involve the periaqueductal grey matter.

TASTE

Afferent nerve fibres carrying taste information are the peripheral processes of neuronal cell bodies in the geniculate ganglion of the facial nerve and in the inferior ganglia of the glossopharyngeal and vagus nerves. Taste from the anterior two-thirds of the tongue, excluding the vallate papillae, and from the

inferior surface of the palate is carried in the sensory root of the facial nerve (nervus intermedius). Taste buds in the vallate papillae, posterior third of the tongue, palatoglossal arches, oropharynx and, to some extent, palate are innervated by the glossopharyngeal nerve. Those in the extreme pharyngeal part of the tongue and the epiglottis are innervated by fibres of the vagus nerve.

On entering the brain stem, these afferent fibres constitute the tractus solitarius, and they terminate in the rostral third of the nucleus solitarius of the medulla. Second-order neurones arising from the nucleus solitarius cross the midline, and many ascend through the brain stem in the dorsomedial part of the medial lemniscus. They terminate in the medial part of the ventral posteromedial nucleus of the thalamus. From the ventral posteromedial nucleus, third-order neurones project through the internal capsule to the anteroinferior part of the sensory cortex and to the limen insulae. Other ascending projections to the hypothalamus have been described that may represent the pathway by which gustatory information reaches the limbic system.

HEARING

The primary afferents of the auditory pathway arise from cell bodies in the spiral ganglion of the cochlea (see Figs. 11.20, 11.23, 11.28, 11.31). The axons constitute the auditory component of the vestibulocochlear nerve, which enters the brain stem at the cerebellopontine angle. Afferent fibres bifurcate and terminate in the dorsal and ventral cochlear nuclei. Onward connections make up the ascending auditory pathway (Fig. 12.15). The dorsal cochlear nucleus projects via the dorsal acoustic stria to the contralateral inferior colliculus. The ventral cochlear nucleus projects via the trapezoid body or the intermediate acoustic stria to relay centres in the superior olivary complex, the nuclei of the lateral lemniscus or the inferior colliculus. The superior olivary complex is dominated by the medial superior olivary nucleus, which receives direct input from the ventral cochlear nucleus on both sides, and is involved in localization of sound by measuring the time difference between afferent impulses arriving from the two ears.

The inferior colliculus consists of a central nucleus and two cortical areas. The dorsal cortex lies dorsomedially, and the external cortex lies ventromedially. Secondary and tertiary fibres ascend in the lateral lemniscus. They converge in the central nucleus, which projects to the ventral division of the medial geniculate body of the thalamus. The external cortex receives

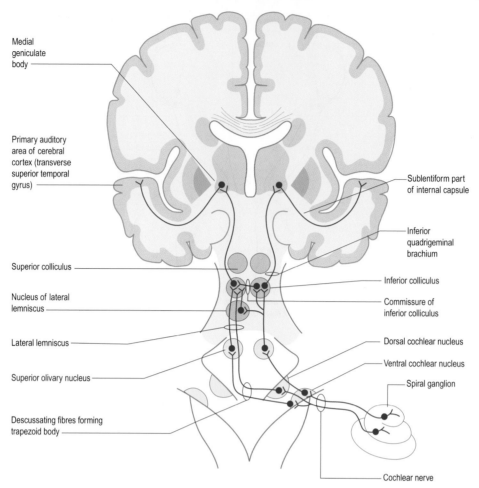

Fig. 12.15 *Ascending auditory pathway.*

both auditory and somatosensory input. It projects to the medial division of the medial geniculate body and, together with the central nucleus, also projects to olivocochlear cells in the superior olivary complex and to cells in the cochlear nuclei. The dorsal cortex receives an input from the auditory cortex and projects to the dorsal division of the medial geniculate body. Connections also run from the nucleus of the lateral lemniscus to the deep part of the superior colliculus, to coordinate auditory and visual responses.

The ascending auditory pathway crosses the midline at several points both below and at the level of the inferior colliculus. However, the input to the central nucleus of the inferior colliculus and higher centres has a clear contralateral dominance. The medial geniculate body is connected reciprocally to the primary auditory cortex, which is located in the superior temporal gyrus, buried in the lateral fissure.

BALANCE

The vestibular sensory pathways are concerned with perception of the position of the head in space and with movement of the head. They also establish important connections for reflex movements governing the equilibrium of the body and the fixity of gaze.

Functionally, the vestibular apparatus is customarily divided into two components: the kinetic labyrinth, which provides information about acceleration and deceleration of the head, and the static labyrinth, which detects the orientation of the head in relation to the pull of gravity. In terms of structure, the kinetic labyrinth consists of the semicircular canals and their ampullary cristae, and the static labyrinth consists of the maculae of the utricle and saccule. However, the saccular macula also responds to head movements, and both maculae can be stimulated by low-frequency sound and may therefore have minor auditory functions (see Fig. 11.28).

Angular acceleration and deceleration of the head cause a counterflow of endolymph in the semicircular canals, which deflects the cupula of each crista and bends the stereocilial and kinocilial bundles. This causes a change in the membrane potential of the receptor cell, which is signalled to the brain as a change in the firing frequency of the vestibular nerve afferents (either an increase or a decrease of the basal resting discharge, depending on the direction of stimulation). When a steady velocity of head movement is reached, the endolymph rapidly adopts the same velocity as the surrounding structures

because of friction with the canal walls, so that the cupula and receptor cells return to their resting state. Because the three semicircular canals are oriented at right angles to each other, all possible directions of acceleration can be detected. In addition, the labyrinths on both sides of the head provide complementary information that is integrated centrally.

In the maculae, the weight of the otoconial crystals creates a gravitational pull on the otoconial membrane and thus on the stereocilial bundles of the sensory cells inserted into its base. Because of this, they are able to detect the static orientation of the head with respect to gravity. They also detect shifts in position according to the extent to which the stereocilia are deflected from the perpendicular. Because the two maculae are set at right angles to each other, and the cells of both maculae are functionally oriented in opposite directions across their striolar boundaries, this system is very sensitive to orientation. Moreover, because the otoconia have a collective inertia or momentum, linear acceleration and deceleration along the antero-posterior axis can be detected by the lag or overshoot of the otoconial membrane with respect to the epithelial surface, and the saccular macula is able to signal these changes of velocity. Similarly, the macular receptors can be stimulated by low-frequency sound, which sets up vibratory movements in the otoconial membrane; however, this appears to require relatively high sound levels. Efferent synapses on the afferent endings of Type I sensory cells and on the bases of Type II cells receive inputs from the brain stem that appear to be inhibitory. They serve to reduce the activity of the afferent fibres either indirectly, in the case of Type I cells, or directly, in the case of Type II cells.

The information gathered by these various receptors is carried to the central nervous system in the vestibular nerve, which enters the brain stem at the cerebellopontine angle and terminates in the vestibular nuclear complex. Neurones in this complex project to motor nuclei in the brain stem and upper spinal cord and to the cerebellum and thalamus. Thalamic efferent projections pass to a cortical vestibular area that is probably located near the intraparietal sulcus in area 2 of the primary somatosensory cortex.

Another major function of the vestibular system is the control of visual reflexes, which allows the fixation of gaze on an object in spite of movements of the head and requires coordinated movements of the eyes, neck and upper trunk. Constant adjustments of the visual axes are achieved chiefly through the MLF, which connects the vestibular nuclear complex with neurones in the oculomotor, trochlear and abducens nuclei and with upper spinal motor neurones (see Fig. 10.26), as well as by the vestibulospinal tracts.

Abnormal activity of the vestibular input or central connections has various effects on these reflexes, such as the production of nystagmus. This can be elicited by a clinical test of vestibular function by syringing the external auditory meatus with water above or below body temperature, a procedure that appears to stimulate the cristae of the lateral semicircular canal directly. Spontaneous high activity in the afferent fibres of the vestibular nerve is seen in Meniere's disease, in which affected patients experience a range of disturbances, including the sensations of dizziness and nausea, the latter reflecting the vestibular input to the vagal reflex pathway.

References

Cagan, R.H. (Ed.), 1989. Neural Mechanisms in Taste. CRC Press, Boca Raton, FL.

Hubel, D.H., 1988. Eye brain and vision. Scientific American Library Series No. 22.

Jonas, J.B., Gusek, G.C., Naumann, G.O., 1988. Optic disc cup and neuroretinal rim size configuration and correlations in normal eyes. Invest. Ophthalmol. Vis. Sci. 29, 1151–1158. *A clinical template of normal range.*

Kandel, E.R., Schwartz, J.H., Jessel, T.M. (Eds.), 2000. Principles of Neural Science, fourth ed. McGraw-Hill, New York.

Oertel, D., Fay, R.R., Popper, A.N. (Eds.), 2002. Integrative Functions in the Mammalian Auditory Pathway. Springer Handbook of Auditory Research, vol. 15. Springer, New York.

Osterberg, G.A., 1935. Topography of the layers of the rods and cones in the human retina. Acta Ophthalmol. (Suppl. 6).

Savino, P.J., Danesh-Meyer, H.V., 2003. Color atlas and synopsis of clinical ophthalmology, Wills Eye Hospital. McGraw-Hill, New York.

Victor, M., Dreyfus, P.M., Mancall, E.L., 1960. Deficiency amblyopia in the alcoholic patient. Arch. Ophthalmol. 64, 1.

Wässle, H., Boycott, B.B., 1991. Functional architecture of the mammalian retina. Physiol. Rev. 71, 447–480. *Unitary cell responses of the various retinal neurones and their connectivity.*

Zeki, S., 1993. A Vision of the Brain. Blackwell Scientific, Oxford.

Chapter 12

Section IV

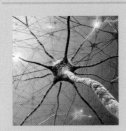

The Cerebellum

Chapter 13   Cerebellum

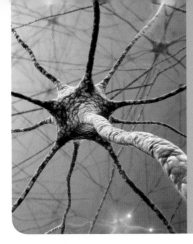

Cerebellum

The cerebellum, the largest part of the hindbrain, is dorsal to the pons and medulla, and its median region is separated from them by the fourth ventricle. It is joined to the brain stem by three pairs of cerebellar peduncles, which contain afferent and efferent fibres. The cerebellum occupies the posterior cranial fossa, where it is covered by the tentorium cerebelli. It is roughly spherical but somewhat constricted in its median region and flattened; its greatest diameter is transverse. In adults, the weight ratio of cerebellum to cerebrum is approximately 1:10; in infants, it is approximately 1:20.

The cerebellum is a central part of the major circuitry that links sensory to motor areas of the brain, and it is required for the coordination of fine movement. In health, it provides corrections during movement, which are the bases for precision and accuracy, and it is critically involved in motor learning and reflex modification. It receives sensory information through spinal, trigeminal and vestibulocerebellar pathways and, via the pontine nuclei, from the cerebral cortex and the tectum. Cerebellar output is mainly to those structures of the brain that control movement.

The basic internal organization of the cerebellum is that of a superficial, highly convoluted cortex (a laminated sheet of neurones and supporting cells) overlying a dense core of white matter. The latter contains deep cerebellar nuclei, which give rise to the efferent cerebellar projections. Although the human cerebellum makes up approximately one-tenth of the entire brain by weight, the surface area of the cerebellar cortex, if unfolded, would be about half that of the cerebral cortex. The great majority of cerebellar neurones are small granule cells; they are so densely packed that the cerebellar cortex contains many more neurones than the cerebral cortex. Unlike the cerebral cortex, where a large number of diverse cell types are arranged differently in different regions, the cerebellar cortex contains a relatively small number of different cell types that are interconnected in a highly stereotypical way. Consequently, one region of the cerebellar cortex looks very much like another.

Disease processes affecting the cerebellum or its connections lead to incoordination. Movements of the eyes, speech apparatus, individual limbs and balance are usually affected, which results in nystagmus, dysarthria, incoordination and ataxia. Although all these movements become defective in widespread disease of the cerebellum or its connections, topographical arrangements within the cerebellum lead to a variety of clinically recognizable disease patterns. Thus, in cerebellar hemisphere disease, the ipsilateral limbs show rhythmical tremor during movement but not at rest. The tremor increases as the target is approached, so reaching and accurate movements of the arm are especially difficult. Diseases that affect the ascending spinocerebellar pathways or the midline vermis have a disproportionate effect on axial structures, leading to severe loss of balance. Lesions of outflow tracts in the superior cerebellar peduncles result in a wide-amplitude, severely disabling, proximal tremor that interferes with all movements and may even disturb posture, leading to rhythmic oscillations of the head or trunk so that the patient is unable to stand or sit without support. However, although cerebellar lesions may initially cause profound motor impairment, a considerable degree of recovery is possible. There are clinical reports that the initial symptoms of large cerebellar lesions (caused by trauma or surgical excision) have improved progressively over time.

Although the basic structure of the cerebellum and its importance for normal movement have long been recognized, many of the details of how it functions remain obscure. The main goal of this chapter is to describe the known structure and connections of the cerebellum.

EXTERNAL FEATURES AND RELATIONS

The cerebellum consists of two large, laterally located hemispheres that are united by a midline vermis (Figs 13.1–13.3). The superior surface of the cerebellum, which would constitute the anterior part of the unrolled cerebellar cortex, is relatively flat. The paramedian sulci are shallow, and the borders between vermis and hemispheres are indicated by kinks in the transverse fissures. The superior surface adjoins the tentorium cerebelli and projects

beyond its free edge. The transverse sinus borders the cerebellum at the point where the superior and inferior surfaces meet. The inferior surface is characterized by a massive enlargement of the cerebellar hemispheres, which extends medially to overlie some of the vermis. Deep paramedian sulci demarcate the vermis from the hemispheres. Posteriorly, the hemispheres are separated by a deep vallecula, which contains the dural falx cerebelli. The inferior cerebellar surface lies against the occipital squama. The shape of the surface facing the brain stem is irregular. It forms the roof of the fourth ventricle and the lateral recesses on each side of it, while the cerebellar peduncles define the diamond shape of the ventricle when viewed from behind. Anterolaterally, the cerebellum lies against the posterior surface of the petrous part of the temporal bone.

The cerebellar surface is divided by numerous curved transverse fissures that separate its folia and give it a laminated appearance. Deeper fissures divide it into lobules. One conspicuous fissure, the horizontal fissure, extends around the dorsolateral border of each hemisphere from the middle cerebellar peduncle to the vallecula, separating the superior and inferior surfaces. Although the horizontal fissure is prominent, it appears relatively late in embryological development and does not mark the boundary between major functional subdivisions of the cortex. The deepest fissure in the vermis is the primary fissure, which curves ventrolaterally around the superior surface of the cerebellum to meet the horizontal fissures. It appears early in embryological development and marks the boundary between the anterior and posterior lobes.

Because the cerebellar cortex has a roughly spherical shape, the true relations between its parts can sometimes be obscured. Thus, the most anterior lobule of the cerebellar vermis, the lingula, lies very close to the most posterior lobule, the nodule. Deep fissures divide the superior vermis into lobules. The lobules of the superior vermis that belong to the anterior lobe are the lingula, central lobule and culmen. The lingula is a single lamina of four or five shallow folia. Its white core is continuous with the anterior medullary velum. It is separated from the central lobule by the precentral fissure. The central lobule and culmen are continuous bilaterally with an adjoining wing (ala) in each hemisphere. The central lobule is separated from the culmen by the preculminary fissure. The culmen (with attached anterior quadrangular lobules) lies between the preculminary and primary fissures.

Between the primary and horizontal fissures are the simple lobule (with attached posterior quadrangular lobules) and the folium (with attached superior semilunar lobules). These two lobule sets are separated by the posterior superior fissure.

From the back forward, the inferior vermis is divided into the tuber, pyramis, uvula and nodule, in that order (see Fig. 13.3C). The tuber is continuous laterally with the inferior semilunar lobules and separated from the pyramis by the lunogracile fissure. The pyramis and attached biventral lobules (containing an intrabiventral fissure) are separated from the uvula and attached cerebellar tonsils by the secondary fissure. Behind the uvula, and separated from it by the median part of the posterolateral fissure, is the nodule. The tonsils are roughly spherical and overhang the foramen magnum on each side of the medulla oblongata.

The nodule and attached flocculi constitute a separate flocculonodular lobe that is separated from the uvula and tonsils by the deep posterolateral fissure. This lobe is richly interconnected with the vestibular nucleus, which is located at the lateral margin of the fourth ventricle.

Functional Divisions

The cerebellum is divided functionally into a body, with inputs mainly from the spinal cord and pontine nuclei, and a flocculonodular lobe, which has strong afferent and efferent connections with the vestibular nuclei (Fig. 13.4). The body is subdivided into a series of regions dominated by their spinal or pontine inputs. The anterior lobe, simple lobule, pyramis and biventral lobules are the main recipients of spinal and trigeminal cerebellar afferents. Pontocerebellar input dominates in the folium, tuber and uvula and in the

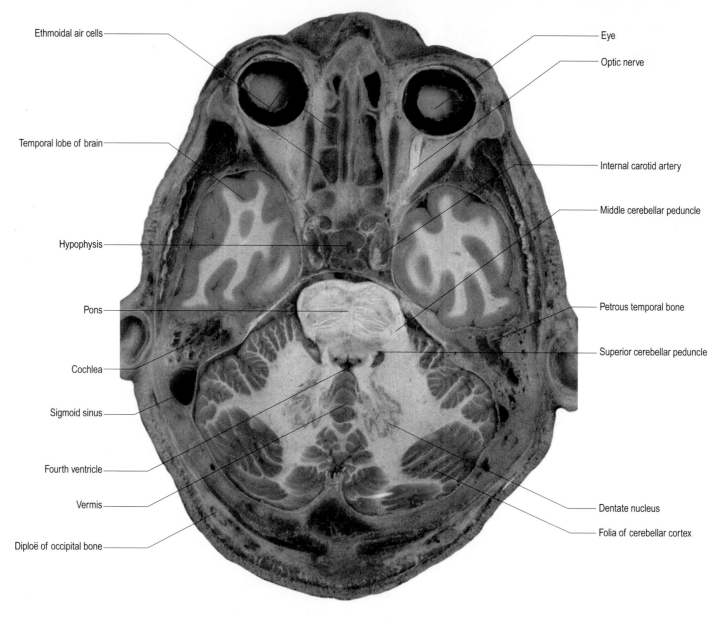

Ethmoidal air cells

Temporal lobe of brain

Hypophysis

Pons

Cochlea

Sigmoid sinus

Fourth ventricle

Vermis

Diploë of occipital bone

Eye

Optic nerve

Internal carotid artery

Middle cerebellar peduncle

Petrous temporal bone

Superior cerebellar peduncle

Dentate nucleus

Folia of cerebellar cortex

Fig. 13.1 *Horizontal section through the cerebellum and brain stem. (Courtesy of Dr. G. J. A. Maart.)*

entire hemisphere, including those regions that receive afferents from the spinal cord.

The mediolateral subdivision of the cerebellum into vermis and hemispheres represents a functional subdivision that is closely related to its output. In mammals, a great increase in the size of the cerebellar hemispheres parallels the development of the cerebral cortex and reflects the importance of the corticopontocerebellar input and of the efferent projections of the cerebellar hemispheres (through the dentate and interposed cerebellar nuclei and the thalamus) to the cerebral cortex.

Cerebellar Peduncles

Three peduncles connect the cerebellum with the rest of the brain (Figs 13.5, 13.6). The middle cerebellar peduncle is the most lateral and by far the largest of the three. It passes obliquely from the basal pons to the cerebellum and is composed almost entirely of fibres arising from the contralateral basal pontine nuclei, with a small addition from nuclei in the pontine tegmentum. The inferior cerebellar peduncle is located medial to the middle peduncle. It consists of an outer, compact fibre tract, the restiform (Latin for 'rope-like') body and a medial, juxtarestiform body. The restiform body is a purely afferent system. It receives the posterior spinocerebellar tract from the spinal cord and the trigeminocerebellar, cuneocerebellar, reticulocerebellar and olivocerebellar tracts from the medulla oblongata. The juxtarestiform body is mainly an efferent system. Apart from primary afferent fibres of the vestibular nerve and secondary afferent fibres from the vestibular nuclei, it is made up almost entirely of efferent Purkinje cell axons from the vestibulocerebellum, on their way to the vestibular nuclei, and the uncrossed fibres from the fastigial nucleus. The crossed fibres from the fastigial nucleus, after

passing dorsal to the superior cerebellar peduncle, enter the brain stem as the uncinate fasciculus at the border of the juxtarestiform and restiform bodies.

The superior cerebellar peduncle contains all the efferent fibres from the dentate, emboliform and globose nuclei and a small fascicle from the fastigial nucleus. It decussates with its opposite number in the caudal mesencephalon, on its way to synapse in the contralateral red nucleus and thalamus. The anterior spinocerebellar tract reaches the upper part of the pontine tegmentum before looping down within this peduncle to join the spinocerebellar fibres entering through the restiform body.

INTERNAL STRUCTURE

The white core of the cerebellum branches in diverging medullary laminae, which occupy the central part of the lobules and are covered by the cerebellar cortex. In a sagittal section through the cerebellum, the highly branched pattern of medullary laminae is known as the arbor vitae. The white core consists of the efferents (Purkinje cell axons) and afferents of the cerebellar cortex. Fibres crossing the midline in the white core of the cerebellum and the anterior medullary velum constitute the cerebellar commissure. This consists of an efferent portion, containing decussating fibres from the fastigial nucleus, and an afferent portion, containing fibres of the restiform body and the middle cerebellar peduncle. (In neuroanatomy, the word 'commissure' may have two meanings. In one sense, a commissure such as the corpus callosum connects homotopic points on the two sides of the brain. However, in the cerebellum, commissural afferent and efferent fibres are simply crossing the midline. The cerebellum has no callosum-like commissure connecting homotopic points on the two sides.)

Chapter 13

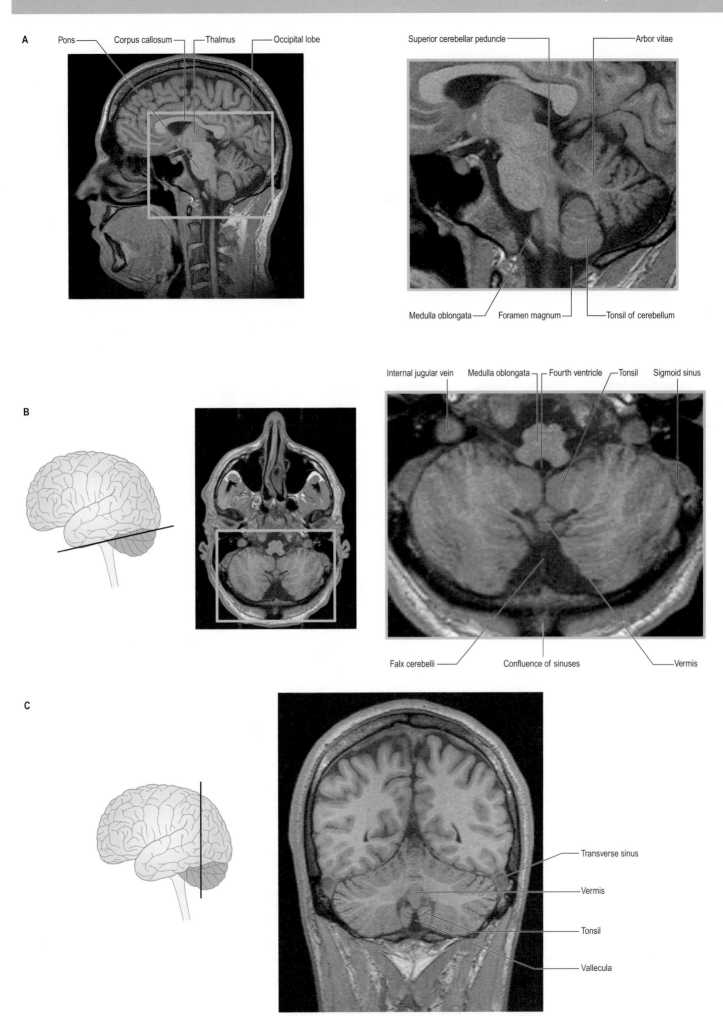

A

Pons — Corpus callosum — Thalmus — Occipital lobe

Superior cerebellar peduncle — Arbor vitae

Medulla oblongata — Foramen magnum — Tonsil of cerebellum

B

Internal jugular vein — Medulla oblongata — Fourth ventricle — Tonsil — Sigmoid sinus

Falx cerebelli — Confluence of sinuses — Vermis

C

Transverse sinus

Vermis

Tonsil

Vallecula

Fig. 13.2 *Magnetic resonance images of the cerebellum of a 16-year-old girl.* **A,** *Sagittal slice.* **B,** *Coronal slice.* **C,** *Axial slice. (Courtesy of Drs. J. P. Finn and T. Parrish, Northwestern University School of Medicine, Chicago, toddp@northwestern.edu.)*

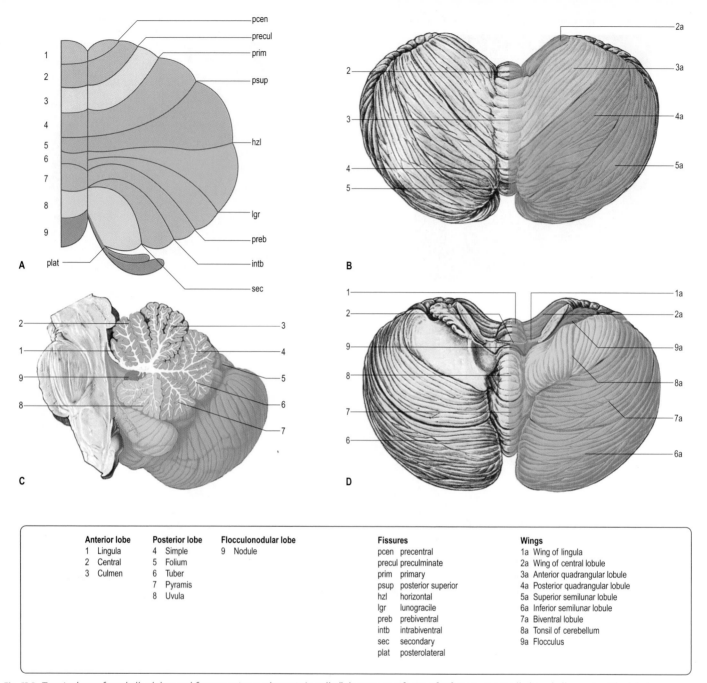

Fig. 13.3 *Terminology of cerebellar lobes and fissures, using a schematic 'unrolled' diagram as a frame of reference.* **A,** *Unrolled cerebellar cortex. The lobules are labelled by numbers, and the fissures between the wings are listed.* **B,** *Cerebellum viewed from above.* **C,** *Median sagittal section of cerebellum. The nodules and wings are numbered and listed.* **D,** *Cerebellum viewed from below.*

Anterior lobe	Posterior lobe	Flocculonodular lobe	Fissures		Wings	
1 Lingula	4 Simple	9 Nodule	pcen	precentral	1a	Wing of lingula
2 Central	5 Folium		precul	preculminate	2a	Wing of central lobule
3 Culmen	6 Tuber		prim	primary	3a	Anterior quadrangular lobule
	7 Pyramis		psup	posterior superior	4a	Posterior quadrangular lobule
	8 Uvula		hzl	horizontal	5a	Superior semilunar lobule
			lgr	lunogracile	6a	Inferior semilunar lobule
			preb	prebiventral	7a	Biventral lobule
			intb	intrabiventral	8a	Tonsil of cerebellum
			sec	secondary	9a	Flocculus
			plat	posterolateral		

Laterally, the medullary laminae merge into a large, central white mass that contains the four cerebellar nuclei: the dentate and the anterior (emboliform) and posterior (globose) interposed and fastigial nuclei (see Fig. 13.4). The dentate nucleus is the most lateral and largest and is an irregularly folded sheet of neurones that encloses a mass of fibres derived mainly from dentate neurones. It resembles a leather purse, the opening of which is directed medially. Fibres stream out through this so-called hilum to form the bulk of the superior cerebellar peduncle. The anterior and posterior interposed and fastigial nuclei lie medial to the dentate nucleus. The anterior interposed nucleus is continuous laterally with the dentate. The posterior interposed nucleus is medial to the anterior nucleus and is continuous with the fastigial nucleus, which is located next to the midline, bordering the fastigium (roof) of the fourth ventricle. Efferent fibres from the interposed nuclei join the superior cerebellar peduncle. A large proportion of the efferent fibres from the fastigial nucleus cross within the cerebellar white matter of the cerebellar commissure. After their decussation, they constitute the uncinate fasciculus (hook bundle), which passes dorsal to the superior cerebellar peduncle to enter the vestibular nuclei of the opposite side (see Fig. 13.6). Uncrossed fastigiobulbar fibres enter the vestibular nuclei by passing along the lateral angle of the fourth ventricle. Some fibres of the fastigial nucleus ascend in the superior cerebellar peduncle.

Cerebellar Cortex

The elements of the cerebellar cortex possess a precise geometrical order, which is arrayed relative to the tangential, longitudinal and transverse planes in individual folia. The cortex contains the terminations of afferent 'climbing' and 'mossy' fibres, five varieties of neurone (granular, stellate, basket, Golgi and Purkinje), neuroglia and blood vessels.

There are three main layers: molecular, Purkinje cell and granular (Fig. 13.7). The main circuit of the cerebellum involves granule cells, Purkinje cells and neurones in the cerebellar nuclei. Granule cells receive the terminals of the mossy fibre afferents (i.e. all afferent systems except the olivocerebellar fibres). The axons of the granule cells ascend to the molecular layer, where they bifurcate into parallel fibres (so called because they are oriented parallel to the transverse fissures and perpendicular to the dendritic trees of the Purkinje cells on which they terminate). Purkinje neurones are large and are the sole output cells of the cerebellar cortex. Their axons terminate in the cerebellar nuclei and vestibular nuclei. In addition to the dense array of parallel fibres, the dendritic trees of Purkinje cells receive terminals from climbing fibres whose neurones of origin are in the inferior olivary nucleus. The cerebellar cortex thus receives two distinct types of input: olivocerebellar climbing fibres, which synapse directly on Purkinje neurones, and mossy fibres, which

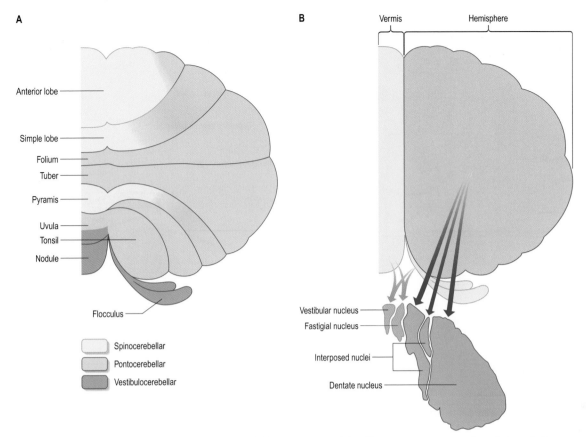

A

Anterior lobe

Simple lobe

Folium

Tuber

Pyramis

Uvula

Tonsil

Nodule

Flocculus

Spinocerebellar

Pontocerebellar

Vestibulocerebellar

B

Vermis   Hemisphere

Vestibular nucleus

Fastigial nucleus

Interposed nuclei

Dentate nucleus

Fig. 13.4 *Diagrams of the flattened cerebellar surface. **A**, Transverse lobular organization of the afferent spino-, ponto- and vestibulocerebellar connections of the cortex. **B**, Longitudinal zonal organization of the vermis and hemispheres with the cerebellar and vestibular nuclei.*

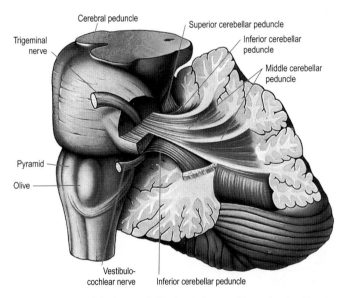

Cerebral peduncle

Trigeminal nerve

Superior cerebellar peduncle

Inferior cerebellar peduncle

Middle cerebellar peduncle

Pyramid

Olive

Vestibulo-cochlear nerve

Inferior cerebellar peduncle

Fig. 13.5 *Dissection of the left cerebellar hemisphere and its peduncles. (Courtesy of Dr. E. B. Jamieson, University of Edinburgh.)*

connect to the Purkinje cells via granular neurones whose axons are the parallel fibres.

Both parallel and climbing fibres excite the Purkinje cells, but they differ greatly in their firing characteristics and their effect on the cells. Purkinje cell axons in turn inhibit their target neurones in the cerebellar nuclei. The cerebellar nuclei project to all the major motor control centres in the brain stem and cerebrum. The stellate, basket and Golgi cells are inhibitory interneurones, which connect the cortical elements in complex geometrical patterns.

The molecular layer is approximately 300 to 400 μm thick. It contains a sparse population of neurones, dendritic arborizations, non-myelinated axons and radial fibres of the neuroglial cells. Purkinje cell dendritic trees extend toward the surface and spread out in a plane perpendicular to the long axis of the cerebellar folia. Purkinje cell dendrites are flattened. The lateral extent of the Purkinje cell dendrites is approximately 30 times greater in the

transverse plane than in a plane parallel to the cerebellar folia. Parallel fibres are the axons of granule cells, the stems of which ascend into the molecular layer, where they bifurcate at T-shaped branches. The two branches extend in opposite directions as parallel fibres along the axis of a folium. Parallel fibres terminate on the dendrites of the Purkinje cells and Golgi cells, which they pass on their way, and on the basket and stellate cells of the molecular layer. Dendritic trees of Golgi neurones reach toward the surface. Unlike the flattened dendritic tree of the Purkinje cell, Golgi cell dendrites span the territory of many Purkinje neurones longitudinally as well as transversely. These dendrites receive synapses from parallel fibres. Some Golgi cell dendrites enter the granular layer, where they contact mossy fibre terminals. The cell bodies of Golgi neurones lie below, in the superficial part of the granular layer. The molecular layer also contains the somata, dendrites and axons of stellate neurones (which are located superficially within the molecular layer) and of basket cells (whose somata lie deeper within the molecular layer). Climbing fibres, which are the terminals of olivocerebellar fibres, ascend through the granular layer to contact Purkinje dendrites in the molecular layer. Radiating branches from large epithelial (Bergmann) glial cells give off processes that surround all neuronal elements, except at the synapses. At the surface of the cerebellum, their conical expansions join to form an external limiting membrane.

The Purkinje cell layer contains the large, pear-shaped somata of the Purkinje cells and the smaller somata of epithelial (Bergmann) glial cells. Clumps of granule cells and occasional Golgi cells penetrate between the Purkinje cell somata.

The granular layer (see Fig. 13.7) is approximately 100 μm thick in the fissures and 400 to 500 μm thick on foliar summits. There are approximately 2.7 million granular neurones per cubic millimetre. It has been estimated that the human cerebellum contains a total of 4.6×10^{10} granule cells and that there are 3000 granule cells for each Purkinje cell.

In summary, the granular layer consists of the somata of granule cells and the start of their axons; dendrites of granule cells; branching terminal axons of afferent mossy fibres; climbing fibres passing through the granular layer en route to the molecular layer; and the somata, basal dendrites and complex axonal ramifications of Golgi neurones. Cerebellar glomeruli are synaptic rosettes consisting of a mossy fibre terminal that forms excitatory synapses on the dendrites of both granule cells and Golgi cells.

Of the five cell types described, the first four are inhibitory, liberating γ-aminobutyric acid (GABA), and the fifth is excitatory, liberating L-glutamate. Figure 13.8 summarizes their main connections.

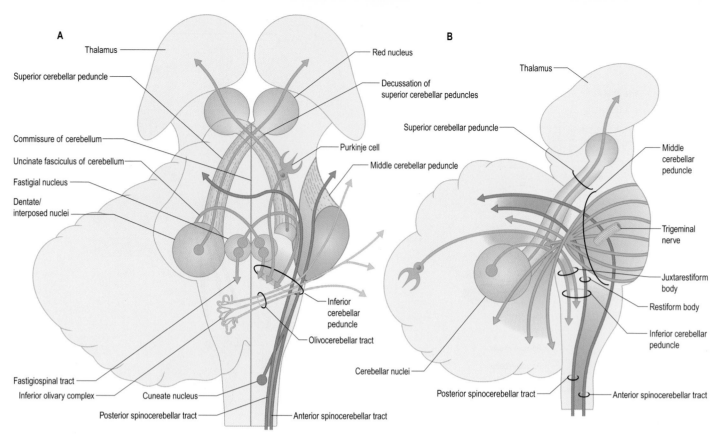

Fig. 13.6 *Diagram illustrating the composition of the cerebellar peduncles.* **A**, *Dorsal view.* **B**, *Lateral view.*

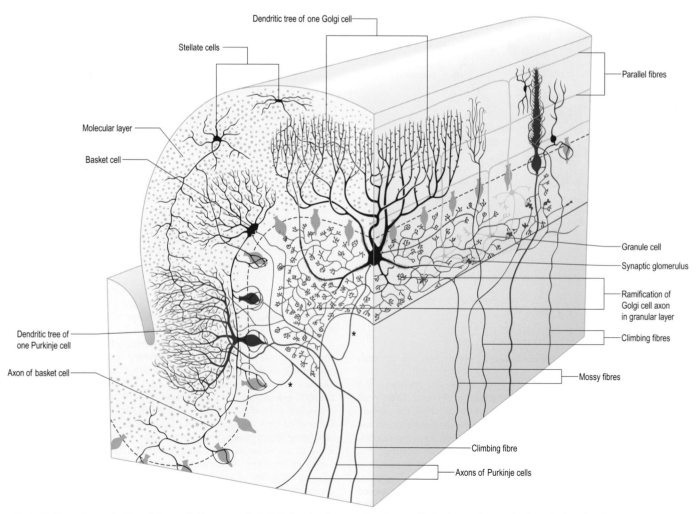

Fig. 13.7 *General organization of the cerebellar cortex. A single folium has been sectioned vertically, both in its longitudinal axis* (right side of the diagram) *and transversely. The two* asterisks *on the left face indicate recurrent collateral branches of Purkinje cell axons.*

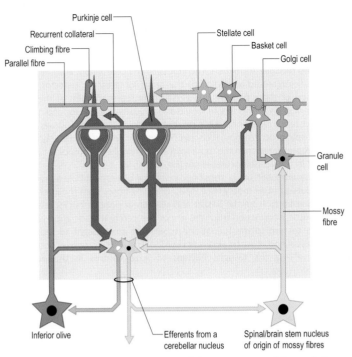

Purkinje cell
Recurrent collateral
Climbing fibre
Parallel fibre
Stellate cell
Basket cell
Golgi cell
Granule cell
Mossy fibre
Inferior olive
Efferents from a cerebellar nucleus
Spinal/brain stem nucleus of origin of mossy fibres

Fig. 13.8 *Diagrammatic representation of the main circuits of the cerebellar cortex. The cortex is indicated by the* grey background.

Purkinje cells have a specific geometry that is conserved in all vertebrate classes (see Fig. 13.7). They are arranged in a single layer between the molecular and granular layers. Individual Purkinje cells are separated by approximately 50 μm transversely and 50 to 100 μm longitudinally. Their somata measure 50 to 70 μm vertically and 30 to 35 μm transversely. The subcellular structure of the Purkinje cell is similar to that of other neurones. One distinguishing feature is subsurface cisterns, often associated with mitochondria, that are present below the plasmalemma of somata and dendrites and may penetrate into the spines. They are intracellular calcium stores, which are important links in the second messenger systems of the cell.

One or sometimes two large primary dendrites arise from the outer pole of a Purkinje cell. From these, an abundant arborization, with several orders of subdivision, extends toward the surface. Branches of each neurone are confined to a narrow sheet in a plane transverse to the long axis of the folium. Proximal first- and second-order dendrites have smooth surfaces with short, stubby spines and are contacted by climbing fibres. Distal branches show a dense array of dendritic spines, which receive synapses from the terminals of parallel fibres. Inhibitory synapses are received from basket and stellate cells and from the recurrent collaterals of Purkinje cell axons, which contact the shafts of the proximal dendrites. The total number of dendritic spines per Purkinje neurone is approximately 180,000.

The axon of a Purkinje cell leaves the inner pole of the soma and crosses the granular layer to enter the subjacent white matter. The initial axon segment receives axo-axonic synaptic contacts from distal branches of basket cell axons. Beyond the initial segment, the axon enlarges, becomes myelinated and gives off collateral branches. The main axon ultimately forms a plexus in one of the cerebellar or vestibular nuclei. The recurrent collateral branches end on other Purkinje cells and on basket and Golgi neurones.

Basket and stellate cells are the neurones of the molecular layer. Their sparsely branched dendritic trees and the ramifications of their axons lie in a plane approximately perpendicular to the long axis of the folium—that is, in the same plane as the Purkinje cell dendritic tree. Stellate cells are located in the superficial molecular layer, and their axons synapse with the shafts of Purkinje cell dendrites. Both stellate and basket cells receive excitatory synapses from parallel fibres passing through their dendritic trees. Basket cells lie in the lower third of the molecular layer. Their somata receive synapses from Purkinje cell recurrent collaterals and from climbing and mossy fibres, as well as from the parallel fibres. Basket cell axons increase in size away from their somata and run deep in the molecular layer just above the Purkinje cells. Continuing for approximately 1 mm, each covers the territories of 10 to 12 Purkinje neurones. Collaterals of the basket cell axons ascend along Purkinje cell dendrites and descend toward Purkinje cell somata and initial axonal segments, forming pericellular networks, or 'baskets,' around them. Branches from each basket cell axon also extend in the direction of the long axis of the folium to an additional three to six rows of Purkinje neurones, flanking the

axon. It follows that as many as 72 Purkinje cell neurones may receive synapses from a single basket neurone.

Most Golgi cell somata occupy the superficial zone of the granular layer, adjoining the Purkinje cell somata. Their dendrites radiate into the molecular layer. Unlike Purkinje cells, the dendritic trees of Golgi cells are not flattened, appearing much the same in transverse and longitudinal foliar section. In both planes they overlap the territories of several neighbouring Purkinje and Golgi cells. Some Golgi dendrites, however, divide in the granular layer and join cerebellar glomeruli, where they receive excitatory synaptic contacts from mossy fibres. The axon of the Golgi cell arises from the base of the cell body or proximal dendrite and immediately divides into a profuse arborization that extends through the entire thickness of the granular layer. The volume of the territory occupied by the axonal ramifications corresponds approximately to that of its dendritic tree in the molecular layer and it overlaps with the axonal arborizations of adjacent Golgi cells. The main synaptic input to Golgi cell dendrites is from parallel fibres in the molecular layer. Purkinje cell recurrent collaterals and mossy and climbing fibres also terminate on their proximal dendrites and, more sparsely, on their somata.

Each granule cell has a spherical nucleus, 5 to 8 μm in diameter, with a mere shell of cytoplasm containing a few small mitochondria, ribosomes and a diminutive Golgi complex. Granule cells give rise to three to five short dendrites that end in claw-like terminals within the synaptic glomeruli. The fine axons of granule cells enter the molecular layer and branch at a T-junction to form parallel fibres passing in opposite directions over a distance of several millimetres. Terminals located along the parallel fibres give them a beaded appearance and are sites of synapses on the dendrites of Purkinje, stellate, basket and Golgi cells in the molecular layer. Most numerous are the synapses with Purkinje dendritic spines. It has been estimated that 250,000 parallel fibres cross a single Purkinje dendritic tree, although every parallel fibre may not synapse with the dendritic tree it crosses.

Two very different excitatory inputs serve the cerebellar cortex: climbing fibres and mossy fibres. Climbing fibres arise only from the inferior olivary nucleus. Olivocerebellar fibres cross the white matter and enter the granular layer, where they branch to form climbing fibres. Each climbing fibre innervates a single Purkinje cell. There are about 10 times as many Purkinje cells as there are cells in the inferior olive, so each olivocerebellar fibre branches into approximately 10 climbing fibres. Individual climbing fibres pass alongside the soma of a Purkinje cell and then branch to make numerous synapses on the short, stubby spines that protrude from the proximal segments of Purkinje cell dendrites.

Mossy fibres take their origin from the spinal cord, trigeminal, dorsal column and reticular nuclei of the medulla and from the pontine tegmentum and basal pons. Like climbing fibres, they are excitatory, but they contrast sharply in their anatomical distribution and physiological properties. As each mossy fibre traverses the white matter, its branches diverge to enter several adjacent folia. Within each folium, these branches expand into grape-like synaptic terminals (mossy fibre rosettes) that occupy the centre of cerebellar glomeruli.

Noradrenergic and serotoninergic fibres form a rich plexus in all layers of the cerebellar cortex. The aminergic fibres are fine and varicose and form extensive cortical plexuses; their release of noradrenaline (norepinephrine) and serotonin is assumed to be non-synaptic, and their effects are paracrine, involving volumes of tissue. The serotoninergic afferents of the cerebellum take their origin from neurones in the medullary reticular formation, other than the raphe nuclei. The noradrenergic, coeruleocerebellar projection, when active, inhibits Purkinje cell firing not by direct action but by β-adrenergic receptor–mediated inhibition of adenylate cyclase in the Purkinje cells. The presence of dopamine in elements of the cerebellar cortex is still disputed. Cerebellar afferents have been traced from dopaminergic cells in the ventral tegmental area, and dopamine D2 and D3 receptors are present in the molecular layer. A similar plexus of thin, choline acetyltransferase–containing fibres is centred on the Purkinje cell layer. The origin of this cholinergic plexus is not known.

The connections of the cerebellum are organized in two perpendicular planes, corresponding to the planar organization of the cerebellar cortex. Efferent connections of the cortex are disposed in parasagittal sheets or bundles that connect longitudinal strips of Purkinje cells with specific cerebellar or vestibular nuclei. The climbing fibre afferents to a Purkinje cell zone from the inferior olive display a similar zonal disposition. Cerebellar output is organized in modules, with a module consisting of one or more Purkinje cell zones, their cerebellar or vestibular target nucleus and their olivocerebellar climbing fibre input. Modular function is determined by the brain stem projections of the cerebellar or vestibular target nucleus. A general feature of the modular organization of the cerebellum is that GABAergic neurones in the cerebellar nuclei project to the subnuclei of the contralateral inferior olive, which give rise to their respective climbing fibre afferents. These recurrent connections are known as nucleo-olivary pathways.

Mossy fibre afferent systems from precerebellar nuclei in the spinal cord and the brain stem terminate in the granular layer of certain lobules in transversely oriented terminal fields. The transverse lobular arrangement of the mossy fibre afferents is enforced by the transverse orientation of the parallel fibres, which are axons of the granule cells and constitute the second link in the mossy fibre–parallel fibre input of the Purkinje cells. Parallel fibres cross and terminate on Purkinje cells belonging to several successive modules as they course through the molecular layer.

Purkinje cells can be activated in two different ways. Granule cell activity generates simple spikes, which resemble the response of other neurones in the brain, whereas activation by a climbing fibre produces a prolonged depolarization on which several spike-like waves are superimposed. The rate of firing of single and complex spikes also differs markedly. Whereas the Purkinje cell may fire simple spikes at a rate of hundreds per second, complex spikes occur at very low frequencies, seldom more than three or four per second.

Purkinje cell activity is regulated by local Golgi, basket and stellate cells. Like Purkinje cells, Golgi cells have a rich dendritic tree that extends through the molecular layer. Unlike Purkinje cells, the Golgi cell dendrites are not restricted to a plane transverse to the folia, and their axons do not leave the cerebellar cortex. Golgi cells regulate firing by presynaptic inhibition of the mossy fibre afferents, so they act as a governor, or rate limiter, of Purkinje cell activity. Stellate and basket cells synapse directly on Purkinje cells and are powerful inhibitors of their activity.

Structural and Functional Cerebellar Localization

Because the cerebellar cortex is largely uniform in microstructure and microcircuitry, it seems likely that its basic mode of operation is also uniform. The most obvious input for this operation is provided by the mossy fibre afferents, which carry information from all levels of the spinal cord, and specialized sensory and motor information relayed from the cerebral cortex and subcortical motor centres. The most obvious output from the cerebellum is directed at motor systems. Purkinje cells are organized in modules, which are discrete, parallel zones that converge on different cerebellar output nuclei coupled to different motor systems in the brain stem, spinal cord and cerebral cortex. Cerebellar function is therefore determined by temporal and spatial factors (e.g. inhibitory interneurones of the cerebellar cortex), which regulate the access of a particular combination of mossy fibre–parallel fibre inputs to an appropriate output. Plastic changes in the response properties of Purkinje cells, in the form of long-term depression of the parallel fibre–Purkinje cell synapses, may also contribute. Short-term and long-term changes in the response properties of Purkinje cells are under the influence of the climbing fibres.

A double, mirrored localization exists in the anterior and posterior cerebellum (Fig. 13.9). The anterior lobe, simple lobule, pyramis and adjoining lobules

of the hemisphere of the posterior lobe all receive branches from the same mossy and climbing fibres and project to the same cerebellar nuclei. The efferent pathways of these regions monitor the activity in the corticospinal tract and in the subcortical motor systems descending from the vestibular nuclei and reticular formation. The inputs to the cerebellum and the outputs from it are organized according to the same somatotopic patterns, but the orientation of these patterns is reversed. The representation of the head is found principally in the simple lobule and caudally in a corresponding region of the posterior lobe. The double representation of the body follows in rough somatotopic order. Vestibular connections of the cerebellum display a similar double representation in the most rostral lobules of the anterior lobe and far caudally in the vestibulocerebellum (Fig. 13.10).

The folium, tuber, uvula, tonsil and posterior biventral lobule all receive an almost pure pontine mossy fibre input. Climbing fibres from the inferior olive and mossy fibres from the basilar and tegmental pontine nuclei relay visual and acoustic information from the respective cerebral association areas and midbrain tectum to the folium and tuber that are thought to represent a vermal visual and acoustic area (see Fig. 13.9). The efferent connections of this area travel via the fastigial nucleus to gaze centres in the pons and midbrain.

CASE 1   CYSTIC ASTROCYTOMA OF THE CEREBELLUM

A 34-year-old woman complains of increasing headache, especially on arising in the morning, accompanied by forceful vomiting, with or without nausea, and blurring of vision. She exhibits papilloedema on funduscopic examination. Her gait is broad based and unsteady, and she has impaired dexterity in the right hand, with virtually unintelligible handwriting and a prominent crescendo intention tremor on the right finger-to-nose test.

Imaging demonstrates a large cystic lesion in the right cerebellar hemisphere, with compression of the fourth ventricle and secondary enlargement of the aqueduct and the lateral ventricles. At surgery, a well-defined mass is found at the margin of the cyst, a so-called mural nodule with the histological characteristic of a low-grade astrocytoma.

Discussion: This patient demonstrates a cerebellar deficit ipsilateral to the cystic astrocytoma in the right cerebellar hemisphere, along with features of secondary hydrocephalus (headache, vomiting, blurring of vision) due to compression of the fourth ventricle. As is generally the case with lesions in a cerebellar hemisphere, the clinical manifestations are ipsilateral to the lesion.

In a young person, the appearance of such a lateralized cerebellar syndrome might initially raise the possibility of von Hippel–Lindau disease, a form of familial neuroectodermal dysplasia characterized by a cerebellar hemangioblastoma (sometimes cystic), typically accompanied by an angiomatous malformation in the retina and sometimes cystic or angiomatous lesions in the liver, pancreas and kidney.

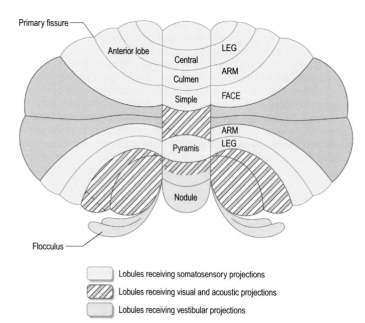

Primary fissure

Anterior lobe

Central

Culmen

Simple

LEG

ARM

FACE

ARM
LEG

Pyramis

Nodule

Flocculus

Lobules receiving somatosensory projections
Lobules receiving visual and acoustic projections
Lobules receiving vestibular projections

Fig. 13.9 *Diagram of localizations in the cerebellar cortex. Somatosensory,* pink; *visual and acoustic,* blue; *vestibular,* yellow.

Afferent Connections of the Cerebellum

Afferent connections of the cerebellum include the mossy fibres and the climbing fibres. Mossy fibre systems terminate bilaterally in transversely oriented 'lobular' areas. The terminations of different mossy fibre systems overlap considerably (see Fig. 13.4). Climbing fibres from different subnuclei of the inferior olive terminate contralaterally, on discrete longitudinal strips of Purkinje cells. This longitudinal pattern closely corresponds with the zonal arrangement in the corticonuclear projection (Fig. 13.11).

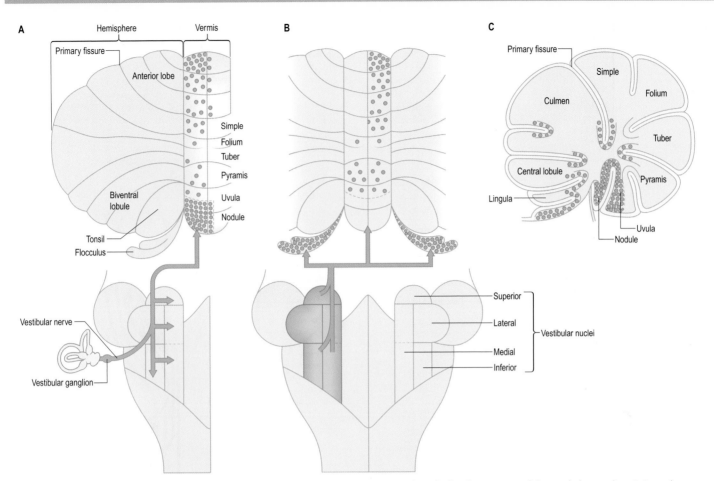

Fig. 13.10 *Vestibulocerebellar mossy fibre projections.* ***A***, *Primary vestibulocerebellar projections from the bipolar neurones of the vestibular ganglion.* ***B***, *Secondary vestibulocerebellar projections from the vestibular nuclei.* ***C***, *Sagittal section showing the distribution of both sets of afferents.*

Spinocerebellar and Trigeminocerebellar Fibres

The spinal cord is connected to the cerebellum through the spinocerebellar and cuneocerebellar tracts and through indirect mossy fibre pathways relayed by the lateral reticular nucleus in the medulla oblongata. These pathways are all excitatory in nature and give collaterals to the interposed and fastigial nuclei before ending on cortical granule cells.

The posterior spinocerebellar tract takes its origin from the posterior thoracic nucleus at the base of the dorsal horn in all thoracic segments of the spinal cord (Fig. 13.12). It enters the inferior cerebellar peduncle, gives collaterals to the cerebellar nuclei and terminates, mainly ipsilaterally, in the vermis and adjoining regions of the anterior lobe and in the pyramis and adjoining lobules of the posterior lobe. The posterior thoracic nucleus receives primary afferents of all kinds from the muscles and joints of the lower limbs, which reach the nucleus via the gracile fasciculus. It also receives collaterals from cutaneous sensory neurones. Accordingly, the tract transmits proprioceptive and exteroceptive information about the ipsilateral lower limbs. Very fast conduction is required to keep the cerebellum informed about ongoing movements. The axons in the posterior spinocerebellar tract are the largest in the central nervous system, measuring 20 μm in external diameter. The upper limb equivalent of the posterior spinocerebellar tract is the cuneocerebellar tract.

The anterior spinocerebellar tract is a composite pathway. It informs the cerebellum about the state of activity of spinal reflex arcs related to the lower limb and lower trunk. Its fibres originate in the intermediate grey matter of the lumbar and sacral segments of the spinal cord (see Fig. 13.12). They cross near their origin and ascend close to the surface as far as the lower midbrain before looping down in the superior cerebellar peduncle. Most fibres cross again in the cerebellar commissure; thus, their distributions to the cerebellar nuclei and cortex appear to be the same as those of the posterior tract.

The rostral spinocerebellar tract originates from cell groups of the intermediate zone and horn of the cervical enlargement. Although considered to be the upper limb and upper trunk counterpart of the anterior spinocerebellar tract, most of its fibres remain ipsilateral throughout their course. It enters the inferior cerebellar peduncle and terminates in the same cerebellar nuclei and folia as the cuneocerebellar tract.

The cuneocerebellar tract contains exteroceptive and proprioceptive components that originate from the cuneate and external cuneate nuclei, respectively. The primary afferents travel in the cuneate fasciculus. The tract itself is predominantly uncrossed and ends in the posterior half of the anterior lobe. Exteroceptive and proprioceptive mossy fibre components of the tract terminate differentially in the apical and basal part of the folia. The exteroceptive component overlaps the pontocerebellar mossy fibre projection in the apices of the folia of the anterior lobe.

Comparable sets of ipsilateral proprioceptive and interoceptive cerebellar projections exist for the extensive territory of the trigeminal brain stem nuclei. These nuclei also project to the ipsilateral inferior olive, relaying there to the contralateral cerebellar cortex and deep nuclei. The cortical representation of the head is directly behind the primary fissure.

Olivocerebellar Fibres

Localization in the Olivocerebellar System: Zones and Microzones — Climbing fibres originate exclusively from the contralateral inferior olivary complex. Projections from the different subnuclei of the inferior olive terminate as climbing fibres on longitudinal strips of Purkinje cells in the cerebellar cortex. Collaterals end on the cerebellar or vestibular target nuclei of these Purkinje cells. A longitudinal zonal arrangement is therefore characteristic of the organization of the olivocerebellar projection (see Fig. 13.11). Moreover, the olivocerebellar projection zones correspond precisely to the corticonuclear projection zones already described. Climbing fibres from the inferior olive are able to modify the cerebellar output in such a way that cells within each subnucleus of the inferior olivary complex monitor the output of a single cerebellar module.

The inferior olivary complex and its climbing fibres can be activated by tactile, proprioceptive, visual and vestibular stimulation and from the sensory, motor and visual cortices and their brain stem relays. A somatotopic arrangement of body parts, matching the olivary projections on to the cerebellar cortex, has been detected in animal experiments.

Olivocerebellar Climbing Fibre Connections — The inferior olivary complex can be subdivided into a convoluted principal olivary nucleus and posterior and medial accessory olivary nuclei. Olivary fibres form the olivocerebellar projection to the contralateral cerebellar cortex and give off collaterals to the lateral vestibular nucleus and to the cerebellar nuclei. Climbing fibres

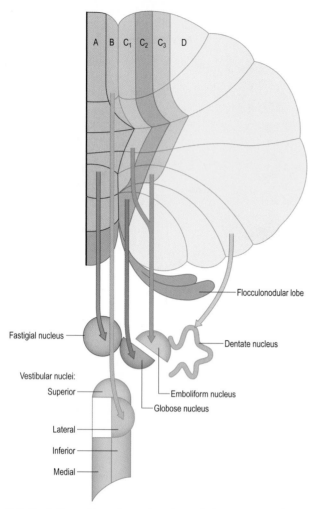

Fig. 13.11 *Cerebellar corticonuclear and corticovestibular projections. The widespread projection from flocculonodular lobe to vestibular nucleus is not arrowed but is indicated in green. (Based on data from Voogd, J., 1964. The Cerebellum of the Cat. Proefschr. Van Gorcum, Assen; and from Voogd, J., Bigaré, F., 1980. Topographic distribution of olivary and corticonuclear fibers in the cerebellum: a review. In: Courville, J., de Mountigny, I., y Latha, R.E. (Eds.), The Inferior Olivary Nucleus. Raven Press, New York, pp. 207–234.)*

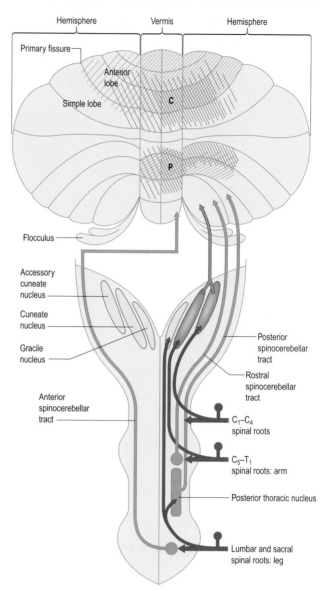

Fig. 13.12 *Spinocerebellar (red) and cuneocerebellar (blue) mossy fibre projections overlap extensively in the culmen (C), pyramis (P) and related intermediate areas of the cortex.*

terminate on longitudinal strips of Purkinje cells. The zonal patterns of the olivocerebellar and Purkinje–nuclear projections correspond precisely. The accessory olivary nuclei project to the vermis and the adjacent hemispheres. The caudal halves of the posterior and medial accessory nuclei innervate the vermis. The caudal part of the posterior accessory nucleus projects to Deiters' nucleus and to the B zone of the anterior vermis. The caudal half of the medial accessory olive gives rise to a projection to the fastigial nucleus and provides climbing fibres to the A zone. The rostral halves of the accessory olives project to the pars intermedia. Climbing fibres from the rostral dorsal accessory olive give collateral projections to the emboliform nucleus and terminate in zones C1 and C3. Zone C2 receives terminals from the rostral medial accessory olive, which provides a collateral projection to the globose nucleus. The principal nucleus projects to the contralateral hemisphere (D zone), and gives collaterals to the dentate nucleus.

The inferior olivary complex receives afferent connections from the spinal cord and from sensory relay nuclei in the brain stem, including the posterior column and sensory trigeminal nuclei. It also receives descending connections from the superior colliculus, parvocellular red nucleus, related nuclei in the midbrain and a GABAergic projection, mainly crossed, from the cerebellar nuclei and certain vestibular nuclei. This latter nucleo-olivary pathway is topically organized. The dentate nucleus projects to the principal nucleus, the emboliform nucleus to the rostral posterior accessory nucleus and the globose nucleus to the rostral medial accessory nucleus. The fastigial nucleus is connected with the caudal medial accessory olive, but the connections are less numerous. The caudal posterior accessory olive receives a nucleo-olivary projection from the lateral vestibular nucleus.

The posterior accessory olive and the caudal half of the medial accessory olive receive an input from the spinal cord and sensory relay nuclei. The middle region of the medial accessory olive receives a projection from the superior colliculus and projects to folium and vermis. The parvocellular red

nucleus and related nuclei project to the olive through the ipsilateral descending central tegmental tracts, which terminate in the rostral half of the medial accessory olive and the principal olive. The parvocellular red nucleus receives converging projections from the cerebellar nuclei and from the motor and premotor cortex. Direct pathways from the cerebral cortex to the inferior olive are sparse. The indirect pathways via the parvocellular red nucleus are much stronger.

Climbing fibres, which terminate in the vestibulocerebellum (flocculus and nodule), are derived from neurones of the medial accessory olive, which receive a strong descending afferent connection from optokinetic centres in the midbrain. Optokinetic information is used by the flocculus in long-term adaptation of compensatory eye movements. Neighbouring neurones are under vestibular control and project to the nodule and the adjoining uvula.

Vestibulocerebellar Fibres

Primary vestibulocerebellar mossy fibres are fibres of the vestibular branch of the vestibulocochlear nerve. They enter the cerebellum with the ascending branch of the vestibular nerve and pass through the superior vestibular nucleus and juxtarestiform body. They terminate, mainly ipsilaterally, in the granular layer of the nodule, caudal part of the uvula, ventral part of the anterior lobe and bottom of the deep fissures of the vermis (see Fig. 13.10A). Secondary vestibulocerebellar mossy fibres arise from the superior vestibular nucleus and the caudal portions of the medial and inferior vestibular nuclei. They terminate bilaterally not only in the same regions that receive primary vestibulocerebellar fibres but also in the flocculus, which lacks a primary vestibulocerebellar projection (see Fig. 13.10B). Some of the mossy fibres from the medial and inferior vestibular nuclei are cholinergic.

Reticulocerebellar Fibres

The lateral reticular nucleus of the medulla oblongata and the paramedian reticular and tegmental reticular nuclei of the pons give rise to mossy fibres. The latter nuclei also supply major collateral projections to the cerebellar nuclei. Spinoreticular fibres terminate in a somatotopic pattern within the entire lateral reticular nucleus, where they overlap with collaterals from the rubrospinal and lateral vestibulospinal tracts and a projection from the cerebral cortex.

The lateral reticular nucleus projects bilaterally to the vermis and hemispheres of the cerebellum. The projection from the dorsal part of the nucleus, which receives collaterals from the rubrospinal tract in addition to spinal afferents, is centred on the ipsilateral hemisphere. The ventral part of the nucleus, which receives a strong projection from the spinal cord and a collateral projection from the lateral vestibulospinal tract, projects bilaterally, mainly to the vermis. The lateral reticular nucleus provides a strong projection to the superior fastigial nucleus, the emboliform nucleus and the medial pole of the globose nucleus.

The paramedian reticular nucleus consists of cell groups at the lateral border of the medial longitudinal fasciculus. It receives fibres from the vestibular nuclei and the interstitiospinal and tectospinal tracts (which descend in the medial longitudinal fasciculus) and from the spinal cord and the cerebral cortex. It projects to the entire cerebellum.

The tegmental reticular nucleus of the pons is located next to the midline in the caudal half of the tegmentum. It receives afferent connections from the cerebral cortex, tectum, nucleus of the optic tract and cerebellar nuclei via the crossed descending branch of the superior cerebellar peduncle. Efferents from the tegmental reticular nucleus reach the cerebellum through the middle cerebellar peduncle. Some terminate superficially in the cortex of the anterior lobe, but many more end in the simple lobule, folium, tuber, vermis and adjoining flocculus. Additional efferents terminate in the caudal fastigial nucleus, dentate nucleus and lateral parts of the globose nucleus.

Pontocerebellar Fibres

The cerebral cortex is the largest single source of fibres that project to the pontine nuclei. Fibres from the pontine nuclei access the cerebellum via the middle cerebellar peduncle, which is the largest afferent system of the human cerebellum. Many corticopontine fibres are collaterals of axons that project to other targets in the brain or spinal cord; it is likely that all corticospinal fibres give off collaterals to the pontine nuclei. Although corticopontine axons arise from lamina V pyramidal cells, the projections from different areas of the cerebral cortex are highly uneven. The areas of cerebral cortex that project to the pontine nuclei are particularly involved in the control of movement. For example, in the case of visual areas, the input arises from extrastriate visual areas in the parietal lobe, whose cells are responsive to movement and function as important links in the visual guidance of movement. Dorsal pontine nuclei receive collateral branches from corticotectal fibres that project to the superior and inferior colliculi from the parietal, temporal and frontal areas of the cerebral cortex, and from tectopontine relays. The onward pontocerebellar projections are to the simple lobule and to the folium and tuber of the vermis.

Fibres of the pontine reticular nuclei are distributed bilaterally, with ipsilateral predominance, to all lobules of the cerebellum other than the lingula and nodule.

More than 90% of fibres in the middle cerebellar peduncle belong to the corticopontocerebellar pathway. Corticopontine fibres travel in the cerebral peduncle. Fibres from the frontal lobe occupy the medial part of the peduncle, and fibres from the parietal, occipital and temporal lobes occupy the lateral part. They synapse on some 20 million neurones in corresponding regions of the basilar pons. The onward pontocerebellar mossy fibre projection is predominantly to the lateral regions of the posterior and anterior lobes, but collaterals are given off to the dentate nucleus (see Fig. 13.4A).

Efferent Connections of the Cerebellum

The output of the cerebellum consists of the inhibitory projections of the Purkinje cells to the cerebellar and vestibular nuclei, and the efferent connections of the cerebellar nuclei to motor centres in the brain stem and, through the thalamus, the motor cortex. Their effects on movement are always indirect, because there are no direct projections from the cerebellar nuclei to motor neurones. Disynaptic connections of the Purkinje cells in the anterior vermis and vestibulocerebellum with motor neurones controlling oculogyric and proximal limb muscles are mediated by the vestibular nuclei. The vermis also influences these motor neurones bilaterally through multisynaptic pathways that involve the fastigial and vestibular nuclei and the reticular formation (Fig. 13.13). The vermis cannot be considered as a single module. Each half of the vermis is composed of several modules (each made up of a longitudinal

Purkinje cell zone and a target nucleus) and their supporting climbing fibre afferent projections.

Each cerebellar hemisphere influences movements of the ipsilateral extremities by way of projections to the dentate and interposed (emboliform and globose) nuclei, which in turn project to the contralateral red nucleus, thalamus and motor cortex (Fig. 13.14).

Corticonuclear and Corticovestibular Fibres

Purkinje cells of each hemivermis project to the ipsilateral fastigial and vestibular nuclei. Purkinje cells of the hemisphere project to the interposed and dentate nuclei. Although the cerebellar cortex is organized in strips of Purkinje cell zones that project to different cerebellar and vestibular nuclei, the borders between these strips are not apparent in the structure of the cortex when it is examined histologically using conventional staining methods. The vermis of the anterior lobe and simple lobule consist of two parallel strips, A and B, of Purkinje cells (see Figs 13.11, 13.13). The medial strip (A zone) projects to the rostral pole of the fastigial nucleus, and the lateral strip (B zone) projects to the lateral vestibular nucleus. The B zone does not continue beyond the simple lobule. The cortex of the entire caudal vermis, which projects to the fastigial nucleus, is included in the A zone. The folium and tuber, which represent a region of the cerebellum that receives a visual input and are involved in the accurate calibration of saccades, project to the caudal pole of the fastigial nucleus. The pyramis, uvula and nodule can be subdivided into several Purkinje cell zones. However, the significance of their connections with the cerebellar and vestibular nuclei is not well

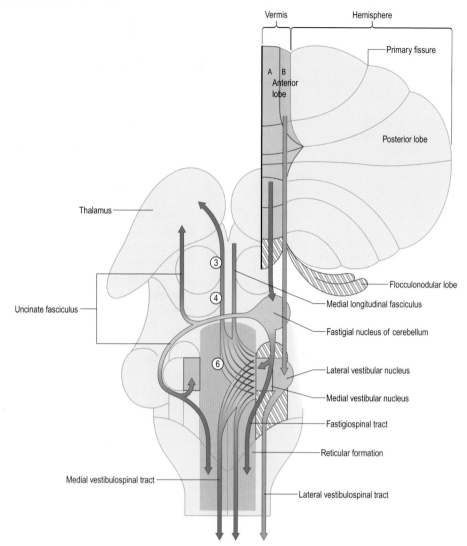

Fig. 13.13 *Efferent connections of the vermis. Connections of the A zones of the vermis and flocculonodular lobe with the fastigial nucleus are indicated, along with those of the B zone with the lateral vestibular nucleus. Some vestibular efferents ascend bilaterally to the ocular motor nuclei and thalamus; others descend to the spinal cord. Motor nuclei of the third (3), fourth (4) and sixth (6) cranial nerves are indicated.*

understood. Corticovestibular projections to the superior, medial and inferior vestibular nuclei, but not to the lateral nucleus, take their origin from the nodule and the adjacent region of the uvula.

The intermediate region consists of two strips of Purkinje cells (C1 and C3 zones), which project to the anterior interposed nucleus. They flank a single zone (C2) that projects to the posterior interposed nucleus (see Figs 13.11, 13.14). The rest of the hemisphere projects to the dentate nucleus. There are indications that the hemisphere can be subdivided into two zones that project to the caudolateral zone and rostromedial parts of the dentate nucleus. The neurones of the caudolateral dentate are generally smaller than those of the rostromedial dentate, and the convolutions are broader. The efferent connections of the flocculus are mainly with the superior, medial and inferior vestibular nuclei and resemble those from the nodule and uvula.

Cerebellovestibular and Cerebelloreticular Fibres

Efferent Connections of the Fastigial Nucleus — The fastigial nucleus is connected bilaterally with the vestibular nuclei and the medullary and pontine reticular formation (see Figs 13.11, 13.14). Smaller crossed connections either ascend to the midbrain and diencephalon or descend into the spinal cord. Small GABAergic neurones give rise to nucleo-olivary fibres, which terminate in the medial accessory olive. The uncinate fasciculus is the major efferent pathway of the fastigial nucleus. Its fibres cross in the rostral part of the cerebellar commissure and pass dorsal to the superior cerebellar peduncle, to enter the vestibular nuclei from their lateral side. Uncrossed fibres enter the vestibular nuclei through the juxtarestiform body (see Fig. 13.6). The distribution of the fastigial projection is bilateral, but with a contralateral preponderance (see Fig. 13.13). Crossed and uncrossed projections end in the medial and inferior vestibular nuclei. They also cross these nuclei to terminate

in the medial reticular formation. Some crossed fibres can be traced caudally into the spinal cord. A small fascicle of crossed fibres from the fastigial nucleus ascends along the superior cerebellar peduncle and is distributed bilaterally to the dorsal tegmentum, central grey matter and deep layers of the superior colliculus and the nuclei of the posterior commissure. Fibres terminate bilaterally in the ventrolateral nucleus and the intralaminar nuclei of the thalamus.

Cerebellovestibular Connections — The relationship between the cerebellum and the vestibular nuclei is complex (see Fig. 13.13). In addition to the vestibulocerebellum (nodule, adjacent folia of the uvula and flocculus), the main vermis and the fastigial nucleus project to the vestibular nuclei. The vestibulocerebellum projects to the superior, medial and inferior vestibular nuclei. Neurones of these nuclei, which receive an input from the vestibular nerve and project to the nuclei controlling eye movements (vestibulo-ocular relay cells), are among the main targets of the Purkinje cells of the nodule and flocculus. Through these connections with vestibulo-ocular relay neurones, the flocculus is involved in the long-term adaptation of compensatory eye movements, the generation of smooth eye movements used to pursue an object and the suppression of the vestibulo-ocular reflex during smooth pursuit. The function of the nodule in the control of eye movement is not as well understood.

The vestibular nuclei are the main source of mossy fibre afferents to the nodule. Their projection to the flocculus is relatively minor. Most mossy fibres that terminate in the flocculus arise from the reticular formation and relay optokinetic and visual information.

The lateral vestibular nucleus, which lacks an input from the labyrinth and receives Purkinje cell axons from the B zone of the anterior vermis, can be regarded as a displaced cerebellar nucleus. It gives rise to the lateral vestibulospinal tract, which descends to all levels of the spinal cord. It is avoided by the efferent pathways from the fastigial nucleus, which terminate more

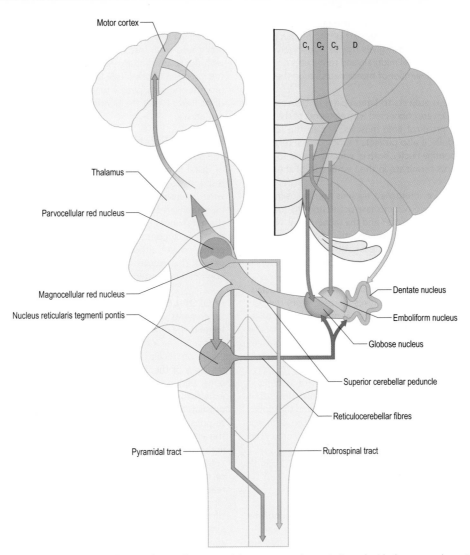

Fig. 13.14 *Efferent connections of the cerebellar hemisphere. Purkinje cell zones and their target nuclei are indicated with the same colours. Efferent fibres from the motor cortex and from the very small magnocellular red nucleus recross and descend to the upper part of the spinal cord.*

ventrally on large neurones in the magnocellular part of the medial vestibular nucleus and in the medial reticular formation. The medial and inferior vestibular nuclei receive a major input from the vestibular nerve. They give rise to bilaterally ascending and descending tracts, which course in the medial longitudinal fasciculus. The ascending tract is composed predominantly of the axons of vestibulo-ocular relay cells. The descending fibres form the medial vestibulospinal tract, which is particularly involved in head righting reflexes when the trunk is tilted.

Fastigial fibres, which terminate in the reticular formation, stimulate the bilaterally descending medullary reticulospinal tracts. The A zone of the vermis exerts a bilateral influence on ventromedially located spinal interneurones and motor neurones that innervate axial, truncal and proximal limb muscles. Some fibres of the uncinate tract descend as far as the cervical cord, where they terminate on the same motor neurones. The B zone exerts an influence on ipsilateral interneurones and motor neurones of the same system through its projection to the lateral vestibular nucleus and the lateral vestibulospinal tract.

The projections of the fastigial nucleus to the thalamus are relatively minor. They are bilateral, as a result of the recrossing of the crossed ascending fibres of the uncinate fasciculus. Their targets include parts of the ventrolateral nucleus and the intralaminar, centrolateral and parafascicular nuclei. Fibres that terminate in the ventrolateral nucleus lie medial to the terminations of fibres from the dentate and interposed nuclei. This region of the ventrolateral nucleus projects to the upper region of the motor cortex and sends collaterals to the medullary reticular formation, which influences ventromedial interneurones and motor neurones in lumbar and sacral segments of the spinal cord via the medullary reticulospinal tracts.

The caudal region of the fastigial nucleus receives Purkinje cell axons from the folium and tuber, an area of the vermis that receives visual inputs. It projects to the contralateral horizontal gaze centre, or paramedian pontine reticular formation, and to the vertical gaze centre, or rostral interstitial

nucleus of the medial longitudinal fascicle, and, bilaterally, to deep layers of the superior colliculus. These projections probably mediate the adaptation of saccades by the vermal visual area.

The cerebellum influences visceromotor systems via the projections of the fastigial nucleus to the parasolitary nucleus (a region bordering the viscerosensory nuclei of the solitary tract), the dorsal visceromotor nucleus of the vagus, the central grey matter, the serotoninergic raphe nuclei of the pons and medulla and the noradrenergic nucleus of the locus coeruleus.

Other pathways from the cerebellar nuclei terminate on precerebellar relay nuclei that give rise to mossy or climbing fibres. Recurrent circuits involving the fastigial nucleus include the nucleus reticularis tegmenti pontis and a projection from the fastigial nucleus to the medial accessory olive. Nucleoolivary projections arise from all the cerebellar nuclei, are crossed and contain GABA as a neurotransmitter. The connections of the fastigial nucleus with the reticular nuclei are excitatory.

Cerebellar nuclei also project to the contralateral interstitial nucleus (of Darkshevich), which lies at the boundary between the midbrain and the diencephalon. This nucleus projects to the medial accessory olive via the central tegmental tract. The fastigial nucleus controls the climbing fibre output of the medial accessory olive, via both its nucleo-olivary projection and its connection to the nucleus of Darkshevich.

Cerebellorubral and Cerebellothalamic Fibres

The axons of neurones in the dentate and interposed nuclei leave the cerebellum in the superior cerebellar peduncle. The superior peduncles, including their nucleo-olivary component, decussate in the caudal midbrain (see Fig. 13.14). Each peduncle then gives off a small descending branch carrying fibres that terminate in the medial reticular formation of the pons and medulla and the pontine tegmental reticular nucleus (see Fig. 13.14). The nucleo-olivary fibres join this descending branch and terminate in the inferior olive in a strictly orderly manner. The ascending branch is distributed to the midbrain and diencephalon, mainly to the red nucleus and thalamus. The anterior interposed nucleus projects to the magnocellular part of the red nucleus. In humans, this projection is very small, and it gives rise to a relatively trivial rubrospinal tract that crosses in the caudal midbrain and terminates on lateral medullary interneurones and a small number of motor neurones in the upper cervical spinal cord.

The anterior interposed nucleus projects to lateral parts of the ventrolateral nucleus of the thalamus, which are connected with elements of the motor cortex projecting to axial and proximal limb muscles, and to the reticular formation of the pons and medulla. It also projects to the pontine tegmental reticular nucleus and to basal pontine nuclei, both of which give rise to mossy fibres. Its nucleo-olivary efferents terminate in the rostral half of the dorsal accessory olive.

The projections of the posterior interposed nucleus are very similar to those of the fastigial nucleus. The two nuclei share projections to the cord, the superior colliculus, the central grey matter and the raphe nuclei. Nucleo-olivary projections from the globose nucleus and the recurrent globose nucleus–interstitial nucleus–inferior olivary nucleus pathway converge on the rostral half of the medial accessory olive. The thalamic projections overlap those from the fastigial and anterior interposed nuclei.

The dentate nucleus projects to the contralateral parvocellular red nucleus and the thalamus. The central tegmental tract takes its origin from the parvocellular red nucleus and terminates on the principal nucleus of the olive. The thalamic projection to the ventrolateral nucleus overlaps those of the other cerebellar nuclei. The inferior and lateral parts of the dentate nucleus project into the most medial region of the ventrolateral nucleus, which in turn projects to the premotor area of the frontal lobe.

The thalamus receives a massive input from other major motor systems, in addition to the input it receives from the cerebellum. In particular, the output of the basal ganglia is relayed to the thalamus by a projection from the globus pallidus. Available evidence suggests that these two great subcortical motor systems terminate on different regions in the ventral thalamus and project to different targets in the motor and premotor cortex.

CEREBELLAR FUNCTIONS
Anticipatory Function

The vermis of the cerebellum is involved in taking anticipatory action to maintain upright posture when objects are picked up. For example, when a book is taken down from a shelf, the first muscle groups to be activated are not the flexors of the shoulder, elbow or fingers but the plantar flexors of the ankle. Contraction of the ankle flexors causes the forefeet to push the lower limbs and trunk backward at the moment the hand grasps the book. Once the lift gets under way, the erector spinae muscles correct for the combined weight of the book and the reaching arm to prevent forward sway of the head and trunk. Labyrinthine receptors simultaneously inform the cerebellum of

any forward movement of the head, and appropriate antigravity thrust is exerted via one or both lateral vestibulospinal tracts. Damage to the vermis may cause total loss of the anticipatory function of the trunk musculature, with the result that any reaching movement may cause the patient to fall in the direction of reach (see later). Damage to the anterior lobe may also compromise the anticipatory function, in this case by deterioration or severance of its linkage with the pontine and medullary reticular nuclei, with resultant gait ataxia.

Postural Fixation

The posterolateral region of the cerebellum is required to prevent oscillation of distal limb parts caused by the viscoelastic properties of the muscles in response to sudden movements. If a volunteer is instructed to exert rapid wrist extension and maintain the extended posture for 2 seconds, electromyographic records taken from the prime movers and antagonists reveal that the antagonists begin to contract before completion of the movement and continue to contract and relax several times in alternating fashion with the prime movers, although with much less force, during the measured fixation period. This 'freeze' control of the wrist can be disrupted by disease of the contralateral posterior lobe, resulting in an action tremor.

Motor Learning

Experiments with monkeys have shown that when a novel motor skill is being learned, the olivocerebellar climbing fibre system becomes active when errors are made. The inferior olivary complex appears to be involved in correction, based on receipt of a copy of the intended movement from collateral branches of the corticospinal tract. Cerebellar output via the superior cerebellar peduncle is also copied on to the parvocellular red nucleus and projected from there to the inferior olive, where it can be compared with the original. Short bursts of climbing fibre activity depress the Purkinje cells responsible for producing the errors. Most human cerebellar disorders involve the anterior or posterior lobe, or both, or their outflows, causing the monitoring system to be lost and learned movements to become clumsy.

Many motor skills require precise timing, which involves an extreme degree of cooperation between prime movers and their antagonists. For example, reading a printed page requires that the scanning eyes snap back to the beginning of a line, time after time. Even small errors may result in dyslexia, whereby slight incoordination of eye movements causes the letters of a word to appear jumbled. Clinical testing of timing can be performed easily by checking the ability to perform rhythmic movements, such as repetitive pronation–supination (Fig. 13.15).

Higher Functions

The cerebellum is currently believed to participate in higher brain functions. This is not unexpected, in view of the two-way linkages (via the thalamus) that exist between the cerebellum and the association and paralimbic areas

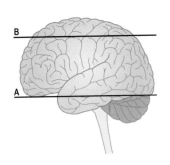

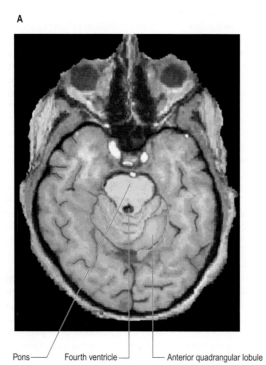

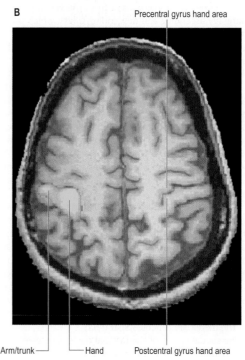

Pons — Fourth ventricle — Anterior quadrangular lobule   Arm/trunk — Hand   Postcentral gyrus hand area

Fig. 13.15 *A* and *B*, *Functional magnetic resonance imaging of a volunteer executing repetitive finger movements of the right hand. The arm–trunk areal activity is attributable to a stabilization function. (Courtesy of Drs. J. P. Finn and T. Parrish, Northwestern University School of Medicine, Chicago.)*

of the cerebral cortex. Its role appears to be one of assistance rather than of generation. For example, during speech, the right posterolateral region of the cerebellum is active bilaterally, which reflects its role in coordinating the muscles involved. However, there is a right-sided predominance, which is consistent with a possible linkage (via the thalamus) with the motor speech area of the left frontal cortex. Moreover, because right lateral cerebellar activity is even greater during functional naming (e.g. 'dig,' 'fly') than during object identification (e.g. 'shovel,' 'airplane'), cognitive as well as motor functions are compromised by cerebellar disorders.

CEREBELLAR DYSFUNCTION

Midline Lesions: Truncal Ataxia

Isolated lesions of the vermis are produced in children by medulloblastomas in the roof of the fourth ventricle. In the recumbent position, there may be no abnormality of motor coordination in the limbs, but there is a progressive inability to stand upright without support, a state known as truncal ataxia. These tumours, which are highly sensitive to radiotherapy, attack the pathway from the vermis to the nuclei of the vestibular nerves. The ataxia reflects malfunction of the linkage between the vermis and the lateral vestibular nucleus, which means that the antigravity support normally driven by the lateral vestibulospinal tract is lost or impaired. Nystagmus can be elicited during visual tracking of the examiner's finger from side to side, reflecting disruption of the labyrinthine connections. Scanning movements of the eye are inaccurate because the vermis no longer controls the gaze centres effectively.

Anterior Lobe Lesions: Gait Ataxia

Disease of the anterior lobe is most often observed in chronic alcoholics and presumably results from prolonged thiamine deficiency. Postmortem studies reveal pronounced shrinkage of the cortex of the anterior lobe. There can be losses of up to 10% of granule cells and 20% of Purkinje cells, and a 30% reduction in the thickness of the molecular layer. The principal anatomical effect is atrophy of the connections between the anterior lobe and interposed nuclei and the reticulospinal pathways involved in normal locomotion. Incoordination of the lower limbs leads to a staggering gait and inability to perform heel-to-toe walking.

A 4-year-old complains of headache, drowsiness and occasional diplopia; he is unsteady on his feet, with frequent falls. Examination demonstrates truncal ataxia, sometimes accompanied by incoordination of the limbs; variable ophthalmoparesis; and papilloedema on funduscopic examination.

Discussion: Medulloblastoma typically presents with a midline cerebellar syndrome, with hydrocephalus and resultant increased intracranial pressure. Clinically, it can be distinguished from ependymoma involving the fourth ventricle by the early appearance of nausea and vomiting in the latter, due to involvement of the fourth floor of the ventricle, including the area postrema. Cranial nerve palsies may appear with either tumour, and increasing intracranial pressure is typical of both.

The predominance of signs suggesting primary involvement of the vermis distinguishes medulloblastoma from cystic (or solid) astrocytoma of the cerebellum, which typically involves a cerebellar hemisphere rather than the vermis (although midline astrocytomas may cause diagnostic confusion).

Tendon reflexes may be depressed in the lower limbs because of the loss of tonic stimulation of fusimotor neurones via the pontine reticulospinal tract. This causes a reduction of monosynaptic reflex activity during walking, which may eventually produce stretching of soft tissues, a phenomenon that can result in hyperextension of the knee joint during standing.

CASE 4   ALCOHOLIC CEREBELLAR DEGENERATION

A middle-aged chronic alcoholic experiences a subacutely evolving disorder of gait, with lurching and frequent falling. Examination demonstrates a broad-based ataxic gait and ataxia with the heel–knee–shin test bilaterally. In contrast, there is little or no evidence of cerebellar deficit involving the upper extremities, and the speech is virtually normal. There is no nystagmus. With the exception of signs of a mild polyneuropathy, the remainder of the examination is normal.

Discussion: The clinical features of a subacute evolving ataxia of the gait and of the legs, with good preservation of cerebellar function in the upper extremities and little if any other deficit, is typical of so-called alcoholic cerebellar degeneration occurring on a background of long-standing poor nutritional intake. The relatively restricted clinical syndrome, affecting primarily gait and the lower extremities, is explained by the observed distribution of lesions in the cerebellar cortex, involving predominantly the superior vermis and anterolateral portion of the cerebellar hemispheres—in accordance with known somatotopic localization in the cerebellar cortex (Fig. 13.16). All neurocellular components of the cerebellar cortex may be involved; Purkinje cells are most liable to damage. Secondary changes may be noted in the deep cerebellar nuclei. In some cases, features of Wernicke's encephalopathy are noted, prompting the suggestion that both disorders reflect a vitamin, perhaps thiamine, deficiency.

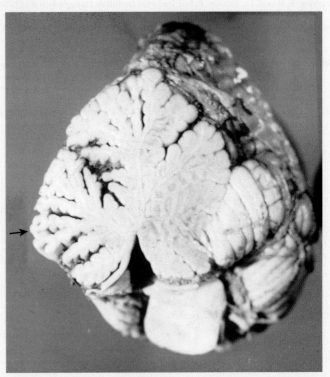

Fig. 13.16 *Alcoholic cerebellar degeneration. Section through the vermis of the cerebellum demonstrating gross atrophy of the superior vermis, in contrast to preservation of the inferior vermis. (From Victor, M., Adams, R.D., Mancall, E.L. A restricted form of cerebellar degeneration occurring in alcoholic patients. Arch. Neurol. 1959; 1(6): 579–688. Copyright © 1959 American Medical Association. All rights reserved.)*

Neocerebellar Lesions: Incoordination of Voluntary Movements

Disease of the neocerebellar cortex, dentate nucleus or white matter of the superior cerebellar peduncle leads to incoordination of voluntary movements, particularly in the upper limbs. When fine purposive movements are attempted, an action tremor or intention tremor develops: the hand and forearm quiver as the target is approached because of faulty agonist–antagonist muscle synergies around the elbow and wrist. The hand may travel past the target (overshoot). The normal smooth trajectory of reaching movements may be replaced by stepped flexions, abductions, and the like (decomposition of movement). Rapid alternating movements performed under command, such as pronation–supination, become irregular as a consequence of loss of the timing function of the cerebellum. The finger-to-nose and heel-to-knee tests are performed with equal clumsiness whether the eyes are open or closed. (This is in contrast to the performance of these tasks in posterior column disease, in which performance is adequate when the eyes are open.) Speech is impaired with regard to both phonation and articulation. Phonation (production of vowel sounds) is uneven and often tremulous, reflecting loss of the smooth contraction of the expiratory muscles. Articulation is slurred (cerebellar dysarthria) because of faulty coordination of the groups of muscles that move the lips, tongue and soft palate and act on the temporomandibular joint. Signs of neocerebellar disorder sometimes originate in the midbrain or pons rather than in the cerebellum itself. Such lesions are usually vascular and interrupt one of the cerebellothalamic pathways (or both, if the decussation of the superior cerebellar peduncles is affected).

'Cerebellar cognitive affective syndrome' is the term used to describe cerebral functional deficits that follow sudden severe damage to the cerebellum, such as after thrombosis of one of the three pairs of cerebellar arteries or surgical removal of a cerebellar tumour. Such patients show cognitive defects in the form of diminished reasoning power, inattention, grammatical errors of speech, poor spatial sense and patchy memory loss. If the vermis is included in the lesion, affective (emotional) symptoms appear, in the form of flatness of affect (dulling of emotional responses) or aberrant emotional behaviour. There may be reduced bloodflow (on positron emission tomography) in one or more of the associated areas linked to the cerebellum by corticoponto-cerebellar fibres.

References

Angevine, J.B., Mancall, E.L., Yakovlev, P., 1961. The human cerebellum: a topographical atlas. Little-Brown, Boston.

Bastian, A.J., Mugnaini, E., Thach, W.T., 1999. Cerebellum. In: Zigmond, M.J., Bloom, F.E., Landis, S.C., Roberts, J.L., Squire, L.R. (Eds.), Fundamental Neuroscience. Academic Press, San Diego, pp. 973–992.

Gebhart, A.L., Petersen, S.E., Thach, W.T., 2002. Role of the posterolateral cerebellum in language. Ann. N. Y. Acad. Sci. 978, 318–333. *One of several studies using functional magnetic resonance imaging to show that the right posterolateral cerebellum is involved in word retrieval and syntax generation.*

Ivry, R.B., Spencer, R.M., Zelaznik, H.N., Diedrichsen, J., 2002. The cerebellum and event timing. Ann. N. Y. Acad. Sci. 978, 302–317.

Jueptner, M., Kruckenberg, M., 2001. Anatomic basis of functional magnetic resonance imaging: motor system. Neuroimaging Clin. N. Am. 11, 203–219.

Rae, C., Haresty, J.A., Dzendrowskyj, T.E., et al, 2002. Cerebellar morphology in developmental dyslexia. Neuropsychologia. 40, 1285–1292.

Schmahmann, J.D., Doyon, J., Toga, A.W., Petrides, M., Evans, A.C., 2000. MRI atlas of the human cerebellum. Harcourt, Orlando.

Schmahmann, J.D., Sherman, J.C., 1998. The cerebellar cognitive affective syndrome. Brain 121, 561–579.

Topka, H., Mescheriakov, S., Boose, A., et al, 1999. A cerebellar-like terminal and postural tremor induced in normal man by transcranial magnetic stimulation. Brain 122, 1551–1562.

Valsamis, M.P., Mancall, E.L., 1973. Toxic cerebellar degeneration. Hum. Pathol. 4, 513–520

Van de Warrenburg, B.P.C., Sinke, R.J., Kremer, B., 2005. Recent advances in hereditary spinocerebellar ataxias. J. Neuropathol. Exp. Neurol. 64, 171–180.

Victor, M., Adams, R.D., Mancall, E.L., 1959. A form of degeneration of the cerebellar cortex observed in chronic alcoholic patients. Arch. Neurol. 1, 579–688.

CASE 5   ATAXIA-TELANGIECTASIA

A 2-year-old girl develops ataxia that becomes increasingly prominent with the passage of time and is associated with slurring of speech and abnormal ocular motility. Myoclonic jerks, dystonic movements and chorea appear with the passage of years. Neurological examination demonstrates superficial telangiectasia involving most prominently the conjunctiva but also the face and ears.

Discussion: This patient suffers from ataxia-telangiectasia. Clinically, this may be the most readily identified form of genetically determined spinocerebellar ataxia, by virtue of the presence of conjunctival telangiectasia, as seen in this child. Abnormal laboratory tests include an elevated α-fetoprotein level, present in a great majority of cases, and decreased IgA and IgG serum levels. Mental and growth retardation are both documented, and a sensory neuropathy may appear. Defective immune responses are found, and recurrent respiratory infections are common.

Anatomically, the disorder is characterized by the loss of both Purkinje and granule cells in the cerebellar cortex. Nerve cell loss is also found in the neuraxis, such as in the dentate and olivary nuclei and elsewhere in the brain stem and spinal cord.

Section V

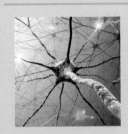

The Cerebrum

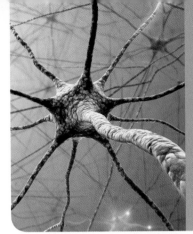

Basal Ganglia

The term basal ganglia denotes a number of subcortical nuclear masses that lie in the inferior part of the cerebral hemisphere, lateral to the thalamus (Figs 14.1, 14.2). They have traditionally been regarded as including the corpus striatum, the claustrum and the amygdaloid complex. More recently, however, the working definition has been narrowed to cover only the corpus striatum and its associated structures in the diencephalon and midbrain. The reasoning behind this change is that these structures form a functional complex involved in the control of movement and motivational aspects of behaviour, whereas the claustrum is of unknown function and the amygdala is more closely related to the limbic system (Ch. 16).

The corpus striatum consists of the caudate nucleus, putamen and globus pallidus (Fig. 14.3). Because of their close proximity, the putamen and globus pallidus were historically considered a single entity, termed the lentiform complex or nucleus. With increasing knowledge of their structure and function, however, it has become clear that the putamen is more correctly considered to be in unity with the caudate nucleus, with which it shares common chemocytoarchitecture and connections. The putamen and caudate nucleus are together referred to as the neostriatum or simply the striatum.

The striatum is considered the principal 'input' structure of the basal ganglia because it receives the majority of afferents from other parts of the neuraxis. Its principal efferent connections are to the globus pallidus and pars reticulata of the substantia nigra. The globus pallidus—in particular, its medial segment— together with the pars reticulata of the substantia nigra (Ch. 10) is regarded as the main 'output' structure because it is the source of massive efferent fibre projections, mostly directed to the thalamus.

Disorders of the basal ganglia are principally characterized by abnormalities of movement, muscle tone and posture. There is a wide spectrum of clinical presentations, ranging from poverty of movement and hypertonia at one extreme (typified by Parkinson's disease) to abnormal involuntary movements (dyskinesias) at the other. The underlying pathophysiological mechanism of these disorders has been much studied in recent years and is better understood than that of any other type of complex neurological dysfunction. This has led to the introduction of new rational strategies for the medical and neurosurgical treatment of movement disorders.

The caudate nucleus is a curved, tadpole-shaped mass. It has a large anterior head, which tapers to a body, and a down-curving tail (Fig. 14.4). The head is covered with ependyma and lies in the floor and lateral wall of the anterior horn of the lateral ventricle, in front of the interventricular foramen. The tapering body is in the floor of the body of the ventricle, and the narrow tail follows the curve of the inferior horn, lying in the ventricular roof in the temporal lobe. Medially, the greater part of the caudate nucleus abuts the thalamus, along a junction marked by a groove, the sulcus terminalis. The sulcus contains the stria terminalis, lying deep to the ependyma (see Fig. 5.3; Fig. 14.5). The stria terminalis forms one margin of the choroid fissure of the lateral ventricle; the hippocampal fimbria and fornix form the other margin. The sulcus terminalis is especially prominent anterosuperiorly (because of the large head and body of the caudate nucleus relative to the tail), where it is accompanied by the thalamostriate vein.

The corpus callosum lies above the head and body of the caudate nucleus. The two are separated laterally by the fronto-occipital bundle and medially by the subcallosal fasciculus, a bundle of axons that caps the nucleus (see Fig. 14.5; Figs 14.6, 14.7). The caudate nucleus is largely separated from the lentiform complex by the anterior limb of the internal capsule (Figs 14.1, 14.6, 14.7). However, the inferior part of the head of the caudate becomes continuous with the most inferior part of the putamen immediately above the anterior perforated substance. This junctional region is sometimes known as the fundus striati (see Fig. 14.6). Variable bridges of cells connect the putamen to the caudate nucleus for most of its length. They are most prominent anteriorly, in the region of the fundus striati and the head and body of the caudate nucleus, where they break up the anterior limb of the internal capsule (see Figs 14.6, 14.7). In the temporal lobe, the anterior part of the tail of the caudate nucleus becomes continuous with the posteroinferior part of the putamen.

The vast bulk of the caudate nucleus and putamen are often referred to as the dorsal striatum. A smaller inferomedial part of the rostral striatum is referred to as the ventral striatum and includes the nucleus accumbens.

The lentiform complex lies deep to the insular cortex, with which it is roughly coextensive, although the two are separated by a thin layer of white matter and the claustrum (see Fig. 14.2; Fig. 14.8). The claustrum splits the insular subcortical white matter to create the extreme and external capsules. The latter separates the claustrum from the putamen (see Figs 16.40, 14.1, 14.2, 14.8). The lentiform complex is separated from the caudate nucleus by the internal capsule.

The lentiform complex consists of the laterally placed putamen and the more medial globus pallidus (pallidum), which are separated by a thin layer of fibres, the lateral or external medullary lamina. The globus pallidus is itself divided into two segments, a lateral (or external) segment and a medial (or internal) segment, separated by an internal (or medial) medullary lamina. The two segments have distinct afferent and efferent connections.

Inferiorly, a little behind the fundus striati, the lentiform complex is grooved by the anterior commissure, which connects inferior parts of the temporal lobes and the anterior olfactory cortex of the two sides (see Fig. 14.6). The area above the commissure is referred to as the dorsal pallidum, and that below it is the ventral pallidum.

STRIATUM

The striatum consists of the caudate nucleus, putamen and ventral striatum, which are all highly cellular and well vascularized. The caudate and putamen are traversed by numerous small bundles of thinly myelinated or nonmyelinated small-diameter axons, which are mostly striatal afferents and efferents. They radiate through the striatal tissue as though converging on, or radiating from, the globus pallidus. The bundles are occasionally referred to by the archaic term 'Wilson's pencils' and they account for the striated appearance of the corpus striatum.

Neurones of both dorsal and ventral striata are mainly medium-sized multipolar cells. They have round, triangular or fusiform somata, mixed with a smaller number of large multipolar cells. The ratio of medium to large cells is at least 20:1. The large neurones have extensive spherical or ovoid dendritic trees up to 600 μm across. The medium-sized neurones also have spherical dendritic trees, approximately 200 μm across, which receive the synaptic terminals of many striatal afferents. The dendrites of both medium and large striatal cells may be either spiny or non-spiny. The most common neurone (usually 75% of the total) is a medium-sized cell with spiny dendrites. These cells use γ-aminobutyric acid (GABA) as their transmitter and also express the genes coding for either enkephalin or substance P/dynorphin. Enkephalinergic neurones appear to express D2 dopamine receptors. Substance P/dynorphin neurones have D1 receptors. These neurones are the major, and perhaps exclusive, source of striatal efferents to the pallidum and substantia nigra pars reticulata. The remaining medium-sized striatal neurones are non-spiny and are intrinsic cells that contain acetylcholinesterase, choline acetyltransferase and somatostatin. Large neurones with spiny dendrites contain acetylcholinesterase and choline acetyltransferase. Most, perhaps all, are intrinsic neurones, as are non-spiny large neurones.

Intrinsic synapses are probably largely asymmetric (Type II), whereas those derived from external sources are symmetric (Type I). The aminergic afferents from the substantia nigra, raphe and locus coeruleus all end as profusely branching axons with varicosities that contain dense-core vesicles (the presumed store of amine transmitters). Many of these varicosities have no conventional synaptic membrane specializations and may release transmitter in a way analogous to that found in peripheral postsynaptic sympathetic axons.

Neuroactive chemicals, whether intrinsic or derived from afferents, are not distributed uniformly in the striatum. For example, serotonin and glutamic acid decarboxylase concentrations are highest caudally, whereas substance P, acetylcholine and dopamine are highest rostrally. However, there is a finer-grain neurochemical organization that informs the view of the striatum as a

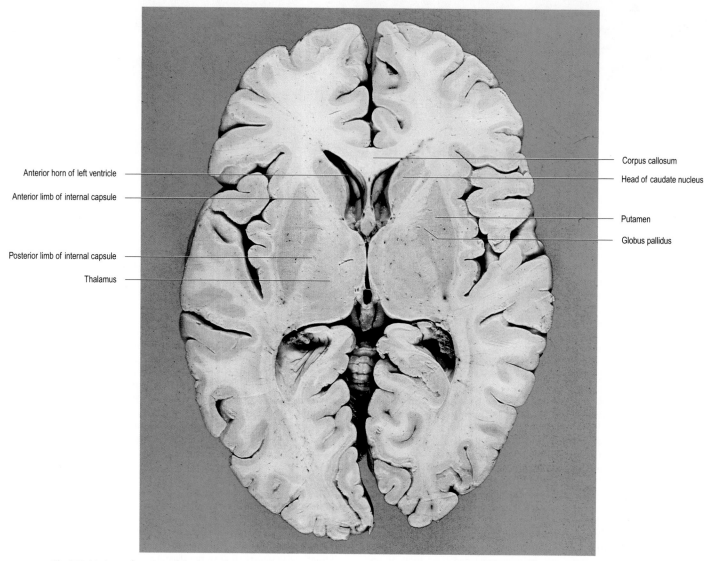

Anterior horn of left ventricle

Anterior limb of internal capsule

Posterior limb of internal capsule

Thalamus

Corpus callosum

Head of caudate nucleus

Putamen

Globus pallidus

Fig. 14.1 *Horizontal section of the brain. (Dissection by E. L. Rees; photograph by Kevin Fitzpatrick on behalf of GKT School of Medicine, London.)*

mosaic of islands or striosomes (sometimes referred to as patches), each 0.5 to 1.5 mm across, packed into a background matrix. Striosomes contain substance P and enkephalin. During development, the first dopamine terminals from the substantia nigra are found in striosomes. Although this exclusivity does not persist after birth, striosomes in the caudate nucleus still contain a higher concentration of dopamine than the matrix does. The latter contains acetylcholine and somatostatin and is the target of thalamostriate axons. Receptors for at least some neurotransmitters are also differentially distributed. For example, opiate receptors are found almost exclusively within striosomes, and muscarinic receptors predominantly so. Moreover, the distribution of neuroactive substances within the striosomes is not uniform. In humans, the striosome–matrix patchwork is less evident in the putamen, where it appears to consist predominantly of matrix, than it is in the caudate nucleus.

All afferents to the striatum terminate in a mosaic manner. The size of a cluster of terminals is usually 100 to 200 μm across. Some afferent terminal clusters are not arranged in register with the clear striosome–matrix distributions seen in nigrostriatal and thalamostriatal axons. In general, afferents from neocortex end in striatal matrix, and those from allocortex end in striosomes. However, the distinction is not absolute. Thus, although afferents from the neocortex arise in layers V and VI, those from the superficial part of layer V end predominantly in striatal matrix, whereas those from deeper neocortex project to striosomes. Striatal cell bodies, which are the sources of efferents, also form clusters, but again, they are not uniformly related to striosomes. For example, the cell bodies of some striatopallidal and striatonigral axons lie clustered within striosomes; others lie outside them, but still in clusters. The neurones and neuropil of the ventral striatum are essentially similar to those of the dorsal striatum, but the striosome–matrix organization is less well defined and seems to consist predominantly of striosomes.

The major connections of the striatum are summarized in Figure 14.9. Although the connections of the dorsal and ventral divisions overlap, a generalization can be made: the dorsal striatum is predominantly connected with

motor and associative areas of the cerebral cortex, whereas the ventral striatum is connected with the limbic system and orbitofrontal and temporal cortices. For both dorsal and ventral striata, the pallidum and substantia nigra pars reticulata are key efferent structures. The fundamental arrangement is the same for both divisions. The cerebral cortex projects to the striatum, which in turn projects to the pallidum and substantia nigra pars reticulata. From these, efferents leave to influence the cerebral cortex (either the supplementary motor area or the prefrontal and cingulate cortices via the thalamus) and the superior colliculus.

The entire neocortex sends glutamatergic axons to the ipsilateral striatum. For a long time, these axons were thought to be collaterals of other cortical efferents, but it is now known that they arise exclusively from small pyramidal cells in layers V and VI. It has also been suggested that some of the cells of origin lie in the supragranular 'cortical association' layers II and III. The projection is organized topographically. The greater part of the input from the cerebral cortex to the dorsal striatum is derived from the frontal and parietal lobes, and that from the occipitotemporal cortex is relatively small. Thus, the orbitofrontal association cortex projects to the inferior part of the head of the caudate nucleus, which lies next to the ventral striatum. The dorsolateral frontal association cortex and frontal eye fields project to the rest of the head of the caudate nucleus, and much of the parietal lobe projects to the body of the nucleus. The somatosensory and motor cortices project predominantly to the putamen. Their afferents establish a somatotopic pattern, in which the lower body is represented laterally and the upper body is represented medially. The motor cortex is unique in sending axons through the corpus callosum to the opposite putamen, where they end with the same spatial ordering. The occipital and temporal cortices project to the tail of the caudate nucleus and to the inferior putamen.

The striatum also receives afferents, which are more crudely spatially organized, from the polysensory intralaminar thalamus. The cerebelloreceptive nucleus centralis lateralis projects to the anterior striatum (especially the

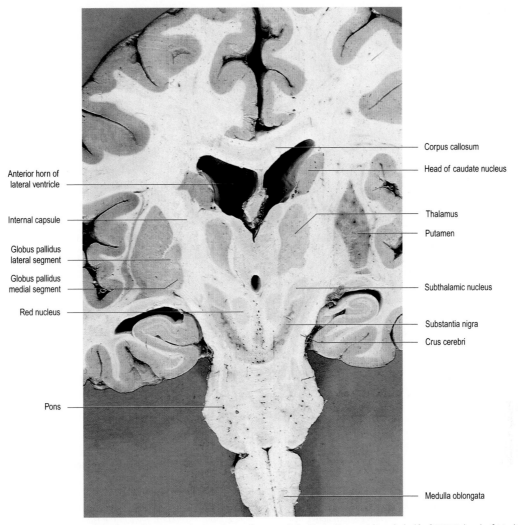

Fig. 14.2 *Oblique coronal section of the brain. (Dissection by E. L. Rees; photograph by Kevin Fitzpatrick on behalf of GKT School of Medicine, London.)*

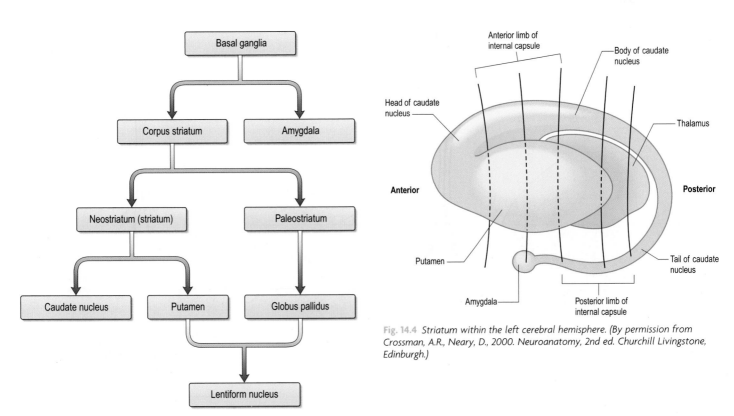

Fig. 14.3 *Relationships of structures forming the basal ganglia.*

Fig. 14.4 *Striatum within the left cerebral hemisphere. (By permission from Crossman, A.R., Neary, D., 2000. Neuroanatomy, 2nd ed. Churchill Livingstone, Edinburgh.)*

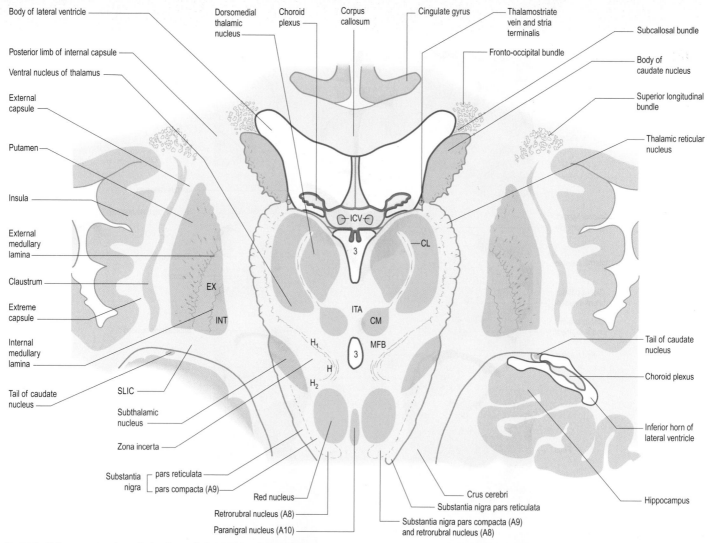

Fig. 14.5 *Oblique section through the diencephalon and basal ganglia. A8, A9, A10, dopaminergic cell groups; CL, centrolateral nucleus of thalamus; CM, centromedian nucleus of thalamus; EX, external pallidal segment; H, H1, H2, subthalamic fields of Forel; ICV, internal cerebral veins in the transverse fissure; INT, internal pallidal segment; ITA, interthalamic adhesion; MFB, median forebrain bundle; SLIC, sublentiform internal capsule; 3, third ventricle.*

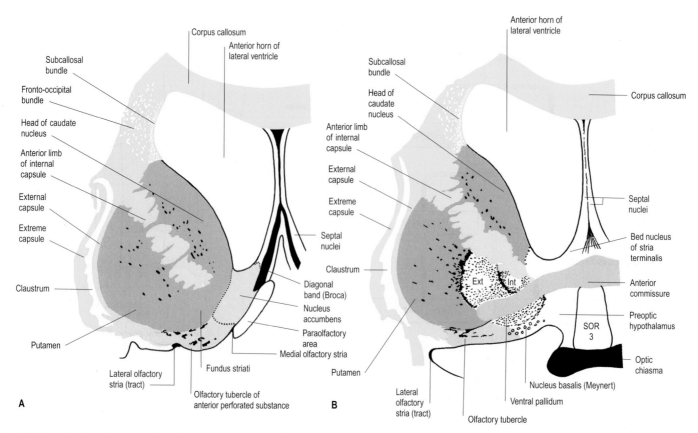

Fig. 14.6 *A and B, Coronal sections through the corpus striatum and anterior perforated substance (A is anterior to B). The pallidum is shown in B. Ext, external segment; Int, internal segment; SOR 3, supraoptic recess of the third ventricle.*

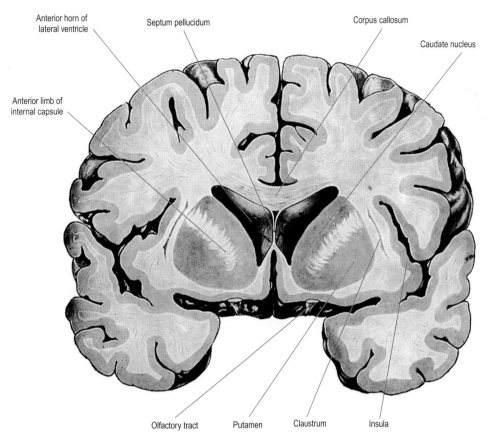

Fig. 14.7 *Posterior aspect of a coronal section through the anterior horn of the lateral ventricles.*

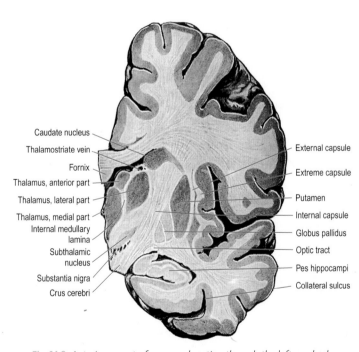

Fig. 14.8 *Anterior aspect of a coronal section through the left cerebral hemisphere.*

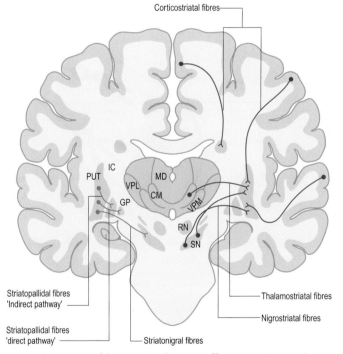

Fig. 14.9 *Connections of the striatum. The major afferent projections to the striatum are shown on the left, and the major efferent projections from the striatum are shown on the right. CM, centromedian nucleus; GP, globus pallidus; IC, internal capsule; MD, medial dorsal nucleus; PUT, putamen; RN, red nucleus; SN, substantia nigra; VPL, ventral posterolateral nucleus of the thalamus; VPM, ventral posteromedial nucleus of the thalamus.*

caudate nucleus), and the cerebello- and pallidoreceptive centromedian nucleus projects to the putamen.

The aminergic inputs to the caudate and putamen are derived from the substantia nigra pars compacta (dopaminergic group A9; Figs 14.10, 14.11), the retrorubral nucleus (dopaminergic group A8; see Fig. 14.5), the dorsal raphe nucleus (serotoninergic group B7; see Fig. 14.10) and the locus coeruleus (noradrenergic group A6). The nigrostriatal input is sometimes referred to as the 'mesostriatal' dopamine pathway. It reaches the striatum by traversing the H fields of the subthalamus. These aminergic inputs appear to modulate the responses of the striatum to cortical and thalamic afferent influences.

Efferents from the striatum pass to both segments of the globus pallidus and to the substantia nigra pars reticulata, where they end in a topically

ordered fashion. Fibres ending in either the lateral or medial pallidal segment originate from different striatal cells (Figs 14.9, 14.12). Those to the lateral pallidum come from neurones that co-localize GABA and enkephalin and give rise to the so-called indirect pathway. This name refers to the fact that these striatal neurones influence the activity of basal ganglia output neurones in the medial pallidum via the intermediary of the subthalamic nucleus. Other striatal neurones, which co-localize GABA and substance P/dynorphin, project

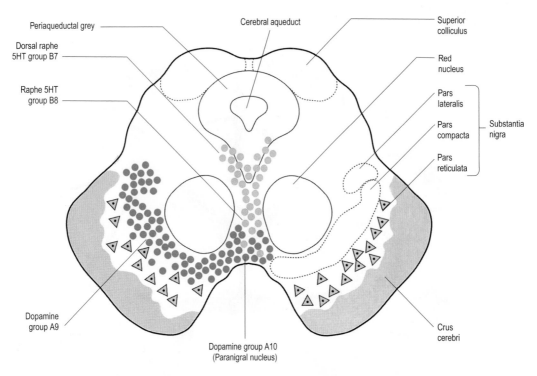

Fig. 14.10 *Transverse section through the midbrain to show the arrangement of dopaminergic cell groups A9 and A10 in the substantia nigra (left) and serotoninergic cell groups B7 and B8 in the raphe.*

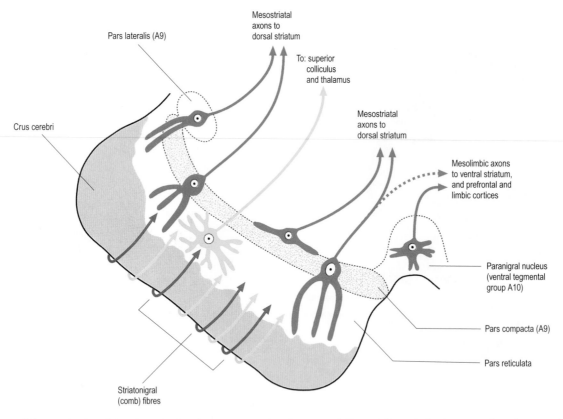

Fig. 14.11 *Scheme of the organization of the substantia nigra in transverse section. Compare with Figure 14.10. Medially, there is no sharp distinction between dopaminergic cells projecting to the dorsal striatum (pars compacta, A9) and those projecting to the ventral striatum and limbic system (paranigral nucleus, A10). Dendrites of dopaminergic neurones intrude into the pars reticulata. Note the distinctive projection systems from the pars reticulata. (From Paxinos (Ed.), 1990. The Human Nervous System, vol. 1, Webster. pp. 889–944. Modified with permission from Elsevier.)*

directly to the medial pallidum and are therefore described as the direct pathway.

A second outflow is established from the striatum to the pars reticulata of the substantia nigra. This also has both direct and indirect components, via the lateral pallidum and subthalamic nucleus (Fig. 14.13). The axons of the direct striatonigral projection constitute the laterally placed 'comb' system, which is spatially quite distinct from the ascending dopaminergic nigrostriatal

pathway. Striatonigral fibres end in a spatially ordered way in the pars reticulata.

The ventral striatum is the primary target of cortical afferents from limbic cortices, including allocortex, and from limbic-associated regions (see Fig. 14.13). Thus, the hippocampus (through the fornix) and the orbitofrontal cortex (through the internal capsule) project to the nucleus accumbens, and the olfactory, entorhinal, anterior cingulate and temporal visual cortices project

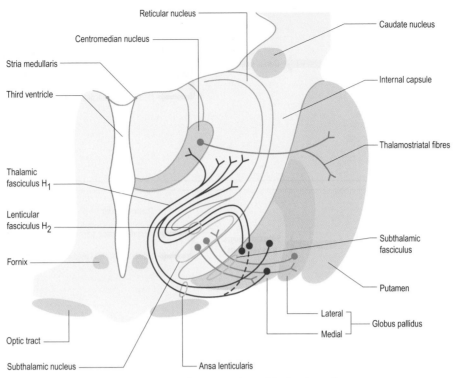

Fig. 14.12 *Major interconnections of the basal ganglia.*

to both the nucleus accumbens and the olfactory tubercle in varying degrees. The tubercle also receives afferents from the amygdala. The contiguities of the cortical areas, which project to the ventral striatum and neighbouring dorsal striatum, emphasize the imprecise nature of the boundaries between the two divisions. All the cortical regions overlap and abut one another, and they project to neighbouring parts of the dorsal striatum as well as to the ventral striatum. The fundus striati and ventromedial caudate nucleus abut the olfactory tubercle and nucleus accumbens (see Fig. 14.6) and receive connections from the orbitofrontal cortex and, to a lesser extent, the lateral prefrontal and anterior cingulate cortices (which also project to the contiguous head of the caudate nucleus).

This continuity of the ventral and dorsal striata, as revealed by the arrangements of corticostriate projections, is reinforced by consideration of the aminergic inputs to the ventral striatum. They are derived from the dorsal raphe (serotoninergic group B7), the locus coeruleus (noradrenergic group A6) and the paranigral nucleus (dopamine group A10), as well as from the most medial part of the substantia nigra pars compacta (group A9; see Figs 14.10, 14.11). The dopamine projections constitute the so-called mesolimbic dopamine pathway, which also projects to the septal nuclei, hippocampus, amygdala and prefrontal and cingulate cortices through the medial forebrain bundle. The lateromedial continuity of cell groups A9 and 10 (see Fig. 14.10) is thus reflected in the relative positions of their ascending fibres in the subthalamus and hypothalamus (the H fields and median forebrain bundle, respectively), as well as in the lateromedial topography of the dorsal and ventral striata (see Fig. 14.6), which in turn have contiguous and overlapping sources of cortical afferents.

As for the dorsal striatum, efferents from the ventral striatum project to the pallidum (in this case, the ventral pallidum) and the substantia nigra pars reticulata (Figs 14.13, 14.14). In the latter case, the connection is both direct and indirect via the subthalamic nucleus. The projections from the pars reticulata are as described for the dorsal system, but axons from the ventral pallidum reach the thalamic mediodorsal nucleus (which projects to the cingulate and prefrontal association cortex) and midline nuclei (which project to the hippocampus). Ventral pallidal axons also reach the habenular complex of the limbic system.

The brain areas beyond the basal nuclei, substantia nigra and subthalamic nucleus, to which both ventral and dorsal systems appear to project, are therefore the prefrontal association and cingulate cortices and the deep superior colliculus.

Nucleus Accumbens

The ventral striatum consists of the nucleus accumbens and the olfactory tubercle. In front of the anterior commissure, much of the grey matter of the anterior perforated substance, and especially the olfactory tubercle, is indistinguishable from and continuous with the fundus striati in terms of cellular

composition, histochemistry and interconnections. The caudate nucleus is continuous medially with the nucleus accumbens (see Fig. 14.6), which abuts the nuclei of the septum, close to the paraolfactory area, the diagonal band of Broca and the fornix.

The nucleus accumbens receives a dopaminergic innervation from the midbrain ventral tegmental area (cell group A10). It is believed to represent the neural substrate for the rewarding effects of several classes of drugs of abuse and is therefore a major determinant of their addictive potential. The experimental observation that the locomotor-activating effects of psychomotor stimulant drugs such as amphetamine and cocaine (which act presynaptically on dopaminergic neurones to enhance dopamine release or block its reuptake, respectively) are dependent on dopamine transmission in the nucleus accumbens led to the hypothesis that the reinforcing or rewarding properties of these drugs are mediated by the mesolimbic dopamine system.

GLOBUS PALLIDUS

The globus pallidus lies medial to the putamen and lateral to the internal capsule. It consists of two segments, lateral (external) and medial (internal), which are separated by an internal medullary lamina and have substantially different connections. Both segments receive large numbers of fibres from the striatum and subthalamic nucleus. The lateral segment projects reciprocally to the subthalamic nucleus as part of the indirect pathway. The medial segment is considered to be a homologue of the pars reticulata of the substantia nigra, with which it shares similar cellular and connectional properties. Together, these segments constitute the main output of the basal ganglia to other levels of the neuraxis, principally to the thalamus and superior colliculus.

The cell density of the globus pallidus is less than one-twentieth that of the striatum. The morphology of the majority of cells is identical in the two segments. They are large multipolar GABAergic neurones that closely resemble those of the substantia nigra pars reticulata. The dendritic fields are discoid, with planes at right angles to incoming striatopallidal axons, each of which potentially contacts many pallidal dendrites *en passant*. This arrangement, coupled with the diameters of the dendritic fields (>500 μm), suggests that a precise topographical organization is unlikely within the pallidum.

Striatopallidal fibres are of two main types. They project to either the lateral or medial pallidal segment. Those projecting to the lateral segment constitute the beginning of the so-called indirect pathway. They use GABA as their primary transmitter and also contain enkephalin. Efferent axons from neurones in the lateral segment pass through the internal capsule in the subthalamic fasciculus and travel to the subthalamic nucleus (see Fig. 15.18).

Striatopallidal axons destined for the medial pallidum constitute the so-called direct pathway. Like the indirect projection, these also use GABA as their primary transmitter, but they also contain substance P/dynorphin, rather

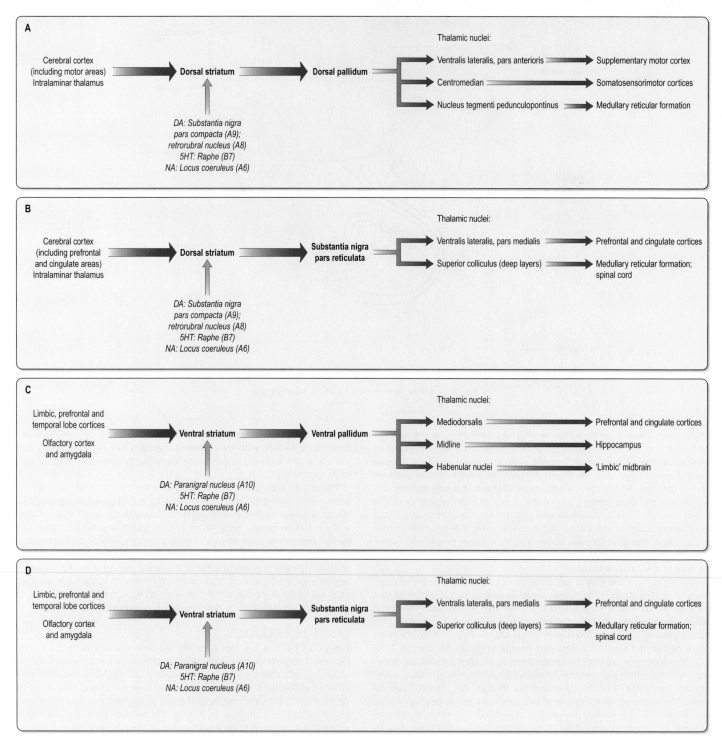

Fig. 14.13 *Schemes of the principal output connections of the basal ganglia derived from dorsal (**A** and **B**) and ventral (**C** and **D**) divisions of the striatum. In each case, pathways established through the pallidum are distinguished from those passing through the substantia nigra pars reticulata. DA, dopamine; 5HT, 5-hydroxytryptamine; NA, noradrenaline (norepinephrine).*

than enkephalin. Efferent axons from the medial pallidal segment project through the ansa lenticularis and fasciculus lenticularis (see Figs 14.12, 15.18). The former runs around the anterior border of the internal capsule, and the latter penetrates the capsule directly. Having traversed the internal capsule, both pathways unite in the subthalamic region, where they follow a horizontal hairpin trajectory and turn upward to enter the thalamus as the thalamic fasciculus. The trajectory circumnavigates the zona incerta and creates the so-called H fields of Forel (see Figs 14.5, 14.14, 15.18). Within the thalamus, pallidothalamic fibres end in the ventral anterior and ventral lateral nuclei and in the intralaminar centromedian nucleus. These, in turn, project excitatory (presumed glutamatergic) fibres primarily to the frontal cortex, including the primary and supplementary motor areas. The medial pallidum also projects fibres caudally to the pedunculopontine nucleus (see Fig. 14.14). This lies at the junction of the midbrain and the pons, close to the superior cerebellar peduncle, and corresponds approximately to the physiologically identified mesencephalic locomotor region.

SUBSTANTIA NIGRA

The substantia nigra is a nuclear complex deep to the crus cerebri in each cerebral peduncle of the midbrain. It consists of a pars compacta and a pars reticulata (see Figs 14.10, 14.11). The pars compacta, together with the smaller pars lateralis, corresponds to dopaminergic cell group A9. With the retrorubral nucleus (group A8), it makes up most of the dopaminergic neurone population of the midbrain and is the source of the mesostriatal dopamine system that projects to the striatum. The pars compacta of each side is continuous with its opposite counterpart through the ventral tegmental dopamine group A10, which is sometimes known as the paranigral nucleus. This is the source of the mesolimbic dopamine system, which supplies the ventral striatum and neighbouring parts of the dorsal striatum, as well as the prefrontal and anterior cingulate cortices. The dopaminergic neurones of the pars compacta (group A9) and paranigral nucleus (ventral tegmental group A10) also contain cholecystokinin or somatostatin.

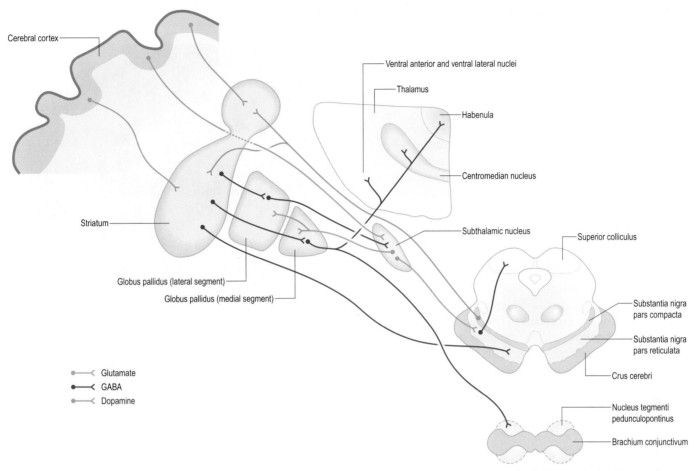

Fig. 14.14 *Transverse section through the basal ganglia showing the principal connections of the globus pallidus with the thalamus and subthalamic nucleus.*

CASE 1   HUNTINGTON'S DISEASE

A 40-year-old woman has been clinically depressed for over 5 years. She has now developed mild memory impairment and progressive cognitive decline. Her family notes that she has become 'jittery,' with frequent random, small-amplitude jerking movements of her limbs, along with facial grimacing. The patient's mother was hospitalized with a diagnosis of schizophrenia, and a sibling committed suicide at age 36 years.

Examination demonstrates a moderately demented woman who exhibits facial grimacing and random choreic movements of her limbs and trunk. Her gait is abnormal, at times alarmingly so, but she does not fall. She exhibits motor impersistence, exemplified, for example, by a so-called serpentine tongue. Ocular saccades are defective.

Discussion: This woman has moderately advanced Huntington's disease (also called Huntington's chorea), characterized anatomically by progressive atrophy of the caudate nucleus and putamen, with neuronal loss involving especially the medium spiny neurones. The major symptoms of Huntington's disease are chorea—an irregular, non-repetitive contraction of muscles, often described as 'dance-like' movements—and neurocognitive changes, initially psychiatric symptoms and eventually progressing to dementia. Cortical atrophy may be advanced, and ventriculomegaly is at times striking, reflecting both cortical and caudate atrophy (Fig. 14.15). Late in the course of the disease, as the striatum is severely affected, the chorea becomes less obvious and the patient may develop a relatively akinetic state. The disease is well recognized as genetically determined, with autosomal

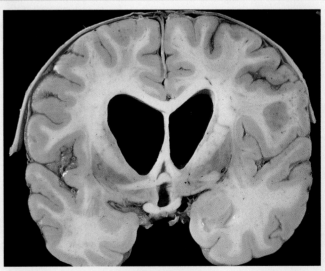

Fig. 14.15 *Huntington's disease. Section through the cerebral hemisphere demonstrating marked atrophy of the caudate nuclei (arrows), with compensatory enlargement of the lateral ventricles.*

dominant inheritance evident in a great majority of cases, characterized by expanded trinucleotide repeats (CAG) on DNA analysis.

Other causes of chorea include post-streptococcal infection (Sydenham's chorea, St. Vitus' dance), pregnancy (chorea gravidarum), polycythemia vera, drug induced (e.g. levodopa), neuroacanthocytosis and a variety of inherited metabolic disorders.

CASE 2 WILSON'S DISEASE

A 22-year-old man develops an increasingly severe tremor of the limbs, sometimes with a distinct wing-beating character, along with dysarthria, an ataxic gait and occasional dystonic features involving the face or limbs. Variable muscular rigidity sometimes interferes with swallowing. Family members describe psychiatric symptoms such as depression and emotional lability preceding the onset of neurological symptoms; he has also exhibited frankly psychotic behaviour.

In addition to the neurological abnormalities predicted by these symptoms, ophthalmic examination demonstrates a yellowish brown Kayser–Fleischer ring involving the corneal limbus, representing a deposition of copper in Descemet's membrane (Fig. 14.16). Imaging demonstrates symmetric ventricular enlargement with widespread atrophic changes, most pronounced in the basal ganglia and thalamus; the putamen is especially involved, with striking vacuolization.

Discussion: This man has Wilson's disease (hepatolenticular degeneration), a progressive familial metabolic disorder reflecting abnormal copper metabolism, with a significant reduction or absence of the protein ceruloplasmin and widespread copper deposition. The liver is typically involved, often with changes suggesting cirrhosis (so-called hobnail liver). Hepatic changes may precede the development of neurological abnormalities. The Kayser–Fleischer ring is often considered the only truly pathognomonic sign in clinical neurology.

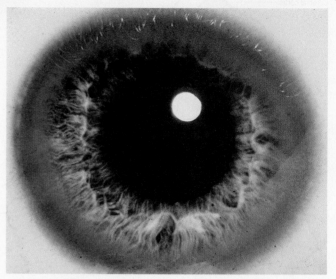

Fig. 14.16 *Wilson's disease (hepatolenticular degeneration). Typical Kayser–Fleischer ring reflecting deposition of copper in Descemet's membrane.*

The pars reticulata contains large multipolar cells that are very similar to those of the pallidum. Together they constitute the output neurones of the basal ganglia system. Their disc-like dendritic trees, like those of the pallidum, are oriented at right angles to afferents from the striatum, probably making *en passant* contacts. Like the striatopallidal axons, of which they may be collaterals, striatonigral axons use GABA and substance P or enkephalin. They distribute differentially in the pars reticulata, such that the enkephalinergic axons terminate in the medial part, whereas substance P axons terminate throughout.

CASE 3 PROGRESSIVE SUPRANUCLEAR PALSY

A 58-year-old man develops a Parkinsonian syndrome, with rigidity and lack of spontaneous movements; on occasion he is observed to have tremor of the hands at rest. He is also experiencing slurring of speech and intermittent difficulty in swallowing. Over time, he exhibits difficulty with ocular motility, primarily with vertical (down) gaze, and he falls frequently. He gradually worsens over the next several years, during which time he develops impairment of mentation, with bradyphrenia and moderate dementia. His overall course is indolent, characterized by increasing motor disability. Death occurs approximately 4 years after the onset of symptoms.

Discussion: This man suffers from progressive supranuclear palsy (Steele–Richardson–Olszewski syndrome), characterized by neuronal degeneration with neurofibrillary tangles and the accumulation of tau protein. Pathological changes may be widespread in the neuraxis but predominate in the pons and midbrain.

The efferent neurones of the pars reticulata are GABAergic. They project to the deep (polysensory) layers of the superior colliculus and to the brain stem reticular formation, including the pedunculopontine nucleus. The pathway from the striatum to the superior colliculus, via the substantia nigra pars reticulata, is thought to function in the control of gaze in a manner analogous to the pathway that initiates general body movement via the pallidum, thalamus and supplementary motor cortex. The uncontrolled or fixed gaze disturbances of advanced Parkinson's disease, progressive supranuclear palsy and Huntington's disease tend to support this.

SUBTHALAMIC NUCLEUS

The subthalamic nucleus is a biconvex, lens-shaped nucleus in the subthalamus of the diencephalon. It lies medial to the internal capsule, immediately rostral to the level at which the latter becomes continuous with the crus cerebri of the midbrain (see Figs 14.2, 14.5, 14.8). Within its substance, small interneurones intermingle with large multipolar cells with dendrites, which extend for about one-tenth the diameter of the nucleus. It is encapsulated dorsally by axons, many of which are derived from the subthalamic fasciculus and carry a major GABAergic projection from the lateral segment of the globus pallidus as part of the indirect pathway. It also receives afferents from the cerebral cortex. The subthalamic nucleus is unique in the intrinsic circuitry of the basal ganglia, in that its cells are glutamatergic. They project excitatory axons to both the globus pallidus and the substantia nigra pars reticulata. Within the pallidum, subthalamic efferent fibres end predominantly in the medial segment, but many also end in the lateral segment.

The subthalamic nucleus plays a central role in the normal function of the basal ganglia and in the pathophysiology of basal ganglia–related disorders. Destruction of the nucleus, which occurs rarely as a result of stroke, results in the appearance of violent, uncontrolled involuntary movements, known as ballism (ballismus). The subthalamic nucleus is also crucially involved in the pathophysiology of Parkinson's disease and is the target of functional neurosurgical therapy for the condition.

PATHOPHYSIOLOGY OF BASAL GANGLIA DISORDERS

The normal functions of the basal ganglia are difficult to summarize succinctly. As far as their role in movement control is concerned, however, a reasonable definition is that they function to promote and support patterns of behaviour

CASE 4 HEMIBALLISMUS

A 69-year-old woman with a small right subcortical intra-cerebral haemorrhage develops rapid, violent, uncontrol-lable flailing movements of her left arm. During the next several days, the movements decrease in amplitude, but she continues to exhibit spontaneous rhythmic 'dancing' movements of her arm.

Discussion: Ballism—or, more commonly, hemiballism (hemiballismus)—is almost always caused by a lesion of the contralateral subthalamic nucleus. The most common cause is a vascular injury, either cerebral infarction or haemorrhage, but it can also be seen with vasculitis (systemic lupus erythematosus), infection (encephalitis), auto-immune disorders (Sydenham's chorea) or tumour. Loss of excitatory output from the subthalamic nucleus results in increased cortical stimulation, with abnormal hyperkinetic movements. Hemiballismus may be considered a severe form of chorea, into which it may evolve. In most cases, the movements are involuntary, spontaneous and irregular, characteristically an uncontrolled 'flinging' of the affected limbs.

and movement that are appropriate in the prevailing circumstances and to inhibit unwanted or inappropriate behaviour and movements. This is exemplified by disorders of the basal ganglia, which are characterized, depending on the underlying pathology, by an inability to initiate and execute wanted movements (as in Parkinson's disease) or an inability to prevent unwanted movements (as in Huntington's disease).

Parkinson's disease is the most common pathological condition affecting the basal ganglia. As noted, it is characterized by akinesia, muscular rigidity and tremor and, due to degeneration of the dopaminergic neurones of the substantia nigra pars compacta, depletion of dopamine levels in the striatum. This has been amply confirmed by postmortem studies. Furthermore, in Parkinsonian patients, positron emission tomography (PET) reveals a deficit of dopamine storage and reuptake, due to a loss of nigrostriatal terminals, but intact dopamine receptors, which are located on the medium spiny neurones, the target of the nigrostriatal pathway.

Dopamine appears to have a dual action on medium spiny striatal neurones. It inhibits those of the indirect pathway and excites those of the direct pathway. Consequently, when dopamine is lost from the striatum, the indirect pathway becomes overactive, and the direct pathway becomes underactive (Fig. 14.18). Overactivity of the striatal projection to the lateral pallidum results in inhibition of pallidosubthalamic neurones and, consequently, overactivity of the subthalamic nucleus. Subthalamic efferents mediate excessive excitatory drive to the medial globus pallidus and substantia nigra pars reticulata. This is exacerbated by underactivity of the GABAergic, inhibitory direct pathway. Overactivity of basal ganglia output then inhibits the motor thalamus and its excitatory thalamocortical connections. Although this description is little more than a first approximation of the underlying pathophysiology, this model of the basis of Parkinsonian symptoms has led to the introduction

CASE 5 PARKINSON'S DISEASE

A middle-aged man finds that he can no longer play tennis with his usual facility. His gait has become somewhat slow and shuffling, and he sometimes experiences defective equilibrium. His wife notes that his posture has become stooped and his speech is often muffled and difficult to understand, tending to fade away during a conversation. His handwriting has become small, at times virtually illegible. The patient admits to having difficulty rising from a chair or turning over in bed. Rapid tremor of the hands has appeared, initially involving only one hand and associated with impaired dexterity in that limb.

Examination demonstrates a stooped posture; widespread but asymmetric cogwheel rigidity; impaired hand dexterity; a distal tremor at repose, lessening with intention; impaired ocular convergence; a masked facies; and a loss of spontaneous movements, with striking difficulty initiating movements. Once instituted, all movements are carried out slowly (bradykinesia). Postural reflexes are defective. His gait is shuffling, with a decidedly propulsive and festinating quality (*marche a petit pas*).

Discussion: This patient exhibits the typical features of Parkinson's disease (true paralysis agitans), with a characteristic combination of hypokinetic (lack of spontaneous movements, bradykinesia, muscle rigidity, impaired dexterity) and hyperkinetic (tremor) signs. Many patients also exhibit bradyphrenia (i.e. slowing of mental processes), and a substantial number become frankly demented.

Parkinsonian symptoms ('Parkinsonism') may appear in a variety of other degenerative disorders, including corticobasal

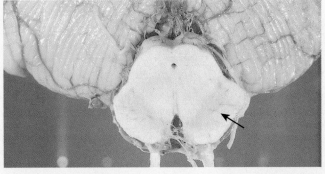

Fig. 14.17 *Parkinson's disease. Section through the midbrain demonstrating depigmentation in the substantia nigra due to loss of melanin* (arrow).

ganglionic degeneration, progressive supranuclear palsy, olivopontocerebellar atrophy, Alzheimer's disease and other dementing illnesses, multiple system atrophy and a host of metabolic derangements secondary to toxic exposure to manganese, carbon monoxide, MPTP (methyl-phenyl-tetrahydro-pyridine) and drugs such as phenothiazines.

Pathological changes in Parkinson's disease predominate in the zona compacta of the substantia nigra (Fig. 14.17), with loss of melanin-containing neurons and the appearance of intracytoplasmic Lewy bodies, representing an accumulation of the protein synuclein and a resultant degeneration of the nigrostriatal pathway and reduction in striatal dopamine. Anatomical changes may in fact be much more widespread, involving a variety of brain stem nuclei as well as the cerebral cortex.

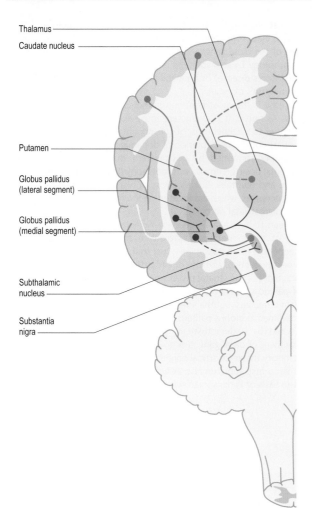

Thalamus

Caudate nucleus

Putamen

Globus pallidus
(lateral segment)

Globus pallidus
(medial segment)

Subthalamic
nucleus

Substantia
nigra

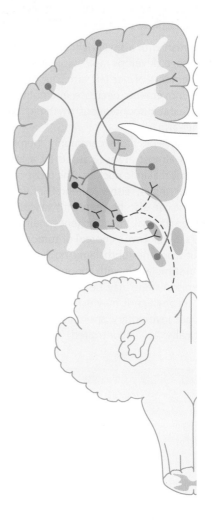

Fig. 14.18 *Pathophysiology of Parkinson's disease. Dotted lines* indicate *dysfunctional pathways. (By permission from Crossman, A.R., Neary, D., 2000. Neuroanatomy, 2nd ed. Churchill Livingstone, Edinburgh.)*

Fig. 14.19 *Pathophysiology of dyskinesias. Dotted lines* indicate dysfunctional *pathways. (By permission from Crossman, A.R., Neary, D., 2000. Neuroanatomy, 2nd ed. Churchill Livingstone, Edinburgh.)*

of new neurosurgical approaches to the treatment of Parkinson's disease, based on lesioning and deep brain stimulation of the medial globus pallidus and subthalamic nucleus (see later).

The current medical treatment for Parkinson's disease relies on levodopa (L-dopa, L-dihydroxyphenylalanine), the immediate metabolic precursor of dopamine; dopamine agonists; or monoamine oxidase inhibitors. Although these drugs usually provide good symptomatic relief for many years, levodopa and, to a lesser extent, dopamine agonists eventually lead to the development of motor complications, including dyskinesias. The involuntary movements that occur as a consequence of long-term treatment of Parkinson's disease resemble those seen in Huntington's disease, tardive dyskinesia and ballism. Experimental evidence suggests that these may share a common neural mechanism (Fig. 14.19). Thus, the indirect pathway becomes underactive, due to the effects of dopaminergic drugs in Parkinson's disease or the degeneration of the striatopallidal projection to the lateral pallidum in Huntington's disease. This leads to physiological inhibition of the subthalamic nucleus by overactive pallidosubthalamic neurones. The involvement of the subthalamic nucleus explains why the dyskinetic movements of levodopa-induced dyskinesia and Huntington's disease resemble those of ballism produced by lesion of the subthalamic nucleus. Underactivity of the subthalamic nucleus removes the excitatory drive from medial pallidal neurones, which are known to be underactive in dyskinesias. Once again, this is an oversimplification. Although it is true that underactivity of the medial globus pallidus is associated with dyskinesias, it is also known that lesions of the globus pallidus alleviate them. This suggests that the dynamic aspects of pallidal and nigral efferent activity are important factors in the generation of dyskinesia.

Another manifestation of basal ganglia dysfunction is dystonia, which is characterized by increased muscle tone and abnormal postures. This may occur as a consequence of levodopa treatment in Parkinson's disease or in inherited disease (e.g. idiopathic torsion or Oppenheim's dystonia). Focal

dystonic syndromes are widely recognized, including blepharospasm (Meige syndrome), torticollis, spastic dysphonia and writer's cramp. The pathophysiological basis of dystonia is unclear. Like dyskinesia, it is probably caused by underactivity of basal ganglia output, so deep brain stimulation of the globus pallidus may be beneficial.

There is evidence that dysfunction of the basal ganglia is involved in other complex, less well-understood behavioural disorders. In animal experiments, lesions of the basal ganglia, especially of the caudate nucleus, induce uncontrollable hyperactivity (e.g. obstinate progression, incessant pacing and other constantly repeated behaviours). Such evidence has led to the notion that the corpus striatum enables the individual to make motor choices and avoid 'stimulus-bound' behaviour. PET studies in humans have shown that sufferers from obsessive-compulsive disorder, which is characterized by repeated ritualistic motor behaviour and intrusive thoughts, exhibit abnormal activity in the prefrontal cortex and caudate nuclei. There have been similar observations in the hyperactive child syndrome. In this respect, it may be significant that the basal ganglia, besides receiving connections from the frontal lobe and limbic cortices, also have an ascending influence on the prefrontal and cingulate cortices through the substantia nigra pars reticulata and dorsomedial and ventromedial thalamus (see Fig. 14.13B–D).

Before the advent of levodopa, neurosurgery for Parkinson's disease was commonplace. The globus pallidus and thalamus were favoured targets for chemical or thermal lesions. Pallidotomy and thalamotomy often improved rigidity and tremor, but they produced little consistent beneficial effect on akinesia. With the introduction of levodopa therapy, which had a profound effect on akinesia, the use of surgical treatment for Parkinson's disease declined. However, it soon became clear that long-term use of levodopa was associated with a number of side effects, such as dyskinesias, 'wearing off' and the 'on–off' phenomenon. More recently, better understanding of the pathophysiology of movement disorders, particularly Parkinson's disease, has stimulated renewed use of neurosurgery to treat movement disorders.

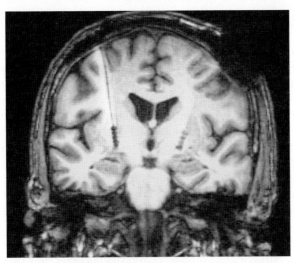

Fig. 14.20 *Magnetic resonance image showing placement of deep brain stimulating electrodes bilaterally in the globus pallidus of a patient with Parkinson's disease. (Courtesy of Professor T. Z. Aziz, Radcliffe Infirmary, Oxford and Charing Cross Hospital, London.)*

In primates that were made Parkinsonian with the neurotoxin MPTP, lesioning the subthalamic nucleus alleviated tremor, rigidity and bradykinesia. This finding raised the possibility that the subthalamic nucleus could be used as a clinical target. Indeed, lesions of the subthalamic nucleus in humans exert a powerful effect in alleviating tremor, rigidity and bradykinesia; however, the likelihood of side effects is not trivial (the subthalamic nucleus is a small structure wrapped by fibres of passage and close to the hypothalamus and internal capsule).

In 1992, Laitinen and colleagues reintroduced pallidotomy for the treatment of end-stage Parkinson's disease but confined the lesions to the

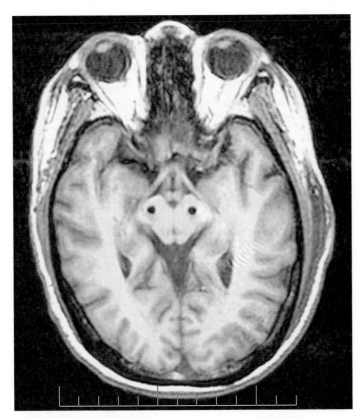

Fig. 14.21 *Magnetic resonance image showing placement of deep brain stimulating electrodes bilaterally in the subthalamic nucleus of a patient with Parkinson's disease. (Courtesy of Professor A. M. Lozano, Toronto Western Hospital.)*

CASE 6 DYSTONIA

A 52-year-old professional pianist is referred by a psychiatrist for evaluation. The patient has played the piano 6 to 8 hours a day, often 7 days a week, since late childhood. He had a successful career as a performer and master-level teacher in a school for performing artists. Three years before assessment, he began complaining of difficulty controlling the movement of his left arm, but only when playing the piano; this was characterized by involuntary pronation of the left forearm and posturing of the hand. He was initially referred for psychiatric evaluation because of anxiety and depression, and it was thought that the movements were the result of a conversion disorder.

Neurological examination is normal. When playing, he exhibits involuntary pronation of the left forearm and extension of the fingers. The diagnosis of an occupational (regional) dystonia is made. Electromyography-guided botulinum toxin injections into the abnormally contracting muscles of the left forearm markedly reduced the movement disorder and allowed him to return to teaching.

Discussion: Dystonia is characterized by involuntary sustained contractions of agonist and antagonist muscles causing twisting, repetitive movements or abnormal postures. The movements can be focal, multifocal or generalized. The focal occupational dystonias are often associated with overuse, as in this patient. Local dystonias such as torticollis, spastic dysphonia and some occupational dystonias may respond to botulinum injections into the involved muscles. Although the exact anatomical change responsible for these disorders is not known, involvement of the basal ganglia is usually assumed.

posteroventral part of the internal pallidal segment. These lesions were found to be extremely reliable in abolishing contralateral rigidity and drug-induced dyskinesias, with slightly less efficacy on tremor and bradykinesia.

The implantation of deep brain electrodes to inhibit cells in the vicinity through high-frequency pulses generated by a pacemaker has been a concept since the early 1970s, but it did not become a widespread reality until the late 1980s, as a result of technological advances. The introduction of this technique, which avoids making permanent lesions, made bilateral surgery safer. There have been numerous reports of the effectiveness of both bilateral pallidal and subthalamic nucleus stimulation (Figs 14.20, 14.21). Subthalamic nucleus stimulation is favoured by most groups because, unlike pallidal stimulation, it allows patients to reduce their anti-Parkinsonian medication.

Serendipity also has a role in such surgery. Clinically, Parkinsonian patients can develop painful dystonic posturing of their limbs, which responds dramatically to bilateral pallidal stimulation. This has led to preliminary studies of bilateral pallidal stimulation for dystonia, with promising results. Because it is believed that pallidal neurones fire at rates below normal in dystonia, this presents a conceptual puzzle, and it is unknown how stimulation works. It appears that the neural mechanism underlying this therapeutic effect on dystonia differs from that in Parkinson's disease and tremor, because in dystonia, the improvement may take weeks to emerge, whereas it is immediate in the case of Parkinson's disease.

CASE 7   RESTLESS LEGS SYNDROME

A 50-year-old married woman presents with a history of insomnia, characterized by difficulty falling asleep and multiple nocturnal awakenings. It began 3 years ago and is increasing in severity; whereas it affected her once a week initially, it now affects her nightly. The resulting daytime sleepiness, anergy and fatigue have begun to interfere with her daytime functioning, including decreased memory for recent events, word-finding difficulties, avoidance of social contact, low mood and decreased job performance. Upon further questioning, she reports an irresistible urge to move both lower extremities beginning at 9 PM and intensifying significantly just after retiring. These are associated with a 'creepy crawly' sensation in her lower extremities, beginning with her calf muscles and generalizing into her hips and abdomen and sometimes into her arms and neck. She obtains temporary relief by stretching her extremities vigorously, rubbing them, using warm soaks or getting out of bed and walking around the house; however, the symptoms return shortly thereafter and awaken her repeatedly after sleep onset. She recalls similar symptoms, transiently, during her last pregnancy. Past medical history is negative, and she is taking no medications. She consumes six caffeinated beverages a day, the last one at 6 PM. Serum tests reveal a low ferritin level of 10 μg/l, yet there is no evidence of anemia. Polysomnography reveals high proportions of stage 1 sleep, diminished proportions of slow-wave sleep, multiple awakenings and arousals and repetitive bursts of electromyographic activity on lower limb leads, each lasting approximately 0.75 second, followed by brief arousal and separated by intervals of 20 seconds.

Discussion: This is a typical case of restless legs syndrome. Core symptoms include an irresistible urge to move the legs, arms or other body parts, with or without uncomfortable or unpleasant sensations in the legs, beginning or worsening during periods of rest or inactivity (lying, sitting). The symptoms are partially or totally relieved by movement (walking, stretching) and are worse in the evening or at night. Associated findings include a positive family history (prevalence in first-degree relatives is three to five times greater than in those without restless legs syndrome), frequent response to dopaminergic therapy, periodic limb movements during sleep or wakefuless, a variable clinical course with frequent exacerbations and remissions, sleep disturbance and a normal neurological examination. Although the pathophysiology of the disorder is not completely understood, some data suggest that restless legs syndrome involves dysfunction in subcortical brain areas, which leads to reduced spinal and possibly cortical inhibition. PET studies have shown small but significant reductions of mean caudate and putamen D2 receptor binding and decreased mean putamen ^{18}F-dopa uptake in patients with restless legs syndrome compared with healthy controls. Recent brain imaging studies have revealed a significant decrease in iron concentrations in iron-rich areas of the brain such as the substantia nigra and, somewhat less significantly, the putamen. The connection between iron and dopamine is an elegantly simple one, as iron is a cofactor for the enzyme tyrosine hydroxylase, which is involved in the synthetic pathway of dopamine from tyrosine. Treatment with iron supplements, although not indicated for restless legs syndrome, can be effective. Two medications used for treatment of this disorder are ropinirole and pramipexole. Sleep hygiene measures, including the avoidance of stimulants such as caffeine close to bedtime, should also be considered.

References

Alexander, G.E., DeLong, M.R., Strick, P.L., 1986. Parallel organization of functionally segregated circuits linking basal ganglia and cortex. Annu. Rev. Neurosci. 9, 357–382. *Landmark publication setting out a conceptual framework for the way the basal ganglia and cerebral cortex process different types of information through largely distinct parallel circuits based on known anatomical connectivity.*

Benarroch, E.E., 2008. Subthalamic nucleus and its connections: anatomic substrate for the network effects of deep brain stimulation. Neurology 70, 1991–1994.

Braak, H., Del Tredici, K., 2008. Nervous system pathology in sporadic Parkinson disease. Neurology 70, 1916–1924.

Crossmann, A.R., 1990. A hypothesis on the pathophysiological mechanisms that underlie levodopa- or dopamine agonist-induced dyskinesia in Parkinson's disease: implications for future strategies in treatment. Mov. Disord. 5, 100–108.

Krack, P., Batir, A., Van Blercom, N., et al., 2003. Five-year follow-up of bilateral stimulation of the subthalamic nucleus in advanced Parkinson's disease. N. Engl. J. Med. 349, 1925–1934. *Reviews the long-term outcome of deep brain stimulation of the subthalamic nucleus in Parkinson's disease.*

Laitinen, L.V., Bergenheim, A.T., Hariz, M.I., 1992. Ventroposterolateral pallidotomy can abolish all Parkinsonian symptoms. Stereotact. Funct. Neurosurg. 58, 14–21. *Key paper that ignited widespread interest in functional neurosurgery for Parkinson's disease.*

Obeso, J.A., Marin, C., Rodriguez-Oroz, C., Blesa, J., Benitiez-Temino, B., Mena-Segovia, J., et al, 2008. The basal ganglia in Parkinson's disease: current concepts and unexplained observations. Ann. Neurol. 64 (Suppl), S30–S46.

Penney J.B., Jr., Young, A.B., 1986. Striatal inhomogeneities and basal ganglia function. Mov. Disord. 1, 3–15. *Landmark publication that introduced some of the basic concepts behind current models of the pathophysiology of Parkinson's disease and Huntington's disease.*

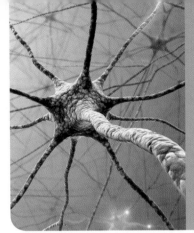

Diencephalon

The diencephalon is part of the prosencephalon (forebrain), which develops from the foremost primary cerebral vesicle and differentiates into a caudal diencephalon and rostral telencephalon. The cerebral hemispheres develop from the sides of the telencephalon, each containing a lateral ventricle. The sites of evagination become the interventricular foramina, through which the two lateral ventricles and midline third ventricle communicate. The diencephalon corresponds largely to the structures that develop lateral to the third ventricle.

The lateral walls of the diencephalon form the epithalamus most superiorly, the thalamus centrally and the subthalamus and hypothalamus most inferiorly. The epithalamus in the mature brain contains the anterior and posterior paraventricular nuclei, the medial and lateral habenular nuclei, the stria medullaris thalami and the pineal gland. The thalamus undergoes proliferation to form numerous nuclear masses that have extensive reciprocal connections with the cerebral cortex. The subthalamic region consists of the subthalamic nucleus, zona incerta and fields of Forel. The subthalamic nucleus is closely related to the basal ganglia and is considered with them in Chapter 14. The hypothalamic rudiment gives rise to most of the subdivisions of the adult hypothalamus.

THALAMUS

The thalamus is an ovoid nuclear mass, approximately 4 cm long, that borders the dorsal part of the third ventricle (Figs 15.1–15.3; see also Fig. 1.10). The narrow anterior pole lies close to the midline and forms the posterior boundary of the interventricular foramen. Posteriorly, an expansion, the pulvinar, extends beyond the third ventricle to overhang the superior colliculus (Fig. 15.4). The brachium of the superior colliculus (superior quadrigeminal brachium) separates the pulvinar above from the medial geniculate body below. A small oval elevation, the lateral geniculate body, lies lateral to the medial geniculate.

The superior (dorsal) surface of the thalamus (see Fig. 15.2) is covered by a thin layer of white matter, the stratum zonale. It extends laterally from the line of reflection of the ependyma (taenia thalami) and forms the roof of the third ventricle. This curved surface is separated from the overlying body of the fornix by the choroid fissure, with the tela choroidea within it. More laterally, it forms part of the floor of the lateral ventricle. The lateral border of the superior surface of the thalamus is marked by the stria terminalis and the overlying thalamostriate vein, which separate the thalamus from the body of the caudate nucleus. Laterally, a slender sheet of white matter, the external medullary lamina, separates the main body of the thalamus from the reticular nucleus. Lateral to this, the thick posterior limb of the internal capsule lies between the thalamus and the lentiform complex.

The medial surface of the thalamus is the superior (dorsal) part of the lateral wall of the third ventricle (see Fig. 5.8). It is usually connected to the contralateral thalamus by an interthalamic adhesion behind the interventricular foramina. The boundary with the hypothalamus is marked by an indistinct hypothalamic sulcus, which curves from the upper end of the cerebral aqueduct to the interventricular foramen. The thalamus is continuous with the midbrain tegmentum, the subthalamus and the hypothalamus.

Internally, the thalamus is divided into anterior, medial and lateral nuclear groups by a vertical Y-shaped sheet of white matter, the internal medullary lamina (Figs 15.5, 15.6). In addition, intralaminar nuclei lie embedded within, and surrounded by, the internal medullary lamina. Midline nuclei either abut the ependyma of the lateral walls of the third ventricle medially or lie adjacent to, and to some extent within, the interthalamic adhesion. Reticular nuclei lie lateral to the main nuclear mass, separated from it by the external medullary lamina.

In general, thalamic nuclei both project to and receive fibres from the cerebral cortex (see Fig. 15.6). The whole cerebral cortex, not only the neocortex but also the phylogenetically older palaeocortex of the piriform lobe and archicortex of the hippocampal formation, are reciprocally connected with the thalamus. The thalamus is the major route by which subcortical

neuronal activity influences the cerebral cortex, and the greatest input to most thalamic nuclei comes from the cerebral cortex.

The projection to the thalamus from the cortex is precisely reciprocal; each cortical area projects in a topographically organized manner to all sites in the thalamus from which it receives an input. Corticothalamic fibres that reciprocate 'specific' thalamocortical pathways arise from modified pyramidal cells of layer VI, whereas those reciprocating 'non-specific' inputs arise from typical pyramidal cells of layer V and may in part be axon collaterals of other cortical–subcortical pathways.

It is customary to consider thalamic nuclei as either 'specific' nuclei, which mediate finely organized and precisely transmitted sensory information to discrete cortical sensory areas, or 'non-specific' nuclei, which are part of a general arousal system. The specific nuclei are further subdivided into relay nuclei and association nuclei. However, many nuclei classified as specific may also send non-specific projections to widespread cortical areas. Similarly, the division of thalamic nuclei into relay and association groups rests on the assumption that relay nuclei receive a major subcortical pathway, whereas association nuclei receive their principal non-cortical input from other thalamic nuclei. There is little evidence of significant intrathalamic connectivity but there are increasing indications of non-cortical afferent pathways linked to so-called association nuclei.

Anterior Group of Thalamic Nuclei

The anterior group of nuclei are enclosed between the arms of the Y-shaped internal medullary lamina and underlie the anterior thalamic tubercle (see Fig. 15.2, 15.6). Three subdivisions are recognized. The largest is the anteroventral nucleus; the others are the anteromedial and anterodorsal nuclei.

The anterior nuclei are the principal recipients of the mammillothalamic tract, which arises from the mammillary nuclei of the hypothalamus. The mammillary nuclei receive fibres from the hippocampal formation via the fornix. The medial mammillary nucleus projects to the ipsilateral anteroventral and anteromedial thalamic nuclei, and the lateral mammillary nucleus projects bilaterally to the anterodorsal nuclei. The nuclei of the anterior group also receive a prominent cholinergic input from the basal forebrain and the brain stem.

The cortical targets of efferent fibres from the anterior nuclei of the thalamus lie largely on the medial surface of the hemisphere (see Fig. 15.6). They include the anterior limbic area (in front of and inferior to the corpus callosum), the cingulate gyrus and the parahippocampal gyrus (including the medial entorhinal cortex and the pre- and para-subiculum). These thalamocortical pathways are reciprocal. There also appear to be minor connections between the anterior nuclei and the dorsolateral prefrontal and posterior areas of the neocortex. The anterior thalamic nuclei are believed to be involved in the regulation of alertness and attention and in the acquisition of memory.

Medial Group of Thalamic Nuclei

The single component of this thalamic region is the mediodorsal or dorsomedial nucleus, which is particularly large in humans. Laterally, it is limited by the internal medullary lamina and intralaminar nuclei (see Figs. 15.5, 15.6). Medially, it abuts the midline parataenial and reuniens (medioventral) nuclei. It can be divided into anteromedial magnocellular and posterolateral parvocellular parts.

The small magnocellular division receives olfactory input from the piriform and adjacent cortex, the ventral pallidum and the amygdala. The mediobasal amygdaloid nucleus projects to the dorsal part of the anteromedial magnocellular nucleus, and the lateral nuclei project to the more central and anteroventral regions. The anteromedial magnocellular nucleus projects to the anterior and medial prefrontal cortex, notably to the lateral posterior and central posterior olfactory areas on the orbital surface of the frontal lobe. In addition, fibres pass to the ventromedial cingulate cortex, and a few pass to the inferior parietal cortex and anterior insula. These cortical connections are reciprocal.

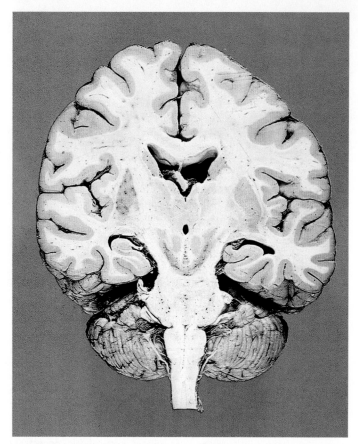

The larger posterolateral parvocellular division connects reciprocally with the dorsolateral and dorsomedial prefrontal cortex, the anterior cingulate gyrus and the supplementary motor area. In addition, efferent fibres pass to the posterior parietal cortex.

The mediodorsal nucleus appears to be involved in a wide variety of higher functions. Damage may lead to a decrease in anxiety, tension, aggression or obsessive thinking. There may also be transient amnesia, with confusion developing over time. Much of the neuropsychology of medial nuclear damage reflects defects in functions similar to those performed by the prefrontal cortex, with which it is closely linked. The effects of ablation of the mediodorsal nuclei parallel, in part, the results of prefrontal lobotomy.

Lateral Group of Thalamic Nuclei

The lateral nuclear complex, lying lateral to the internal medullary lamina, is the largest major division of the thalamus (see Fig. 15.6). It is divided into dorsal and ventral tiers of nuclei. The lateral dorsal nucleus, lateral posterior nucleus and pulvinar lie dorsally. The lateral and medial geniculate nuclei lie inferior to the pulvinar, near the posterior pole of the thalamus. The ventral tier nuclei are the ventral anterior, ventral lateral and ventral posterior nuclei.

Ventral Anterior Nucleus

The ventral anterior (VA) complex lies at the anterior pole of the ventral nuclear group. It is limited anteriorly by the reticular nucleus and posteriorly by the ventral lateral nucleus, and it lies between the external and internal medullary laminae. It consists of a principal part (VApc) and a magnocellular part (VAmc). The subcortical connections to this region are largely ipsilateral from the internal segment of the globus pallidus and the pars reticulata of the substantia nigra. The terminal fields from these origins do not overlap. Fibres from the globus pallidus end in VApc. The substantia nigra projects to VAmc. Corticothalamic fibres from premotor cortex (area 6) terminate in VApc, and fibres from the frontal eye field (area 8) terminate in VAmc. The VA thalamus does not appear to receive fibres directly from the motor cortex. The efferent projections from VA are incompletely known. Some pass to intralaminar thalamic nuclei, and others project to widespread regions of the frontal lobe and to the anterior parietal cortex. Their functions are unclear. The VA thalamus appears to play a central role in the transmission of the cortical 'recruiting response,' a phenomenon in which stimulation of the

Fig. 15.1 *Dorsal half of a brain sectioned in an oblique coronal plane that passes through the cerebral hemispheres, diencephalon, midbrain, pons and medulla oblongata, to show the general disposition of the main structures, some of which are labelled in Figure 15.3. Compare also with Figure 1.10. (Photograph by Kevin Fitzpatrick on behalf of GKT School of Medicine, London.)*

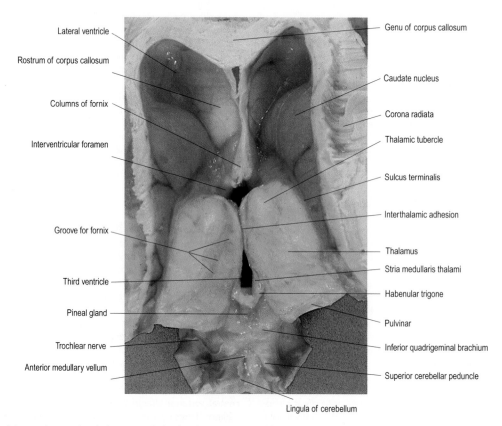

Lateral ventricle

Rostrum of corpus callosum

Columns of fornix

Interventricular foramen

Groove for fornix

Third ventricle

Pineal gland

Trochlear nerve

Anterior medullary vellum

Genu of corpus callosum

Caudate nucleus

Corona radiata

Thalamic tubercle

Sulcus terminalis

Interthalamic adhesion

Thalamus

Stria medullaris thalami

Habenular trigone

Pulvinar

Inferior quadrigeminal brachium

Superior cerebellar peduncle

Lingula of cerebellum

Fig. 15.2 *Dorsal aspect of the caudate nuclei, thalami, pineal gland and tectum, revealed by removal of most of the corpus callosum, the body of the fornix and the tela choroidea.*

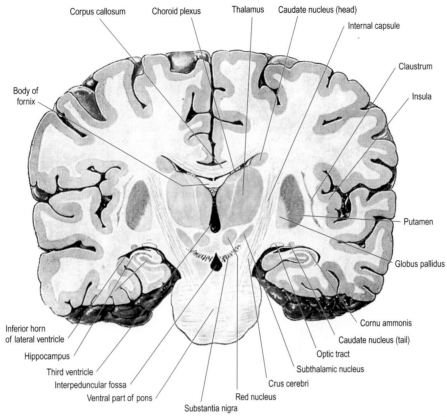

Fig. 15.3 *Coronal section of the brain showing the principal parts of the diencephalon and basal ganglia. Compare with Figure 1.10.*

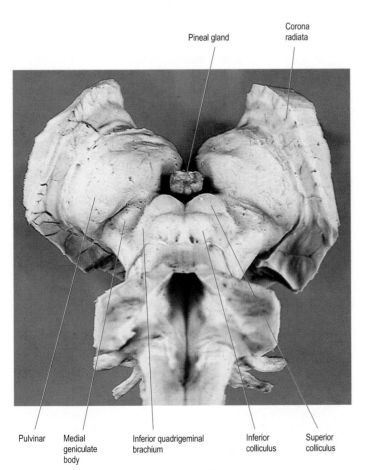

Fig. 15.4 *Oblique view of the dorsal aspect of the brain stem and thalamus. (Photograph by Kevin Fitzpatrick on behalf of GKT School of Medicine, London.)*

thalamus can initiate long-lasting, high-voltage repetitive negative electrical waves over much of the cerebral cortex.

Ventral Lateral Nucleus

The ventral lateral (VL) thalamus consists of two major divisions with distinctly different connections and functions. The anterior division, or pars oralis (VLo), receives topographically organized fibres from the internal segment of the ipsilateral globus pallidus. The posterior division, or pars caudalis (VLc), receives topographically organized fibres from the contralateral deep cerebellar nuclei. Additional subcortical projections have been reported from the spinothalamic tract and the vestibular nuclei. Numerous cortical afferents to both VLo and VLc originate from precentral motor cortical areas, including areas 4 and 6.

The VLo nucleus sends efferent fibres to the supplementary motor cortex on the medial surface of the hemisphere and to the lateral premotor cortex. The VLc nucleus projects efferent fibres to the primary motor cortex, where they end in a topographically arranged fashion. The head region of area 4 receives fibres from the medial part of VLc, and the leg region receives fibres from lateral VLc.

Responses can be recorded in the VL thalamus during both passive and active movement of the contralateral body. The topography of its connections and recordings made within the nucleus suggest that VLc contains a body representation comparable with that in the ventral posterior nucleus. Stereotaxic surgery of the VL nucleus is sometimes used in the treatment of essential tremor. In the past, thalamotomy was used extensively for the treatment of Parkinson's disease; however, the internal segment of the globus pallidus and the subthalamic nucleus are now the preferred neurosurgical targets for Parkinson's disease.

Ventral Posterior Nucleus

The ventral posterior (VP) nucleus is the principal thalamic relay for the somatosensory pathways. It is thought to consist of two major divisions, the ventral posterolateral (VPl) and ventral posteromedial (VPm) nuclei. The VPl nucleus receives the medial lemniscal and spinothalamic pathways, and the VPm nucleus receives the trigeminothalamic pathway. Connections from the vestibular nuclei and lemniscal fibres terminate along the ventral surface of the VP nucleus.

There is a well-ordered topographical representation of the body in the VP nucleus. The VPl is organized so that sacral segments are represented laterally and cervical segments medially. The latter abut the face area of

A

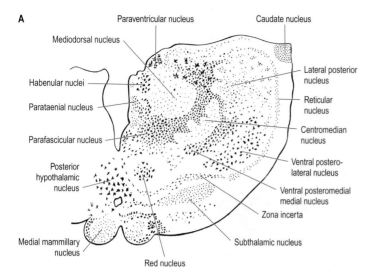

Paraventricular nucleus
Caudate nucleus
Mediodorsal nucleus
Lateral posterior nucleus
Habenular nuclei
Reticular nucleus
Parataenial nucleus
Centromedian nucleus
Parafascicular nucleus
Ventral postero-lateral nucleus
Posterior hypothalamic nucleus
Ventral posteromedial medial nucleus
Zona incerta
Medial mammillary nucleus
Subthalamic nucleus
Red nucleus

B

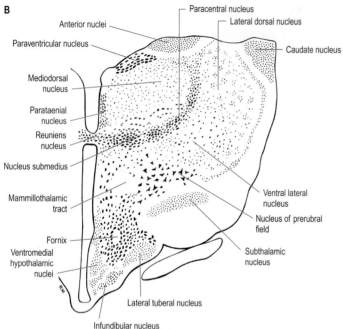

Paracentral nucleus
Anterior nuclei
Lateral dorsal nucleus
Paraventricular nucleus
Caudate nucleus
Mediodorsal nucleus
Parataenial nucleus
Reuniens nucleus
Nucleus submedius
Ventral lateral nucleus
Mammillothalamic tract
Nucleus of prerubral field
Fornix
Subthalamic nucleus
Ventromedial hypothalamic nuclei
Lateral tuberal nucleus
Infundibular nucleus

Fig. 15.5 *Coronal sections through the diencephalon showing the main nuclear aggregations of nerve cell bodies.* **A,** *At the level of the mammillary bodies.* **B,** *At the level of the tuber cinereum. Note the variations in cell size, shape and packing density, which characterize the nuclear masses of the thalamus, subthalamus and hypothalamus at these levels.*

representation (trigeminal territory) in VPm. Taste fibres synapse anteriorly and ventromedially within the VPl nucleus.

At a more detailed level, single body regions are represented as curved lamellae of neurones, parallel to the lateral border of the VP nucleus, such that there is a continuous overlapping progression of adjacent receptive fields from dorsolateral to ventromedial. Considerably less change in location of receptive field on the body is seen when passing anteroposteriorly through the nucleus. Although not precisely dermatomal in nature, these curvilinear lamellae of cells probably derive from afferents related to a few adjacent spinal segments. There is considerable distortion of the body map within the nucleus, reflecting the differences in the density of peripheral innervation in different body regions; for example, many more neurones respond to stimulation of the hand than of the trunk. Within a single lamella, neurones in the anterodorsal part of the nucleus respond to deep stimuli, including movement of joints, tendon stretch and manipulation of muscles. Most ventrally, neurones once again respond to deep stimuli, particularly tapping. Intervening cells within a single lamella respond only to cutaneous stimuli. This organization has been confirmed by recordings made in the human VP nucleus.

Single lemniscal axons have an extended anteroposterior terminal zone within the nucleus. Rods of cells running the length of the anteroposterior, dorsoventrally oriented lamellae respond with closely similar receptive field properties and locations, derived from a small bundle of lemniscal afferents. It appears, therefore, that each lamella contains the complete representation of a single body part (e.g. a finger). Lamellae consist of multiple narrow rods

of neurones, oriented anteroposteriorly, each of which receives input from the same small region of the body represented within the lamella and from the same type of receptors. These thalamic 'rods' form the basis for both place- and modality-specific input to columns of cells in the somatic sensory cortex. Spinothalamic tract afferents to the VPl nucleus terminate throughout the nucleus. The neurones from which these axons originate appear to be mainly of the 'wide dynamic range' class, with responses to both low-threshold mechanoreceptors and high-threshold nociceptors. A smaller proportion are solely high-threshold nociceptors. Some neurones respond to temperature changes. There is evidence that spinothalamic tract neurones carrying nociceptive and thermal information terminate in a distinct nuclear area, identified as the posterior part of the ventral medial nucleus (VMpo).

The VP nucleus projects to the primary somatic sensory cortex of the postcentral gyrus and to the second somatic sensory area in the parietal operculum. VMpo projects to the insular cortex. Within the primary sensory cortex, the central cutaneous core of the VP nucleus projects solely to area 3b; dorsal and ventral to this, a narrow band of cells projects to both area 3b and area 1. The most dorsal and ventral deep stimulus receptive cells project to areas 3a and 2. The whole nucleus projects to the second somatic sensory area.

Medial Geniculate Nucleus

The medial geniculate nucleus, which is a part of the auditory pathway (Ch. 12), is located within the medial geniculate body, a rounded elevation situated posteriorly on the ventrolateral surface of the thalamus and separated from the pulvinar by the superior quadrigeminal brachium. It receives fibres travelling in the inferior quadrigeminal brachium. Three major subnuclei—medial, ventral and dorsal—are recognized within it. The inferior brachium separates the medial (magnocellular) nucleus, which consists of sparse, deeply staining neurones, from the lateral nucleus, which is made up of medium-sized, densely packed and darkly staining cells. The dorsal nucleus overlies the ventral nucleus and expands posteriorly; therefore, it is sometimes known as the posterior nucleus of the medial geniculate. It contains small to medium-sized, pale-staining cells, which are less densely packed than those of the lateral nucleus. The ventral nucleus receives fibres from the central nucleus of the ipsilateral inferior colliculus via the inferior quadrigeminal brachium and also

SUPEROLATERAL SURFACE OF HEMISPHERE

MEDIAL SURFACE OF HEMISPHERE

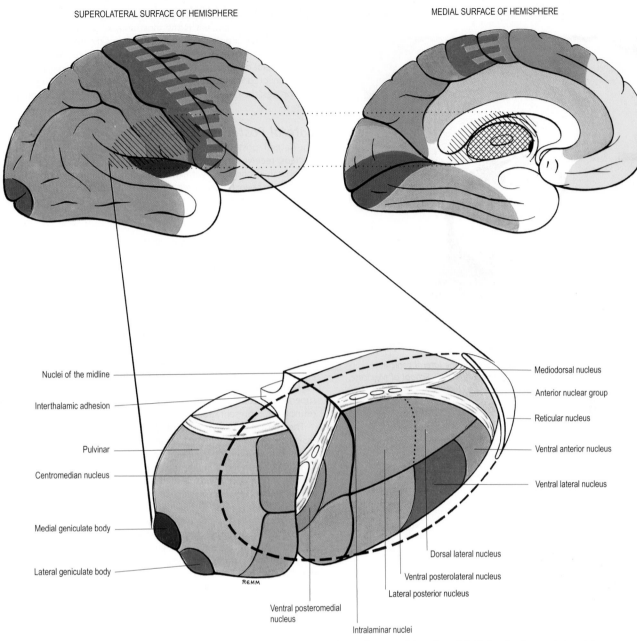

Nuclei of the midline

Interthalamic adhesion

Pulvinar

Centromedian nucleus

Medial geniculate body

Lateral geniculate body

REMM

Mediodorsal nucleus

Anterior nuclear group

Reticular nucleus

Ventral anterior nucleus

Ventral lateral nucleus

Dorsal lateral nucleus

Ventral posterolateral nucleus

Lateral posterior nucleus

Ventral posteromedial nucleus

Intralaminar nuclei

Fig. 15.6 *Main nuclear masses of the thalamus* (viewed from the lateral aspect in the lower illustration) *have been labelled and colour-coded, and the same colours have been used to indicate the areas of cerebral neocortex interconnected with these nuclei. The lack of colour in the centromedian, intralaminar and reticular nuclei and in restricted areas of the frontal and temporal lobes is not related to the colour code.*

from the contralateral inferior colliculus. The nucleus contains a complete tonotopic representation. Low-pitched sounds are represented laterally, and progressively higher-pitched sounds are encountered as the nucleus is traversed from lateral to medial. The dorsal nucleus receives afferents from the pericentral nucleus of the inferior colliculus and from other brain stem nuclei of the auditory pathway. A tonotopic representation has not been described in this subdivision, and cells within the dorsal nucleus respond to a broad range of frequencies. The magnocellular medial nucleus receives fibres from the inferior colliculus and from the deep layers of the superior colliculus. Neurones within the magnocellular subdivision may respond to modalities other than sound. However, many cells respond to auditory stimuli, usually to a wider range of frequencies than do neurones in the ventral nucleus. Many units show evidence of binaural interaction, with the leading effect arising from stimuli in the contralateral cochlea. The ventral nucleus projects primarily to the primary auditory cortex. The dorsal nucleus projects to auditory areas surrounding the primary auditory cortex. The magnocellular division projects diffusely to auditory areas of the cortex and to adjacent insular and opercular fields.

Lateral Geniculate Nucleus

The lateral geniculate body, which is part of the visual pathway (Ch. 12), is a small ovoid ventral projection from the posterior thalamus (Fig. 15.7). The

superior quadrigeminal brachium enters the posteromedial part of the lateral geniculate body dorsally, lying between the medial geniculate body and the pulvinar.

The lateral geniculate nucleus is an inverted, somewhat flattened U-shaped nucleus and is laminated. Its internal organization is usually described on the basis of six laminae, although seven or eight may be present. The laminae are numbered 1 to 6, from the innermost ventral to the outermost dorsal (Fig. 15.8). Laminae 1 and 2 consist of large cells, the magnocellular layers, whereas layers 4 to 6 have smaller neurones, the parvocellular laminae. The apparent gaps between laminae are called the interlaminar zones. Most ventrally, an additional superficial, or S, lamina is recognized.

The lateral geniculate nucleus receives a major afferent input from the retina. The contralateral nasal retina projects to laminae 1, 4 and 6, whereas the ipsilateral temporal retina projects to laminae 2, 3 and 5. The parvocellular laminae receive axons predominantly of X-type retinal ganglion cells, which are slowly conducting cells with sustained responses to visual stimuli. The faster conducting, rapidly adapting Y-type retinal ganglion cells project mainly to magnocellular laminae 1 and 2 and give off axonal branches to the superior colliculus. A third type of retinal ganglion cell—the W cell, which has large receptive fields and slow responses—projects to both the superior colliculus and the lateral geniculate nucleus and terminates particularly in the interlaminar zones and in the S lamina.

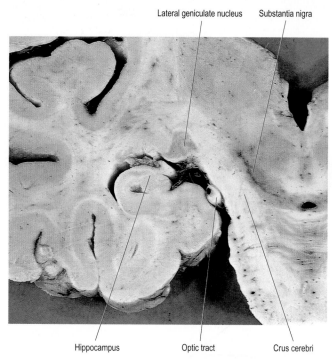

Lateral geniculate nucleus   Substantia nigra

Hippocampus   Optic tract   Crus cerebri

Fig. 15.7 *Coronal section through the brain showing the lateral geniculate nucleus. (Photograph by Kevin Fitzpatrick on behalf of GKT School of Medicine, London.)*

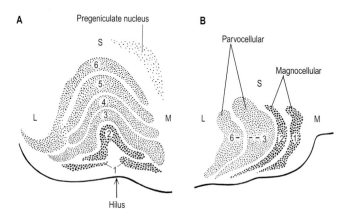

A Pregeniculate nucleus

B

Parvocellular

Magnocellular

S

6

5

4

3

2

1

Hilus

Fig. 15.8 *Coronal sections through the lateral geniculate nucleus near its central region (A) and its posterior pole (B). L, lateral; M, medial; S, superior. (Photograph by Kevin Fitzpatrick on behalf of GKT School of Medicine, London.)*

The lateral geniculate nucleus is organized in a visuotopic manner and contains a precise map of the contralateral visual field. The vertical meridian is represented posteriorly, the peripheral anteriorly, the upper field laterally, and the lower field medially (Ch. 12). Similar precise point-to-point representation is also found in the projection of the lateral geniculate nucleus to the visual cortex. Radially arranged inverted pyramids of neurones in all laminae respond to a single small area of the contralateral visual field and project to a circumscribed area of cortex. The termination of geniculocortical axons in the visual cortex is considered in detail in Chapter 16.

Aside from retinal afferents, the lateral geniculate nucleus receives a major corticothalamic projection, the axons of which ramify densely in the interlaminar zones. The major part of this projection arises from the primary visual cortex, Brodmann's area 17, but smaller projections from extrastriate visual areas pass to the magnocellular and S laminae. Other afferents include fibres from the superficial layer of the superior colliculus (which terminate in the interlaminar zone between laminae 1 and 2 or 2 and 3 and around lamina S), noradrenergic fibres from the locus coeruleus, serotoninergic afferents from the midbrain raphe nuclei and cholinergic fibres from the pontine and mesencephalic reticular formation.

The efferent fibres of the lateral geniculate nucleus pass principally to the primary visual cortex (area 17) in the banks of the calcarine sulcus. It is possible that additional small projections pass to extrastriate visual areas in the occipital lobe, possibly arising primarily in the interlaminar zones.

Lateral Dorsal Nucleus

The lateral dorsal nucleus is the most anterior of the dorsal tier of lateral nuclei. Its anterior pole lies within a splitting of the internal medullary lamina. Posteriorly, it merges with the lateral posterior nucleus. Subcortical afferents to the lateral dorsal nucleus are from the pretectum and superior colliculus. It is connected with the cingulate, retrosplenial and posterior parahippocampal cortices; the presubiculum of the hippocampal formation; and the parietal cortex.

Lateral Posterior Nucleus

The lateral posterior nucleus, which lies dorsal to the ventral posterior nucleus, receives its subcortical afferents from the superior colliculus. It is reciprocally connected with the superior parietal lobe. Additional connections have been reported with the inferior parietal, cingulate and medial parahippocampal cortices.

Pulvinar

The pulvinar corresponds to the posterior expansion of the thalamus, which overhangs the superior colliculus. It has three major subdivisions: the medial, lateral and inferior pulvinar nuclei. The medial pulvinar nucleus is dorsomedial and consists of compact, evenly spaced neurones. The inferior pulvinar nucleus lies laterally and inferiorly and is traversed by bundles of axons in the mediolateral plane, an arrangement that confers a fragmented appearance of horizontal cords or sheets of cells separated by fibre bundles. The inferior pulvinar nucleus lies most inferiorly and laterally and is a more homogeneous collection of cells.

The subcortical afferents to the pulvinar are uncertain. Medial and lateral pulvinar nuclei may receive fibres from the superior colliculus. It has been suggested that the inferior pulvinar nucleus receives fibres both from the superior colliculus and directly from the retina and that it contains a complete retinotopic representation.

The cortical targets of efferent fibres from the pulvinar are widespread. In essence, the medial pulvinar nucleus projects to association areas of the parietotemporal cortex, whereas lateral and inferior pulvinar nuclei project to visual areas in the occipital and posterior temporal lobes. Thus, the inferior pulvinar nucleus connects with the striate and extrastriate cortex in the occipital lobe and with visual association areas in the posterior part of the temporal lobe. The lateral pulvinar nucleus connects with extrastriate areas of the occipital cortex, posterior parts of the temporal association cortex and the parietal cortex. The medial pulvinar nucleus connects with the inferior parietal cortex, the posterior cingulate gyrus and widespread areas of the temporal lobe, including the posterior parahippocampal gyrus and the perirhinal and entorhinal cortices. It also has extensive connections with prefrontal and orbitofrontal cortices. Similarly, the lateral pulvinar nucleus may also connect with the rostromedial prefrontal cortex.

Little is known of the functions of the pulvinar. The inferior pulvinar nucleus contains a complete retinotopic representation, and lateral and medial pulvinar nuclei also contain visually responsive cells. However, the latter nucleus, at least, is not purely visual; other modality responses can be recorded, and some cells may be polysensory. Given the complex functions of the association areas to which they project, particularly in the temporal lobe (e.g. perception, cognition, memory), it is likely that the role of the pulvinar in modulating these functions is equally complex.

Anteriorly, the major subdivisions of the pulvinar blend into a poorly differentiated region within which several nuclear components have been recognized, including the anterior or oral pulvinar, the suprageniculate limitans and the posterior nuclei. The connectivity of this complex is not well understood. It is recognized that different components receive subcortical afferents from the spinothalamic tract and the superior and inferior colliculi. Cortical connections centre primarily on the insula and adjacent parts of the parietal operculum posteriorly. Stimulation of this region has been reported to elicit pain, and large lesions may alleviate painful conditions. Similarly, excision of its cortical target in the parietal operculum, or small infarcts in this cortical region, may result in hypoalgesia.

Intralaminar Nuclei

The intralaminar nuclei are collections of neurones within the internal medullary lamina of the thalamus. Two groups of nuclei are recognized. The anterior (rostral) group is subdivided into central medial, paracentral and central lateral nuclei. The posterior (caudal) intralaminar group consists of the centromedian and parafascicular nuclei. The designations central medial and centromedian can lead to confusion, but they are an accepted part of the terminology of thalamic nuclei in common usage. The centromedian nucleus is much larger, is considerably expanded in humans in comparison with other species and is importantly related to the globus pallidus, deep cerebellar nuclei and motor cortex. Anteriorly, the internal medullary lamina separates the mediodorsal nucleus from the ventral lateral complex. It is occupied by the paracentral nucleus laterally and the central medial nucleus ventromedially, as the two laminae converge toward the midline. A little more posteriorly, the central lateral nucleus appears dorsally in the lamina as the latter splits to enclose the lateral dorsal nucleus. More posteriorly, at the level of the ventral posterior nucleus, the lamina splits to enclose the ovoid centromedian nucleus. The smaller parafascicular nucleus lies more medially.

The anterior intralaminar nuclei (i.e. central medial, paracentral and central lateral) have reciprocal connections with widespread cortical areas. There is some evidence of areal preference. Thus, the central lateral nucleus projects mainly to parietal and temporal association areas, the paracentral nucleus to the occipitotemporal and prefrontal cortex and the central medial nucleus to the orbitofrontal and prefrontal cortex and to the cortex on the medial surface. In contrast, the posterior nuclei (i.e. centromedian and parafascicular) have more restricted connections, principally with the motor, premotor and supplementary motor areas. Both anterior and posterior intralaminar nuclei also project to the striatum. Many cells throughout the anterior nuclei have branched axons, which pass to both the cortex and the striatum. Dual projections are less frequent in the posterior nuclei. The thalamostriate projection is topographically organized. The posterior intralaminar nuclei receive a major input from the internal segment of the globus pallidus. Additional afferents come from the pars reticulata of the substantia nigra, the deep cerebellar nuclei, the pedunculopontine nucleus of the midbrain and possibly the spinothalamic tract. The anterior nuclei have widespread subcortical afferents. The central lateral nucleus receives afferents from the spinothalamic tract, and all component nuclei receive fibres from the brain stem reticular formation, the superior colliculus and several pretectal nuclei. Afferents to all intralaminar nuclei from the brain stem reticular formation include a prominent cholinergic pathway.

The precise functional role of the intralaminar nuclei is unclear. They appear to mediate cortical activation from the brain stem reticular formation and play a part in sensorimotor integration. Damage to the intralaminar nuclei may contribute to thalamic neglect—that is, the unilateral neglect of stimuli originating from the contralateral body or extrapersonal space. This may arise particularly from unilateral damage to the centromedian–parafascicular complex. The latter has been targeted in humans for the neurosurgical control of pain and epilepsy. Bilateral injury to the posterior intralaminar nuclei leads to akinetic mutism, with apathy and loss of motivation. A second syndrome associated with damage involving the intralaminar nuclei is that of unilateral motor neglect, in which there is contralateral paucity of spontaneous movement and motor activity.

Midline Nuclei

There is considerable divergence among authors as to which elements of the medial diencephalon constitute the nuclei of the midline thalamic group. In this chapter, the midline group of nuclei includes those medial thalamic structures ventral to the central medial nucleus—that is, the rhomboid and reuniens nuclei, together with the parataenial nuclei more dorsolaterally.

The midline nuclei receive subcortical afferent fibres from the hypothalamus, the periaqueductal grey matter of the midbrain, the spinothalamic tract and the medullary and pontine reticular formations. They are the major thalamic target of ascending noradrenergic and serotoninergic axons from the locus coeruleus and raphe nuclei, respectively, and they also receive a cholinergic input from the midbrain. Efferents from the midline nuclei pass to the hippocampal formation, the amygdala and the nucleus accumbens. Additional thalamocortical axons reach the cingulate and possibly the orbitofrontal cortex. The dual cortical and basal nuclear relationship of these nuclei has often led to their being considered part of the intralaminar system. The cortical projections are reciprocal. The relationships of the midline nuclei clearly identify them as part of the limbic system. There is some evidence that they may play a role in memory and arousal and, pathologically, may be important in the regulation of seizure activity.

Reticular Nucleus

The reticular nucleus is a curved lamella of large, deeply staining fusiform cells that wraps around the lateral margin of the thalamus, separated from it by the external medullary lamina. Anteriorly, it curves around the rostral pole of the thalamus to lie between it and the prethalamic nuclei, notably the bed nucleus of the stria terminalis. The nucleus is so named because it is crisscrossed by bundles of fibres that, as they pass between the thalamus and cortex, produce a reticular appearance.

The nucleus is thought to receive collateral branches of corticothalamic, thalamocortical and probably thalamostriatal and pallidothalamic fibres as they traverse it. It receives an additional, probably cholinergic, afferent pathway from the nucleus cuneiformis of the midbrain. Broadly speaking, the afferents from the cortex and thalamus are topographically arranged. The

reticular nucleus contains visual, somatic and auditory regions, each with a crude topographical representation of the sensorium concerned. Cells within these regions respond to visual, somatic or auditory stimuli with a latency, suggesting that these properties arise from activation by thalamocortical axon collaterals. Only in areas where representations abut do cells show modality convergence.

The efferent fibres from the reticular nucleus pass into the body of the thalamus and are GABAergic. The projections into the main thalamic nuclei broadly, but not entirely, reciprocate the thalamoreticular connections. There may also be projections to the contralateral dorsal thalamus. The reticular nucleus is believed to function in gating information relayed through the thalamus.

HYPOTHALAMUS

The hypothalamus consists of only 4 cubic centimetres of neural tissue, or 0.3% of the total brain. Nevertheless, it contains the integrative systems that, via the autonomic and endocrine effector systems, control fluid and electrolyte balance, food ingestion and energy balance, reproduction, thermoregulation and immune and many emotional responses.

The hypothalamus extends from the lamina terminalis to a vertical plane posterior to the mammillary bodies, and from the hypothalamic sulcus to the base of the brain beneath the third ventricle. It lies beneath the thalamus and anterior to the tegmental part of the subthalamus and the mesencephalic tegmentum (see Figs 15.5, 5.8, 15.10). Laterally, it is bordered by the anterior part of the subthalamus, internal capsule and optic tract. Structures in the floor of the third ventricle reach the pial surface in the interpeduncular fossa (Fig. 15.9). From anterior to posterior, they are the optic chiasma, tuber cinereum, tuberal eminences and infundibular stalk, mammillary bodies and posterior perforated substance. The last lies in the interval between the diverging crura cerebri, pierced by small central branches of posterior cerebral arteries. Within it is the small interpeduncular nucleus, which receives terminals of the fasciculus retroflexus of both sides and has other connections with the mesencephalic reticular formation and mammillary bodies.

The mammillary bodies are smooth, hemispherical, pea-sized eminences lying side by side, anterior to the posterior perforated substance. Each has nuclei enclosed in white fascicles derived largely from the fornix. The tuber cinereum, between the mammillary bodies and the optic chiasma, is a convex mass of grey matter. From it, the median, conical, hollow infundibulum becomes continuous ventrally with the posterior lobe of the pituitary. Around the base of the infundibulum is the median eminence, which is demarcated by a shallow tubero-infundibular sulcus.

Hypothalamic lesions have long been linked with widespread and bizarre endocrine syndromes and with metabolic, visceral, motor and emotional disturbances. The hypothalamus has major interactions with the neuroendocrine system and the autonomic nervous system, integrating responses to both internal and external afferent stimuli with the complex analysis of the world provided by the cerebral cortex.

The hypothalamus controls the endocrine system in a variety of ways: through magnocellular neurosecretory projections to the posterior pituitary, through parvocellular neurosecretory projections to the median eminence (these control the endocrine output of the anterior pituitary and thereby the peripheral endocrine organs) and via the autonomic nervous system. The posterior pituitary neurohormones vasopressin and oxytocin are primarily involved in the control of osmotic homeostasis and various aspects of reproductive function, respectively. Through its effects on the anterior pituitary, the hypothalamus influences the thyroid gland (thyroid-stimulating hormone [TSH]), suprarenal cortex (adrenocorticotropic hormone [ACTH]), gonads (luteinizing hormone [LH], follicle-stimulating hormone [FSH], prolactin), mammary gland (prolactin) and the processes of growth and metabolic homeostasis (growth hormone [GH]).

The hypothalamus influences both parasympathetic and sympathetic divisions of the autonomic nervous system. In general, parasympathetic effects predominate when the anterior hypothalamus is stimulated; sympathetic effects depend more on the posterior hypothalamus.

Stimulation of the anterior hypothalamus and paraventricular nucleus can cause decreased blood pressure and decreased heart rate. Stimulation in the anterior hypothalamus induces sweating and vasodilatation (and thus heat loss) via projections that pass through the medial forebrain bundle to autonomic centres in the brain stem and cord. Damage to the anterior hypothalamus (e.g. during surgery for suprasellar extensions of pituitary tumours) can result in an uncontrollable rise in body temperature. Projections to the ventromedial hypothalamus conjointly regulate food intake. Stimulation in the posterior part of the hypothalamus induces sympathetic arousal with vasoconstriction, piloerection, shivering and increased metabolic heat production. Circuitry mediating shivering is located in the dorsomedial posterior hypothalamus. This does not imply the existence of discrete parasympathetic and

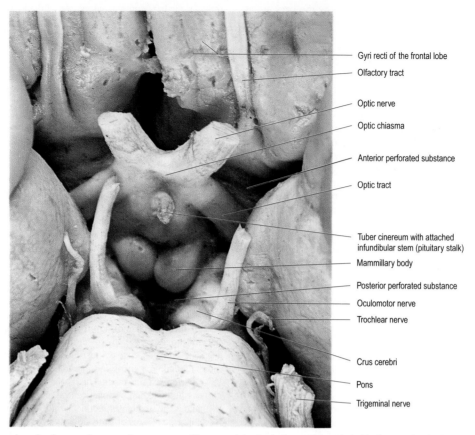

Gyri recti of the frontal lobe

Olfactory tract

Optic nerve

Optic chiasma

Anterior perforated substance

Optic tract

Tuber cinereum with attached
infundibular stem (pituitary stalk)

Mammillary body

Posterior perforated substance

Oculomotor nerve

Trochlear nerve

Crus cerebri

Pons

Trigeminal nerve

Fig. 15.9 *Interpeduncular fossa and surrounding structures. (Photograph by Kevin Fitzpatrick on behalf of GKT School of Medicine, London.)*

sympathetic 'centres.' Stimuli in many different parts of the hypothalamus can cause profound changes in heart rate, cardiac output, vasomotor tone, peripheral resistance, differential bloodflow in organs and limbs, frequency and depth of respiration, motility and secretion in the alimentary tract, erection and ejaculation.

Hypothalamic Nuclei

The hypothalamus contains a number of neuronal groups that have been classified on phylogenetic, developmental, cytoarchitectonic, synaptic and histochemical grounds into named nuclei, many of which are not clearly delineated, especially in the adult. Although it contains a few large myelinated tracts, many of the connections are diffuse and unmyelinated, and the precise paths of many afferent, efferent, and intrinsic connections are uncertain.

The hypothalamus can be divided anteroposteriorly into chiasmatic (supraoptic), tuberal (infundibulo-tuberal) and posterior (mammillary) regions and mediolaterally into periventricular, intermediate (medial) and lateral zones. Between the intermediate and lateral zones is a paramedian plane that contains the prominent myelinated fibres of the column of the fornix, the mammillothalamic tract and the fasciculus retroflexus. For this reason, some authors group the periventricular and intermediate zones as a single medial zone. These divisions are artificial, and functional systems cross them. The main nuclear groups and myelinated tracts are illustrated in Figures 15.10 and 15.11.

The periventricular zone of the hypothalamus borders the third ventricle. In the anterior wall of the ventricle is the vascular organ of the lamina terminalis (organum vasculosum), which is continuous dorsally with the median preoptic nucleus and subfornical organ. On each side in the chiasmatic region are part of the preoptic nucleus; the small, sexually dimorphic suprachiasmatic nucleus; and periventricular neurones, which are medial to and blend with the paraventricular nucleus. In the tuberal region, the periventricular cell group expands around the base of the third ventricle to form the arcuate nucleus, which overlies the median eminence. In the posterior region, the narrow periventricular zone is continuous laterally with the posterior hypothalamic area and behind that with midbrain periaqueductal grey matter. The periventricular zone also contains a prominent periventricular fibre system.

Suprachiasmatic Nucleus

Although it contains only a few thousand neurones, the suprachiasmatic nucleus is a remarkable structure. It appears to be the neural substrate for

day–night cycles in motor activity, body temperature, plasma concentration of many hormones, renal secretion, sleeping and waking and many other variables. Lesions of the suprachiasmatic region lead to a disordered sleep–wake cycle.

The suprachiasmatic nucleus has two principal subdivisions. Retinal fibres terminate in a ventrolateral subdivision, characterized by neurones immunoreactive for vasoactive intestinal polypeptide (VIP). This appears to be a general input zone, which also receives afferents from the midbrain raphe and parts of the lateral geniculate nucleus of the thalamus. The dorsomedial subdivision has relatively sparse afferent innervation and characteristically contains parvocellular neurones immunoreactive for arginine vasopressin. Neurones within the suprachiasmatic nuclei that receive direct retinal input do not respond to pattern, movement or colour. Instead, they operate as luminance detectors, responding to the onset and offset of light, and their firing rates vary in proportion to light intensity, thereby synchronizing to the light–dark cycle.

The nucleus receives glutamatergic afferents from retinal ganglion cells that entrain the rhythm to the light–dark cycle, but these are not essential for the production of the rhythm, which persists in the blind. The suprachiasmatic nucleus contains many different neurotransmitters, including vasopressin, VIP, neuropeptide Y and neurotensin. Axons from the suprachiasmatic nuclei pass to many other hypothalamic nuclei, including the paraventricular, ventromedial, dorsomedial and arcuate nuclei.

The suprachiasmatic nucleus also influences the activity of preganglionic sympathetic neurones at the C8–T1 level. These project to superior cervical ganglion neurones, which in turn project to the pineal gland. In the pineal gland, which contains modified photoreceptors, circadian variation in the postganglionic sympathetic input causes parallel variation in pineal N-acetyltransferase activity and thus pineal melatonin production. The role of the pineal gland in humans is uncertain. Pineal tumours can influence reproductive development, and the administration of melatonin has been advocated to alleviate jet lag.

Parvocellular neurosecretory neurones lie within the periventricular zone, in particular the medial parvocellular part of the paraventricular nucleus and the arcuate nucleus. The arcuate nucleus is median in the postinfundibular part of the tuber cinereum. It extends forward into the median eminence and almost encircles the infundibular base but does not meet anteriorly, where the infundibulum adjoins the median part of the optic chiasma. Its numerous neurones are all small and round in coronal section, and oval or fusiform in

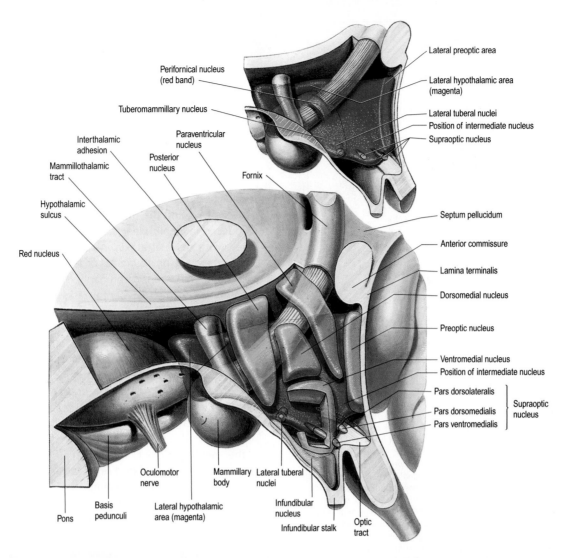

Fig. 15.10 *Hypothalamic region of the left cerebral hemisphere viewed from the medial aspect and dissected to display the major hypothalamic nuclei. In the upper diagram, the medially placed nuclear groups have been removed; in the lower diagram, both lateral and medial groups are included. Lateral to the fornix and the mammillothalamic tract is the lateral hypothalamic region (magenta), in which the tuberomammillary nucleus is situated posteriorly and the lateral preoptic nucleus rostrally. Surrounding the fornix is the perifornical nucleus (red band), which joins the lateral hypothalamic area with the posterior hypothalamic nucleus. The medially placed nuclei (yellow) fill in much of the region between the mammillothalamic tract and the lamina terminalis, but they also project caudally to the tract. The lateral tuberal nuclei (blue) are situated ventrally, largely in the lateral hypothalamic area. The supraoptic nucleus (green) may form three separate parts. The intermediate nuclei form three groups between the supraoptic and paraventricular nuclei (Modified from Nauta, W.J.H., Haymaker, W., 1969. Hypothalamic nuclei and fiber connections. In: Haymaker, W., Anderson, E., Nauta, W.J.H. (Eds.), The Hypothalamus. Charles C Thomas, Springfield, Ill. By permission of Charles C Thomas Publisher, Ltd., Springfield, Illinois.)*

sagittal section. No glial layer intervenes between the nucleus and the ependymal tanycytes lining the infundibular recess of the third ventricle. Circadian variation in the secretion of all anterior pituitary hormones suggests that projections from the suprachiasmatic nucleus must reach parvocellular neurosecretory neurones. Afferents from the limbic system probably mediate the widespread effects of stress, and serotonin and noradrenaline from the brain stem influence the output of most anterior pituitary hormones. The axons of parvocellular neurones converge on the infundibulum, forming a tubero-infundibular tract, which ends on the capillary loops that form the hypophysial portal vessels.

Neurones producing growth hormone–releasing hormone (GHRH) are largely restricted to the arcuate nucleus. Some extend dorsally into the periventricular nucleus and laterally into the retrochiasmatic area. Their fibres run through the periventricular region to the neurovascular zone of the median eminence. The neurones receive afferent information from glucose receptors in the ventromedial nucleus. Inputs from the hippocampal–amygdala–septal complex could explain the release of GH during stress. In humans, midline defects such as septo-optic dysplasia are associated with defective GH secretion. Dopamine has a stimulatory effect.

Neurones producing somatostatin (GH release-inhibiting hormone) are located in the periventricular nucleus. GHRH and somatostatin are secreted in intermittent (3- to 5-hour) reciprocal pulses, but the origin of the pulses is unclear. A large pulse of GH is secreted at the onset of slow-wave sleep. Somatostatin also inhibits the release of pituitary TSH.

Neurones producing GHRH and projecting to the median eminence are also located in the periventricular and arcuate nuclei. Other GHRH-producing neurones are found in the periventricular preoptic area, but these appear to project to the vascular organ of the lamina terminalis. LH and FSH are secreted in circhoral (hourly) pulses, which are stimulated by GHRH, and are influenced by central monoamine and γ-aminobutyric acid (GABA), by oestrogen and progesterone acting indirectly through other neurones, by corticotropin-releasing factor and by endogenous opioids.

Corticotropin-releasing hormone neurones are located primarily in parvocellular paraventricular neurones. They are profoundly stimulated by neurogenic (limbic input) and hypoglycaemic (ventromedial nucleus) stress and are also controlled by negative feedback by cortisol.

Thyrotropin-releasing hormone (TRH) neurones are more widely distributed in the periventricular, ventromedial and dorsomedial nuclei. TRH release is influenced by core temperature, sensed in the anterior hypothalamus, and by negative feedback of thyroid hormones. It stimulates the release of pituitary TSH and also acts to excite cold-sensitive and inhibit warm-sensitive neurones in the preoptic area.

Other tubero-infundibular arcuate neurones contain neuropeptide Y and neurotensin. Arcuate neurones containing pro-opiomelanocortin peptides project to the periventricular nucleus rather than to the median eminence.

In addition to these peptide-containing cells, dopamine neurones in the arcuate nucleus (A12 group) have terminals in the median eminence and infundibulum. Dopamine acts as the principal prolactin–release inhibiting hormone

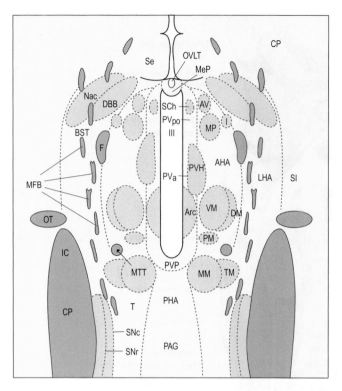

Fig. 15.11 *Schematic horizontal section to show the major cell groups and tracts in and around the hypothalamus. AHA, anterior hypothalamic area; Arc, arcuate nucleus; AV, anteroventral preoptic nucleus; BST, bed nucleus of stria terminalis; CP, caudate nucleus and putamen; DBB, nucleus of diagonal band; DM, dorsomedial nucleus; LHA, lateral hypothalamic area; MeP, median preoptic nucleus; MM, medial mammillary body; MP, medial preoptic nucleus; Nac, nucleus accumbens; OVLT, vascular organ of the lamina terminalis; PAG, periaqueductal grey matter; PHA, posterior hypothalamic area; PM, posteromedial nucleus; PV, periventricular nucleus (PVa, anterior part; PVP, posterior part; PVpo, preoptic part); PVH, paraventricular (hypothalamic) nucleus; SCh, suprachiasmatic nucleus; Se, septal cortex; SI, substantia innominata; SNc, substantia nigra pars compacta; SNr, substantia nigra pars reticularis; T, midbrain tegmentum; TM, tuberomammillary nucleus; VM, ventromedial nucleus. Fibre tracts (shaded): CP, cerebral peduncle; F, fornix; IC, internal capsule; MFB, medial forebrain bundle; MTT, mammillothalamic tract; OT, optic tract. (Modified from Swanson, L.W., 1991. Biochemical switching in hypothalamic circuits mediating responses to stress. Prog. Brain Res. 87, 181–200. With permission from Elsevier.)*

and also inhibits the secretion of TSH (likewise, TSH acts as a prolactin-releasing hormone). Noradrenergic terminals are found in the median eminence, where they may act largely in a paracrine manner.

The intermediate zone of the hypothalamus contains the best differentiated nuclei. These are the paraventricular and supraoptic nuclei; 'intermediate' nuclear groups, which show sexual dimorphism; ventromedial and dorsomedial nuclei; mammillary body; and tuberomammillary nuclei. Magnocellular neurosecretory neurones are found in the supraoptic and paraventricular nuclei and as isolated clusters of cells between them.

Supraoptic and Paraventricular Nuclei

The supraoptic nucleus, curved over the lateral part of the optic chiasma, contains a uniform population of large neurones. Behind the chiasma, a thin plate of cells in the floor of the brain forms the retrochiasmatic part.

Supraoptic neurones synthesize vasopressin, and they all appear to project to the neurohypophysis. The magnocellular vasopressin neurones can detect as little as 1% increase in the osmotic pressure of the blood and stimulate the release of vasopressin from the posterior pituitary. A fall in blood volume or blood pressure of greater than 5% to 10% stimulates the release of vasopressin and the urge to drink via volume receptors in the walls of the great veins and atria and baroreceptors in the carotid sinus. These project via the vagus and glossopharyngeal nerves to the nucleus tractus solitarius and thence to the magnocellular nuclei. A biochemical defect in vasopressin production, or interruption of the supraoptico-hypophysial pathway (e.g. due to a head injury), can cause cranial diabetes insipidus.

The paraventricular nucleus extends from the hypothalamic sulcus downward across the medial aspect of the column of the fornix, its ventrolateral angle reaching toward the supraoptic nucleus. Its neurones are more diverse.

CASE 2   WERNICKE'S ENCEPHALOPATHY

A 62-year-old man, a chronically undernourished alcoholic, complains of double vision. During the following week, unsteadiness of gait and mild mental confusion appear. Progression of these symptoms prompts hospitalization. Examination demonstrates a confused and disoriented man who exhibits bilateral sixth nerve palsies, coarse nystagmus on gaze to either side and a striking ataxia of gait. A diagnosis of acute Wernicke's encephalopathy is made, and he is treated with parenteral thiamine. During the next week, the ophthalmoparesis disappears, and the nystagmus, though lingering, is much reduced in amplitude. His gait slowly improves, but he is left with residual ataxia. As his sensorium clears under treatment, a profound disorder of memory becomes evident, characterized primarily by a striking inability to form new memories. Mental tasks that are not memory dependent are, for the most part, intact.

Discussion: This man exhibits a classic Wernicke-Korsakoff syndrome due to thiamine deficiency. Anatomically, the ophthalmoparesis reflects reversible lesions involving the brain stem oculomotor complex bilaterally in the midbrain or pons, and the nystagmus is due to lesions involving the vestibular nuclei. The truncal ataxia is related to observed lesions involving the superior vermis of the cerebellum. The anatomical substrate of the memory defect, the Korsakoff component of the disorder, in all likelihood reflects bilateral subtotal tissue necrosis, which may be haemorrhagic, involving the mammillary bodies or thalamus (Fig. 15.12). Despite vigorous therapy with thiamine, the memory problem may persist indefinitely, posing a major functional disability.

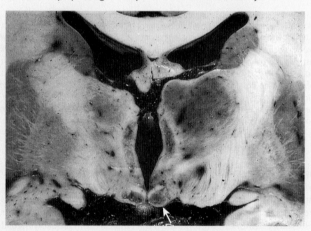

Fig. 15.12 *Wernicke's encephalopathy. Section at the level of the mammillary bodies in a case of Wernicke's encephalopathy shows subacute necrotic changes in the mammillary bodies (arrow), with enlargement of the third ventricle and non-haemorrhagic periventricular lesions. (From Victor, M., Adams, R.D., Collins, G.H., 1971. The Wernicke's-Korsakoff Syndrome. F.A. Davis, Philadelphia.)*

Magnocellular neurones, which project to the neurohypophysis, tend to lie laterally; parvocellular neurones, which project to the median eminence and infundibulum, lie more medially; and intermediate-sized neurones, which may project caudally, lie posteriorly. The axons of the paraventricular magnocellular neurones pass toward the supraoptic nucleus (paraventriculo-hypophysial tract), where they join axons of supraoptic neurones to form a supraoptico-hypophysial tract. This runs down the infundibulum, superficially, and into the neural lobe, where the axons are distended and branch repeatedly around the capillaries. Vasopressin and oxytocin are produced by separate neurones. Vasopressin neurones tend to cluster in the ventrolateral part of the paraventricular nucleus, and oxytocin cells lie around them.

The hypothalamus is essential for the control of pituitary oxytocin, gonadotropin and prolactin secretion. The release of oxytocin from neurosecretory nerve terminals in the neurohypophysis induces contraction of both the uterus, at term, and the myoepithelial cells that surround the mammary gland alveoli. Two neuroendocrine reflexes are involved. Stretching of the cervix of the uterus during childbirth stimulates a multisynaptic afferent pathway that passes via the pelvic plexus, anterolateral column and brain stem to the magnocellular oxytocin neurones (the Ferguson reflex). This is a positive feedback mechanism that is terminated by the birth of the child. The milk ejection reflex involves stimulation (by suckling) of the intercostal nerves, which innervate the nipples, and a similar central pathway. It can be both conditioned to a baby's cry and inhibited by stress.

At the tuberal level, the ventromedial nucleus is well defined by a surrounding neurone-poor zone, but the dorsomedial nucleus above it is much less distinct. The ventromedial nucleus contains neurones receptive to plasma levels of glucose and other nutrients and receives visceral somatic afferents via the nucleus tractus solitarius. The lateral hypothalamus receives olfactory afferents, which act as important food signals. Both areas receive extensive inputs from limbic structures. Stimulation and lesion experiments, together with human case studies, suggest that the ventromedial nuclei act together as a 'satiety centre.' Bilateral ventromedial nucleus damage promotes overeating (hyperphagia), and restricting food intake may provoke rage-like outbursts. The resultant obesity is usually coupled with hyposexuality (Fröhlich's syndrome). Interestingly, in infants, ventromedial damage can lead to emaciation despite apparent normal feeding. Experimental lesions in the lateral hypothalamus promote hypophagia or aphagia, whereas stimulation can prolong feeding, supporting the concept of a lateral hypothalamic 'feeding centre.'

The ventromedial nucleus, lateral hypothalamic area and paraventricular nucleus also influence intermediate metabolism through the autonomic and endocrine systems. These appear to complement the effects on feeding behaviour. Thus, ventromedial stimulation facilitates glucagon release and increases glycogenolysis, gluconeogenesis and lipolysis, whereas lateral hypothalamic stimulation causes insulin release and opposite metabolic effects. Lesions of the ventromedial nucleus also cause increased vagal and decreased sympathetic tone.

The medial mammillary nuclei, which form the bulk of the mammillary bodies, are very prominent. The composition of a lateral mammillary nucleus is controversial, although a group of larger cells can be distinguished along the lateral border of the medial mammillary nucleus. Lateral to this lies the tuberomammillary nucleus, which gives rise to widespread axons that diffusely innervate the entire cerebral cortex, hypothalamus and brain stem.

The lateral zone of the hypothalamus forms a continuum that runs from the preoptic nucleus through the lateral hypothalamic area to the posterior hypothalamus. In the tuberal region, the lateral tuberal nuclei are large and well defined and surrounded by fine fibres.

Connections of the Hypothalamus

The hypothalamus has afferent and efferent connections with the rest of the body via two (possibly three) distinct routes: neural connections, the blood stream and (probably) the cerebrospinal fluid.

Some hypothalamic neurones have specific receptors that sense the temperature, osmolarity, glucose, free fatty acid and hormone content of the blood. Neurosecretory neurones secrete neurohormones into the blood. These control the anterior pituitary and act on organs such as the kidney, breast, uterus and blood vessels. Some of these neural connections, especially those to the mammillary bodies, form discrete myelinated fascicles; most, however, are diffuse and unmyelinated, and their origin and termination are uncertain. Most pathways are multisynaptic, which means that the majority of synapses on any hypothalamic neurone are derived from hypothalamic interneurones.

Broadly, neural inputs to the hypothalamus are derived from the ascending visceral and somatic sensory systems, the visual and olfactory systems and numerous tracts from the brain stem, thalamus, 'limbic' structures and neocortex. Efferent neural projections are reciprocal to most of these sources; in particular, they impinge on and control the central origins of autonomic nerve fibres. The hypothalamus therefore exerts control via the autonomic and endocrine systems and through its connections to the telencephalon.

Afferent Connections

The hypothalamus receives visceral, gustatory and somatic sensory information from the spinal cord and brain stem. It receives largely polysynaptic projections from the nucleus tractus solitarius, probably directly and indirectly via the parabrachial nucleus and medullary noradrenergic cell groups

(ventral noradrenergic bundle); collaterals of lemniscal somatic afferents (to the lateral hypothalamus); and projections from the dorsal longitudinal reticular formation. Many enter via the medial forebrain bundle (see Fig. 15.11) and periventricular fibre system. Others converge in the midbrain tegmentum, forming the mammillary peduncle to the mammillary body.

The major forebrain inputs to the hypothalamus are derived from structures in the limbic system, including the hippocampal formation, amygdala and septum, and from the piriform lobe and adjacent neocortex. These connections, which are reciprocal, form prominent fibre systems: the fornix, stria terminalis and ventral amygdalofugal tracts.

The hippocampal formation, in particular the subiculum and CA1, is reciprocally connected to the hypothalamus by the fornix, a complex tract that also contains commissural connections. As the fornix curves ventrally toward the anterior commissure, it is joined by fascicles from the cingulate gyrus, indusium griseum and septal areas. It divides around the anterior commissure into pre- and postcommissural parts. The precommissural fornix is distributed to the septum and preoptic hypothalamus, and the septum in turn sends numerous fibres to the hypothalamus. The postcommissural fornix passes ventrally and posteriorly through the hypothalamus to the medial mammillary nucleus. In its course, it gives off many fibres to the medial and lateral hypothalamic nuclei.

The amygdala innervates most hypothalamic nuclei anterior to the mammillary bodies. Its corticomedial nucleus innervates preoptic and anterior hypothalamic areas and the ventromedial nucleus. The central nuclei project to the lateral hypothalamus. The fibres reach the hypothalamus by two routes. The short ventral amygdalofugal path passes medially over the optic tract, beneath the lentiform complex, to reach the hypothalamus. The long, curved stria terminalis runs parallel to the fornix, separated from it by the lateral ventricle; it passes through the bed nucleus of the stria terminalis and is then distributed to the anterior hypothalamus via the medial forebrain bundle.

Olfactory afferents reach the hypothalamus largely via the nucleus accumbens and septal nuclei, and most terminate in the lateral hypothalamus. Visual afferents leave the optic chiasma and pass dorsally into the suprachiasmatic nucleus. No auditory connections have been identified, although it is clear that such stimuli influence hypothalamic activity. However, many hypothalamic neurones respond best to complex sensory stimuli, suggesting that sensory information reaching the neocortex has converged and been processed by the amygdala, hippocampus and neocortex. Neocortical corticohypothalamic afferents to the hypothalamus are poorly defined but probably arise from frontal and insular cortices. Some may relay in the mediodorsal thalamic nucleus and project into the hypothalamus via the periventricular route. Other direct corticohypothalamic fibres may end in lateral, dorsomedial, mammillary and posterior hypothalamic nuclei, but all these connections are questionable.

Like the rest of the forebrain, the hypothalamus also receives diffuse aminergic inputs from the locus coeruleus (noradrenaline, or norepinephrine) and the raphe nuclei (serotonin, or 5-hydroxytryptamine [5-HT]). In addition, it receives a cholinergic input from the ventral tegmental ascending cholinergic pathway; a noradrenergic input to dorsomedial, periventricular, paraventricular, supraoptic and lateral hypothalamic nuclei from the ventral tegmental noradrenergic bundle; and dopamine fibres from the mesolimbic dopaminergic system. Group A11 innervates the medial hypothalamic nuclei, and groups A13 and A14 supply the dorsal and rostral hypothalamic nuclei. Many of these fibres also run in the medial forebrain bundle.

The medial forebrain bundle is a loose grouping of fibre pathways that mostly run longitudinally through the lateral hypothalamus (see Fig. 15.11). It connects forebrain autonomic and limbic structures with the hypothalamus and brain stem, receiving and giving small fascicles throughout its course. It contains descending hypothalamic afferents from the septal area and orbitofrontal cortex, ascending afferents from the brain stem and efferents from the hypothalamus.

Efferent Connections

Hypothalamic efferents include reciprocal paths to the limbic system, descending polysynaptic paths to autonomic and somatic motor neurones and neural and neurovascular links with the pituitary.

Septal areas and the amygdaloid complex have reciprocal hypothalamic connections along the paths described earlier. The medial preoptic and anterior hypothalamic areas give short projections to nearby hypothalamic groups. The ventromedial nucleus has more extensive projections that pass via the medial forebrain bundle to the bed nucleus of the stria terminalis, basal nucleus of Meynert, central nucleus of the amygdala and midbrain reticular formation. The posterior hypothalamus projects largely to midbrain central grey matter. Some tuberal and posterior lateral hypothalamic neurones project directly to the entire neocortex and appear to be essential for maintaining cortical arousal, but the topography of these projections is unclear.

CASE 3 NARCOLEPSY

A 25-year-old graduate student presents with the complaint of excessive daytime fatigue, interfering with social and occupational function, beginning at age 17. She also reports difficulties with memory, concentration and attention and diffuse headaches in association with sleepiness. Colleagues and teachers have reported that she repeatedly falls asleep in class. The patient confirms a long-standing history of momentary 'blackout spells' while sedentary, not usually preceded by a premonitory subjective sense of sleepiness; these spells have also occurred while driving, resulting in a few episodes of veering into the adjoining lane. In addition, she reports automatisms, wherein she types illegibly on the computer as she falls asleep. Upon questioning, she reports vivid dreams during sleep, usually with a threatening content and associated with an inability to move to extricate herself from the imagined danger. She also recalls rare episodes of cataplexy—the sudden onset of weakness in her facial muscles after laughter or anger. On one occasion, she collapsed in a store when she lost all motor ability in both legs for a few minutes; she was rushed to the emergency room and released within a few hours, with no positive findings. She maintains regular bedtimes, obtaining 8 hours of sleep each night. She naps for 2 hours a day on weekends, finding naps to be refreshing; naps are associated with dreams.

Past medical and psychiatric histories are negative, and she takes no medications. She consumes two caffeinated beverages in the morning, which allows her to function at a nominal cognitive level in the morning. Serum laboratory tests, including TSH, are within normal limits. The Epworth Sleepiness Scale (ESS) score is 19, which is elevated. Polysomnography reveals high proportions of stages 1 and 2 sleep; diminished proportions of slow-wave sleep; multiple awakenings and arousals, most prominently during rapid eye movement (REM) sleep; and a short REM latency of 67 minutes. The apnoea-hypopnoea index is within normal limits at 1.2. Multiple sleep latency testing performed during the day following the nocturnal polysomnogram reveals a mean sleep latency of 2.5 minutes and three sleep-onset REM episodes.

Discussion: This case illustrates narcolepsy with cataplexy. Consistent with the diagnosis are the symptoms of excessive daytime somnolence with consequent sleep attacks, a high ESS score, cataplexy, hypnagogic hallucinations and sleep paralysis. The mean sleep latency score of less than 8 minutes in conjunction with two or more sleep-onset REM episodes, in the context of no other sleep, medical, or neurological pathology, confirms the diagnosis of narcolepsy.

Although the cause of human narcolepsy is unknown, recent studies have demonstrated an enhanced pattern of gliosis, as visualized through glial fibrillary acidic protein–labelled astrocytes in the hypothalamus and, to a lesser extent, the thalamus of narcoleptic brains compared with those of controls. Gliosis is thought to be the basis of the destruction of hypocretin or orexin neurones in the perifornical area of the posterior hypothalamus; under normal conditions, these neurones have widespread projections throughout the human central nervous system, with dense innervations of the hypothalamus, histaminergic tuberomammillary nucleus, noradrenergic locus coeruleus, serotoninergic raphe nuclei, dopaminergic ventral tegmental area, midline thalamus and nucleus of the diagonal band–nucleus basalis complex of the forebrain. This pattern of projections from the hypocretin neurones is thought to play an important role in arousal and maintenance of the awake state. The cause of the destruction of hypocretin neurones is unknown, but a high association between the human leukocyte antigen (HLA) allele DQB1*0602 and narcolepsy suggests a common genetic pathophysiological mechanism for the disorder. Because most other HLA-associated disorders are autoimmune in nature (e.g. multiple sclerosis, myasthenia gravis, systemic lupus erythematosus), narcolepsy may be an autoimmune disorder as well.

Hypothalamic neurones projecting to autonomic neurones are found in the paraventricular nucleus (oxytocin and vasopressin neurones), perifornical and dorsomedial nuclei (atrial natriuretic peptide neurones), lateral hypothalamic area (α-melanocyte-stimulating hormone neurones) and zona incerta (dopamine neurones). These fibres run through the medial forebrain bundle into the tegmentum, ventrolateral medulla and dorsal lateral funiculus of the spinal cord. In the brain stem, fibres innervate the parabrachial nucleus, nucleus ambiguus, nucleus of the solitary tract and dorsal motor nucleus of the vagus. In the spinal cord, they end on sympathetic and parasympathetic preganglionic neurones in the intermediolateral column. Both oxytocin- and vasopressin-containing fibres can be traced to the most caudal spinal autonomic neurones.

The medial mammillary nucleus gives rise to a large ascending fibre bundle that diverges into mammillothalamic and mammillotegmental tracts (see Fig. 15.11). The mammillothalamic tract ascends through the lateral hypothalamus to reach the anterior thalamic nuclei, where massive projections radiate to the cingulate gyrus. The mammillotegmental tract curves inferiorly into the midbrain, ventral to the medial longitudinal fasciculus, and is distributed to the tegmental reticular nuclei.

Pituitary Gland

The pituitary gland, or hypophysis cerebri, is a reddish grey ovoid body approximately 12 mm in transverse diameter and 8 mm in anteroposterior diameter, weighing approximately 500 mg (see Fig. 5.8; Fig. 15.13). It is continuous with the infundibulum, a hollow, conical inferior process from the tuber cinereum of the hypothalamus. It lies within the pituitary fossa of the sphenoid bone, where it is covered superiorly by a circular diaphragma sellae of dura mater. The latter is pierced centrally by an aperture for the infundibulum and separates the anterior superior aspect of the pituitary from the optic chiasma. The pituitary is flanked by the cavernous sinuses and their contents. Inferiorly, it is separated from the floor of the pituitary fossa by a venous sinus that communicates with the circular sinus. The meninges blend with the pituitary capsule and are not separate layers.

The pituitary has two major parts—neurohypophysis and adenohypophysis—which differ in their origin, structure and function. The neurohypophysis is a diencephalic downgrowth connected with the hypothalamus. The adenohypophysis is an ectodermal derivative of the stomatodeum. Both include parts of the infundibulum (whereas the older terms 'anterior lobe' and 'posterior lobe' do not). The infundibulum has a central infundibular stem that contains neural hypophysial connections and is continuous with the median eminence of the tuber cinereum. Thus, the neurohypophysis includes the median eminence, infundibular stem and neural lobe or pars posterior. Surrounding the infundibular stem is the pars tuberalis, a component of the adenohypophysis. The main mass of the adenohypophysis can be divided into the pars anterior (pars distalis) and the pars intermedia, which are separated in fetal and early postnatal life by the hypophysial cleft, a vestige of Rathke's pouch, from which it develops. Although usually obliterated in childhood, remnants may persist in the form of cystic cavities near the adenoneurohypophysial frontier, sometimes invading the neural lobe. The human pars intermedia is rudimentary. It may be partially displaced into the neural lobe, so it has been included in the anterior and posterior parts by different observers. Apart from this equivocation, which is of little significance in view of the exiguous status of

Habenular Nuclei and Stria Medullaris

The habenular nuclei lie posteriorly at the dorsomedial corner of the thalamus, immediately deep to the ependyma of the third ventricle, with the stria medullaris thalami above and lateral. The medial habenular nucleus is a densely packed, deeply staining mass of cholinergic neurones, whereas the lateral nucleus is more dispersed and paler staining. The habenulo-interpenduncular tract, or fasciculus retroflexus, emerges from the ventral margin of the nuclei and courses ventrally, skirts the inferior zone of the thalamic mediodorsal nucleus and traverses the superomedial region of the red nucleus to reach the interpeduncular nucleus. The habenular nuclear complex is limited laterally by a fibrous lamina that enters the habenulo-interpeduncular tract. Posteriorly, the nuclei of the two sides and the internal medullary laminae are linked across the midline by the habenular commissure. The tela choroidea of the third ventricle usually arises from the ependyma at the superolateral corner of the medial habenular nucleus.

Afferent fibres to the habenular nuclei travel in the stria medullaris from the prepiriform cortex bilaterally, the basal nucleus of Meynert and the hypothalamus. Afferents from the internal segment of the globus pallidus ascend through the thalamus and may be collaterals of pallidothalamic axons. Additional inputs come from the pars compacta of the substantia nigra, the midbrain raphe nuclei and the lateral dorsal tegmental nucleus. The afferent pathways mostly end in the lateral habenular nucleus. The only identified afferent fibres to the medial habenular nucleus come from the septofimbrial nucleus.

The medial habenular nucleus sends efferent fibres to the interpeduncular nucleus of the midbrain. The lateral habenular nucleus sends fibres to the raphe nuclei and the adjacent reticular formation of the midbrain, to the pars compacta of the substantia nigra and the ventral tegmental area and to the hypothalamus and basal forebrain.

The main habenular outflow reaches the interpeduncular nucleus, mediodorsal thalamic nucleus, mesencephalic tectum and reticular formation, the largest component constituting the habenulo-interpeduncular tract to the interpeduncular nucleus. The latter provides relays to the midbrain reticular formation, from which tectotegmentospinal tracts and dorsal longitudinal fasciculi connect with autonomic preganglionic neurones controlling salivation and gastric and intestinal secretory activity and motility and with motor nuclei for mastication and deglutition.

The stria medullaris crosses the superomedial thalamic aspect, skirts medial to the habenular trigone and sends many fibres into the ipsilateral habenula. Other fibres cross in the anterior pineal lamina and decussate, as the habenular commissure, to reach the contralateral habenula. Some fibres are really commissural and interconnect the amygdaloid complexes and hippocampal cortices. They are accompanied by crossed tectohabenular fibres. Serotonin-containing fibres from the ventral ascending tegmental serotoninergic bundle, which join the habenulo-interpeduncular tract to reach the nuclei, may control neurones of the habenulopineal tract and thus influence innervation of pinealocytes. Similarly, habenular nuclear afferents from the dorsal ascending the tegmental noradrenergic bundle may influence pinealocytes.

Little is known of the physiological functions of the habenular nuclei. It has been suggested that they are involved in the control of sleep mechanisms. Although the human habenula is relatively small, it is a focus of integration of diverse olfactory, visceral and somatic afferent paths. Lesions that include this area of the medial diencephalon indicate that it plays a role in the regulation of visceral and neuroendocrine functions. Ablation of the habenula causes extensive changes in metabolism and in endocrine and thermal regulation.

Posterior Commissure

The posterior commissure, which is of unknown constitution in humans, is a small fasciculus that decussates in the posterior pineal lamina. Various small nuclei are associated with it. Among these are the interstitial nuclei of the posterior commissure, the nucleus of Darkshevich in the periaqueductal grey matter, and the interstitial nucleus of Cajal near the upper end of the oculomotor complex, closely linked with the medial longitudinal fasciculus. Fibres from all these nuclei and the fasciculus cross in the posterior commissure. It also contains fibres from thalamic and pretectal nuclei and the superior colliculi, together with fibres that connect the tectal and habenular nuclei. The destinations and functions of many of these fibres are obscure.

Pineal Gland

The pineal gland, or epiphysis cerebri (see Fig. 5.8; Fig. 15.19), is a small, reddish grey organ occupying a depression between the superior colliculi. It is inferior to the splenium of the corpus callosum, from which it is separated by the

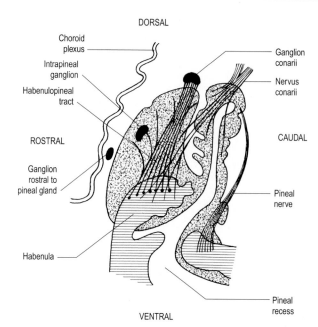

Fig. 15.19 *Principal neural pathways described in connection with the human fetal pineal gland.*

tela choroidea of the third ventricle and the contained cerebral veins. It is enveloped by the lower layer of the tela, which is reflected from the gland to the tectum. The pineal is approximately 8 mm long. Its base, directed anteriorly, is attached by a peduncle, which divides into inferior and superior laminae that are separated by the pineal recess of the third ventricle and contain the posterior and habenular commissures, respectively. Aberrant commissural fibres may invade the gland but do not terminate near parenchymal cells.

Septa extend into the pineal gland from the surrounding pia mater. They divide the gland into lobules and carry blood vessels and fine unmyelinated sympathetic axons. The gland has a rich blood supply. The pineal arteries are branches of the medial posterior choroidal arteries, which are branches of the posterior cerebral artery. Within the gland, branches of the arteries supply fenestrated capillaries whose endothelial cells rest on a tenuous and sometimes incomplete basal lamina. The capillaries drain into numerous pineal veins, which open into the internal cerebral veins or the great cerebral vein.

Postganglionic adrenergic sympathetic axons (derived from the superior cervical ganglion) enter the dorsolateral aspect of the gland from the region of the tentorium cerebelli as the nervus conarii, which may be single or paired. The nerve lies deep to the endothelium of the wall of the straight sinus. It is associated with blood vessels and parenchymal cells within the pineal.

The pineal gland contains cords and clusters of pinealocytes, associated with astrocyte-like neuroglia. Neuroglia are the main cellular component of the pineal stalk. Pinealocytes are highly modified neurones. They contain multiple synaptic ribbons, randomly distributed between adjacent cells, and are coupled by gap junctions. Two or more processes extend from each cell body and end in bulbous expansions near capillaries or, less frequently, on ependymal cells of the pineal recess. These terminal expansions contain rough endoplasmic reticulum, mitochondria and dense-core vesicles that store melatonin. Melatonin and its precursor serotonin are synthesized from tryptophan by the pinealocytes and secreted into the surrounding network of fenestrated capillaries.

The pineal is an endocrine gland of major regulatory importance. It modifies the activity of the adenohypophysis, neurohypophysis, endocrine pancreas, parathyroids, adrenal cortex, adrenal medulla and gonads. Its effects are largely inhibitory. Indolamine and polypeptide hormones secreted by pinealocytes are believed to reduce the synthesis and release of hormones by the pars anterior, either by acting directly on its secretory cells or by indirectly inhibiting the production of hypothalamic releasing factors. Pineal secretions may reach their target cells via the cerebrospinal fluid or the blood stream. Some pineal indolamines, including melatonin and enzymes for their biosynthesis (e.g. serotonin, *N*-acetyltransferase), show circadian rhythms in concentration. The level rises during darkness and falls during the day, when secretion may be inhibited by sympathetic activity. It is thought that the intrinsic

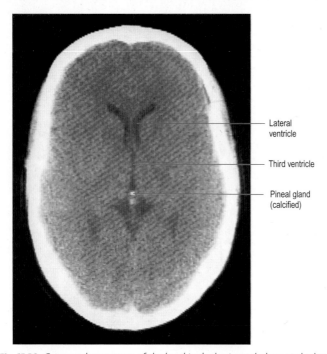

Lateral
ventricle

Third ventricle

Pineal gland
(calcified)

Fig. 15.20 *Computed tomogram of the head in the horizontal plane at the level of the pineal gland. (Courtesy of Shaun Gallagher, GKT School of Medicine, London; photograph by Sarah-Jane Smith.)*

rhythmicity of an endogenous circadian oscillator in the suprachiasmatic nucleus of the hypothalamus governs cyclical pineal behaviour.

From the second decade, calcareous deposits accumulate in pineal extracellular matrix, where they are deposited concentrically as corpora arenacea or 'brain sand' (Fig. 15.20). Calcification is often detectable in skull radiographs, where it can be a useful indicator of a space-occupying lesion if the gland is significantly displaced from the midline.

References

Benarroch, E.E., 2008. The midline and intralaminar thalamic nuclei-anatomic and functional specificity and implications in neurologic disease. Neurology 71, 944–949.

Jones, E.G., 1985. The Thalamus. Plenum Press, New York, pp. 403–411. *Describes the nomenclature and connections of thalamic nuclei.*

Macchi, G., Jones, E.G., 1997. Toward an agreement on terminology of nuclear and subnuclear divisions of the motor thalamus. J. Neurosurg. 86, 670–685. *Compares the different nomenclatures for motor thalamic nuclei in humans and monkeys and proposes a common terminology.*

Nasreddine, Z.S., Saver, J.L., 1997. Pain after thalamic stroke: right diencephalic predominance and clinical features in 180 patients. Neurology 48, 1196–1199.

Nieuwenhuys, R., 1985. Chemoarchitecture of the Brain. Springer-Verlag, Berlin. *Describes the connections and neurochemistry of the hypothalamus.*

Schmahmann, J.D., 2003. Vascular syndromes of the thalamus. Stroke. 2264–2278.

Victor, M., Adams, R.D., Collins, G.H., 1971. The Wernicke-Korsakoff syndrome. FA Davis Company, Philadelphia.

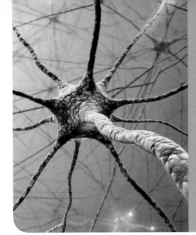

Cerebral Hemispheres

The cerebral hemispheres are the largest part of the human brain. They each have a highly convoluted external cortex, beneath which lies an extensive internal mass of white matter that contains the basal ganglia. Each hemisphere also contains a lateral ventricle, continuous with the third ventricle through the interventricular foramen. The two hemispheres are linked by the commissural fibres of the corpus callosum.

The cerebral hemisphere contains primary motor and sensory areas. These represent the highest level at which motor activities are controlled and the highest level to which general and special sensory systems project, providing the neural substrate for the conscious experience of sensory stimuli. Association areas are modality specific and also multimodal, and they enable complex analysis of the internal and external environments and of the individual's relationship to the external world. Parts of the hemisphere, termed the limbic system, have an ancient lineage. They are concerned with memory and the emotional aspects of behaviour, providing an affective patina to conscious experience and interfacing with subcortical areas, such as the hypothalamus, through which widespread physiological activities are integrated. Other areas, primarily within the frontal region, are concerned with the highest aspects of cognitive function and contribute to personality, foresight and planning.

The cerebral cortex is often divided into a phylogenetically old allocortex, consisting of the archicortex and palaeocortex, and a newer neocortex.

The cerebral hemispheres are separated by a deep median cleft, the great longitudinal fissure, which contains a crescentic fold of dura mater, the falx cerebri. Each cerebral hemisphere presents superolateral, medial and inferior surfaces or aspects.

The superolateral surface follows the concavity of the cranial vault. The medial surface is flat and vertical, separated from its fellow by the great longitudinal fissure and falx cerebri. The inferior (basal) surface is irregular and divided into orbital and tentorial regions. The orbital part of the frontal lobe is concave and lies above the orbital and nasal roofs. The tentorial region is the inferior surface of the temporal and occipital lobes. Anteriorly, it is adapted to its half of the middle cranial fossa; posteriorly, it lies above the tentorium cerebelli, which is interposed between it and the superior surface of the cerebellum. The anterior and posterior hemispheric extremities are the frontal and occipital poles, respectively, and the temporal pole is the anterior extremity of the temporal lobe.

GYRI, SULCI, AND LOBES

The surface of the cerebral hemisphere exhibits a complex pattern of convolutions, or gyri, which are separated by furrows of varying depth known as fissures, or sulci. Some of these are consistently located; others less so. In part, they provide the basis for dividing the hemisphere into lobes. The frontal, parietal, temporal and occipital lobes correspond approximately in surface extent to the cranial bones from which they take their names. The insula is a cortical region hidden within the depths of the lateral fissure by overhanging parts (opercula) of the frontal, parietal and temporal lobes. A complex of gyri on the medial aspect of the hemisphere makes up the limbic lobe.

The area of the cerebral cortex is approximately 2200 square centimetres. Its convoluted nature increases the cortical volume to three times what it would be if the surface were smooth.

On the superolateral cerebral surface, two prominent furrows—the lateral (Sylvian) fissure and the central sulcus—are the main features that determine its surface divisions (Figs 16.1, 16.3). The lateral fissure is a deep cleft on the lateral and inferior surfaces. It separates the frontal and parietal lobes above from the temporal lobe below. It has a short stem that divides into three rami. The stem commences inferiorly at the anterior perforated substance, extending laterally between the orbital surface of the frontal lobe and the anterior pole of the temporal lobe and accommodating the sphenoparietal venous sinus. Upon reaching the lateral surface of the hemisphere, it divides into anterior horizontal, anterior ascending and posterior rami. The anterior ramus runs forward for 2.5 cm or less into the inferior frontal gyrus, and

the ascending ramus ascends for an equal distance into the same gyrus. The posterior ramus is the largest. It runs posteriorly and slightly upward, across the lateral surface of the hemisphere for approximately 7 cm, and turns up to end in the parietal lobe. Its floor is the insula, and it accommodates the middle cerebral vessels.

The central sulcus (see Figs 16.1, 16.3) is the boundary between the frontal and parietal lobes. It starts in or near the superomedial border of the hemisphere, a little behind the midpoint between the frontal and occipital poles. It runs sinuously downward and forward for 8 to 10 cm to end a little above the posterior ramus of the lateral sulcus, from which it is always separated by an arched gyrus. Its general direction makes an angle of approximately 70° with the median plane. It demarcates the primary motor and somatosensory areas of the cortex, located in the precentral and postcentral gyri, respectively.

The superior frontal gyrus, above the superior frontal sulcus, is continuous over the superomedial margin with the medial frontal gyrus. It may be incompletely divided. The middle frontal gyrus is between the superior and inferior frontal sulci. The inferior frontal gyrus is below the inferior frontal sulcus and is invaded by the anterior and ascending rami of the lateral fissure. In the left hemisphere, the areas around these rami make up the motor speech area (Broca's; areas 44 and 45).

The medial cerebral surface (Figs 16.2, 16.4) lies within the great longitudinal fissure. The commissural fibres of the corpus callosum lie in the depths of the fissure. The curved anterior part of the corpus callosum is the genu, continuous below with the rostrum and narrowing rapidly as it passes back to the upper end of the lamina terminalis. The genu continues above into the trunk or body, the main part of the commissure, which arches up and back to a thick, rounded posterior extremity, the splenium. The bilateral vertical laminae of the septum pellucidum are attached to the concave surfaces of the trunk, genu and rostrum, occupying the interval between them and the fornix. In front of the lamina terminalis, and almost coextensive with it, is the paraterminal gyrus, a narrow triangle of grey matter separated from the rest of the cortex by a shallow posterior paraolfactory sulcus. A short vertical sulcus, the anterior paraolfactory sulcus, may occur a little anterior to the paraterminal gyrus. The cortex between these two sulci is the subcallosal area (paraolfactory gyrus).

The anterior region of the medial surface is divided into outer and inner zones by the curved cingulate sulcus, starting below the rostrum and passing first forward, then up and finally backward, conforming to the callosal curvature. Its posterior end turns up to the superomedial margin approximately 4 cm behind its midpoint and is posterior to the upper end of the central sulcus. The outer zone, except for its posterior extremity, is part of the frontal lobe; it is subdivided into anterior and posterior areas by a short sulcus that ascends from the cingulate sulcus above the midpoint of the corpus callosum. The larger anterior area is the medial frontal gyrus, and the posterior is the paracentral lobule. The superior end of the central sulcus usually invades the paracentral lobule posteriorly, and the precentral gyrus is continuous with the lobule. This area is concerned with movements of the contralateral lower limb and perineal region; clinical evidence suggests that it exercises voluntary control over defecation and micturition.

The zone under the cingulate sulcus is the cingulate gyrus. Starting below the rostrum, this gyrus follows the callosal curve, separated by the callosal sulcus. It continues around the splenium to the inferior surface and then into the parahippocampal gyrus through the narrow isthmus.

The posterior region of the medial surface is traversed by the parieto-occipital and calcarine sulci. These two deep sulci converge anteriorly to meet a little posterior to the splenium. The parieto-occipital sulcus marks the boundary between the parietal and occipital lobes. It starts on the superomedial margin of the hemisphere approximately 5 cm anterior to the occipital pole, sloping down and slightly forward to the calcarine sulcus. The calcarine sulcus starts near the occipital pole. Although usually restricted to the medial surface, its posterior end may reach the lateral surface. Directed anteriorly, it joins the parieto-occipital sulcus at an acute angle behind the splenium.

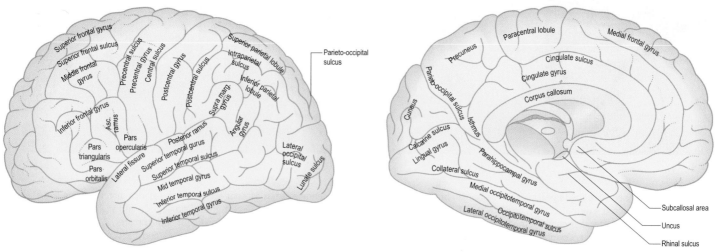

Fig. 16.1 *Lateral aspect of the left cerebral hemisphere indicating the major gyri and sulci.*

Fig. 16.2 *Sagittal section of the brain, with the brain stem removed, showing the medial aspect of the left cerebral hemisphere.*

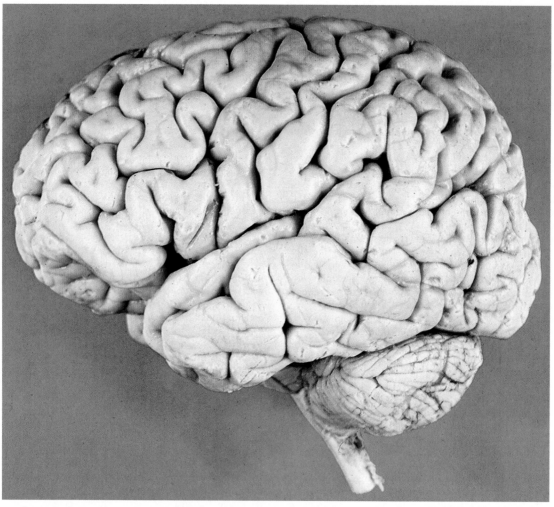

Fig. 16.3 *Left lateral aspect of the brain. (Dissection by E. L. Rees; photograph by Kevin Fitzpatrick on behalf of GKT School of Medicine, London.)*

Continuing forward, it crosses the inferomedial margin of the hemisphere and forms the inferolateral boundary of the isthmus, which connects the cingulate with the parahippocampal gyrus. The visual cortex lies above and below the posterior part of the calcarine sulcus, behind the junction with the parieto-occipital sulcus. The calcarine is deep and produces an elevation, the calcar avis, in the wall of the posterior horn of the lateral ventricle.

The area posterior to the upturned end of the cingulate sulcus, and anterior to the parieto-occipital sulcus, is the precuneus. It forms the medial surface of the parietal lobe with the part of the paracentral lobule behind the central sulcus. The medial surface of the occipital lobe is formed by the cuneus, a wedge of cortex bounded in front by the parieto-occipital sulcus, below by the calcarine sulcus and above by the superomedial margin.

The inferior cerebral surface is divided by the stem of the lateral fissure into a small anterior part and a larger posterior part (Figs 1.8, 16.5, 16.6). The anterior part is the orbital region of the inferior surface. It is transversely concave and lies above the cribriform plate of the ethmoid, the orbital plate of the frontal and the lesser wing of the sphenoid. A rostrocaudal olfactory sulcus traverses the region near its medial margin, overlapped by the olfactory bulb and tract. The medial strip thus demarcated is the gyrus rectus. The rest of this surface bears irregular orbital sulci, generally H-shaped, that divide it into the anterior, medial, posterior and lateral orbital gyri.

The larger posterior region of the inferior cerebral surface is partly superior to the tentorium as well as to the middle cranial fossa and is traversed by the anteroposterior collateral and occipitotemporal sulci (see Figs 16.2, 16.4). The

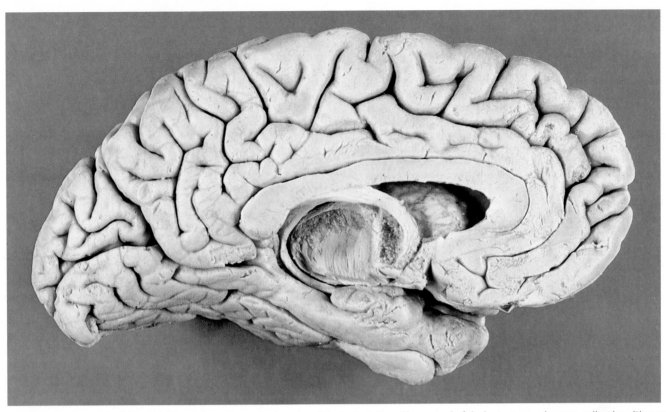

Fig. 16.4 *Medial surface of the left cerebral hemisphere after sagittal section of the brain, followed by removal of the brain stem and septum pellucidum. (Photograph by Kevin Fitzpatrick on behalf of GKT School of Medicine, London.)*

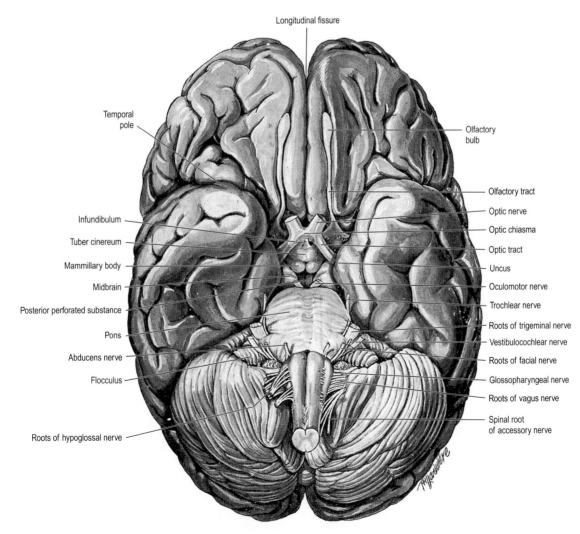

Longitudinal fissure

Temporal pole

Olfactory bulb

Olfactory tract

Optic nerve

Infundibulum

Optic chiasma

Tuber cinereum

Optic tract

Mammillary body

Uncus

Midbrain

Oculomotor nerve

Posterior perforated substance

Trochlear nerve

Roots of trigeminal nerve

Pons

Vestibulocochlear nerve

Abducens nerve

Roots of facial nerve

Flocculus

Glossopharyngeal nerve

Roots of vagus nerve

Spinal root of accessory nerve

Roots of hypoglossal nerve

Fig. 16.5 *Basal aspect of the brain.*

collateral sulcus starts near the occipital pole and extends anteriorly and parallel to the calcarine sulcus, separated from it by the lingual gyrus. Anteriorly, it may continue into the rhinal sulcus, but the two are usually separate. The rhinal sulcus (fissure) runs forward in the line of the collateral sulcus, separating the temporal pole from the hook-shaped uncus postero-medial to it. This sulcus is the lateral limit of the piriform lobe (Fig. 16.7).

The occipitotemporal sulcus is parallel to the collateral sulcus and lateral to it. It usually does not reach the occipital pole and is frequently divided.

The lingual gyrus, between the calcarine and collateral sulci, passes into the parahippocampal gyrus. The parahippocampal gyrus begins at the isthmus, where it is continuous with the cingulate gyrus, and passes forward, medial to the collateral and rhinal sulci. Anteriorly, the parahippocampal gyrus continues into the uncus, its medial edge lying lateral to the midbrain. The uncus is the anterior end of the parahippocampal gyrus and is the posterolateral boundary of the anterior perforated substance. It is part of the piriform lobe

of the olfactory system, which is phylogenetically one of the oldest parts of the cortex.

The medial occipitotemporal gyrus extends from the occipital to the temporal poles. It is limited medially by the collateral and rhinal sulci and laterally by the occipitotemporal sulcus. The lateral occipitotemporal gyrus is continuous, around the inferolateral margin of the hemisphere, with the inferior temporal gyrus.

CEREBRAL CORTEX

The microscopic structure of the cerebral cortex is an intricate blend of nerve cells and fibres, neuroglia and blood vessels. The principal cell types are described first, followed by their laminar organization within the cortex.

Microstructure

The neocortex essentially consists of three neuronal cell types. The most abundant are pyramidal cells. Non-pyramidal cells, also called stellate or granule cells, are divided into spiny and non-spiny neurones. All types have been subdivided on the basis of size and shape (Fig. 16.8).

Pyramidal cells (Fig. 16.9) have a flask-shaped or triangular cell body ranging from 10 to 80 μm in diameter. The soma gives rise to a single thick apical dendrite and multiple basal dendrites. The apical dendrite ascends toward the cortical surface, tapering and branching, to end in a spray of terminal twigs in the most superficial lamina, the molecular layer. From the basal surface of the cell body, dendrites spread more horizontally, for distances up to 1 mm for the largest pyramidal cells. Like the apical dendrite, the basal dendrites branch profusely along their length. All pyramidal cell dendrites are studded with myriad dendritic spines. These become more numerous as the distance from the parent cell soma increases. A single slender axon arises from the axon hillock, which is usually situated centrally on the basal surface of the pyramidal neurone. Ultimately, in the vast majority of (if not all) cases, the axon leaves the cortical grey matter to enter the white matter. Pyramidal cells are thus, perhaps universally, projection neurones. They appear to use excitatory amino acids, either glutamate or aspartate, exclusively as their neurotransmitters.

Spiny stellate cells are the second most numerous cell type in the neocortex and, for the most part, occupy lamina IV. They have relatively small multipolar cell bodies, commonly 6 to 10 μm in diameter. Several primary dendrites, profusely covered in spines, radiate for varying distances from the cell body. Their axons ramify within the grey matter, predominantly in the

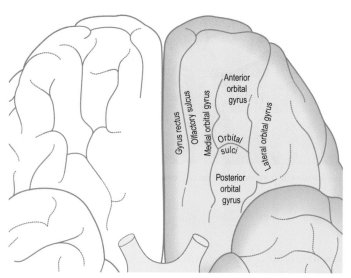

Fig. 16.6 *Orbital surface of the left frontal lobe.*

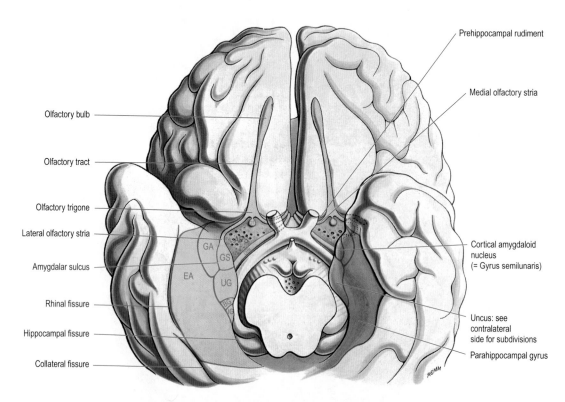

Fig. 16.7 *Inferior aspect of the brain with the brain stem removed. The right temporal pole has been displaced laterally to expose underlying structures. Structures related to the olfactory and limbic systems are coloured blue. The uncus is divided into three areas: the intralimbic gyrus (IG), the band of Giacomini (BG) and the uncinate gyrus (UG). The lateral olfactory stria continues into the gyrus semilunaris (GS), which is bordered laterally by the gyrus ambiens (GA). Farther lateral is the entorhinal area (EA), which is the rostral extension of the parahippocampal gyrus. APS, anterior perforated substance; DBB, diagonal band of Broca; OT, olfactory tubercle. (After Kuhlenbeck; from Haymaker, W., Anderson, E., Nauta, W.J.H. (Eds.), The Hypothalamus. Charles C Thomas, Springfield, Ill. By permission of Charles C Thomas Publishers, Ltd., Springfield, Ill.)*

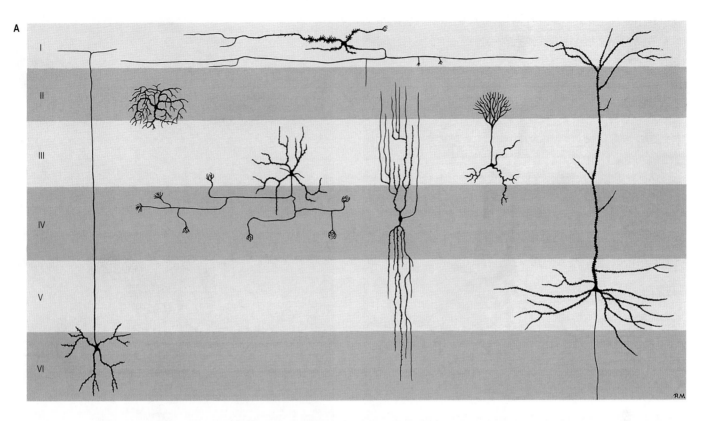

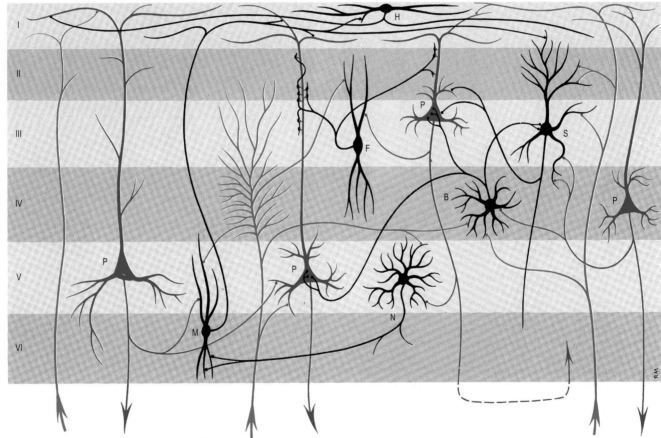

Fig. 16.8 *A, Characteristic neocortical neurones. Shown from left to right are the Martinotti (M), neurogliaform (N), basket (B), horizontal (H), fusiform (F), stellate (S) and pyramidal (P) types of neurone. B, The most frequent types of neocortical neurone, showing typical connections with one another and with afferent fibres (blue). Neurones limited to the cortex in their distribution are indicated in black. Efferent neurones are in magenta. The right and left afferent fibres are association or corticocortical connections; the central afferent is a specific sensory fibre. Neurones are shown in their characteristic lamina, but many have somata in more than one layer.*

vertical plane. Spiny stellate cells are likely to use glutamate as their neurotransmitter.

The smallest group comprises the heterogeneous non-spiny or sparsely spinous stellate cells. All are interneurones, and their axons are confined to grey matter. In morphological terms, this is not a single class of cell but a multitude of different forms, including basket, chandelier, double bouquet,

neurogliaform, bipolar-fusiform and horizontal cells. Various types may have horizontally, vertically or radially ramifying axons.

Neurones with mainly horizontally dispersed axons include basket and horizontal cells. Basket cells have a short, vertical axon that rapidly divides into horizontal collaterals; these end in large terminal sprays synapsing with the somata and proximal dendrites of pyramidal cells. The cell bodies of

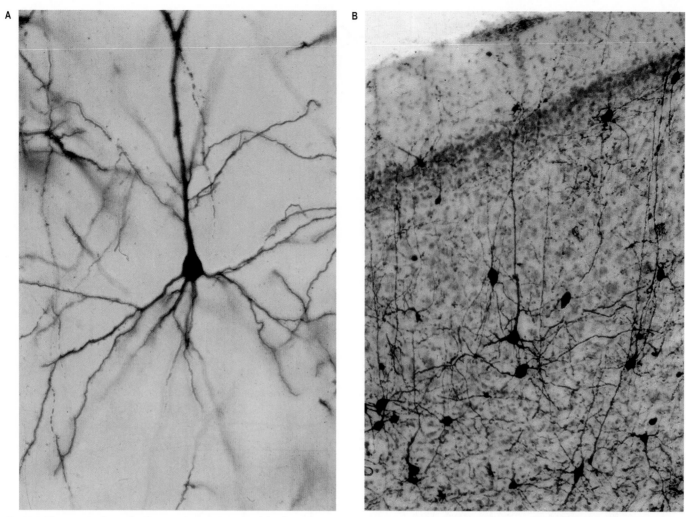

Fig. 16.9 *Neurones in the cerebral cortex.* ***A,*** *A single pyramidal cell stands out among many unstained elements.* ***B,*** *Isolated Golgi-stained neurones are prominent among the Nissl-stained cortical elements. (Preparations provided by A. R. Lieberman, Department of Anatomy, University College, London.)*

horizontal cells lie mainly at the superficial border of lamina II and occasionally deep in lamina I (the molecular or plexiform layer). They are small and fusiform, and their dendrites spread short distances in two opposite directions in lamina I. Their axons often stem from a dendrite, then divide into two branches that travel away from each other for great distances in the same layer.

Neurones with an axonal arborization that is predominantly perpendicular to the pial surface include chandelier, double bouquet and bipolar-fusiform cells. Chandelier cells have a variable morphology, although most are ovoid or fusiform, and their dendrites arise from the upper and lower poles of the cell body. The axonal arborization, which emerges from the cell body or a proximal dendrite, is characteristic and identifies these neurones. A few cells in the more superficial laminae (II and IIIa) have descending axons; deeper cells (laminae IIIc and IV) have ascending axons, and intermediate neurones (IIIb) often have both. The axons ramify close to the parent cell body and terminate in numerous vertically oriented strings that run alongside the axon hillocks of the pyramidal cells with which they synapse. Double bouquet (or bitufted) cells are found in laminae II and III, and their axons traverse laminae II and V. Generally, these neurones have two or three main dendrites that give rise to superficial and deep dendritic tufts. A single axon usually arises from the oval or spindle-shaped cell soma and rapidly divides into ascending and descending branches. These branches collateralize extensively, but the axonal arbor is confined to a perpendicularly extended yet horizontally confined cylinder, 50 to 80 μm across. Bipolar cells are ovoid, with a single ascending dendrite and a single descending dendrite that arise from the upper and lower poles, respectively. These primary dendrites branch sparsely. Their branches run vertically to produce a narrow dendritic tree, rarely more than 100 μm across, which may extend through most of the cortical thickness. Commonly, the axon originates from one of the primary dendrites and rapidly branches to form a vertically elongated, horizontally confined axonal arbor that closely parallels the dendritic tree in extent.

The principal recognizable neuronal type is the neurogliaform or spiderweb cell. These small spherical cells, 10 to 12 μm in diameter, are found mainly in

laminae II to IV, depending on the cortical area. Seven to 10 thin dendrites typically radiate from the cell soma, some branching once or twice to form a spherical dendritic field measuring 100 to 150 μm in diameter. The slender axon arises from the cell body or a proximal dendrite. Almost immediately, it branches profusely within the vicinity of the dendritic field (and usually somewhat beyond it), to form a spherical axonal arbor up to 350 μm in diameter.

The majority of non-spiny or sparsely spinous non-pyramidal cells probably use γ-aminobutyric acid (GABA) as their principal neurotransmitter. This is almost certainly the case for basket, chandelier, double bouquet, neurogliaform and bipolar cells. Some are also characterized by the coexistence of one or more neuropeptides, including neuropeptide Y, vasoactive intestinal polypeptide (VIP), cholecystokinin, somatostatin and substance P. Acetylcholine is present in a subpopulation of bipolar cells, which may also be GABAergic and contain VIP.

Laminar Organization

The most apparent microscopic feature of the neocortex stained for cell bodies or for fibres is its horizontal lamination. Its value for understanding cortical functional organization is debatable, but the use of cytoarchitectonic descriptions to identify regions of cortex is common.

Typical neocortex is described as having six layers or laminae lying parallel to the surface (Figs 16.10–16.12).

Lamina I — The molecular or plexiform layer is cell sparse, containing only scattered horizontal cells and their processes enmeshed in a compacted mass of tangential, principally horizontal axons and dendrites. These are afferent fibres, which arise from outside the cortical area, together with intrinsic fibres from cortical interneurones and the apical dendritic arbors of virtually all pyramidal neurones of the cerebral cortex. In histological sections stained to show myelin, layer I appears as a narrow horizontal band of fibres.

Lamina II — The external granular lamina contains a varying density of small neuronal cell bodies. These include both small pyramidal and non-pyramidal cells; the latter may predominate. Myelin fibre stains show mainly vertically arranged processes traversing the layer.

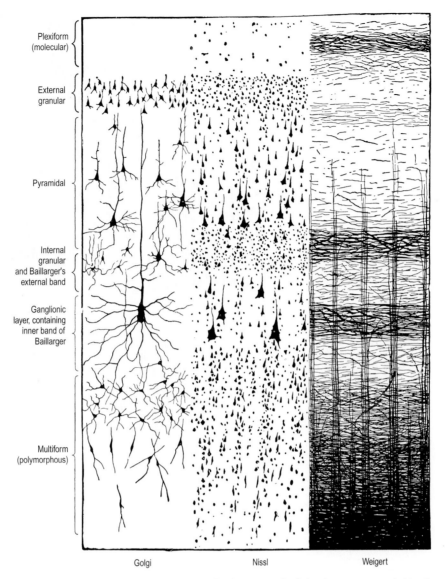

Fig. 16.10 *Layers of the cerebral cortex. The three vertical columns represent the disposition of cellular elements as revealed by the staining techniques of Golgi (impregnating whole neurones), Nissl (staining cell bodies) and Weigert (staining nerve fibres).*

Lamina III — The external pyramidal lamina contains pyramidal cells of varying sizes, together with scattered non-pyramidal neurones. The pyramidal cells are smallest in the most superficial part of the layer and largest in the deepest part. This lamina is frequently subdivided into IIIa, IIIb and IIIc, with IIIa the most superficial and IIIc the deepest. As in layer II, myelin stains reveal a mostly vertical organization of fibres.

Lamina IV — The internal granular lamina is usually the narrowest of the cellular laminae. It contains densely packed small, round cell bodies of non-pyramidal cells, notably spiny stellate cells and some small pyramidal cells. In myelin stained sections, a prominent band of horizontal fibres (outer band of Baillarger) is seen within the lamina.

Lamina V — The internal pyramidal (ganglionic) lamina typically contains the largest pyramidal cells in any cortical area, although actual sizes vary considerably from area to area. Scattered non-pyramidal cells are also present. In myelin stains, the lamina is traversed by ascending and descending vertical fibres and also contains a prominent central band of horizontal fibres (inner band of Baillarger).

Lamina VI — The multiform (or fusiform-pleomorphic) layer consists of neurones with an assortment of shapes, including recognizable pyramidal, spindle, ovoid and many other variably shaped somata. Typically, most cells are small to medium-sized. This lamina blends gradually with the underlying white matter, and a clear demarcation of its deeper boundary is not always possible.

Neocortical Structure

Five regional variations are described in neocortical structure (see Fig. 16.11). Although all are said to develop from the same six-layered pattern, two types—granular and agranular—are regarded as virtually lacking certain laminae and are referred to as heterotypical. Homotypical variants, in which all six laminae are found, are called frontal, parietal and polar—names that link them with specific cortical regions in a somewhat misleading manner (e.g. the frontal type also occurs in parietal and temporal lobes).

The agranular type has diminished or absent granular laminae (II and IV) but always contains scattered stellate somata. Large pyramidal neurones are found in the greatest densities in agranular cortex, which is typified by the numerous efferent projections of pyramidal cell axons. Although it is often equated with motor cortical areas such as the precentral gyrus (area 4), agranular cortex also occurs elsewhere, such as in areas 6, 8 and 44 and parts of the limbic system.

In the granular type of cortex, the granular layers are maximally developed and contain densely packed stellate cells, among which small pyramidal neurones are dispersed. Laminae III and IV are poorly developed or unidentifiable. This type of cortex is particularly associated with afferent projections. However, it does have efferent fibres, derived from the scattered pyramidal cells, although they are less numerous than elsewhere. Granular cortex occurs in the postcentral gyrus (somatosensory area), striate area (visual area) and superior temporal gyrus (acoustic area) and in small parts of the parahippocampal gyrus. Despite its very high density of stellate cells, especially in the striate area, it is the second thinnest of the five main types. In the striate cortex, the external band of Baillarger (lamina IV) is well defined as the stria (white line) of Gennari.

The other three types of cortex are intermediate forms. In the frontal type, large numbers of small and medium-sized pyramidal neurones appear in laminae III and V, and the granular layers (II and IV) are less prominent. The

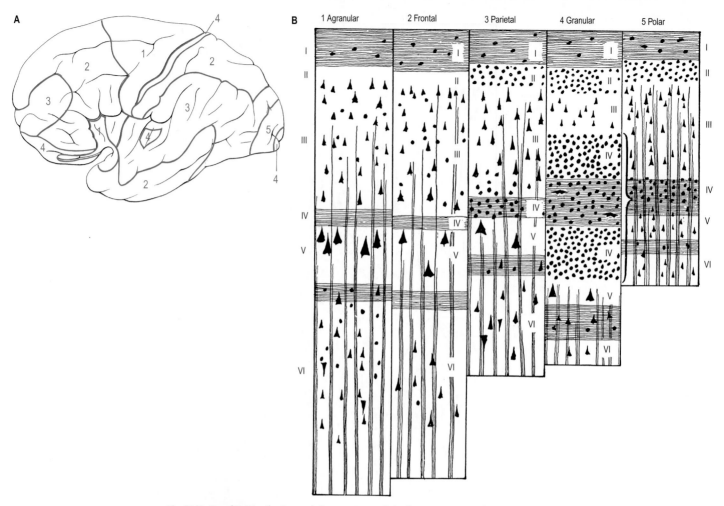

Fig. 16.11 *A and B, Distribution and characteristics of the five major types of cerebral cortex.*

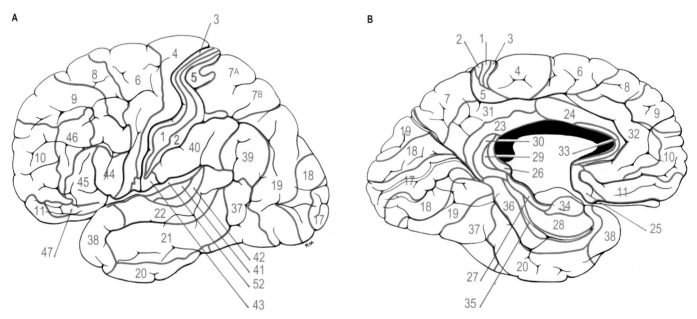

Fig. 16.12 *Lateral (A) and medial (B) surfaces of the left cerebral hemisphere depicting Brodmann's areas.*

relative prominence of these major forms of neurone vary reciprocally wherever this form of cortex exists.

The parietal type of cortex contains pyramidal cells, which are mostly smaller than in the frontal type. The granular laminae are, on the contrary, wider and contain more stellate cells. This kind of cortex occupies large areas in the parietal and temporal lobes. The polar type is classically identified with small areas near the frontal and occipital poles. It is the thinnest form of cortex. All six laminae are represented, but the pyramidal layer (III) is reduced in thickness and not as extensively invaded by stellate

cells as in the granular type of cortex. In both polar and granular types, the multiform layer (VI) is more highly organized than in other types.

For almost 100 years it has been customary to refer to discrete cortical territories not only by their anatomical location in relation to gyri and sulci but also in relation to their cytoarchitectonic characteristics as originally descried by Brodmann (see Fig. 16.12). Some of the areas so defined (e.g. the primary sensory and motor cortices) have clear relevance in terms of anatomical connections and functional significance; others less so.

Overview of Cortical Connectivity

All neocortical areas have axonal connections with other cortical areas on the same side (ipsilateral corticocortical or association connections) and on the opposite side (contralateral corticocortical or commissural connections) and with subcortical structures.

The primary somatosensory, visual and auditory areas give rise to ipsilateral corticocortical connections to the association areas of the parietal, occipital and temporal lobes, respectively, which then progressively project toward the medial temporal limbic areas, notably the parahippocampal gyrus, entorhinal cortex and hippocampus. Thus, the first somatosensory area (SI) projects to the superior parietal cortex (Brodmann's area 5), which in turn projects to the inferior parietal cortex (area 7). From there, connections pass to cortex in the walls of the superior temporal sulcus, to the posterior parahippocampal gyrus and into limbic cortex. Similarly, the primary visual cortex (area 17) projects to the parastriate cortex (area 18), which in turn projects to the peristriate region (area 19). Information then flows to inferotemporal cortex (area 20), to cortex in the walls of the superior temporal sulcus, to medial temporal areas in the posterior parahippocampal gyrus and to limbic areas. The auditory system shows a similar progression from primary auditory cortex to temporal association cortex and finally to the medial temporal lobe.

In addition to this stepwise outward progression from sensory areas through posterior association cortex, connections occur at each stage with parts of the frontal cortex. Thus, taking the somatosensory system as an example, primary somatosensory cortex (SI) in the postcentral gyrus is reciprocally connected with primary motor cortex (area 4) in the precentral gyrus. As the next step in the outward progression, the superior parietal lobule (area 5) is interconnected with the premotor cortex (area 6), which in turn is connected with area 7 in the inferior parietal lobule. This has reciprocal connections with prefrontal association cortex on the lateral surface of the hemisphere (areas 9 and 46) and with temporal association areas, which connect with more anterior prefrontal association areas and, ultimately, with orbitofrontal cortex. Similar stepwise links exist between areas on the visual and auditory association pathways in the occipitotemporal lobe and areas of the frontal association cortex. The connections between sensory and association areas are reciprocal.

All neocortical areas are connected with subcortical regions, although the density of these connections varies among areas. First among these are connections with the thalamus (Ch. 15). All areas of the neocortex receive afferents from more than one thalamic nucleus, and all such connections are reciprocal. The vast majority of (if not all) cortical areas project to the striatum, tectum, pons and brain stem reticular formation. Additionally, all cortical areas are reciprocally connected with the claustrum; the frontal cortex connects with the anterior part, and the occipital lobe with the posterior part.

All cortical areas receive a topographically organized cholinergic projection from the basal forebrain, which is profoundly affected by the neurodegenerative processes of Alzheimer's disease. Similarly, noradrenergic fibres pass to all cortical areas from the locus coeruleus, as do serotoninergic fibres from the midbrain raphe nuclei, histaminergic fibres from the posterior hypothalamus and dopaminergic fibres from the ventral midbrain.

Different cortical areas have widely different afferent and efferent connections. Some have connections that are unique, such as the corticospinal motor projection (corticospinal tract) from pyramidal cells in a restricted area around the central sulcus.

Widely separated but functionally interconnected areas of cortex share common patterns of connections with subcortical nuclei and within the neocortex. For example, contiguous zones of the striatum, thalamus, claustrum, cholinergic basal forebrain, superior colliculus and pontine nuclei connect with anatomically widely separated areas in the prefrontal and parietal cortices, which are themselves interconnected. In contrast, other cortical regions that are functionally distinct (e.g. areas in the temporal and parietal cortices) do not share such contiguity in their subcortical connections. (See Case 12.)

Cortical Lamination and Cortical Connections

The cortical laminae represent, to some extent, horizontal aggregations of neurones with common connections. This is most clearly seen in the lamination of cortical efferent (pyramidal) cells. The internal pyramidal lamina, layer V, gives rise to corticosubcortical fibres, notably corticostriate, corticobulbar, corticopontine and corticospinal axons. In addition, a significant proportion of feedback corticocortical axons arise from cells in this layer, as do some corticothalamic fibres. Layer VI, the multiform lamina, is the major source of corticothalamic fibres. Supragranular pyramidal cells—predominantly in layer III, but also in layer II—give rise primarily to both ipsilateral (association) and contralateral (commissural) corticocortical pathways. Short corticocortical fibres arise more superficially, and long corticocortical (both association and commissural) axons come from cells in the deeper parts of layer III. Major afferents to a cortical area tend to terminate in layers I, IV and VI. Quantitatively,

fewer projections end either in the intervening laminae II, III and V or sparsely throughout the depth of the cortex. Numerically, the major single input to a cortical area tends to have its main termination field in layer IV. This pattern of termination is seen in the major thalamic input to visual cortex and somatosensory cortex. In general, non-thalamic subcortical afferents to the neocortex, which are shared by widespread areas, tend to terminate throughout all cortical layers, but the laminar pattern of their endings still varies considerably from area to area.

Columns and Modules

Experimental physiological and connectional studies have demonstrated the internal organization of the cortex, which is at right angles to the pial surface, with vertical columns or modules running through the depth of the cortex. The term 'column' refers to the observation that all cells encountered by a microelectrode penetrating and passing perpendicularly through the cortex respond to a single peripheral stimulus, a phenomenon first identified in the somatosensory cortex. In the visual cortex, narrow (50 μm) vertical strips of neurones respond to a bar stimulus of the same orientation (orientation columns), and wider strips (500 μm) respond preferentially to stimuli detected by one eye (ocular dominance columns). Adjacent orientation columns aggregate within an ocular dominance column to form a hypercolumn, responding to all orientations of stimulus for both eyes for one point in the visual field. Similar functional columnar organization has been described in widespread areas of neocortex, including the motor cortex and so-called association areas.

Frontal Lobe

The frontal lobe is the rostral region of the hemisphere, anterior to the central sulcus and above the lateral fissure. On the superolateral surface, extending onto the medial surface, is the precentral gyrus, running parallel to the central sulcus and limited anteriorly by the precentral sulcus. The area of the frontal lobe anterior to the precentral sulcus is divided into the superior, middle and inferior frontal gyri (see Figs 16.1, 16.2). In front of these gyri lies the frontal pole. The ventral surface of the frontal lobe overlies the bony orbit and is the orbitofrontal cortex. The medial surface extends from the frontal pole anteriorly to the paracentral lobule behind. It consists of the medial frontal cortex and the anterior cingulate cortex.

Primary Motor Cortex

The primary motor cortex (MI) corresponds to the precentral gyrus (area 4). It is the area of cortex with the lowest threshold for eliciting contralateral muscle contraction by electrical stimulation. The primary motor cortex contains a detailed, topographically organized map (motor homunculus) of the opposite body half, with the head represented most laterally and the legs and feet represented on the medial surface of the hemisphere in the paracentral lobule (Fig. 16.13). A striking feature is the disproportionate representation of body parts in relation to their physical size. Thus, large areas represent the muscles of the hand and face, which are capable of finely controlled or fractionated movements.

The cortex of area 4 is agranular, and layers II and IV are difficult to identify. The most characteristic feature is the presence in lamina V of some extremely large pyramidal cell bodies, Betz cells, which may approach 80 μm in diameter. The axons of these neurones project into the corticospinal and corticobulbar tracts.

The major thalamic connections of area 4 are with the ventral posterolateral nucleus, which in turn receives afferents from the deep cerebellar nuclei. The ventral posterolateral nucleus also contains a topographical representation of the contralateral body, which is preserved in its point-to-point projection to area 4, where it terminates largely in lamina IV. Other thalamic connections of area 4 are with the centromedian and parafascicular nuclei. These seem to provide the only route through which output from the basal ganglia, via the thalamus, reaches the motor cortex; this appears to be the case, because the projection of the internal segment of the globus pallidus to the ventrolateral nucleus of the thalamus is confined to the anterior division, and there is no overlap with cerebellothalamic territory. The anterior part of the ventrolateral nucleus projects to the premotor and supplementary motor areas of cortex, with no projection to area 4.

The ipsilateral somatosensory cortex (SI) projects in a topographically organized way to area 4, and the connection is reciprocal. The projection to the motor cortex arises in areas 1 and 2, with little or no contribution from area 3b. Fibres from SI terminate in layers II and III of area 4, where they contact mainly pyramidal neurones. Evidence suggests that neurones activated monosynaptically by fibres from SI, as well as those activated polysynaptically, make contact with layer V pyramidal cells, which give rise to corticospinal fibres, including Betz cells. Movement-related neurones in the motor cortex that can be activated from SI tend to have a late onset of activity, mainly during the execution of movement. It has been suggested that this pathway

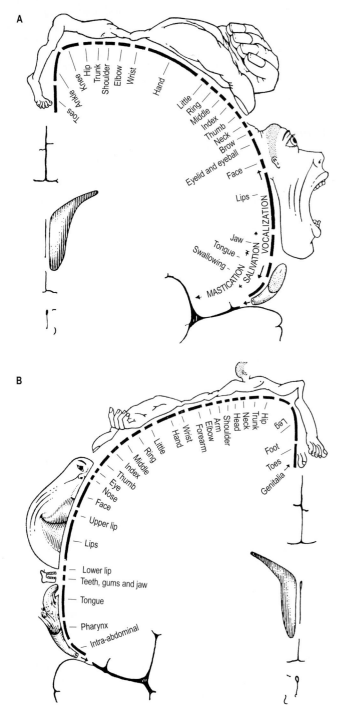

A

B

Fig. 16.13 *A, The motor homunculus showing proportional somatotopic representation in the main motor area. B, The sensory homunculus showing proportional somatotopic representation in the somaesthetic cortex. (After Penfield, W., Rasmussen, T., 1950. The Cerebral Cortex of Man. Macmillan, New York.)*

plays a role primarily in the making of motor adjustments during a movement. Additional ipsilateral corticocortical fibres to area 4 from behind the central sulcus come from the second somatosensory area (SII).

Neurones in area 4 are responsive to peripheral stimulation and have receptive fields similar to those in the primary sensory cortex. Cells located posteriorly in the motor cortex have cutaneous receptive fields, whereas more anteriorly situated neurones respond to stimulation of deep tissues.

The motor cortex receives major frontal lobe association fibres from the premotor cortex and the supplementary motor area, as well as fibres from the insula. It is probable that these pathways modulate motor cortical activity in relation to the preparation, guidance and temporal organization of movements. Area 4 sends fibres to, and receives fibres from, its contralateral counterpart and also projects to the contralateral supplementary motor cortex.

Apart from its contribution to the corticospinal tract, the motor cortex has diverse subcortical projections. The connections to the striatum and pontine nuclei are heavy. It also projects to the subthalamic nucleus. The motor cortex

sends projections to all nuclei in the brain stem, which are themselves the origin of descending pathways to the spinal cord—namely, the reticular formation, red nucleus, superior colliculus, vestibular nuclei and inferior olivary nucleus.

Corticospinal Tract — The corticospinal or pyramidal tract provides direct control by the cerebral cortex over motor centres of the spinal cord. A homologous pathway to the brain stem, the corticobulbar or corticonuclear projection, fulfills a similar function in relation to motor nuclei of the brain stem. The corticospinal tract does not originate solely from the motor cortex but is conveniently considered in conjuction with it.

The percentage of corticospinal fibres that arise from the primary motor cortex may actually be quite small, probably in the range of 20% to 30%. They arise from pyramidal cells in layer V and give rise to the largest-diameter corticospinal axons. There is also a widespread origin from other parts of the frontal lobe, including the premotor cortex and the supplementary motor area. Many axons from the frontal cortex, notably the motor cortex, terminate in the ventral horn of the spinal cord. In cord segments mediating dexterous hand and finger movements, they terminate in the lateral part of the ventral horn, in close relationship to motor neuronal groups. A small percentage establish direct monosynaptic connections with α motor neurones.

Between 40% and 60% of pyramidal tract axons arise from parietal areas, including area 3a, area 5 of the superior parietal lobe, and SII in the parietal operculum. The majority of parietal fibres to the spinal cord terminate in the deeper layers of the dorsal horn.

Corticomotor neuronal cells are active in relation to agonist muscle force of contraction; their relation to amplitude of movement is less clear. Their activity precedes the onset of electromyographic activity by 50 to 100 milliseconds, suggesting a role for cortical activation in generating rather than monitoring movement.

Premotor Cortex

Immediately in front of the primary motor cortex lies Brodmann's area 6 (Fig. 16.14). Area 6 extends onto the medial surface, where it becomes contiguous with area 24 in the cingulate gyrus, anterior and inferior to the paracentral lobule. A number of functional motor areas are contained in this cortical region. Lateral area 6, the area over most of the lateral surface of the hemisphere, corresponds to the premotor cortex. The premotor cortex is divided into dorsal and ventral areas on functional grounds and on the basis of ipsilateral corticocortical association connections.

The major thalamic connections of the premotor cortex are with the anterior division of the ventrolateral nucleus and with the centromedian, parafascicular and centrolateral components of the intralaminar nuclei. Subcortical projections to the striatum and pontine nuclei are prominent, and this area also projects to the superior colliculus and the reticular formation. Both dorsal and ventral areas contribute to the corticospinal tract. Commissural connections are with the contralateral premotor, motor and superior parietal (area 5) cortices. Ipsilateral corticocortical (association) connections with area 5 in the superior parietal cortex and inferior parietal area 7b are common to both dorsal and ventral subdivisions of the premotor cortex, and both send a major projection to the primary motor cortex. The dorsal premotor area also receives fibres from the posterior superior temporal cortex and projects to the supplementary motor cortex. The frontal eye field (area 8) projects to the dorsal subdivision. Perhaps the greatest functionally significant difference in connectivity between the two premotor area subdivisions is that the dorsal premotor area receives from the dorsolateral prefrontal cortex, whereas the ventral subdivision receives from the ventrolateral prefrontal cortex. All these association connections are either likely or known to be reciprocal.

Neuronal activity in the premotor cortex in relation to both preparation for movement and movement itself has been extensively studied experimentally. Direction selectivity for movement is a common feature of many neurones. In behavioural tasks, neurones in the dorsal premotor cortex show anticipatory activity and task-related discharge as well as direction selectivity, but little or no stimulus-related changes. The dorsal premotor cortex is probably important in establishing a motor set or intention, contributing to motor preparation in relation to internally guided movement. In contrast, ventral premotor cortex is related more to the execution of externally (especially visually) guided movements in relation to a specific external stimulus.

Frontal Eye Field

The frontal eye field lies predominantly within Brodmann's area 8, anterior to the superior premotor cortex (Fig. 16.15). It receives its major thalamic projection from the parvocellular mediodorsal nucleus, with additional afferents from the medial pulvinar, the ventral anterior nucleus and the suprageniculate–limitans complex. It connects with the paracentral nucleus of the intralaminar group. The thalamocortical pathways to the frontal eye field form part of a pathway from the superior colliculus, the substantia nigra and

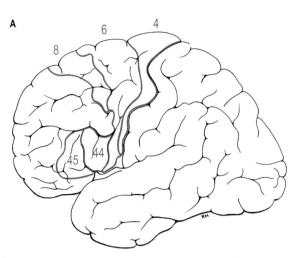

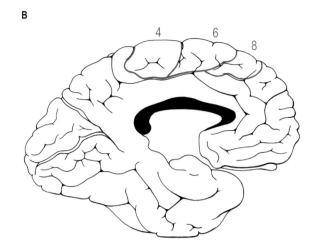

Fig. 16.14 *Lateral (A) and medial (B) surfaces of the left cerebral hemisphere showing the approximate correspondence of Brodmann's areas to the primary motor cortex (area 4), premotor areas (areas 6 and 8) and motor speech areas (areas 44 and 45).*

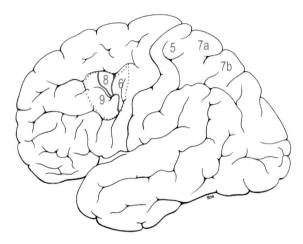

Fig. 16.15 *Lateral surface of the left cerebral hemisphere showing the frontal eye field, corresponding to parts of Brodmann's areas 6, 8 and 9. The perimeter of this area is delineated by an interrupted line to indicate the uncertainty of its precise extent.*

the dentate nucleus of the cerebellum. The frontal eye field has extensive ipsilateral corticocortical connections, receiving fibres from several visual areas in the occipital, parietal and temporal lobes, including the medial temporal area (V5) and area 7a. There is also a projection from the superior temporal gyrus, which is auditory rather than visual in function. From within the frontal lobe, the frontal eye field receives fibres from the ventrolateral and dorsolateral prefrontal cortices. It projects to the dorsal and ventral premotor cortices and to the medial motor area, probably to the supplementary eye field adjacent to the supplementary motor area proper. It projects prominently to the superior colliculus, the pontine gaze centre within the pontine reticular formation and other oculomotor-related nuclei in the brain stem. As its name implies, it is important in the control of eye movements. Destructive lesions of the frontal eye field cause ipsilateral conjugate deviation of the eyes, whereas stimulation, such as with an epileptic discharge, induces contralateral deviation.

Supplementary Motor Cortex

The supplementary motor area (MII) lies medial to area 6 and extends from the most superolateral part to the medial surface of the hemisphere. Area 24 in the cingulate gyrus adjacent to area 6 contains several motor areas, which are termed cingulate motor areas. An additional functional subdivision, the pre–supplementary motor area, lies anterior to the supplementary motor area on the medial surface of the cortex. For purposes of this discussion, these additional medial motor areas are included with the supplementary motor cortex.

The supplementary motor area receives its major thalamic input from the anterior part of the ventral lateral nucleus, which in turn is the major recipient of fibres from the internal segment of the globus pallidus. Additional thalamic afferents are from the ventral anterior nucleus; the intralaminar nuclei, notably the centrolateral and centromedial nuclei; and the mediodorsal nucleus. The

CASE 1 GAZE DEVIATION

A 75-year-old, right-handed man with a long history of hypertension and hypercholesterolemia is admitted to the hospital after awakening with left-sided weakness. He is mildly confused but awake and able to answer questions. The visual fields are full to confrontation. Head and eyes are deviated to the right, and he has a left hemiplegia and left hemihypaesthesia. Magnetic resonance imaging (MRI) shows a large ischaemic infarct in the territory of the right middle cerebral artery.

Subsequent examinations continue to document head and eye deviations to the right. The vestibulo-ocular ('doll's eye') reflex induces only very transient eye movements to the left of midline. Four days after admission, the head deviation has improved significantly, as has spontaneous eye movement to the left of the midline. Thereafter, the patient is increasingly able to direct his gaze to the left.

Discussion: Acute destructive (ischaemic) cerebral hemispheric lesions involving the frontal ('adversive') eye field are well known to produce ipsilateral eye deviation, with a markedly impaired ability to direct voluntary gaze past the midline to the opposite side on command. Over a period of several days, the gaze deviation generally improves and ultimately resolves. This is in contrast to an irritative lesion (e.g. a focal seizure), which induces deviation of the head and eyes to the opposite side.

connections with the thalamus are reciprocal. The supplementary motor cortex receives connections from widespread regions of the ipsilateral frontal lobe, including the primary motor cortex; the dorsal premotor area; the dorsolateral and ventrolateral prefrontal, medial prefrontal and orbitofrontal cortex; and the frontal eye field. These connections are reciprocal, but the major ipsilateral efferent pathway is to the motor cortex. Parietal lobe connections of the supplementary motor cortex are with superior parietal area 5 and possibly inferior parietal area 7b. Contralateral connections are with the supplementary motor area and motor and premotor cortices of the contralateral hemisphere. Subcortical connections, other than with the thalamus, pass to the striatum, subthalamic nucleus, pontine nuclei, brain stem reticular formation and inferior olivary nucleus. The supplementary motor area makes a substantial contribution to the corticospinal tract, contributing as much as 40% of the fibres from the frontal lobe.

The supplementary motor area contains a representation of the body in which the leg is posterior and the face anterior, with the upper limb between them. Its role in the control of movement involves primarily complex tasks, which require temporal organization of sequential movements and retrieval of motor memory. The consequences of damage to the supplementary motor area bear some striking similarities to the effects of basal ganglia dysfunction; akinesia is common, and there may be problems with the performance of sequential, complex movements. Stimulation of the supplementary motor area in conscious patients has been reported to elicit the sensation of an urge to move or the feeling that a movement is about to occur. A region anterior to the supplementary motor area for face representation is important in vocalization and speech production.

Prefrontal Cortex

The prefrontal cortex on the lateral surface of the hemisphere comprises predominantly Brodmann's areas 9, 46 and 45 (see Figs 16.12, 16.14, 16.15). In non-human primates, two subdivisions of the lateral prefrontal cortex are recognized: a dorsal area equivalent to area 9 and perhaps including the superior part of area 46, and a ventral area consisting of the inferior part of area 46 and area 45. Areas 44 and 45 are particularly notable in humans because, in the dominant hemisphere, they constitute the motor speech area (Broca's area; see Case 12). Both the dorsolateral and ventrolateral prefrontal areas receive their major thalamic afferents from the mediodorsal nucleus, and there are additional contributions from the medial pulvinar, the ventral anterior nucleus and the paracentral nucleus of the anterior intralaminar group. The dorsolateral area receives long association fibres from the posterior and middle superior temporal gyrus, including auditory association areas; from parietal area 7a; and from much of the middle temporal cortex. From within the frontal lobe it also receives projections from the frontal pole (area 10) and from the medial prefrontal cortex (area 32) on the medial surface of the hemisphere. It projects to the supplementary motor area, the dorsal premotor cortex and the frontal eye field. All these thalamic and corticocortical connections are reciprocal. Commissural connections are with the homologous area and with the contralateral inferior parietal cortex. The ventrolateral prefrontal area receives long association fibres from areas 7a and 7b of the parietal lobe, auditory association areas of the temporal operculum, the insula and the anterior part of the lower bank of the superior temporal sulcus. From within the frontal lobe it receives fibres from the anterior orbitofrontal cortex and projects to the frontal eye field and the ventral premotor cortex. It connects with the contralateral homologous area via the corpus callosum. These connections are probably all reciprocal.

The cortex of the frontal pole (area 10) receives thalamic input from the mediodorsal nucleus, the medial pulvinar and the paracentral nucleus. It is reciprocally connected with the cortex of the temporal pole, the anterior orbitofrontal cortex and the dorsolateral prefrontal cortex. The orbitofrontal cortex connects with the mediodorsal, anteromedial, ventral anterior, medial pulvinar, paracentral and midline nuclei of the thalamus. Cortical association pathways come from the inferotemporal cortex, the anterior superior temporal gyrus and the temporal pole. Within the frontal lobe, it has connections with the medial prefrontal cortex, the ventrolateral prefrontal cortex and medial motor areas. Commissural and other connections follow the general pattern for all neocortical areas.

The medial prefrontal cortex is connected with the mediodorsal, ventral anterior, anterior medial pulvinar, paracentral, midline and suprageniculate–limitans nuclei of the thalamus. It receives fibres from the anterior cortex of the superior temporal gyrus. Within the frontal lobe, it has connections with the orbitofrontal cortex and the medial motor areas of the dorsolateral prefrontal cortex.

Information on the detailed functions of the subregions of the prefrontal cortex is sparse. The dorsolateral prefrontal cortex is important for spatial processing of afferent information and for the organization of self-ordered working memory tasks, including verbal working memory. The ventrolateral prefrontal cortex is concerned with the mnemonic processing of objects.

Evidence from surgical lesions (prefrontal lobotomy) or pathological damage suggests a role for the prefrontal cortex in the appreciation or understanding of time, the normal expression of emotions (affect) and the ability to predict the consequences of actions. Both hemispheres interact in these functions, so deficits following unilateral damage may be relatively slight. The medial prefrontal cortex as a whole is important in auditory and visual associations, and widespread changes in prefrontal activation are associated with calculating, thinking and decision making.

Parietal Lobe

The parietal lobe lies posterior to the central sulcus. On the medial aspect of the hemisphere, its boundary with the occipital lobe is clearly demarcated by the deep parieto-occipital sulcus. On the lateral aspect of the hemisphere, its boundaries with the occipital and temporal lobes are less distinct and somewhat arbitrary. The inferior boundary is the posterior ramus of the lateral fissure and its imaginary posterior prolongation.

The lateral aspect of the parietal lobe is divided into three areas by postcentral and intraparietal sulci (see Fig. 16.1). The postcentral sulcus, often divided into upper and lower parts, is posterior and parallel to the central sulcus. Inferiorly, it ends above the posterior ramus of the lateral fissure. The postcentral gyrus or primary somatosensory cortex lies between the central and postcentral sulci. Posterior to the postcentral sulcus there is a large area, subdivided by the intraparietal sulcus. It usually starts in the postcentral sulcus near its midpoint and extends posteroinferiorly across the parietal lobe, dividing it into superior and inferior parietal lobules. Posteriorly, its occipital ramus extends into the occipital lobe, joining the transverse occipital sulcus at right angles.

The superior parietal lobule, between the superomedial margin of the hemisphere and the intraparietal sulcus, is continuous anteriorly with the postcentral gyrus around the upper end of the postcentral sulcus; posteriorly, it often joins the arcus parieto-occipitalis, surrounding the lateral part of the parieto-occipital sulcus.

The inferior parietal lobule, below the intraparietal sulcus and behind the lower part of the postcentral sulcus, is divided into three parts. The anterior part is the supramarginal gyrus, which arches over the upturned end of the lateral fissure. It is continuous anteriorly with the lower part of the postcentral gyrus and posteroinferiorly with the superior temporal gyrus. The middle part of the inferior parietal lobule, called the angular gyrus, arches over the end of the superior temporal sulcus and is continuous posteroinferiorly with the middle temporal gyrus. The posterior part of the inferior parietal lobule arches over the upturned end of the inferior temporal sulcus onto the occipital lobe, forming an arcus temporo-occipitalis.

Somatosensory Cortex

The postcentral gyrus corresponds to the primary somtosensory cortex (SI; Brodmann's areas 3a, 3b, 1 and 2). Area 3a lies most anteriorly, apposing area 4, the primary motor cortex of the frontal lobe; area 3b is buried in the posterior wall of the central sulcus; area 1 lies along the posterior lip of the central sulcus; and area 2 occupies the crown of the postcentral gyrus.

The primary somatosensory cortex contains within it a topographical map of the contralateral half of the body. The face, tongue and lips are represented inferiorly; the trunk and upper limbs are represented on the superolateral aspect and the lower limbs on the medial aspect of the hemisphere, giving rise to the familiar 'homunculus' map (see Fig. 16.13).

The somatosensory properties of SI depend on its thalamic input from the ventral posterior nucleus of the thalamus, which in turn receives the medial lemniscal, spinothalamic and trigeminothalamic pathways. The nucleus is

CASE 3 PARIETAL LOBE DISEASE

A 68-year-old right-handed hypertensive woman is admitted to the hospital following the abrupt development of a left hemiparesis and a hemisensory syndrome characterized primarily by impaired proprioception on the left side. When seen acutely, the patient denies her motor deficit (anosognosia) and in fact denies the very existence of her paretic side (hemisomatotopagnosia). With sensory testing, she ignores (neglects) the left side of her body, as demonstrated with double simultaneous stimulation, and fails to attend to the left side of space. She is mentally confused.

Discussion: This woman exhibits a serious disorder of the body scheme (body image) as a result of an acute (vascular) lesion (infarction) involving primarily the right (non-dominant) parietal cortex. Impaired proprioception and at least some degree of mental confusion are characteristic components of the clinical syndrome. Within several days of onset, the hemisomatotopagnosia disappears, and she becomes increasingly aware of the existence of her hemiparesis. The sensory inattention may persist indefinitely.

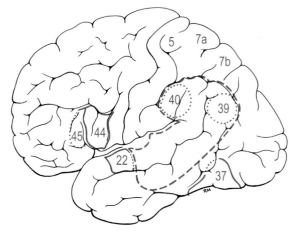

Fig. 16.16 *Lateral surface of the left hemisphere showing the motor speech areas (44 and 45) and areas 5, 7a and 7b. Wernicke's area is variously depicted by different authorities and is tentatively indicated here by the large parietotemporal area enclosed by the* dotted line *and including areas 39 and 40. Some consider areas 22 and 37 to be auditory and visuo-auditory areas, respectively, associated with speech and language.*

divided into a ventral posterolateral part, which receives information from the trunk and limbs, and a ventral posteromedial part, in which the head is represented. Within the ventral posterior nucleus, neurones in the central core respond to cutaneous stimuli, and those in the most dorsal anterior and posterior parts, which arch as a 'shell' over this central core, respond to deep stimuli. This is reflected in the differential projections to SI: the cutaneous central core projects to 3b, the deep tissue–responsive neurones send fibres to areas 3a and 2 and an intervening zone projects to area 1. Within the ventral posterior nucleus, anteroposterior rods of cells respond with similar modality and somatotopic properties. They appear to project to restricted focal patches in SI of approximately 0.5 mm, which form narrow strips mediolaterally along SI. The laminar termination of thalamocortical axons from the ventral posterior nucleus is different in the separate cytoarchitectonic subdivisions of SI. In areas 3a and 3b these axons terminate mainly in layer IV and the adjacent deep part of layer III, whereas in areas 1 and 2 they end in the deeper half of layer III, avoiding lamina IV. Additional thalamocortical fibres to SI arise from the intralaminar system, notably the centrolateral nucleus.

There is a complex internal connectivity within SI. An apparently stepwise hierarchical progression of information processing occurs from area 3b through area 1 to area 2. Outside the postcentral gyrus, SI has ipsilateral corticocortical association connections with a second somatosensory area (SII); area 5 in the superior parietal lobe; area 4, the motor cortex, in the precentral gyrus; and the supplementary motor cortex in the medial part of area 6 of the frontal lobe.

SI has reciprocal commissural connections with its contralateral homologue, with the exception that the cortices containing the representation of the distal extremities are relatively devoid of such connections. Callosal fibres in SI arise mainly from the deep part of layer III and terminate in layers I to IV. Callosally projecting pyramidal cells receive monosynaptic thalamic and commissural connections.

SI has reciprocal subcortical connections with the thalamus and claustrum and receives afferents from the basal nucleus of Meynert, the locus coeruleus and the midbrain raphe. It has other prominent subcortical projections. Corticostriatal fibres, arising in layer V, pass mainly to the putamen of the same side. Corticopontine and corticotectal fibres from SI arise in layer V. SI projects to the main pontine nuclei and to the pontine tegmental reticular nucleus. In addition, axons arising in SI pass to the dorsal column nuclei and the spinal cord. Corticospinal pyramidal cells are found in layer V of SI. The topographical representation in the cortex is preserved in terms of the spinal segments to which different parts of the postcentral gyrus project. Thus, the arm representation projects to the cervical enlargement, the leg representation to the lumbosacral enlargement and so on. Within the grey matter of the spinal cord, fibres from SI terminate in the dorsal horn, Rexed's laminae III to

V. Fibres from areas 3b and 1 end more dorsally, and those from area 2 more ventrally.

The second somatosensory area (SII) lies along the upper bank of the lateral fissure, posterior to the central sulcus. SII contains a somatotopic representation of the body, with the head and face most anteriorly, adjacent to SI, and the sacral regions most posteriorly. SII is reciprocally connected with the ventral posterior nucleus of the thalamus in a topographically organized fashion. Some thalamic neurones probably project to both SI and SII via axon collaterals. Other thalamic connections of SII are with the posterior group of nuclei and with the intralaminar central lateral nucleus. SII also projects to laminae IV to VII of the dorsal horn of the cervical and thoracic spinal cord, the dorsal column nuclei, the principal trigeminal nucleus and the periaqueductal grey matter of the midbrain.

Within the cortex, SII is reciprocally connected with SI in a topographically organized manner and projects to the primary motor cortex. SII also projects in a topographically organized way to the lateral part of area 7 (area 7b) in the superior parietal lobe, and it makes connections with the posterior cingulate gyrus. Across the corpus callosum, both right and left SII areas are interconnected, although distal limb representations are probably excluded. There are additional callosal projections to SI and area 7b.

Experimental studies show that neurones in SII respond particularly to transient cutaneous stimuli, such as brush strokes or tapping, which are characteristic of the responses of Pacinian corpuscles in the periphery. They show little response to maintained stimuli.

Superior and Inferior Parietal Lobules

Posterior to the postcentral gyrus, the superior part of the parietal lobe is composed of areas 5, 7a and 7b (see Fig. 16.12; Fig. 16.16). Area 5 receives a dense feed-forward projection from all cytoarchitectonic areas of SI in a topographically organized manner. The thalamic afferents to this area come from the lateral posterior nucleus and from the central lateral nucleus of the intralaminar group. Ipsilateral corticocortical fibres from area 5 go to area 7, the premotor and supplementary motor cortices, the posterior cingulate gyrus and the insular granular cortex. Commissural connections between area 5 on both sides tend to avoid the areas of representation of the distal limbs. The response properties of cells in area 5 are more complex than in SI, with larger receptive fields and evidence of submodality convergence. Area 5 contributes to the corticospinal tract.

In non-human primates, the inferior parietal lobe is area 7. In humans, this area is more superior, and areas 39 and 40 intervene inferiorly. The counterparts of the latter areas in monkeys are unclear, and there is little experimental evidence of their connections and functions. Their role in human cerebral processing is discussed later. In the monkey, area 7b receives somatosensory inputs from area 5 and SII. Connections pass to the posterior cingulate gyrus (area 23), insula and temporal cortex. Area 7b is reciprocally connected with area 46 in the prefrontal cortex and the lateral part of the premotor cortex. Commissural connections of area 7b are connected with the contralateral homologous area and with SII, the insular granular cortex and area 5. Thalamic connections are with the medial pulvinar nucleus and the intralaminar paracentral nucleus.

In monkeys, area 7a is not related to the cortical pathways for somatosensory processing; instead, it forms part of a dorsal cortical pathway for spatial vision. The major ipsilateral corticocortical connections to area 7a are derived from visual areas in the occipital and temporal lobes. In the ipsilateral hemisphere, area 7a has connections with the posterior cingulate cortex (area 24) and with areas 8 and 46 of the frontal lobe. Commissural connections are with its contralateral homologue. Area 7a is connected with the medial pulvinar and intralaminar paracentral nuclei of the thalamus. In experimental studies, neurones within area 7a are visually responsive. They relate largely to peripheral vision, respond to stimulus movement and are modulated by eye movement.

Injury of the superior parietal cortex in humans can lead to the inability to recognize the shapes of objects by touch (astereognosis) and a variety of disorders reflecting breakdown of the body scheme or body image, such as difficulty assimilating spatial perception of the body (amorphosynthesis) and sensory neglect of the contralateral body (asomatognosia), which causes a variety of syndromes, including so-called dressing apraxia (see Case 3). More complex perceptional disturbances follow damage of the inferior parietal cortex, including areas 39 and 40. These include difficulties with language, because Wernicke's speech area includes parts of the inferior parietal lobe of the dominant hemisphere (see Fig. 16.16 and Case 12), and dyscalculia if the dominant hemisphere is involved. Contralateral sensory neglect extends to the extracorporeal space and includes the visual appreciation of the world, such as the omission of one side (usually the left) of a drawing when a patient is asked to copy a sketch of a clock face. Difficulties with complex orientation in space, such as map reading, are also seen.

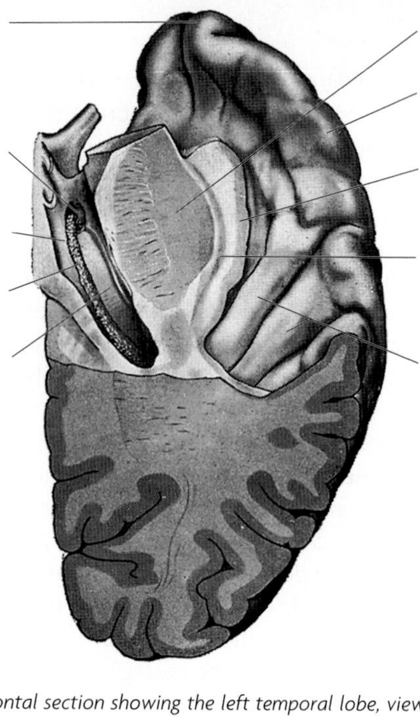

Fig. 16.17 *Horizontal section showing the left temporal lobe, viewed from below.*

CASE 4   GERSTMANN'S SYNDROME

A 72-year-old right-handed man with a history of hypertension, a remote myocardial infarction, and dyslipidemia awakens on the morning of admission and experiences trouble talking—speaking 'gibberish' according to his wife. On examination in the hospital, he is noted to have a fluent aphasia, with language functioning returning to normal after several hours. However, he now exhibits an inability to correctly identify specific fingers on the examiner's hands, left–right confusion, inability to write dictated words without dyslexia, and dyscalculia for simple arithmetic.

MRI of the brain with diffusion imaging reveals an area of acute infarction in the region of the left posterior temporal and parietal region.

Discussion: Gerstmann's syndrome consists of finger agnosia, left–right confusion, dysgraphia and dyscalculia. These four signs only uncommonly appear in isolation. Gerstmann's syndrome has long been thought to be characteristic of lesions, usually vascular, involving the angular and supramarginal gyri of the dominant, thus usually left, hemisphere.

Temporal Lobe

The temporal lobe is inferior to the lateral fissure. It is limited behind by an arbitrary line from the preoccipital incisure to the parieto-occipital sulcus, which meets the superomedial margin of the hemisphere approximately 5 cm from the occipital pole. Its lateral surface is divided into three parallel gyri by two sulci.

The superior temporal sulcus begins near the temporal pole and slopes slightly up and backward, parallel to the posterior ramus of the lateral sulcus. Its end curves up into the parietal lobe. The inferior temporal sulcus is subjacent and parallel to the superior and is often broken into two or three short sulci. Its posterior end also ascends into the parietal lobe, posterior and parallel to the upturned end of the superior sulcus.

Thus, the lateral surface is divided into three parallel gyri: superior (area 22), middle (area 21) and inferior (area 20) temporal gyri. The temporal pole

(area 38) lies in front of the termination of these gyri. Along its superior margin, the superior temporal gyrus is continuous with gyri in the floor of the posterior ramus of the lateral sulcus. These vary in number and extend obliquely anterolaterally from the circular sulcus around the insula as transverse temporal gyri of Heschl (Fig. 16.17). The anterior transverse temporal gyrus and adjoining part of the superior temporal gyrus are auditory in function and are considered to be Brodmann's area 42. The anterior gyrus is approximately area 41.

Cortex of the medial temporal lobe includes major subdivisions of the limbic system, such as the hippocampus and entorhinal cortex. Areas of neocortex adjacent to these limbic regions are grouped together as medial temporal association cortex. The temporal and frontal lobes are expanded enormously in humans. This poses the problem of relating physiological and anatomical studies of non-human primates to human brain topography. In general, the commonly studied Old World monkeys lack a middle temporal gyrus.

CASE 5   TEMPORAL LOBE EPILEPSY

A 27-year-old right-handed woman complains of intermittently smelling odors, usually unpleasant, occasionally accompanied by unpleasant tastes. There is no recognized external source for these hallucinatory phenomena. During several such episodes she has briefly lost the ability to speak. She also describes an associated sense of depersonalization. Observers have noted lip-smacking and chewing movements during these episodes. On at least two occasions these abnormalities have been followed by a generalized seizure. She admits to having frequent déjà vu experiences since her late teens.

Discussion: This patient is experiencing repetitive complex partial seizures (so-called uncinate or psychomotor seizures). Clinically, the seizure focus is presumed to be in the vicinity of the uncus, amygdala or insula in her dominant (left) hemisphere. The location of the focus is confirmed by the appearance of anterior temporal spikes in the electroencephalogram.

Imaging demonstrates a solid anterior temporal tumour; following surgical resection, she is virtually seizure free.

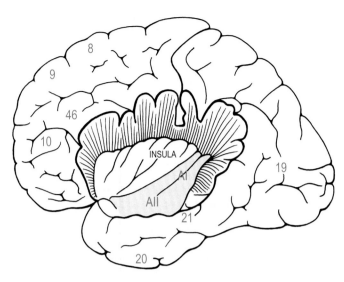

Fig. 16.18 *Lateral aspect of the left cerebral hemisphere. The opercula have been cut away to expose the insula and the adjoining anterior and posterior transverse temporal gyri and their continuity with the superior temporal gyrus.*

Auditory Cortex

The temporal operculum houses the primary auditory cortex, AI (Fig. 16.18). This is coextensive with granular area 41 in the transverse temporal gyri. Surrounding areas constitute auditory association cortex. The primary auditory cortex is reciprocally connected with all subdivisions of the medial geniculate nucleus and may receive additional thalamocortical projections from the medial pulvinar. The geniculocortical fibres terminate densely in layer IV. AI contains a tonotopic representation of the cochlea in which high frequencies are represented posteriorly and low frequencies anteriorly. Single-cell responses are to single tones of a narrow frequency band. Cells in single vertical electrode penetrations share an optimal frequency response.

The auditory cortex interconnects with prefrontal cortex, although the projections from AI are small. In general, posterior parts of the operculum project to areas 8 and 9. Central parts project to areas 8, 9 and 46. More anterior regions project to areas 9 and 46, to area 12 on the orbital surface of the hemisphere and to the anterior cingulate gyrus on the medial surface. Contralateral corticocortical connections are with the same and adjacent regions in the other hemisphere. Onward connections of the auditory association pathway converge with those of the other sensory association pathways in cortical regions within the superior temporal sulcus.

Injury of the auditory cortex in humans produces a variety of manifestations, including cortical deafness, verbal auditory agnosia and non-verbal auditory agnosia. The markedly bilateral nature of the auditory pathway means that noticeable deficits occur only when there is bilateral damage. Damage of the temporoparietal junction has effects on auditory selective attention.

Evidence suggests that area 21 in humans, the middle temporal cortex, is polysensory and that it connects with auditory, somatosensory and visual cortical association pathways. The auditory association areas of the superior temporal gyrus project in a complex, ordered fashion to the middle temporal gyrus, as does the parietal cortex. The middle temporal gyrus connects with the frontal lobe—the most posterior parts project to the posterior prefrontal cortex, areas 8 and 9, and the intermediate regions connect more anteriorly with areas 19 and 46. Farther forward, the middle temporal region has connections with anterior prefrontal areas 10 and 46 and with anterior orbitofrontal areas 11 and 14. The most anterior middle temporal cortex is connected with the posterior orbitofrontal cortex, area 12, and with the medial surface of the frontal pole. Farther forward, this middle temporal region projects to the temporal pole and the entorhinal cortex. Thalamic connections are with the pulvinar nuclei and the intralaminar group. Other subcortical connections follow the general pattern for all cortical areas. Some projections (e.g. to the pons), particularly from anteriorly in the temporal lobe, are minimal. Physiological responses of cells in this middle temporal region show a convergence of different sensory modalities, and some of these neurones are involved in facial recognition. In line with this complexity, lesions of the temporal lobe in humans can lead to considerable disturbance of intellectual function, particularly when the dominant hemisphere is involved. These disturbances can include visuospatial difficulties, prosopagnosia, hemiagnosia and severe sensory dysphasia.

CASE 6   PROSOPAGNOSIA

A 32-year-old man is riding his motorcycle without a helmet when he loses control of the vehicle and is thrown to the ground. He suffers a closed head injury and remains comatose for 3 weeks. During rehabilitation, he is unable to identify his family when shown pictures of them; however, when they come to visit he recognizes them by their voices. Brain MRI reveals diffuse cortical trauma and a right medial temporal haemorrhage.

Discussion: This man is suffering from prosopagnosia, sometimes called 'face blindness.' This rare disorder is usually caused by brain injury (right posterior cerebral artery stroke, brain trauma, neurodegenerative disease), but it can also be congenital. It is a form of visual agnosia, in that sufferers' fine visual discrimination is usually intact, such that they are able to read and can identify facial features (e.g. beard, eyeglasses), but they cannot recognize a person's face. In severe cases, patients with prosopagnosia cannot recognize themselves in a mirror. The neuronal pathways for face recognition are complex, but cerebral localization for prosopagnosia is likely the right inferior temporo-occipital area, specifically the fusiform gyrus, the inferior occipital gyrus or both. Lesions of these regions have been shown to produce prosopagnosia; however, it has also been observed with other right-sided or, in some cases, bilateral cortical injury.

The inferior temporal cortex, area 20, is a higher visual association area. The posterior inferior temporal cortex receives major ipsilateral corticocortical fibres from occipitotemporal visual areas, notably V4. It contains a coarse retinotopic representation of the contralateral visual field and sends a major feed-forward pathway to the anterior part of the inferior temporal cortex. The anterior inferior temporal cortex projects onto the temporal pole and to paralimbic areas on the medial surface of the temporal lobe. Additional ipsilateral association connections of the inferior temporal cortex are with the anterior middle temporal cortex, in the walls of the superior temporal gyrus and with visual areas of the parietotemporal cortex. Frontal lobe connections are with area 46 in the dorsolateral prefrontal cortex (posterior inferior temporal) and with the orbitofrontal cortex (anterior inferior temporal). The posterior area also connects with the frontal eye fields. Reciprocal thalamic connections are with the pulvinar nuclei; the posterior part is related mainly to the inferior and lateral nuclei, and the anterior part to the medial and adjacent lateral pulvinar. Intralaminar connections are with the paracentral and central medial nuclei. Other subcortical connections conform to the general pattern of all cortical regions. Callosal connections are between corresponding areas and the adjacent visual association areas of each hemisphere.

The cortex of the temporal pole receives feed-forward projections from widespread areas of temporal association cortex that are immediately posterior to it. The dorsal part receives predominantly auditory input from the anterior part of the superior temporal gyrus. The inferior part receives visual input from the anterior area of the inferior temporal cortex. Other ipsilateral connections are with the anterior insular, posterior and medial orbitofrontal and medial prefrontal cortices. The temporal pole projects onward into limbic and paralimbic areas. Thalamic connections are mainly with the medial pulvinar nucleus and with intralaminar and midline nuclei. Other subcortical connections are the same as for the cortex in general, although some projections, such as to the pontine nuclei, are very small. Physiological responses of cells here and in more medial temporal cortex correspond particularly to behavioural performance and to the recognition of high-level aspects of social stimuli.

Nuclei of the amygdala (see later) project to, and receive fibres from, neocortical areas, predominantly of the temporal lobe and possibly the inferior parietal cortex. The density of these pathways increases toward the temporal pole.

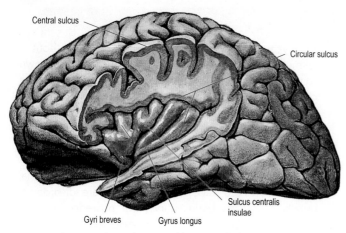

Fig. 16.19 *The insula, exposed by removal of the opercula.*

Labels: Central sulcus; Circular sulcus; Gyri breves; Gyrus longus; Sulcus centralis insulae

Insula

The insula lies deep in the floor of the lateral fissure; it is almost surrounded by a circular sulcus and is overlapped by adjacent cortical areas, the opercula (see Figs 16.17–16.20). The frontal operculum is between the anterior and ascending rami of the lateral fissure, forming a triangular division of the inferior frontal gyrus. The frontoparietal operculum, between ascending and posterior rami of the lateral fissure, consists of the posterior part of the inferior frontal gyrus, the lower ends of the precentral and postcentral gyri and the lower end of the anterior part of the inferior parietal lobule. The temporal operculum, below the posterior ramus of the lateral fissure, is formed by superior temporal and transverse temporal gyri. Anteriorly, the inferior region of the insula adjoins the orbital part of the inferior frontal gyrus.

When the opercula are removed, the insula appears as a pyramidal area, its apex beneath and near the anterior perforated substance, where the circular sulcus is deficient (see Figs 16.19, 16.20). The medial part of the apex is termed the limen insulae (gyrus ambiens). A central insular sulcus, which slants posterosuperiorly from the apex, divides the insular surface into a large anterior part and a small posterior part. The anterior part is divided by shallow sulci into three or four short gyri, whereas the posterior part is one long gyrus, often divided at its upper end. The cortex of the insula is continuous with that of its opercula in the circular sulcus. The insula is approximately coextensive with the subjacent claustrum and putamen.

Cytoarchitectonically, three zones are recognized within the insula. Anteriorly, and extending caudally into the central insula, the cortex is agranular. It is surrounded by a belt of dysgranular cortex in which laminae II and III can be recognized; this in turn is surrounded by an outer zone of homotypical granular cortex that extends to the caudal limit of the insula.

Thalamic afferents to the insula come from subdivisions of the ventral posterior nucleus and medial geniculate body, the oral and medial parts of the pulvinar, the suprageniculate–limitans complex, the mediodorsal nucleus and the nuclei of the intralaminar and midline groups. It appears that the anterior (agranular) cortex is connected predominantly with the mediodorsal and ventroposterior nuclei, whereas the posterior (granular) cortex is connected predominantly with the pulvinar and the ventral posterior nuclei. The other nuclear groups appear to connect with all areas.

Ipsilateral cortical connections of the insula are diverse. Somatosensory connections are with SI, SII and surrounding areas; area 5 of the superior parietal lobe; and area 7b of the inferior parietal lobe. The insular cortex also has connections with the orbitofrontal cortex. Several auditory regions in the temporal lobe interconnect with the posterior granular insula and the dysgranular cortex more anteriorly. Connections with visual areas are virtually absent. The anterior agranular cortex of the insula appears to have connections primarily with olfactory, limbic and paralimbic structures, including, most prominently, the amygdala. Little is known about the functions of the human insula. However, the somatosensory functions of the posterior part are clearly present in humans, and the anterior insular cortex appears to have a role in olfaction and taste. The insula also seems to be a key station in the discriminative touch pathway, which passes via SII, at least for the somatosensory pathway. The posterior region of the insula has been implicated in language functions, which raises the possibility that higher-order auditory association pathways may pass via areas in the insula.

Claustrum

The claustrum (see Figs 16.35, 16.42) is a thin sheet of grey matter lying deep to the insula. It is approximately coextensive with the insula, from which it is separated by the extreme capsule. Medially, the claustrum is separated from the putamen by the external capsule. It is thickest anteriorly and inferiorly, where it becomes continuous with the anterior perforated substance, amygdala and prepiriform cortex. In animals, it has reciprocal, topographically organized connections with many regions of the neocortex. Little is known about the connections and functional significance of the claustrum in the human brain.

Occipital Lobe

The occipital lobe lies behind an arbitrary line joining the preoccipital incisure and the parieto-occipital sulcus. The transverse occipital sulcus descends from the superomedial margin of the hemisphere, behind the parieto-occipital sulcus, and is joined about its midpoint by the intraparietal sulcus. The lateral occipital sulcus divides the lobe into superior and inferior occipital gyri (see Figs 16.1, 16.2). The lunate sulcus, when present, lies just in front of the occipital pole. It is placed vertically and is occasionally joined to the calcarine sulcus. Its lips separate striate from peristriate areas; the parastriate area is buried in the sulcus between the other two striate areas. The lunate sulcus is posterior to the gyrus descendens, which is behind the superior and inferior occipital gyri. Curved superior and inferior polar sulci often appear near the ends of the lunate sulcus. The superior polar sulcus arches up onto the medial occipital surface near the upper limit of the lunate sulcus. The inferior polar sulcus arches down and forward onto the inferior cerebral surface from the lower limit of the lunate sulcus. These polar sulci enclose semilunar extensions of the striate area and indicate the extent of the visual cortex associated with the macula.

The occipital lobe comprises almost entirely Brodmann's areas 17, 18 and 19. Area 17, the striate cortex, is the primary visual cortex (V1). A host of other distinct visual areas resides in the occipital and temporal cortices. Functional subdivisions V2, V3 (dorsal and ventral) and V3A lie within Brodmann's area 18. Other functional areas at the junction of the occipital cortex with the parietal or temporal lobe lie wholly or partly in area 19.

The primary visual cortex is located mostly on the medial aspect of the occipital lobe and is coextensive with the subcortical nerve fibre stria of Gennari in layer IV; hence, its alternative name, the striate cortex. It occupies the upper and lower lips and depths of the posterior part of the calcarine sulcus and extends into the cuneus and lingual gyrus (Fig. 16.21). Posteriorly, it is limited by the lunate sulcus and by polar sulci above and below this sulcus. It extends to the occipital pole.

The primary visual cortex receives afferent fibres from the lateral geniculate nucleus (see Figs 15.7, 15.8) via the optic radiation. The latter curves posteriorly and spreads through the white matter of the occipital lobe. Its fibres terminate in strict point-to-point fashion in the striate area. The cortex of each hemisphere receives impulses from two half retinae, which represent the contralateral half of the binocular visual field. Superior and inferior retinal quadrants are connected with corresponding areas of the striate cortex. Thus, the superior retinal quadrants (representing the inferior half of the visual field) are connected with the visual cortex above the calcarine sulcus, and the inferior retinal quadrants (representing the upper half of the visual field) are connected with the visual cortex below the calcarine sulcus. The peripheral parts of the retinae activate the most anterior parts in the visual cortex. The macula impinges on a disproportionately large posterior part.

The striate cortex is granular. Layer IV, bearing the stria of Gennari, is commonly divided into three sublayers. Passing from superficial to deep, these are IVA, IVB (which contains the stria), and IVC. The densely cellular IVC is further subdivided into a superficial IVCα and a deep IVCβ. Layer IVB contains only sparse, mainly non-pyramidal neurones. The input to area 17 from the lateral geniculate nucleus terminates predominantly in layers IVA and IVC. Other thalamic afferents, from the inferior pulvinar nucleus and the intralaminar group, pass to layers I and VI. Geniculocortical fibres terminate in alternating bands. Axons from geniculate laminae, which receive information from the ipsilateral eye (laminae II, III and V), are segregated from those of laminae receiving input from the contralateral eye (laminae I, IV and VI). Neurones within layer IVC are monocular; that is, they respond to stimulation of either the ipsilateral or contralateral eye, but not both. This horizontal segregation forms the anatomical basis of the ocular dominance column, in that neurones encountered in a vertical strip from pia to white matter exhibit a preference for stimulation of one eye or the other, even though they are binocular outside layer IV. The other major functional basis for the columnar organization of the visual cortex is the orientation column: that is, an electrode passing through the depth of the cortex at right angles to the plane from pia to white matter encounters neurones that all respond preferentially to either a stationary or a moving straight line of a given orientation within the visual field. Cells with simple, complex and hypercomplex receptive fields occur in area 17. Simple cells respond optimally to lines in a narrowly defined position. Complex cells respond to a line anywhere within a receptive field, but with

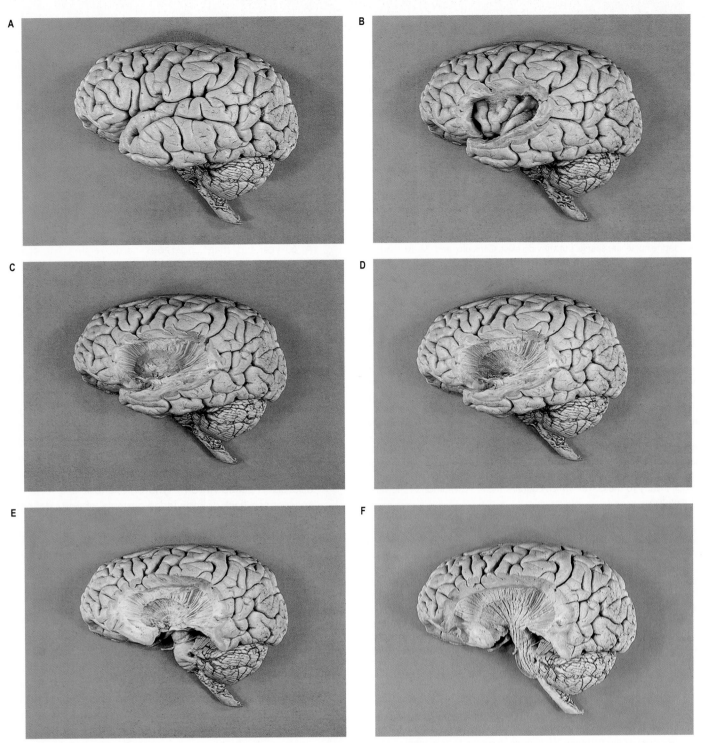

Fig. 16.20 *Series of dissections of the left cerebral hemisphere at progressively deeper levels to demonstrate the insula and subjacent structures.* **A,** *Intact brain.* **B,** *Cortical gyri of the insula exposed by removal of the frontal, temporal and parietal opercula.* **C,** *Removal of the insular cortex, extreme capsule, claustrum and external capsule to expose the lateral aspect of the putamen.* **D,** *Removal of the lentiform complex to display fibres of the internal capsule.* **E,** *Removal of part of the temporal lobe to show the internal capsule fibres converging on the crus cerebri of the midbrain.* **F,** *Removal of the optic tract and superficial dissection of the pons and upper medulla, emphasizing the continuity of the corona radiata, internal capsule, crus cerebri, longitudinal pontine fibres and medullary pyramid.* (*Dissections by E. L. Rees; photographs by Kevin Fitzpatrick on behalf of GKT School of Medicine, London.*)

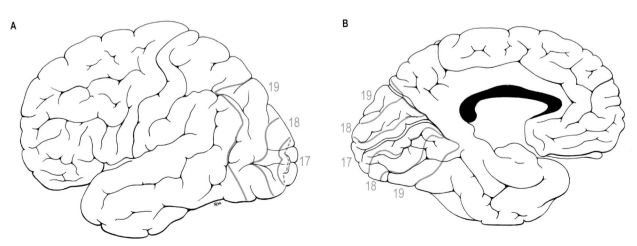

Fig. 16.21 *Lateral (A) and medial (B) surfaces of the left cerebral hemispheres showing the visual areas in the occipital lobe. The striate, parastriate and peristriate areas correspond approximately to Brodmann's areas 17, 18 and 19, respectively, and to visual areas V1, V2 and V3.*

a specific orientation. Hypercomplex cells are similar to complex cells, except that the length of the line or bar stimulus is critical for an optimal response. There is a relationship between the complexity of response and the position of cells in relation to the cortical laminae. Simple cells are mainly in layer IV, and complex and hypercomplex cells predominate in either layers II and III or layers V and VI.

Ipsilateral corticocortical fibres pass from area 17 to a variety of functional areas in areas 18 and 19 and in the parietal and temporal cortices. Fibres from area 17 pass to area 18 (which contains visual areas V2, V3 and V3a); area 19 (which contains V4); the posterior intraparietal and parieto-occipital areas; and parts of the posterior temporal lobe, middle temporal area and medial superior temporal area. Subcortical efferents of the striate cortex pass to the superior colliculus, pretectum and parts of the brain stem reticular formation. Projections to the striatum (notably the tail of the caudate nucleus) and to the pontine nuclei are sparse, but they do exist. Geniculo- and claustrocortical projections are reciprocated by prominent descending projections, which arise in layer VI.

The second visual area (V2) occupies much of area 18 but is not coextensive with it. It contains a complete retinotopic representation of the visual hemifield, which is a mirror image of that in area 17; the vertical meridian is represented most posteriorly along the border between areas 17 and 18. The major ipsilateral corticocortical feed-forward projection to V2 comes from V1. Feed-forward projections from V2 pass to several other visual areas (and are reciprocated by feedback connections), including the third visual area (V3) and its various subdivisions (see later), the fourth visual area (V4), areas in the temporal and parietal association cortices and the frontal eye fields. Thalamic afferents to V2 come from the lateral geniculate nucleus, the inferior and lateral pulvinar nuclei and parts of the intralaminar group of nuclei. Additional subcortical afferents are the same as for cortical areas in general. Subcortical efferents arise predominantly in layers V and VI. They pass to the thalamus, claustrum, superior colliculus, pretectum, brain stem reticular formation, striatum and pons. As in area 17, the callosal connections of V2 are restricted predominantly to the cortex, which contains the representation of the vertical meridian.

The third visual area (V3) is a narrow strip adjoining the anterior margin of V2, probably still within Brodmann's area 18. V3 has been subdivided into dorsal (V3/V3d) and ventral (VP/V3v) regions on the basis of its afferents from area V1, myeloarchitecture, callosal and association connections and receptive field properties. The dorsal subdivision receives from V1, whereas the ventral does not. Functionally, the dorsal part shows less wavelength selectivity, greater direction selectivity and smaller receptive fields than the ventral subdivision. Both areas receive a feed-forward projection from V2 and are interconnected by association fibres. Another visual area, V3a, lies anterior to the dorsal subdivision of V3. It receives afferent association connections from V1, V2, V3/V3d and VP/V3v, and it has a complex and irregular topographical organization. All subdivisions project to diverse visual areas in the parietal, occipital and temporal cortices, including V4, and to the frontal eye fields.

The fourth visual area (V4) lies within area 19 anterior to the V3 complex. It receives a major ipsilateral feed-forward projection from V2. Colour selectivity as well as orientation selectivity may be transmitted to V4, and bilateral damage causes achromatopsia. V4 is more complex than a simple colour discrimination area because it is also involved in the discrimination of orientation, form and movement. It sends a feed-forward projection to the inferior temporal cortex and receives a feedback projection. It also connects with other visual areas that lie more dorsally in the temporal lobe and in the parietal lobe. Thalamocortical connections are with the lateral and inferior pulvinar and the intralaminar nuclei. Other subcortical connections conform to the general pattern for all cortical areas. Callosal connections are with the contralateral V4 and other occipital visual areas.

A fifth visual area, V5 or the middle temporal area, is found in non-human primates toward the posterior end of the superior temporal sulcus. It receives ipsilateral association connections from areas V1, V2, V3 and V4 in a topographically organized way. Other lesser projections are received from widespread visual areas in the temporal and parieto-occipital lobes and from the frontal eye fields. V5 is primarily a movement detection or discrimination area and contains a high proportion of movement-sensitive, direction-selective cells. Feed-forward projections go to surrounding temporal and parietal areas and to the frontal eye field. Thalamic connections are with the lateral and inferior pulvinar and intralaminar group of nuclei. Other connections follow the general pattern of all neocortical areas.

Current concepts of visual processing in inferior temporal and temporoparietal cortices suggest that two parallel pathways (dorsal and ventral) emanate from the occipital lobe. The dorsal pathway, concerned primarily with visuospatial discrimination, projects from V1 and V2 to the superior temporal and surrounding parietotemporal areas and ultimately to area 7a of the parietal cortex. Damage to these pathways disrupts motion perception and causes optic ataxia and may also disrupt the learning of visuospatial tasks. V4 is a key relay station for the ventral pathway, which is related to perception and object recognition. Its connections pass sequentially along the inferior temporal gyrus in a feed-forward manner, from V4 to posterior, intermediate and then anterior inferior temporal cortices. Ultimately, they feed into the temporal polar and medial temporal areas and interface with the limbic system.

CASE 7   CORTICAL BLINDNESS AND ANTON'S SYNDROME

A 65-year-old man undergoes cardioversion for atrial fibrillation. Two days later he is observed walking into objects in his hospital room. He insists that he can see, but he is unable to count fingers, read or identify objects presented to him. Pupillary light reactions are intact, and ocular motility is normal. Brain MRI demonstrates bilateral occipital lobe infarcts.

Discussion: The inability to see because of bilateral injury to the occipital lobes is termed cortical blindness and it is caused by a loss of the brain's ability to process visual information. Normal pupillary light reflexes argue against a peripheral (retinal, optic nerve) cause of blindness in such circumstances. In rare cases of cortical blindness, patients insist that they can see and confabulate when asked to describe objects in their environment. This disorder is called Anton's syndrome, and it is a form of anosognosia (lack of knowledge or denial of one's deficit). Cortical blindness is usually caused by cerebral ischaemia from bilateral embolic strokes or from hypotension with cerebral hypoperfusion, but it can also result from closed head injury.

CASE 8   BALINT'S SYNDROME

A 49-year-old woman suffers severe blood loss with resultant hypovolemic shock following a motor vehicle accident. She required cardiopulmonary resuscitation at the accident scene. Several days later, her doctors notice that although she is able to see, she has difficulty identifying objects in her room. She can see the clock but is unable to tell the time. She cannot feed herself because she cannot correctly reach for the food. On examination, she has diminished voluntary eye movements in all planes. She cannot recognize more than one object at a time. MRI reveals bilateral parieto-occipital infarctions.

Discussion: Balint's syndrome is an uncommon disorder caused by bilateral injury to the parietal and occipital cortices. Typical symptoms of Balint's syndrome include optic apraxia, the inability to voluntarily change visual fixation; optic ataxia, the inability to accurately reach for a point in space; and simultagnosia, the inability to recognize more than one object in the visual field. Causes of this curious syndrome include cerebral ischaemia from hypotension, with border zone infarcts, as in this patient; bilateral embolic strokes; neurodegenerative diseases, such as Alzheimer's disease or posterior cortical atrophy; and brain tumour.

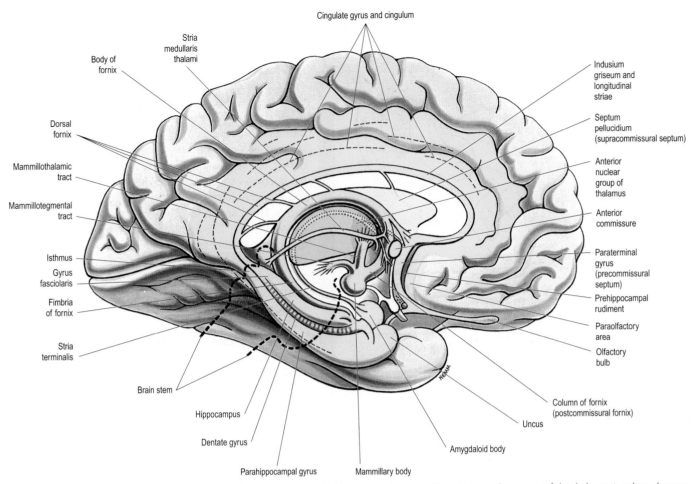

Fig. 16.22 *Medial aspect of the left cerebral hemisphere demonstrating some limbic structures* (yellow). *The anterior nuclear group of the thalamus is coloured* orange, *and the rest of the thalamus is* magenta. *The approximate position of the brain stem is outlined in a* heavy interrupted line.

Limbic Lobe

The limbic lobe includes large parts of the cortex on the medial wall of the hemisphere, principally the subcallosal, cingulate and parahippocampal gyri (Fig. 16.22). It also includes the hippocampal formation, which consists of the hippocampus proper (Ammon's horn or cornu ammonis), the dentate gyrus, the subicular complex (subiculum, presubiculum, parasubiculum) and the entorhinal cortex (area 28). There is a close relationship between these phylogenetically old cortical structures and the termination of the olfactory tract in the frontal and medial temporal lobes.

On the basis of emotional disturbances displayed by patients who presented with damage to the hippocampus and cingulate gyrus, Papez (1937) described a closed circuit (the Papez circuit) that links the hippocampus with the cingulate cortex, via the mammillary bodies and anterior thalamus. He proposed that emotional expression is organized in the hippocampus, experienced in the cingulate gyrus and expressed via the mammillary bodies. The hypothalamus was thought to be the site where hippocampal processes gain access to the autonomic outflow that controls the peripheral expression of emotional states. The Papez circuit is now widely accepted as being involved with cognitive processes, including mnemonic functions and spatial short-term memory.

The term 'limbic system' has become popular to describe the limbic lobe along with the closely associated subcortical nuclei, including the amygdala, septum, hypothalamus, habenula, anterior thalamic nuclei and parts of the basal ganglia.

The cingulate gyrus can be divided rostrocaudally into several cytoarchitectonically discrete areas: the prelimbic (area 32) and infralimbic (area 25) cortices, the anterior cingulate cortex (areas 23 and 24) and part of the posterior cingulate or retrosplenial cortex (area 29). The cingulate gyrus, which is related to the medial surfaces of the frontal lobe, contains specific motor areas and has extensive connections with neocortical areas of the frontal lobe. The cingulate gyrus on the medial surface of the parietal lobe has equally extensive connections with somatosensory and visual association areas of the parietal, occipital and temporal lobes. These afferents to the cingulate gyrus are predominantly from neocortical areas on the lateral surface of the hemisphere. Within the cingulate cortex, most projections pass caudally, ultimately into the posterior parahippocampal gyrus. Through

this system, afferents from widespread areas of association cortex converge on the medial temporal lobe and hippocampal formation. There are other parallel stepwise routes to these targets through cortical areas on the lateral surface.

The cingulate gyrus is the area that shows the most consistent pain-evoked changes in synaptic activity related to regional cerebral bloodflow as measured by either positron emission tomography (PET) or functional magnetic resonance imaging (fMRI) (Derbyshire et al 1997). It must be remembered that pain evokes a multidimensional response in the brain, including cognitive, emotional, autonomic and motor components, so it is not always possible to assign specific functions to parts of the brain that generate PET or fMRI signals in response to pain Peyron, Laurent and Garcia-Larrea 2000). However, in many experimental paradigms, a combination of signals from the cingulate gyrus, somatosensory area SII and insula appears to be involved in the conscious appreciation of nociception and neuropathic pain.

The complex parahippocampal gyrus includes areas 27, 28 (entorhinal cortex), 35, 36, 48 and 49 and temporal cortical fields. The rich interconnections within the cingulate and parahippocampal cortices, and with the hippocampal formation, are schematically represented in Figure 16.23. Only a few are described in detail here. In monkeys, the infralimbic cortex (area 25) has been shown to project to areas 24a and 24b. Area 25 also has reciprocal connections with the entorhinal cortex. Projections between paralimbic area 32 and the limbic cortex (anterior, retrosplenial and entorhinal cortex) are somewhat less prominent. Areas 24 and 29 are connected with the paralimbic posterior cingulate area 23. The strong connections between subicular and entorhinal areas are discussed in the context of the hippocampal formation itself. Reference to Figure 16.23 emphasizes the way the pro-isocortical cingulate and related areas (32, 24c, 23, 29d, 35b, 36) interface between the limbic-archicortex and peri-archicortex and widespread areas of the neocortex. This pattern of cortical connection—outward from the hippocampus via the entorhinal cortex to the perirhinal cortex, caudal parahippocampal gyrus and posterior cingulate gyrus—has enormous functional importance as far as the hippocampus is concerned, as discussed later. The parahippocampal gyrus projects to virtually all association areas of the cortex in primates and also provides the major funnel through which polymodal sensory inputs converge on the hippocampus.

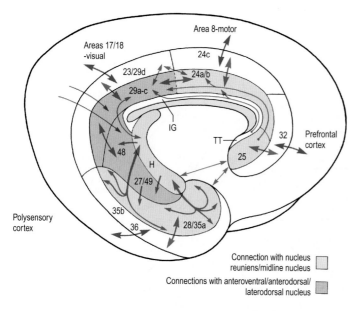

Areas 17/18 -visual

Area 8-motor

24c

23/29d

24a/b

29a-c

IG

TT

32 Prefrontal cortex

48

25

27/49

H

Polysensory cortex

35b

36

28/35a

Connection with nucleus reuniens/midline nucleus ☐

Connections with anteroventral/anterodorsal/ laterodorsal nucleus ▨

Fig. 16.23 Left limbic cortex illustrating the major interconnections between areas as well as connections with major thalamic areas and extralimbic cortex. (Redrawn from Lopes da Silva, F.H., Witter, M.P., Beoijinga, P.H., et al., 1990. Anatomic organization and physiology of the limbic cortex. Physiol. Rev. 70, 453–511, by permission from the American Physiological Society.)

Olfactory Pathways

The olfactory pathways include the olfactory nerves, olfactory bulb and olfactory tract, together with its central connections in the frontal and temporal lobes. These are primarily described in Chapter 12. The close association of these structures with limbic regions is shown in Figure 16.7.

Hippocampal Formation

The hippocampal formation includes the dentate gyrus, hippocampus, subicular complex and entorhinal cortex.

The hippocampus lies above the subiculum and medial parahippocampal gyrus, forming a curved elevation, approximately 5 cm long, along the floor of the inferior horn of the lateral ventricle (Fig. 16.25). Its anterior end is expanded, and its margin there may have two or three shallow grooves that give it a paw-like appearance, the pes hippocampi. The ventricular aspect is convex. It is covered by ependyma, beneath which fibres of the alveus converge medially on a longitudinal bundle of fibres, the fimbria of the fornix (Fig. 16.26). Passing medially from the collateral sulcus, the neocortex of the parahippocampal gyrus merges with the transitional juxtallocortex of the subiculum. The latter curves superomedially to the inferior surface of the dentate gyrus, then laterally to the laminae of the hippocampus. The curvature continues, first superiorly, then medially above the dentate gyrus, and ends pointing toward the centre of the superior surface of the dentate gyrus. The dentate gyrus is a crenated strip of cortex related inferiorly to the subiculum, laterally to the hippocampus and, more medially, to the fimbria of the fornix (Figs 16.26, 16.27). The form of the fimbria is quite variable, but medially, it is separated from the crenated medial margin of the dentate gyrus by the fimbriodentate sulcus (Fig. 16.28). The hippocampal sulcus, of variable depth, lies between the dentate gyrus and the subicular extension of the parahippocampal gyrus. Posteriorly, the dentate gyrus is continuous with the gyrus fasciolaris and thus with the indusium griseum. Anteriorly, it continues into the notch of the uncus, turning medially across its inferior surface, as the tail of the dentate gyrus (band of Giacomini) and vanishes on the medial aspect of the uncus (see Fig. 16.27). The tail separates the inferior surface of the uncus into an anterior uncinate gyrus and posterior intralimbic gyrus.

The trilaminar cortex of the dentate gyrus is the least complex of the hippocampal fields. Its major cell type is the granule cell, found in the dense granule cell layer. Granule cells (approximately 9×10^6 in the human dentate gyrus) have unipolar dendrites that extend into the overlying molecular layer, which receives most of the afferent projections to the dentate gyrus (primarily from the entorhinal cortex). The granule cell and molecular layers are sometimes referred to as the fascia dentata. The polymorphic layer, or hilus of the dentate gyrus, contains cells that give rise primarily to ipsilateral association fibres. They remain within the dentate gyrus and do not extend into other hippocampal fields.

The hippocampus is trilaminar archicortex. It consists of a single pyramidal cell layer, with plexiform layers above and below it. It can be divided into three distinct fields: CA1, CA2 and CA3 (Figs 16.28, 16.29). Field CA3 borders the hilus of the dentate gyrus at one end, and field CA2 at the other. Field CA3 pyramidal cells are the largest in the hippocampus, and the whole pyramidal cell layer in this field is about 10 cells thick. The most important feature of pyramidal cells in CA3 is that they receive the mossy fibre input from dentate granule cells on their proximal dendrites. The border between CA3 and CA2 is not well marked because the pyramidal cells of the former appear to extend under the border of the latter for some distance. The CA2 field has the most compact layer of pyramidal cells. It completely lacks a mossy fibre input from dentate granule cells and receives a major input from the supramammillary region of the hypothalamus. Field CA1 is usually described as the most complex of the hippocampal subdivisions, and its appearance varies along its transverse and rostrocaudal axes. The CA1–CA2 border is not sharp, and at its other end, CA1 overlaps the subiculum for some distance. The thickness of the pyramidal cell layer varies from 10 to more than 30 cells. Approximately 10% of neurones in this field are interneurones.

It is common to describe several strata within the layers of the hippocampus (see Figs 16.28, 16.29). Starting from the ventricular aspect, these are the alveus (containing subicular and hippocampal pyramidal cell axons converging on the fimbria of the fornix), stratum oriens (mainly the basal dendrites of pyramidal cells and some interneurones), stratum pyramidalis, stratum lucidum

CASE 10   HERPES ENCEPHALITIS

A 26-year-old woman is brought to the emergency room because of agitation and bizarre behaviour of 3 days' duration. She previously complained of malaise and headache and has a history of anxiety and depression. Her general physical examination is normal. She makes occasional inappropriate, sexually explicit comments during the examination, as well as provocative sexually oriented displays. She remains agitated, with repeated emotional outbursts, and ultimately needs to be restrained. There are no focal neurological deficits on examination.

Routine laboratory investigations are negative. A CT scan is unremarkable. A lumbar puncture yields cerebrospinal fluid containing 25 lymphocytes per high-power field, a glucose level of 54 mg/dl and a protein content of 60 mg/dl. Electroencephalogram reveals independent bitemporal periodic lateralizing epileptiform discharges and mild generalized background slowing. MRI demonstrates an area of hyperintensity on diffusion-weighted imaging in the left temporal lobe. The cerebrospinal fluid polymerase chain reaction is positive for herpes simplex. She is treated with acyclovir.

The patient's behaviour gradually improves, but short-term memory deficits become apparent and persist, and she has visual agnosia.

Discussion: Herpes encephalitis is characterized by behavioural and personality changes. Aphasia may be present. The clinical syndrome may resemble the changes encountered in the Klüver-Bucy experimental model following bilateral temporal lobectomy. Anatomically, medial temporal structures are most consistently involved (Fig. 16.24). Lesions may be more widespread, however, involving orbital frontal and cingulate gyri. Many patients exhibit a marked memory deficit as a residual finding.

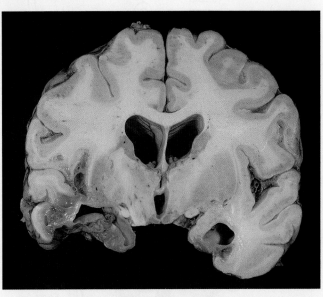

Fig. 16.24 *Herpes simplex encephalitis demonstrating selective involvement of the medial temporal lobes bilaterally. (Courtesy of John S. Woodard, MD.)*

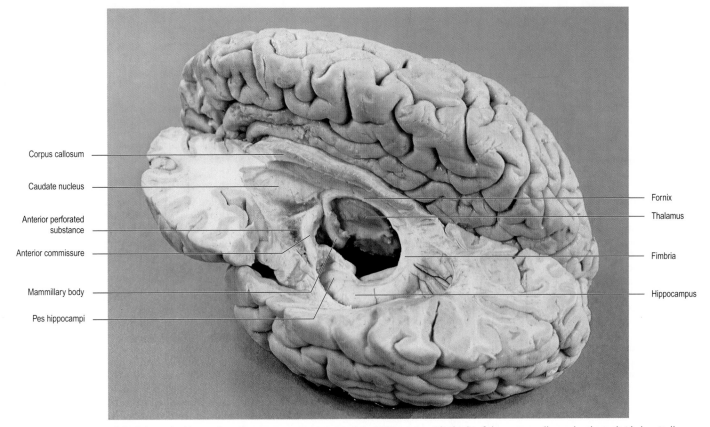

Corpus callosum

Caudate nucleus

Anterior perforated substance

Anterior commissure

Mammillary body

Pes hippocampi

Fornix

Thalamus

Fimbria

Hippocampus

Fig. 16.25 *Dissection of the left cerebral hemisphere demonstrating structures of the limbic system. The body of the corpus callosum has been divided sagitally. The frontal, temporal and occipital lobes have been sectioned horizontally, and their superior parts removed. The left lentiform complex and thalamus have been removed, and the floor of the inferior horn of the lateral ventricle opened. (Dissection by A. M. Seal; photograph by Kevin Fitzpatrick on behalf of GKT School of Medicine, London.)*

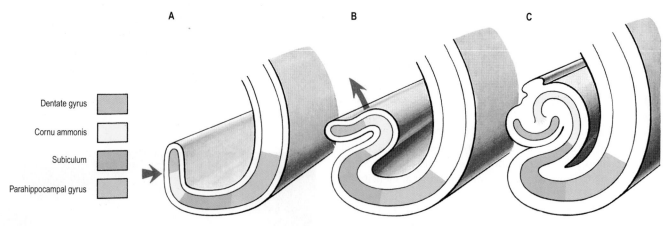

Fig. 16.26 *A–C, Coronal sections of the temporal lobe and inferior horn of the lateral ventricle illustrating the hippocampus and related structures. This series of diagrams is intended to assist in understanding the relative positions of the dentate gyrus, cornu ammonis, subiculum and parahippocampal gyrus in the floor of the inferior horn.*

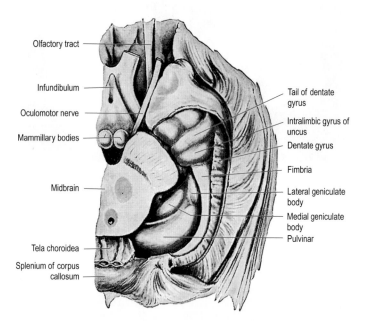

Fig. 16.27 *Basal aspect of the brain dissected to display the dentate gyrus, uncus and fimbria on the left.*

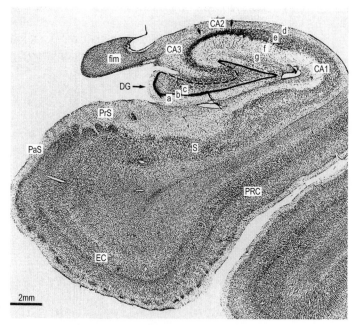

Fig. 16.28 *Coronal, thionin-stained section of the human hippocampal formation. a, molecular layer of the dentate gyrus; b, granule cell layer of the dentate gyrus; c, plexiform layer of the dentate gyrus; CA1–CA3, fields of the hippocampus; d, stratum oriens layer of the hippocampus; DG, dentate gyrus; e, pyramidal cell layer of the hippocampus; EC, entorhinal cortex; f, stratum radiatum of the hippocampus; fim, fimbria; g, stratum lacunosum-molecular of the hippocampus; PaS, parasubiculum; PRC, perirhinal cortex; PrS, presubiculum; S, subiculum. (Photomicrograph courtesy of David Amaral.)*

(containing mossy fibres that make contact with the proximal dendrites of pyramidal cells in field CA3), stratum radiatum and stratum lacunosum-moleculare. The stratum lucidum is not as prominent in humans as it is in other primates, and it is not present in fields CA1 and CA2.

In the stratum radiatum and stratum oriens, CA3 and CA2 cells receive associational connections from other rostrocaudal levels of the hippocampus, as well as afferents from subcortical structures such as the septal nuclei and supramammillary region. The projections from pyramidal cells of fields CA3 and CA2 to CA1, often called Schaffer collaterals, also terminate in the stratum radiatum and stratum oriens. The projections from the entorhinal cortex to the dentate gyrus (the perforant pathway) travel in the stratum lacunosum-moleculare, where they make synaptic contact *en passant* with the distal apical dendrites of hippocampal pyramidal cells.

The subicular complex is generally subdivided into the subiculum, presubiculum and parasubiculum (see Figs 16.28, 16.29). The major subcortical projections of the hippocampal formation (to the septal nuclei, mammillary nuclei, nucleus accumbens and anterior thalamus), and those to the entorhinal cortex, all arise from pyramidal neurones of the subicular complex. The subiculum consists of a superficial molecular layer containing apical dendrites of subicular pyramidal cells, a pyramidal cell layer that is approximately 30 cells thick and a deep polymorphic layer. The presubiculum is medial to the subiculum and is distinguished by a densely packed superficial layer of pyramidal cells. There is a plexiform layer superficial to this dense cell layer. Cells deep to it are regarded as either a medial extension of the subiculum or a lateral extension of the deep layers of the entorhinal cortex. The parasubiculum also has a superficial plexiform layer and a primary cell layer. It forms the boundary between the subicular complex as a whole and the entorhinal cortex. The cell layers deep to the parasubiculum are indistinguishable from the deep layers of the entorhinal cortex.

The entorhinal cortex (Brodmann's area 28; see Figs 16.7, 16.28, 16.29) extends rostrally to the anterior limit of the amygdala. Caudally, it overlaps a portion of the hippocampal fields. The more primitive levels of the entorhinal cortex (below the amygdala) receive projections from the olfactory bulb. More caudal regions do not generally receive primary olfactory inputs.

The entorhinal cortex is divisible into six layers and is quite distinct from other neocortical regions. Layer I is acellular and plexiform. Layer II is a narrow cellular layer that consists of islands of large pyramidal and stellate cells. These cell islands are a distinguishing feature of the entorhinal cortex. They form small bumps on the surface of the brain that can be seen by the naked eye (verrucae hippocampae) and indicate the boundaries of the entorhinal cortex. Layer III consists of medium-sized pyramidal cells. There is no internal granular layer (another classic feature of entorhinal cortex); in its place is an acellular region of dense fibres called the lamina dissecans, which is sometimes called layer IV. Layers III and V are apposed in regions where the lamina dissecans is absent. Layer V consists of large pyramidal cells five or six deep. Layer VI is readily distinguishable from layer V only close to the border with the perirhinal cortex. Its cells continue around the angular bundle (subcortical white matter deep to the subicular complex, made up largely of perforant path axons) to lie beneath the pre- and parasubiculum.

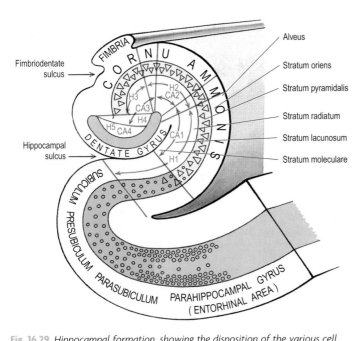

Fig. 16.29 *Hippocampal formation, showing the disposition of the various cell fields. Dentate gyrus, pink; hippocampus proper (cornu ammonis), yellow; areas of the subicular complex, green; entorhinal cortex, blue. CA1–CA3, hippocampal cell fields.*

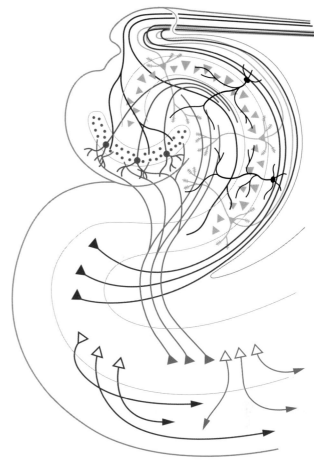

Fig. 16.30 *Neuronal organization and connections of the dentate gyrus, hippocampus (cornu ammonis), subiculum and parahippocampal gyrus. Cell somata, dendrites and axons of the pyramidal neurones of the cornu ammonis are yellow; the axons form the efferent hippocampal fibres of the alveus and fimbria. Afferent fibres to the cornu ammonis from the fimbria are purple; afferents from the entorhinal cortex via the perforant path are blue; basket neurones are black; neurones of the dentate gyrus and their axons, which form the mossy fibres of the hippocampus, are magenta; and subicular efferents to the fornix via the alveus are green.*

Glutamate or aspartate appears to be the major excitatory transmitter in three pathways in the hippocampal formation—namely, the perforant pathway, which arises in the entorhinal cortex and terminates primarily in the dentate gyrus; the mossy fibres, which run from the dentate granule cells to the pyramidal cells of the CA3 field; and the Schaffer collaterals of CA3 pyramidal cells, which terminate on CA1 pyramidal cells.

GABAergic neurones are found in the deep portions of the granule cell layer in the dentate gyrus (basket cells). The highest concentration of GABA receptors is found in the molecular layer of the dentate gyrus. In the hippocampus proper, GABAergic cells are found mostly in the stratum oriens but also in the pyramidal cell layer and stratum radiatum.

There are many peptide-containing neurones in the hippocampal formation. Granule cells in the dentate gyrus appear to contain the opioid peptide dynorphin, which is also present in mossy fibres running to the CA3 field. Enkephalin, or a related peptide, may be present in fibres arising in the entorhinal cortex. There is a dense plexus of somatostatin-immunoreactive fibres in the molecular layer of the dentate gyrus and also in the stratum lacunosum-moleculare of the hippocampus. The polymorphic layer of the dentate gyrus, stratum oriens of the hippocampus and deep layers of the entorhinal cortex all contain somatostatin-immunoreactive neurones. VIP-immunoreactive neurones are plentiful in many hippocampal fields, especially in the superficial layers of the entorhinal cortex. Cells containing cholecystokinin (CCK) immunoreactivity are found in the hilar region of the dentate gyrus; in all layers of the hippocampus, especially in the pyramidal cell layer; and throughout the subicular complex and entorhinal cortex. There are also substantial plexuses of CCK-immunoreactive fibres in the stratum lacunosum-moleculare, subicular complex and entorhinal cortex. Hippocampal CCK-immunoreactive cells may give rise to extrinsic projections (e.g. to the lateral septum and medial mammillary nucleus), because CCK-immunoreactive fibres are found in the fimbria or fornix.

The dentate gyrus is the point of entry into the hippocampal circuitry. It receives fibres via the perforant path projections from layers II and III of the entorhinal cortex. The axons terminate in the outer two thirds of the molecular layer of the dentate gyrus, on the dendritic spines of granule cells. These cells project heavily via their mossy fibres onto the proximal dendrites of CA3 pyramidal cells. The latter give rise, via the so-called Schaffer collaterals, to a projection that terminates mainly in the stratum radiatum of the CA1 hippocampal field. The CA1 field projects heavily to the subicular complex, which projects to the entorhinal cortex.

The subiculum, rather than the hippocampus, projects to the mammillary complex, whereas the hippocampus gives rise principally to efferents destined for the septal complex. Summaries of hippocampal circuitry and connections are shown schematically in Figure 16.30.

The medial septal complex and the supramammillary area of the posterior hypothalamus are the two major sources of subcortical afferents to the hippocampal formation. There are also projections from the amygdaloid complex

and claustrum (to the subicular complex and entorhinal cortex), as well as monoaminergic projections from the ventral tegmental area, the mesencephalic raphe nuclei and the locus coeruleus. The noradrenergic and serotoninergic projections reach all hippocampal fields but are especially dense in the dentate gyrus.

The projections from the septal complex arise in the medial septal and vertical limb nuclei of the diagonal band. They travel via the dorsal fornix, fimbria, and supracallosal striae and take a ventral route through the amygdaloid complex. These projections reach all hippocampal fields, but the most prominent terminations are in the dentate gyrus, field CA3, presubiculum, parasubiculum and entorhinal cortex. Many of these medial septal or diagonal band neurones are GABAergic or cholinergic, and they form part of the topographically organized basal forebrain cholinergic system (cell groups Ch1 and Ch2).

Neurones in the supramammillary area also provide significant innervation of the hippocampal formation. They arrive partly through the fornix and partly through a ventral route, and they terminate most heavily in the dentate gyrus and fields CA2 and CA3 of the cornu ammonis.

All divisions of the anterior thalamic nuclear complex and the associated lateral dorsal nucleus project to the hippocampal formation and are directed predominantly to the subicular complex. Some midline thalamic nuclei, particularly the parataenial, central medial and reuniens nuclei, also project to the hippocampal formation, especially to the entorhinal cortex.

In humans, the fornix contains approximately 1.2 million fibres. Cells in the CA3 field project bilaterally to the lateral nucleus of the septal complex, via the precommissural fornix. They give rise to the Schaffer collaterals to CA1 cells and to the commissural projections to the contralateral hippocampus. Neurones in the subicular complex and entorhinal cortex give rise to projections to the nucleus accumbens and to parts of the caudate nucleus and putamen. The subicular complex gives rise to the major postcommissural fibre system of the fornix. The presubiculum, in particular, projects to the anterior thalamic nuclear complex (anteromedial, anteroventral and laterodorsal nuclei). Both the subiculum and the presubiculum provide the major extrinsic input to the mammillary complex. Both the lateral and the medial mammillary nuclei receive afferents from the subicular complex.

Several fields in the temporal lobe neocortex, especially TF and TH of the parahippocampal gyrus, the dorsal bank of the superior temporal gyrus, the perirhinal cortex (Brodmann's area 35) and the temporal polar cortex, together with the agranular insular cortex and posterior orbitofrontal cortex, all project to the entorhinal cortex. Projections to the entorhinal cortex also arise from the dorsolateral prefrontal cortex (Brodmann's areas 9, 10, 46), the medial frontal cortex (Brodmann's areas 25, 32), the cingulate cortex (Brodmann's areas 23, 24) and the retrosplenial cortex. The subicular complex receives direct cortical inputs, such as from the temporal polar cortex, perirhinal cortex, parahippocampal gyrus, superior temporal gyrus and dorsolateral prefrontal cortex. The entorhinal cortex projects to the perirhinal cortex as well as to the temporal polar cortex and caudal parahippocampal and cingulate gyri. In monkeys, the subicular complex also projects to a number of cortical areas, including the perirhinal cortex, parahippocampal gyrus, caudal cingulate gyrus, and medial frontal and medial orbitofrontal cortices.

Septum

The septum is a midline and paramedian structure (see Figs 14.6, 16.22). Its upper portion corresponds largely to the bilateral laminae of fibres, sparse grey matter and neuroglia known as the septum pellucidum, which separates the lateral ventricles. Below this, the septal region is made up of four main nuclear groups: dorsal, ventral, medial and caudal. The dorsal group is essentially the dorsal septal nucleus, the ventral group consists of the lateral septal nucleus, the medial group contains the medial septal nucleus and the nucleus of the diagonal band of Broca and the caudal group contains the fimbrial and triangular septal nuclei.

The major afferents to the region terminate primarily in the lateral septal nucleus. They include fibres carried in the fornix that arise from hippocampal fields CA3 and CA1 and the subiculum. There are also afferents arising from the preoptic area; anterior, paraventricular and ventromedial hypothalamic nuclei; and lateral hypothalamic area. The lateral septum receives a rich monoaminergic innervation, including noradrenergic afferents from the locus coeruleus and medullary cell groups (A1, A2), serotoninergic afferents from the midbrain raphe nuclei and dopaminergic afferents from the ventral tegmental area (A10).

Projections from the lateral septum run to the medial and lateral preoptic areas, anterior hypothalamus, and supramammillary and midbrain ventral tegmental area via the medial forebrain bundle. There is also a projection to the medial habenular nucleus and to some midline thalamic nuclei via the stria medullaris thalami, which runs on the dorsomedial wall of the third ventricle. The projections from the habenula via the fasciculus retroflexus to the interpeduncular nucleus and adjacent ventral tegmental area in the midbrain provide a route through which forebrain limbic structures can influence midbrain nuclear groups.

A large proportion of the medial septal or diagonal band neurones are cholinergic or GABAergic. They project to the hippocampal formation and cingulate cortex.

Amygdala

The amygdaloid nuclear complex is made up of lateral, central and basal nuclei that lie in the dorsomedial temporal pole, anterior to the hippocampus, and close to the tail of the caudate nucleus (see Fig. 16.22). Collectively, the nuclei form the ventral, superior and medial walls of the tip of the inferior horn of the lateral ventricle. The amygdala is partly continuous above with the inferomedial margin of the claustrum. Fibres of the external capsule and substriatal grey matter, including the cholinergic magnocellular nucleus basalis (of Meynert), incompletely separate it from the putamen and globus pallidus. Laterally, it is close to the optic tract. It is partly deep to the gyrus semilunaris, gyrus ambiens and uncinate gyrus (see Fig. 16.7).

The lateral nucleus has dorsomedial and ventrolateral subnuclei. The central nucleus has medial and lateral subdivisions. The basal nucleus is commonly divided into a dorsal magnocellular basal nucleus, an intermediate parvocellular basal nucleus and a ventral band of darkly staining cells usually referred to as the paralaminar basal nucleus because it borders the white matter ventral to the amygdaloid complex. The accessory basal nucleus lies medial to the basal nuclear divisions. It is usually divided into dorsal magnocellular and ventral parvocellular parts. The lateral and basal nuclei are often referred to collectively as the basolateral area (nuclear group) of the amygdaloid complex.

CASE 11   ALZHEIMER'S DISEASE

A 64-year-old man is brought for evaluation by his family because of impaired memory noted in the past 6 months. He has been unable to keep up with the demands of his business, has made a number of unfortunate decisions reflecting faulty judgment and has found it necessary to turn control of the family finances over to his wife. He has become increasingly apathetic and withdrawn, removing himself from his customary active social life.

On examination, he appears apathetic, with little spontaneous speech. He responds to direct questions and challenges slowly and incompletely. He has impaired memory for both recent and remote events, can no longer carry out simple arithmetic calculations, has a shortened attention span and is unable to explain proverbs or similarities in an abstract manner. He becomes intermittently agitated and is often delusional. With the exception of a mild, predominantly dysnomic form of aphasia and the occasional appearance of Parkinsonian signs, such as bradykinesia and rigidity, the remainder of the neurological examination is normal. A reversion to primitive reflex levels (e.g. forced grasping) may be evident.

Discussion: This man demonstrates the typical devastating, progressive clinical abnormalities of Alzheimer's disease, probably the most common dementing illness of middle and later life (to be distinguished from diffuse Lewy body disease, vascular dementia, and normal-pressure hydrocephalus, for example). Ultimately, much of the cerebral grey matter is involved, with typical neuropathological alterations and neurofibrillary changes reflecting intracellular accumulation of the protein tau, amyloid-containing senile plaques, deposition of amyloid in small vessel walls and neuronal vacuolization and loss. The earliest morphological changes are found in the medial temporal lobe and in the basal nucleus (of Meynert), with secondary loss of acetylcholine transferase, especially in the neocortex, reflecting the degeneration of cholinergic projections from the basal nucleus (Fig. 16.31).

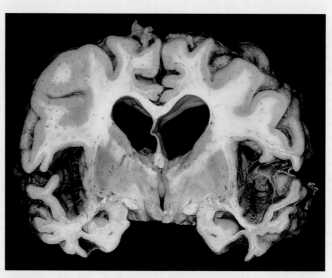

Fig. 16.31 Alzheimer's disease, demonstrating marked cortical atrophy with enlargement of the lateral ventricles (hydrocephalus ex vacuo) and gaping of the Sylvian fissures. (Courtesy of John S. Woodard, MD.)

It has been suggested that the basolateral complex of nuclei (lateral, basal, accessory basal) shares several characteristics with the cortex and that it may be considered a quasi-cortical structure. Although it lacks a laminar structure, it has direct, often reciprocal, connections with adjacent temporal and other areas of cortex, and it projects to the motor or premotor cortex. It receives a direct cholinergic and non-cholinergic input from the magnocellular corticopetal system in the basal forebrain and has reciprocal connections with the mediodorsal thalamus. The distribution of small peptidergic neurones in the basolateral nuclear complex (e.g. those containing neuropeptide Y, somatostatin and CCK) are also similar in form and density to those found in the adjacent temporal lobe cortex. Projection neurones from this part of the amygdala appear to utilize, at least in part, the excitatory amino acids glutamate and aspartate as transmitters. Moreover, they project to the ventral striatum rather than to hypothalamic and brain stem sites. Thus, it may be appropriate to consider this part of the amygdaloid complex as a polymodal cortex-like area that is separated from the cerebral cortex by fibres of the external capsule.

The central nucleus is present through the caudal half of the amygdaloid complex, lying dorsomedial to the basal nucleus. It is divided into medial and lateral parts. The medial part, which contains larger cells than the lateral part, resembles the adjacent putamen. The medial and central nuclei appear to have an extension across the basal forebrain, as well as within the stria terminalis, which merges with the bed nucleus of the stria terminalis. This extensive nuclear complex, sometimes referred to as the 'extended amygdala,' is illustrated in Figure 16.32. It can be considered a macrostructure formed by the centromedial amygdaloid complex (medial nucleus, medial and lateral parts of the central nucleus), the medial bed nucleus of the stria terminalis and the cell columns that traverse the sublenticular substantia innominata, which lies between them. It has been suggested that portions of the medial nucleus accumbens may be included in the extended amygdala.

A consistent feature of the intrinsic connections among amygdaloid nuclei is that they arise primarily in lateral and basal nuclei and terminate in central and medial nuclei, which suggests a largely unidirectional flow of information. In brief, the lateral nucleus projects to all divisions of the basal nucleus, accessory basal nucleus, and paralaminar and anterior cortical nuclei and less heavily to the central nucleus. The lateral nucleus receives few afferents from other nuclei. The magnocellular, parvocellular and intermediate parts of the basal nucleus project to the accessory basal, central (especially the medial part) and medial nuclei, as well as to the periamygdaloid cortex and the amygdalohippocampal area. The accessory basal nucleus projects densely to the central nucleus, especially its medial division, as well as to the medial and

cortical nuclei. Its major intra-amygdaloid afferents arise from the lateral nucleus. The medial nucleus projects to the accessory basal, anterior cortical and central nuclei, as well as to the periamygdaloid cortex and amygdalohippocampal area; afferents arise especially from the lateral nucleus. The intrinsic connections of the cortical nucleus are not well understood. The posterior part of the cortical nucleus projects to the medial nucleus, but it has been difficult to differentiate this projection from that arising in the amygdalohippocampal area. The central nucleus projects to the anterior cortical nucleus and the various cortical transition zones. It forms an important focus for afferents from many of the amygdaloid nuclei, especially the basal and accessory basal nuclei, and it has major extrinsic connections.

The organization of the extensive subcortical and cortical interconnections and connections of the amygdala are consistent with a role in emotional behaviour. It receives highly processed unimodal and multimodal sensory information from the thalamus and sensory and association cortices, olfactory information from the bulb and piriform cortex and visceral and gustatory information relayed via brain stem structures and the thalamus. Its projections reach widespread areas of the brain, including the endocrine and autonomic domains of the hypothalamus and brain stem. In a functional sense, the limbic–amygdala complex is strategically placed between the cerebral cortex and hypothalamus, serving to effectively modulate an organism's response to changes within the environment via hypothalamic and neuroendocrine mechanisms, as well as motor responses via the brain stem.

Afferent Connections — The heaviest brain stem projection to the amygdala arises in the peripeduncular nucleus. The parabrachial nuclei also project to the central nucleus. The amygdala receives a rich monoaminergic innervation. The noradrenergic projection arises primarily from the locus coeruleus; serotoninergic fibres arise from the dorsal and, to some extent, median raphe nuclei; and the dopaminergic innervation arises primarily in the midbrain ventral tegmental area (A10). The basal and parvocellular accessory basal nuclei, the amygdalohippocampal area and nucleus of the lateral olfactory tract receive a very dense cholinergic innervation arising from the magnocellular nucleus basalis of Meynert.

The amygdala has rich interconnections with allocortical, juxtallocortical and, especially, neocortical areas. In addition to direct projections from the olfactory bulb to the nucleus of the lateral olfactory tract, anterior cortical nucleus and periamygdaloid cortex (piriform cortex), there are associational connections between all parts of the primary olfactory cortex and these same superficial amygdaloid structures. The amygdaloid complex has particularly extensive and rich connections with many areas of the neocortex in unimodal and polymodal regions of the frontal, cingulate, insular and temporal neocortices.

The anterior temporal lobe provides the largest proportion of the cortical input to the amygdala, predominantly to the lateral nucleus. Rostral parts of the superior temporal gyrus, which may represent unimodal auditory association cortex, project to the lateral nucleus. There are also projections from polymodal sensory association cortices of the temporal lobe, including the perirhinal cortex (areas 35 and 36), the caudal half of the parahippocampal gyrus, the dorsal bank of the superior temporal sulcus and both the medial and lateral areas of the cortex of the temporal pole.

The CA1 field of the hippocampus and adjacent subiculum, and possibly the entorhinal cortex, project to the amygdala, mainly to the parvocellular basal nucleus.

The rostral insula projects heavily to the lateral, parvocellular basal and medial nuclei. The caudal insula, which is reciprocally connected with the second somatosensory cortex, also projects to the lateral nucleus, thus providing a route by which somatosensory information reaches the amygdala. The caudal orbital cortex projects to the basal, magnocellular accessory basal and lateral nuclei. The medial prefrontal cortex projects to the magnocellular divisions of the accessory and basal nuclei.

Efferent Connections — The central nucleus provides the major relay for projections from the amygdala to the brain stem and receives many of the return projections. It projects to the periaqueductal grey matter, ventral tegmental area, substantia nigra pars compacta, peripeduncular nucleus and tegmental reticular formation (midbrain); parabrachial nuclei (pons); and nucleus of the solitary tract and dorsal motor nucleus of the vagus (medulla).

The central nucleus is the major relay for amygdaloid projections to the hypothalamus. Amygdaloid fibres reach the bed nucleus of the stria terminalis primarily via the stria terminalis, but also via the ventral amygdalofugal pathway. In general, central and basal nuclei project to the lateral part of the bed nucleus, whereas medial and posterior cortical nuclei project to the medial bed nucleus. Anterior cortical and medial nuclei project largely to the medial preoptic area and anterior medial hypothalamus, including the paraventricular and supraoptic nuclei. There is a particularly prominent projection to the ventromedial and premammillary nuclei. The amygdala projects to the rostrocaudal extent of the lateral hypothalamus. The majority of the fibres

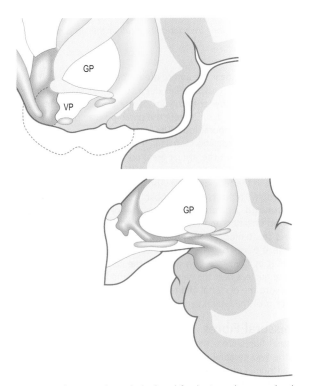

Fig. 16.32 *Coronal section through the basal forebrain and temporal pole, illustrating the relationship among the striatum* (yellow), *globus pallidus (dorsal globus pallidus, GP; ventral pallidum, VP), extended amygdala* (blue) *and magnocellular corticopetal basal forebrain system* (magenta). *Note that the medial part of the nucleus accumbens–olfactory tubercle area* (green) *may be a mixed zone of the ventral striatopallidal system and the extended amygdala.*

originate in the central nucleus and run principally in the ventral amygdalofu-gal pathway and medial forebrain bundle.

There is a rich projection to the mediodorsal nucleus of the thalamus, which gives access to the prefrontal cortex and also complements direct projections from the amygdala to the same cortical domain. The projection to the mediodorsal nucleus arises from most amygdaloid nuclei, but particularly from the lateral, basal and accessory basal nuclei and the periamygdaloid cortex. The major termination of amygdaloid afferents is in the medial magnocellular part of the mediodorsal nucleus, especially rostrally. This part of the mediodorsal nucleus projects to the identical medial and orbital prefrontal cortical areas that receive amygdaloid afferents directly. However, this projection to the mediodorsal nucleus is not reciprocated. The central and medial nuclei project not to the mediodorsal nucleus but to the midline nuclei, especially the nucleus centralis and nucleus reuniens.

The parvocellular division of the basal nucleus, magnocellular accessory basal nucleus (but not the magnocellular basal nucleus) and central nucleus all project to basal forebrain cholinergic cell groups, notably the nucleus basalis of Meynert and the horizontal limb nucleus of the diagonal band.

The striatum, and particularly the nucleus accumbens, receives prominent projections from the amygdaloid complex. The basal and accessory basal nuclei are the most important contributors to this projection. The ventral striatum sends many fibres to the ventral pallidum, which in turn projects to the mediodorsal nucleus of the thalamus. Thus, the ventral striatopallidal system provides a second route through which the amygdala can influence mediodorsal thalamic–prefrontal cortical processes.

The lateral magnocellular accessory basal and parvocellular basal nuclei contribute the largest proportion of efferents to the hippocampal formation. The main projection is from the lateral nucleus to the rostral entorhinal cortex, but many fibres also terminate in the hippocampus proper and the subiculum. There appears to be marked polarity in amygdalohippocampal connections—the amygdala has a greater influence on hippocampal processes than *vice versa*.

The amgygdaloid nuclear complex projects to widely dispersed neocortical fields. Amygdalocortical projections originate principally in the basal nucleus and, to a smaller extent, in the lateral and cortical nuclei.

The amygdala projects to virtually all levels of the visual cortex in both the temporal and occipital lobes. The largest component of these projections arises from the magnocellular basal nucleus. The amygdala also reciprocates projections to the auditory cortex in the rostral half of the superior temporal gyrus. Projections to the polymodal sensory areas of the temporal lobe generally reciprocate the amygdalopetal projections. Efferents from the lateral and accessory basal nuclei are directed to the temporal pole, particularly the medial perirhinal area.

The insular cortex is heavily innervated by the amygdaloid medial and anterior cortical nuclei. The orbital cortex and medial frontal cortical areas 24, 25 and 32, including parts of the anterior cingulate gyrus, also receive a heavy projection. Areas 8, 9, 45 and 46 of the dorsolateral prefrontal cortex, as well as the premotor cortex (area 6), receive a patchy innervation. The basal nucleus is an important source of these projections, which are augmented by contributions from the accessory basal (magnocellular and parvocellular divisions) and lateral nuclei.

Lesions of the Amygdala — The amygdala is important in evaluating the significance of environmental events, particularly the association between environmental stimuli and reinforcement. Such stimulus–reward associations are markedly impaired following lesions of the amygdala, such as Klüver-Bucy syndrome. (See Cases 5, 10.)

WHITE MATTER OF CEREBRAL HEMISPHERE

The nerve fibres that make up the white matter of the cerebral hemispheres are categorized on the basis of their course and connections. They may be association fibres, which link different cortical areas in the same hemisphere; commissural fibres, which link corresponding cortical areas in the two hemispheres; or projection fibres, which connect the cerebral cortex with the corpus striatum, diencephalon, brain stem and spinal cord.

Association Fibres

Association fibres may be either short association (arcuate or U) fibres, which link adjacent gyri, or long association fibres, which connect more widely separated gyri (Figs 16.33, 16.34). Short association fibres may be entirely intracortical. Many pass subcortically between adjacent gyri; some merely pass from one wall of a sulcus to the other.

Long association fibres are grouped into bundles, such as uncinate fasciculus, cingulum, superior longitudinal fasciculus, inferior longitudinal fasciculus and fronto-occipital fasciculus. The uncinate fasciculus connects the motor speech (Broca's) area and orbital gyri of the frontal lobe with the cortex in the temporal pole. The fibres follow a sharply curved course across the stem

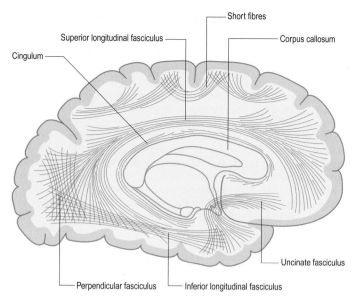

Fig. 16.33 *Principal association fibres of the cerebral hemisphere.*

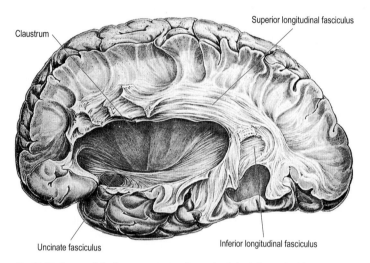

Fig. 16.34 *Some of the long association fasciculi of the left cerebral hemisphere.*

of the lateral sulcus, near the anteroinferior part of the insula. The cingulum is a long, curved fasciculus that lies deep to the cingulate gyrus. It starts in the medial cortex below the rostrum of the corpus callosum, follows the curve of the cingulate gyrus, enters the parahippocampal gyrus and spreads into the adjoining temporal lobe. The superior longitudinal fasciculus is the largest of the long association fasciculi. It starts in the anterior frontal region and arches back, above the insular area, contributing fibres to the occipital cortex (areas 18 and 19). It curves down and forward, behind the insular area, to spread out in the temporal lobe. The inferior longitudinal fasciculus starts near the occipital pole. Its fibres, probably derived mostly from areas 18 and 19, sweep forward, separated from the posterior horn of the lateral ventricle by the optic radiation and tapetal commissural fibres; they are distributed throughout the temporal lobe. The fronto-occipital fasciculus starts at the frontal pole. It passes back deep to the superior longitudinal fasciculus, separated from it by the projection fibres in the corona radiata. It lies lateral to the caudate nucleus near the central part of the lateral ventricle. Posteriorly, it fans out into the occipital and temporal lobes, lateral to the posterior and inferior horns of the lateral ventricle.

Commissural Fibres

Commissural fibres cross the midline, many of them linking corresponding areas in the two cerebral hemispheres. By far the largest commissure is the corpus callosum. Others include the anterior, posterior and habenular commisures and the commissure of the fornix.

Corpus Callosum

The corpus callosum is the largest fibre pathway of the brain (Figs. 16.2, 16.4, 16.35, 16.36). It links the cerebral cortex of the two cerebral hemispheres, and it roofs much of the lateral ventricles. It forms an arch approximately 10 cm

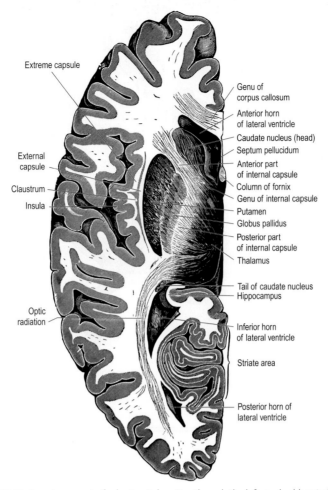

Fig. 16.42 *Superior aspect of a horizontal section through the left cerebral hemisphere.*

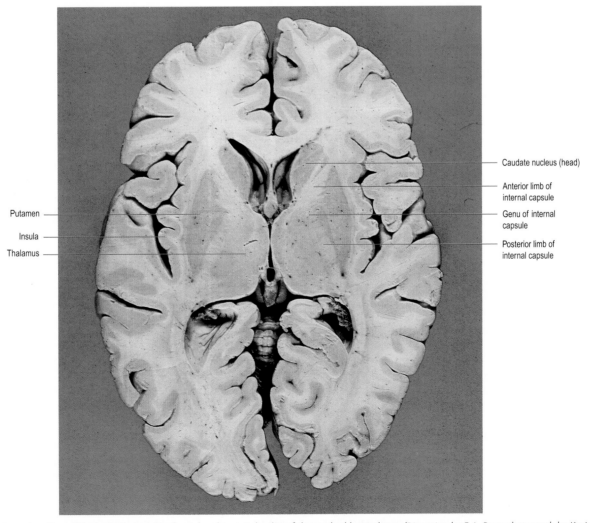

Fig. 16.43 *Horizontal section of the brain through the frontal and occipital poles of the cerebral hemispheres. (Dissection by E. L. Rees; photograph by Kevin Fitzpatrick on behalf of GKT School of Medicine, London.)*

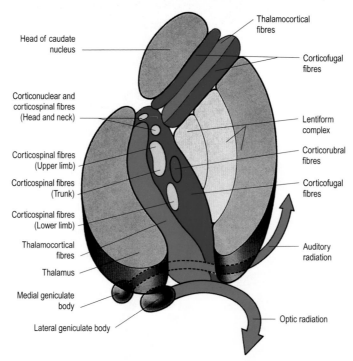

Fig. 16.44 *Horizontal section through the internal capsule illustrating its main fibre components. Descending motor fibres, yellow; corticofugal fibres to the thalamus and pons, red; ascending fibres, blue. (From Truex, R.C. [Ed.], Strong and Elwyn's Human Neuroanatomy, 4th ed. London: Baillière Tindall and Cox, London; and Kretschmann, H.-J., 1998. Localization of the corticospinal fibres in the internal capsule in man. J. Anat. [Lond.] 160, 219–225.)*

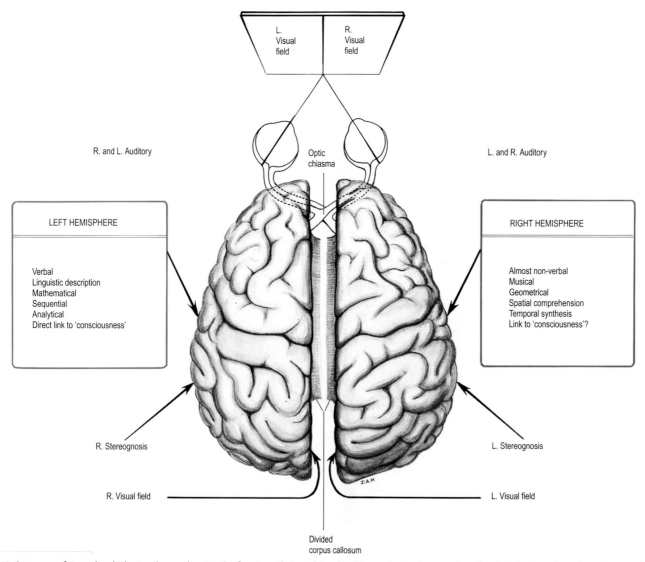

Fig. 16.45 *Summary of Sperry's split-brain schema, showing the functions that are lateralized to one hemisphere or the other. Split-brain patients have been studied by presenting stimuli selectively to one or the other hemisphere and comparing the subject's responses with them. For instance, a stimulus presented briefly to one visual field or placed in one hand is accessible only to the opposite hemisphere (because the projections are contralateral and all commissural connections have been severed). Objects in the right visual field or right hand are recognized and named easily by the 'verbal' left hemisphere. In contrast, patients cannot name, and appear to lack knowledge of, objects placed in the left visual field or left hand, because these are available only to the 'non-verbal' right hemisphere. However, the object has undoubtedly been identified correctly, because the person can later pick it out from a selection of objects. These functional specializations are relative and apply to people with left hemisphere language representation. Subsequent studies have added more detail and complexity. Overall, split-brain work has been central in establishing the extent and nature of functional asymmetries, and its importance was highlighted by Sperry's 1981 Nobel Prize. (From Sperry, R.W., 1984. Consciousness, personal identity and the divided brain. Neuropsychologia 17, 153–166, modified with permission from Elsevier; and Sperry, R.W., 1974. Lateral specialization in the surgically separated hemisphere. In: Schmidt, F.O., Worden, F.G. (Eds.), The Neurosciences. Third Study Program. MIT Press, Cambridge, Mass., pp. 5–19.)*

impairment with left hemisphere lesions led to the more general concept of a dominant left hemisphere and a minor right hemisphere.

Much information on the lateralization of cerebral function has come from studying patients in whom the corpus callosum was divided (commissurotomy) to treat intractable epilepsy and rare subjects who lack part or all of the corpus callosum. Commissurotomy produces the 'split-brain' syndrome (Fig. 16.45), supporting the notion that abilities or functions are predominantly associated with one hemisphere or the other. Knowledge of such lateralization of function has been advanced more recently by functional brain imaging techniques such as PET.

The left hemisphere usually prevails for verbal and linguistic functions, mathematical skills and analytical thinking. The right hemisphere is mostly non-verbal; it is more involved in spatial and holistic or gestalt thinking, in many aspects of music appreciation and in some emotions. Memory also shows lateralization: verbal memory is primarily a left hemisphere function, and non-verbal memory is represented in the right hemisphere. These asymmetries are relative, not absolute, and they vary in degree according to the function and the individual. Moreover, they apply primarily to right-handed individuals. Those persons with a left-hand preference or mixed handedness make up a heterogeneous group that generally shows reduced or anomalous lateralization rather than a simple reversal of the situation in right-handers. For example, speech representation can occur in either or both hemispheres. Women show less functional asymmetry, on average, than men.

Certain cerebral anatomical asymmetries are apparent at both the macroscopic and histological levels. One of the most notable is in the planum temporale, which is usually larger on the left side than the right (Fig. 16.46). Probably as a result of this size difference, the lateral fissure is longer and more horizontal in the left hemisphere; this observation, together with the orientation of the overlying vasculature, provides a surface marker of temporal lobe asymmetry. The limits of asymmetry in the superior temporal lobe

remain uncertain but appear to include Heschl's gyrus and some other structures adjacent to (and sometimes considered an extension of) the planum temporale.

There is evidence that planum temporale asymmetry originates almost entirely from right–left differences in the size of a cytoarchitectonic subfield called Tpt (see Fig. 16.46). Subtle asymmetries in the superior temporal lobe have been demonstrated in terms of overall size and shape, sulcal pattern and cytoarchitecture, as well as at the neuronal level. It seems reasonable to assume that these differences underlie some of the functional asymmetry for language representation.

Asymmetries in areal size, cytoarchitecture or neurocytology occur elsewhere in the cerebral cortex as well as subcortically. For example, many brains have a wider right frontal pole and a wider left occipital pole. Brodmann's area 45 in the inferior frontal lobe, corresponding to Broca's area, contains a population of large pyramidal neurones that are found only on the left side. The cortical surface surrounding the central sulcus is larger in the left hemisphere, especially in the areas containing the primary somatosensory and motor maps of the arm, suggesting that one cerebral manifestation of hand preference is a larger amount of neural circuitry in the relevant parts of the cortex. Histological asymmetries are also found in areas that are not usually considered to be closely related to either language or handedness. The left entorhinal cortex has significantly more neurones than the right.

The most interesting clinical implications of cerebral asymmetry occur when disturbed lateralization appears to be inherent in the nature or even the cause of a disorder. This relationship is most striking in schizophrenia. A number of studies suggest that the disease is associated with a failure to develop normal structural and functional cerebral asymmetry and that its pathology is characterized by a greater affliction of the left than the right hemisphere. Other putative neurodevelopmental disorders, including dyslexia and autism, may also be associated with asymmetric cerebral abnormalities.

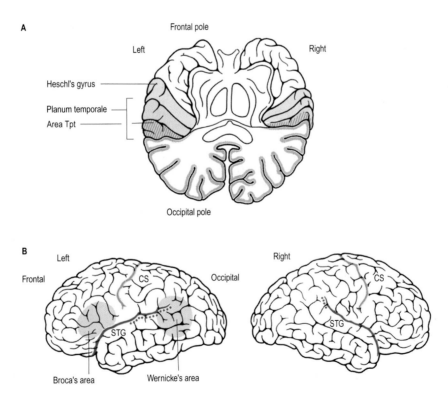

Fig. 16.46 *Examples of anatomical asymmetries in the cerebral cortex. **A**, Horizontal section showing the exposed upper surface of the temporal lobes. The planum temporale (stippled in red) forms the upper posterior part of the temporal lobe, bordered anteriorly by Heschl's gyrus (stippled in blue), laterally by the Sylvian fissure and posteriorly by the end of the Sylvian fissure. The brain shown here demonstrates marked asymmetry in size of the planum temporale, which is larger on the left in a majority of brains. This brain also shows asymmetry of Heschl's gyrus. The asymmetric length of the lateral border of the planum temporale underlies the asymmetries in the Sylvian fissure itself (see also **B**). Asymmetry of the planum temporale arises mostly from differences in the size of the cytoarchitectonic field Tpt (shaded in green). Tpt forms much of the posterior part of the planum temporale, although it also extends onto the lateral surface of the posterior superior temporal gyrus. **B**, Lateral views of the left and right hemispheres emphasizing differences between the two Sylvian fissures (red). Compared with the left hemisphere, the right Sylvian fissure is shorter and turns upward. This reflects planum temporale asymmetries (represented by adjacent red stippling). The approximate locations of Broca's and Wernicke's areas in the left hemisphere are indicated. However, much of Wernicke's area is buried within the sulcal folds and is not visible on a lateral view. CS, central sulcus; STG, superior temporal gyrus. (Adapted from Geschwind, N., Levitsky, W., 1968. Human brain. Science 161, 186–187, by permission from AAAS.)*

CASE 15   CREUTZFELDT-JAKOB DISEASE

A 65-year-old man first began to exhibit impaired judgment, anxiety and fatigue 18 months previously. He then developed a progressive dementia. His symptoms gradually worsened and became associated with severe recent and then remote memory problems. Abrupt myoclonic jerks of the upper extremities appeared several weeks before his neurological evaluation.

Neurological examination now confirms dementia with evidence of marked memory loss, impairment of executive functions, dyscalculia, visuospatial disturbances and visual agnosia. Increased muscle tone is evident in all four extremities, along with generalized hyperreflexia with bilateral extensor plantar responses (Babinski's sign). Frequent myoclonic jerks of the upper extremities and left lower extremities are seen; his gait is unsteady, with impaired postural reflexes.

MRI demonstrates ventriculomegaly and increased signal intensity on T2-weighted, FLAIR and diffusion-weighted images in the basal ganglia of both hemispheres. Electroencephalogram shows a generalized periodic pattern of sharp waves at intervals of 0.7 to 1 second in duration. A cerebrospinal fluid immunoassay demonstrates a 14-3-3 protein.

Discussion: The combination of history, neurological examination and diagnostic test results points strongly to a diagnosis of Creutzfeldt-Jakob disease, a human prion disease and one of the so-called transmissible spongiform encephalopathies. Anatomically, the disorder involves grey matter diffusely throughout the neuraxis, with remarkable devastation, especially of the cerebral cortex, but ultimately involving the entire central nervous system (Fig. 16.47).

Presence of the 14-3-3 protein coupled with the clinical course strongly supports the diagnosis of Creutzfeldt-Jakob disease. A periodic electroencephalographic pattern with intervals of 0.5 to 2 seconds is also characteristic of the disease, although it generally appears very late in the course of the illness.

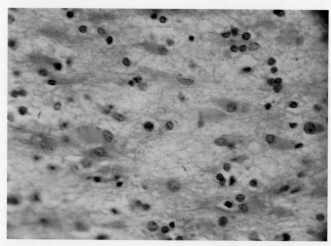

Fig. 16.47 *Creutzfeldt-Jakob disease. There is striking loss of neurones in the cerebral cortex, with a brisk astrocytic response and microcavitation (spongiform encephalopathy).*

References

Alheid, G.F., Heimer, L., 1988. New perspectives in basal forebrain organization of special relevance for neuropsychiatric disorders: the striatopallidal, amygdaloid and corticopetal components of the substantia innominata. Neuroscience 27, 1–39. *Provides evidence that the region of the substantia innominata in the basal forebrain is composed of parts of three forebrain structures: the ventral striatopallidal system, the extended amygdala and the magnocellular corticopetal system.*

Budson, A.E., Price, B.H., 2005. Memory dysfunction. N. Engl. J. Med. 352, 692–699.

Derbyshire, S.W., Jones, A.K., Gyulai, F., Clark, S., Townsend, D., Firestone, L.L., 1997. Pain processing during three levels of noxious stimulation produces differential patterns of central activity. Pain 73, 431–445.

Galpern, W.R., Lang, A.E., 2006. Interface between tauopathies and synucleinopathies: a tale of two proteins. Ann. Neurol. 59, 449–458.

Geschwind, M.D., Shu, H., Haman, A., Sejvar, J.J., Miller, B.L., 2008. Rapidly progressive dementia. Ann. Neurol. 64, 97–108.

Josephs, K.A., 2008. Frontotemporal dementia and related disorders: deciphering the enigma. Ann. Neurol. 64, 4–14.

Marlowe, W.B., Mancall, E.L., Thomas, J.J., 1975. Complete Kluver-Bucy syndrome in man. Cortex. 11, 53–59.

Papez, J.W., 1937. A proposed mechanism of emotion. Arch. Neurol. Psychiatry 38, 725–743. *Classic description of the mechanism of human emotion.*

Passingham, R.E., 1993. The Frontal Lobes and Voluntary Action. Oxford University Press, Oxford.

Penfield, W., Rasmussen, T., 1950. The Cerebral Cortex of Man. Macmillan, New York. *Classic description of the organization of sensory and motor homunculi in the human cerebral cortex.*

Peyron, R., Laurent, B., Garcia-Larrea, L., 2000. Functional imaging of brain responses to pain: A review and meta-analysis. Neurophysiol. Clin. 30, 263–288.

Sperry, R.W., 1974. Lateral specialization in the surgically separated hemisphere. In: Schmidt, F.O., Worden, F.G. (Eds.), The Neurosciences: Third study program. MIT Press, Cambridge, Mass, pp. 5–19.

Sperry, R.W., 1984. Consciousness, personal identity and the divided brain. Neuropsychologia. 17, 153–166.

Victor, M., Angevine, J.G., Fisher, C.M., Mancall, E.L., 1961. Memory loss with lesions of hippocampal formation. Arch. Neurol. 5, 244.

Section VI

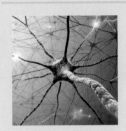

The Peripheral and Autonomic Nervous Systems

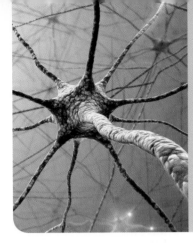

Cervical Plexus

The cervical plexus is formed by the ventral rami of the upper four cervical nerves, and it supplies some neck muscles, the diaphragm and areas of skin on the head, neck and chest (Figs 17.1–17.3; see also Fig. 11.10). It is situated in the neck opposite a line drawn down the side of the neck from the root of the auricle to the level of the upper border of the thyroid cartilage. It is deep to the internal jugular vein, the deep fascia and sternocleidomastoid, and anterior to scalenus medius and levator scapulae. Each ramus, except the first, divides into ascending and descending parts that unite in communicating loops. From the first loop (C2 and C3), superficial branches supply the head and neck; cutaneous nerves of the shoulder and chest arise from the second loop (C3 and C4). Muscular and communicating branches arise from the same nerves. The branches are superficial or deep. The superficial branches perforate the cervical fascia to supply the skin, whereas the deep branches generally supply the muscles. The superficial branches either ascend (lesser occipital, great auricular and transverse cutaneous nerves) or descend (supraclavicular nerves). The deep branches form medial and lateral series.

LESSER OCCIPITAL NERVE

The lesser occipital nerve is derived mainly from the second cervical nerve (although fibres from the third cervical nerve sometimes contribute). It curves around the accessory nerve and ascends along the posterior margin of the sternocleidomastoid. Near the cranium it perforates the deep fascia and passes up onto the scalp behind the auricle. It supplies the skin and connects with the great auricular and greater occipital nerves and the auricular branch of the facial nerve. Its auricular branch supplies the skin on the upper third of the medial aspect of the auricle and connects with the posterior branch of the great auricular nerve. The auricular branch is occasionally derived from the greater occipital nerve.

It has been suggested that compression or stretching of the lesser occipital nerve contributes to cervicogenic headache.

GREAT AURICULAR NERVE

The great auricular nerve is the largest ascending branch of the cervical plexus. It arises from the second and third cervical rami, encircles the posterior border of the sternocleidomastoid, perforates the deep fascia and ascends on the muscle beneath platysma with the external jugular vein. It passes to the parotid gland, dividing into anterior and posterior branches. The anterior branch is distributed to the facial skin over the parotid gland, connecting in the gland with the facial nerve. The posterior branch supplies the skin over the mastoid process and on the back of the auricle (except its upper part); a filament pierces the auricle to reach the lateral surface, where it is distributed to the lobule and concha. The posterior branch communicates with the lesser occipital nerve, the auricular branch of the vagus nerve and the posterior auricular branch of the facial nerve.

TRANSVERSE CUTANEOUS (CERVICAL) NERVE OF THE NECK

The transverse cutaneous nerve arises from the second and third cervical rami, curves around the posterior border of the sternocleidomastoid near its midpoint and runs obliquely forward, deep to the external jugular vein, to the anterior border of the muscle. It perforates the deep cervical fascia and divides under platysma into ascending and descending branches that are distributed to the anterolateral areas of the neck. The ascending branches ascend to the submandibular region, forming a plexus with the cervical branch of the facial nerve beneath platysma. Some branches pierce platysma and are distributed to the skin of the upper anterior areas of the neck. The descending branches pierce platysma and are distributed anterolaterally to the skin of the neck, as low as the sternum.

SUPRACLAVICULAR NERVES

The supraclavicular nerves arise from a common trunk formed from rami from the third and fourth cervical nerves and emerge at the posterior border of

the sternocleidomastoid. Descending under platysma and the deep cervical fascia, the trunk divides into medial, intermediate and lateral (posterior) branches, which diverge to pierce the deep fascia a little above the clavicle. The medial supraclavicular nerves run inferomedially across the external jugular vein and the clavicular and sternal heads of the sternocleidomastoid to supply the skin as far as the midline and as low as the second rib. They supply the sternoclavicular joint. The intermediate supraclavicular nerves cross the clavicle to supply the skin over pectoralis major and deltoid down to the level of the second rib, next to the area of supply of the second thoracic nerve. Overlap between these nerves is minimal. The lateral supraclavicular nerves descend superficially across trapezius and the acromion, supplying the skin of the upper and posterior parts of the shoulder.

DEEP BRANCHES—MEDIAL SERIES
Communicating Branches

Communicating branches pass from the loop between the first and second cervical rami to the vagus and hypoglossal nerves and to the sympathetic trunk. The hypoglossal branch later leaves the hypoglossal nerve as a series of branches—namely, the meningeal, superior root of ansa cervicalis and nerves to thyrohyoid and geniohyoid. A branch also connects the fourth and

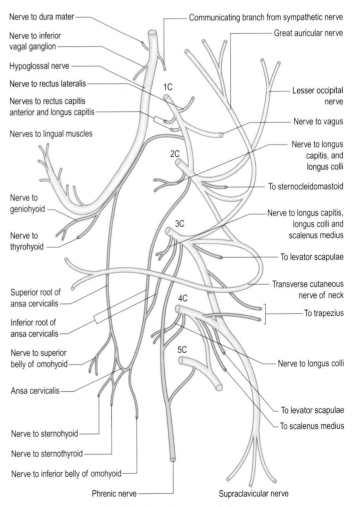

Fig. 17.1 *Plan of the cervical plexus.*

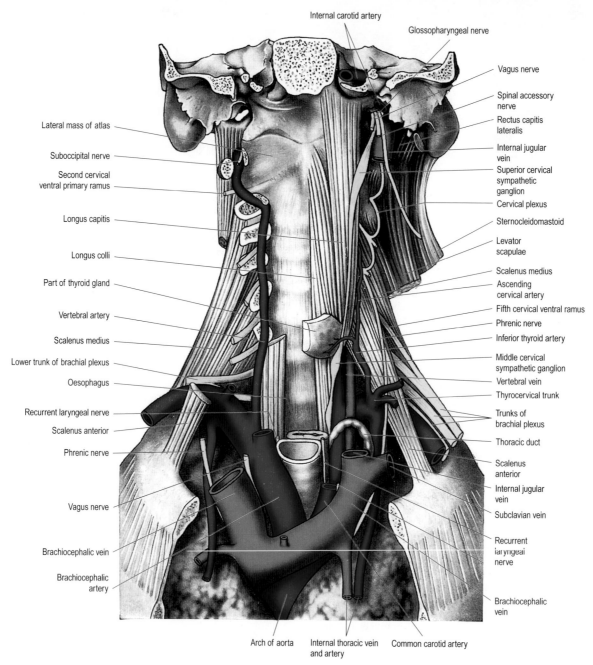

Fig. 17.2 *Dissection showing the prevertebral region and superior mediastinum. On the right the costal elements of the upper six cervical vertebrae have been removed to expose the cervical part of the vertebral artery. On the left most of the deep relations of the common carotid artery and the internal jugular vein are exposed.*

fifth cervical rami. The first four cervical ventral rami each receive a grey ramus communicans from the superior cervical sympathetic ganglion.

The superior root of the ansa cervicalis (descendens hypoglossi; see Fig. 17.1) leaves the hypoglossal nerve where it curves around the occipital artery and then descends anterior to or in the carotid sheath. It contains only fibres from the first cervical spinal nerve. After giving a branch to the superior belly of omohyoid, it is joined by the inferior root of the ansa from the second and third cervical spinal nerves. The two roots form the ansa cervicalis (ansa hypoglossi), from which branches supply sternohyoid, sternothyroid and the inferior belly of omohyoid. Another branch descends anterior to the vessels into the thorax to join the cardiac and phrenic nerves.

Muscular Branches

Muscular branches supply rectus capitis lateralis (C1), rectus capitis anterior (C1, C2), longus capitis (C1–3) and longus colli (C2–4). The inferior root of the ansa cervicalis and the phrenic nerve are additional muscular branches.

Inferior Root of Ansa Cervicalis

The inferior root of the ansa cervicalis (nervus descendens cervicalis) is formed by the union of branches from the second and third cervical rami (see

Fig. 17.1). It descends on the lateral side of the internal jugular vein, crosses it a little below the middle of the neck and continues forward to join the superior root anterior to the common carotid artery, forming the ansa cervicalis (ansa hypoglossi), from which all infrahyoid muscles except the thyrohyoid are supplied. The inferior root comes from the second and third cervical ventral rami in approximately 75% cases, from the second to fourth in 15% and from the third alone in 5%. Occasionally, it may be derived either from the second alone or from the first to third.

Phrenic Nerve

The phrenic nerve arises chiefly from the fourth cervical ventral ramus, but it also has contributions from the third and fifth. It is formed at the upper part of the lateral border of scalenus anterior and descends almost vertically across its anterior surface behind the prevertebral fascia. It descends posterior to the sternocleidomastoid, the inferior belly of omohyoid (near its intermediate tendon), the internal jugular vein, transverse cervical and suprascapular arteries and, on the left, the thoracic duct. At the root of the neck it runs anterior to the second part of the subclavian artery, from which it is separated by the scalenus anterior (according to some accounts, on the left side the nerve passes anterior to the first part of the subclavian artery), and posterior

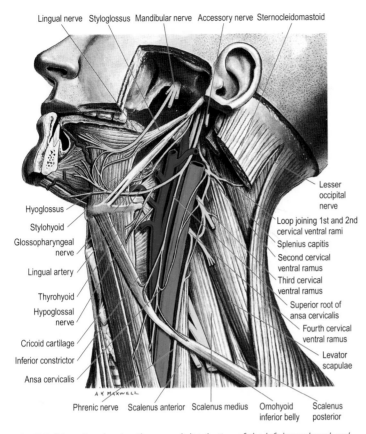

Lingual nerve Styloglossus Mandibular nerve Accessory nerve Sternocleidomastoid

Hyoglossus

Stylohyoid

Glossopharyngeal nerve

Lingual artery

Thyrohyoid

Hypoglossal nerve

Cricoid cartilage

Inferior constrictor

Ansa cervicalis

Lesser occipital nerve

Loop joining 1st and 2nd cervical ventral rami

Splenius capitis

Second cervical ventral ramus

Third cervical ventral ramus

Superior root of ansa cervicalis

Fourth cervical ventral ramus

Levator scapulae

A K MAXWELL

Phrenic nerve   Scalenus anterior   Scalenus medius   Omohyoid inferior belly   Scalenus posterior

Fig. 17.3 *Dissection showing the general distribution of the left hypoglossal and lingual nerves and the position and constitution of some parts of the cervical plexus on the left side.*

to the subclavian vein. The phrenic nerve enters the thorax by crossing medially in front of the internal thoracic artery.

In the neck, each nerve receives variable filaments from the cervical sympathetic ganglia or their branches and may also connect with internal thoracic sympathetic plexuses.

Accessory Phrenic Nerve
The accessory phrenic nerve is composed of fibres from the fifth cervical ventral ramus that run in a branch of the nerve to subclavius. This lies lateral to the phrenic nerve and descends posterior (occasionally anterior) to the subclavian vein. The accessory phrenic nerve usually joins the phrenic nerve near the first rib, but it may not do so until near the pulmonary hilum or beyond. The accessory phrenic nerve may be derived from the fourth or sixth cervical ventral rami or from the ansa cervicalis.

DEEP BRANCHES—LATERAL SERIES
Communicating Branches
Lateral deep branches of the cervical plexus (C2–4) may connect with the spinal accessory nerve within the sternocleidomastoid, in the posterior triangle or beneath trapezius.

Muscular Branches
Muscular branches are distributed to the sternocleidomastoid (C2–4), trapezius (C2 and possibly C3), levator scapulae (C3, C4) and scalenus medius (C3, C4). Branches to the trapezius cross the posterior triangle obliquely below the spinal accessory nerve.

References
Berkovitz, B.K.B., Kirsch, C., Moxham, B.J., Alusi, G., Cheeseman, T., 2002. Interactive Head and Neck. Primal Pictures, London.

Wilson-Pauwels, L., Akesson, E.J., Stewart, P.A., 1998. Cranial Nerves: Anatomy and Clinical Comments. Decker, Toronto.

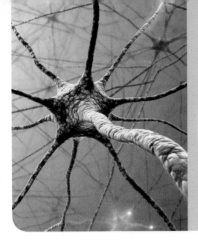

Brachial Plexus

OVERVIEW OF THE BRACHIAL PLEXUS

The brachial plexus is a union of the ventral rami of the lower four cervical nerves and the greater part of the first thoracic ventral ramus (Figs 18.1, 18.2). The fourth ramus usually gives a branch to the fifth, and the first thoracic frequently receives one from the second. These ventral rami are the roots of the plexus; they are almost equal in size but variable in their mode of junction. Contributions to the plexus by C4 and T2 vary. When the branch from C4 is large, that from T2 is frequently absent and the branch from T1 is reduced, forming a 'prefixed' type of plexus. If the branch from C4 is small or absent, the contribution from C5 is reduced, that from T1 is larger and there is always a contribution from T2; this arrangement constitutes a 'postfixed' type of plexus.

Close to their exit from the intervertebral foramina, the fifth and sixth cervical ventral rami receive grey rami communicantes from the middle cervical sympathetic ganglion, and the seventh and eighth rami receive grey rami from the cervicothoracic ganglion. The first thoracic ventral ramus receives a grey ramus from, and contributes a white ramus to, the cervicothoracic ganglion.

The most common arrangement of the brachial plexus is as follows: the fifth and sixth rami unite at the lateral border of scalenus medius as the upper trunk; the eighth cervical and first thoracic rami join behind scalenus anterior as the lower trunk; the seventh cervical ramus becomes the middle trunk. The three trunks incline laterally, and either just above or behind the clavicle, each bifurcates into anterior and posterior divisions. The anterior divisions of the upper and middle trunks form a lateral cord that lies lateral to the axillary artery. The anterior division of the lower trunk descends at first behind and then medial to the axillary artery and forms the medial cord, which often receives a branch from the seventh cervical ramus. Posterior divisions of all three trunks form the posterior cord, which is at first above and then behind the axillary artery. The posterior division of the lower trunk is much smaller than the others and contains few, if any, fibres from the first thoracic ramus. It is frequently derived from the eighth cervical ramus before the trunk is formed.

OVERVIEW OF THE PRINCIPAL NERVES

Axillary Nerve (C5, C6)

The axillary nerve is a branch of the posterior cord of the brachial plexus. It winds posteriorly around the neck of the humerus together with the circumflex humeral vessels and supplies the deltoid and teres minor and an area of skin over the deltoid region (Fig. 18.3).

Radial Nerve (C5–8, T1)

The radial nerve is the continuation of the posterior cord of the brachial plexus (Fig. 18.4). In the upper arm it lies in the spiral groove of the humerus, where it is accompanied by the profunda brachii artery and its venae comitantes. It enters the posterior (extensor) compartment and supplies triceps, then reenters the anterior compartment of the arm by piercing the lateral intermuscular septum. At the level of the lateral epicondyle it gives off the posterior interosseous nerve, which passes between the two heads of the supinator and enters the extensor compartment of the forearm. The posterior interosseous nerve supplies these muscles. The radial nerve itself continues into the forearm in the anterior compartment deep to the brachioradialis. It terminates by supplying the skin over the posterior aspect of the thumb, index, middle fingers and radial half of the ring finger.

Musculocutaneous Nerve (C5–7)

The musculocutaneous nerve is formed from the continuation of the lateral cord of the brachial plexus. It pierces the coracobrachialis; supplies it, biceps and brachialis; then continues into the forearm as the lateral cutaneous nerve of the forearm (Fig. 18.5).

Median Nerve (C6–8, T1)

The median nerve is formed by the union of the terminal branch of the lateral and medial cords of the brachial plexus (Fig. 18.6). It has no branches in the upper arm. It enters the forearm between the two heads of pronator teres and gives off the anterior interosseous nerve, which supplies all the flexor muscles of the forearm except for flexor carpi ulnaris and the ulnar half of flexor digitorum profundus. The median nerve itself passes deep to the flexor retinaculum at the wrist. On entering the palm, it gives off motor branches to the thenar muscles and the radial two lumbricals and cutaneous branches to the palmar aspect of the thumb, index and middle fingers and the radial half of the ring finger.

Ulnar Nerve (C7, C8, T1)

The ulnar nerve is the continuation of the medial cord of the brachial plexus (Fig. 18.7). Like the median nerve, it has no branches in the upper arm. It enters the posterior compartment of the upper arm midway down its length by piercing the medial intermuscular septum and passes behind the medial epicondyle of the humerus to enter the forearm. It passes to the wrist deep to flexor carpi ulnaris, giving branches to this muscle and to the ulnar half of flexor digitorum profundus. Just proximal to the wrist it gives off a dorsal cutaneous branch that supplies the skin over the dorsal aspect of the little finger and the ulnar half of the ring finger. The ulnar nerve crosses into the palm superficial to the flexor retinaculum in Guyon's canal. It divides into a motor branch, which supplies the hypothenar muscles, the intrinsics (apart from the radial two lumbricals) and adductor pollicis, and cutaneous branches, which supply the skin of the palmar aspect of the little finger and ulnar half of the ring finger.

Dermatomes

Our knowledge of the extent of individual dermatomes, especially in the limbs, is based largely on clinical evidence (Fig. 18.8). The dermatomes of the upper limb arise from spinal nerves C5–8 and T1. C7 supplies the central part of the hand. Considerable overlap exists between adjacent dermatomes innervated by nerves derived from consecutive spinal cord segments.

Myotomes

Each spinal nerve originally supplies the musculature derived from its own myotome. Where myotomal derivatives remain entities, they retain their original segmental supply. When derivatives from adjoining myotomes fuse, the resulting muscles do not always retain a nerve supply from each corresponding spinal nerve. Because muscles develop in situ, in the mesodermal cores of the developing limbs, it is impossible to identify their original segments by a developmental study. Most limb muscles are innervated by neurones from more than one segment of the spinal cord. Tables 18.1 to 18.4 summarize the predominant segmental origins of the nerve supply for each of the upper limb muscles and for movements taking place at the joints of the upper limb; damage to these segments or to their motor roots results in maximal paralysis.

Reflexes

Biceps Jerk (C5, C6) — The elbow is flexed to a right angle and slightly pronated. A finger is placed on the biceps tendon and struck with a percussion hammer; this should elicit flexion and slight supination of the forearm.

Triceps Jerk (C6–8) — The arm is supported at the wrist and flexed to a right angle. The triceps is struck with a percussion hammer just proximal to the olecranon; this should elicit extension of the elbow.

Radial Jerk (C7, C8) — The radial jerk is a periosteal, not a tendon, reflex. The elbow is flexed to a right angle, and the forearm is placed in the mid position. The radial styloid is struck with the percussion hammer. This elicits contraction of brachioradialis, which causes flexion of the elbow.

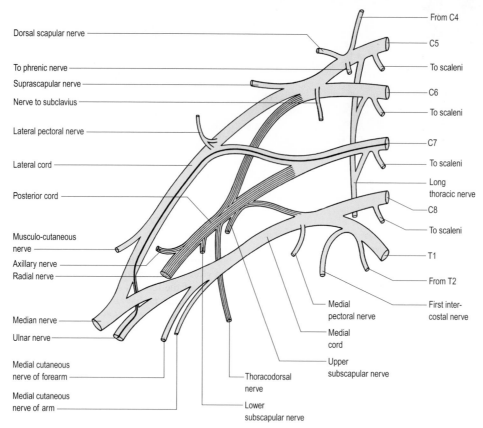

Dorsal scapular nerve

To phrenic nerve
Suprascapular nerve
Nerve to subclavius

Lateral pectoral nerve

Lateral cord

Posterior cord

Musculo-cutaneous
nerve
Axillary nerve
Radial nerve

Median nerve
Ulnar nerve

Medial cutaneous
nerve of forearm

Medial cutaneous
nerve of arm

From C4
C5
To scaleni
C6
To scaleni
C7
To scaleni
Long
thoracic nerve
C8
To scaleni
T1
From T2
First inter-
costal nerve

Medial
pectoral nerve

Medial
cord

Upper
subscapular nerve

Thoracodorsal
nerve

Lower
subscapular nerve

Fig. 18.1 *Plan of the brachial plexus. The posterior division of the trunks and their derivatives are shaded; the fibres from C7 that enter the ulnar nerve are shown as a heavy black line. C4 to C8 and T1 and T2 indicate the ventral rami of these cervical and thoracic spinal nerves.*

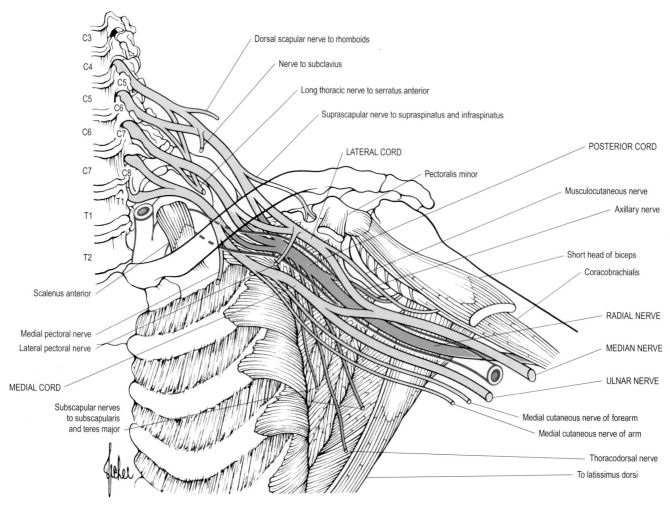

C3
C4
C5
C5
C6
C6
C7
C7
C8
T1
T1
T2

Scalenus anterior

Medial pectoral nerve
Lateral pectoral nerve

MEDIAL CORD

Subscapular nerves
to subscapularis
and teres major

Dorsal scapular nerve to rhomboids

Nerve to subclavius

Long thoracic nerve to serratus anterior

Suprascapular nerve to supraspinatus and infraspinatus

LATERAL CORD

Pectoralis minor

POSTERIOR CORD

Musculocutaneous nerve

Axillary nerve

Short head of biceps
Coracobrachialis

RADIAL NERVE

MEDIAN NERVE

ULNAR NERVE

Medial cutaneous nerve of forearm
Medial cutaneous nerve of arm

Thoracodorsal nerve
To latissimus dorsi

Fig. 18.2 *Diagram of the brachial plexus, its branches and the muscles they supply. (From Aids to the Examination of the Peripheral Nervous System, 4th ed. 2000. Saunders, London.)*

320

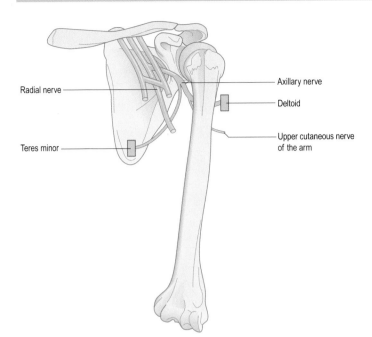

Fig. 18.3 *Motor and sensory branches of the axillary nerve. (From Aids to the Examination of the Peripheral Nervous System, 4th ed. 2000. Saunders, London. With permission of Guarantors of Brain.)*

MUSCLE INNVERVATION AND FUNCTION

Table 18.1 provides the following information about the innervation and functions of muscles in the upper limb:

Movements — At the central nervous level of control, muscles are recognized not as individual actuators but as components of movement. Muscles may contribute to several types of movement, acting variously as prime movers, antagonists, fixators or synergists. For example, in the movement of the scapula around the thorax, serratus anterior acts as an antagonist of trapezius, but in the forward rotation of the scapula, the two muscles combine as prime movers. Moreover, a muscle that crosses two joints can produce more than one movement. Even a muscle that acts across one joint can produce a combination of movements, such as flexion with medial rotation or extension with adduction. Some muscles have therefore been included in more than one place in Table 18.1, but even these listings are not exhaustive.

Nerve Roots — The spinal roots listed as contributing to muscle innervation vary in different texts; this is a reflection of the often unreliable nature of available information. The most positive identifications have been obtained by electrically stimulating spinal roots and recording the evoked electromyographic activity in the muscles. This is a laborious process, however, and data of this quality are in limited supply. Much of the information in Table 18.1 is based on neurological experience gained in examining the effects of lesions, and some of it is far from new.

Major and Minor Contributions — Spinal roots have been given the same shading in Table 18.1 when they innervate a muscle to a similar extent or when differences in their contribution have not been described. Heavy shading indicates roots from which there is known to be a dominant contribution. From a clinical viewpoint, some of these roots may be regarded as innervating the muscle almost exclusively: for example, deltoid by C5, brachioradialis by C6, triceps by C7. Minor contributions have been retained in the table to increase its utility in other contexts, such as electromyography and comparative anatomy.

Clinical Testing — For diagnostic purposes, it is neither necessary nor possible to test every muscle, and the experienced neurologist can cover every clinical possibility with a much shorter list. In Table 18.1, red has been used to highlight those muscles or movements that have diagnostic value. The emphasis here is on the differentiation of lesions at different root levels. Other lists could be developed to differentiate between lesions at the level of the root, plexus or peripheral nerve; at different sites along the length of a nerve; or between different peripheral nerves. The preferred criteria for including a given muscle in such a list are that it is visible and palpable, that its action is isolated or can be isolated by the examiner, that it is innervated by one peripheral nerve or (predominantly) one root, that it has a clinically elicitable reflex and that it is useful in differentiating among different nerves, roots or lesion levels.

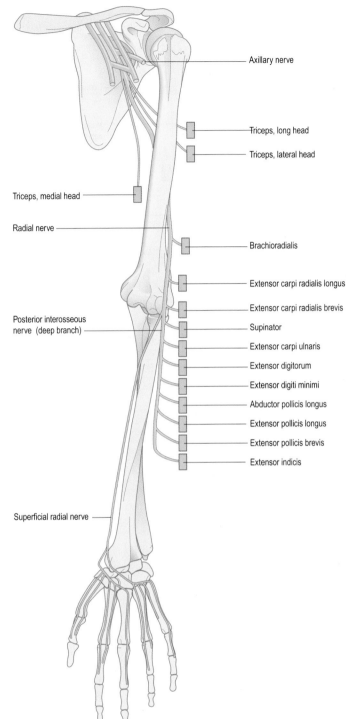

Fig. 18.4 *Motor and sensory branches of the radial nerve. Variation exists in the cutaneous innervation of the dorsal aspects of the digits. Here, the radial nerve is shown supplying all five digits. The dorsum of the ring and little fingers is frequently innervated by the dorsal branch of the ulnar nerve. (From Aids to the Examination of the Peripheral Nervous System, 4th ed. 2000. Saunders, London. With permission of Guarantors of Brain.)*

DETERMINATION OF A LESION'S LOCATION

In clinical practice it is necessary to test only a relatively small number of muscles to determine the location of a lesion. For example, abduction of the arm might test shoulder abduction, a C5 root lesion, the axillary nerve or deltoid.

Any muscle to be tested must satisfy a number of criteria. It should be visible, so that wasting or fasciculation can be observed and the muscle's consistency with contraction can be felt. It should have an isolated action, so that its function can be tested separately. The muscle tested should help differentiate between lesions at different levels in the neuraxis and in peripheral nerves, or between peripheral nerves. It should be tested in such a way

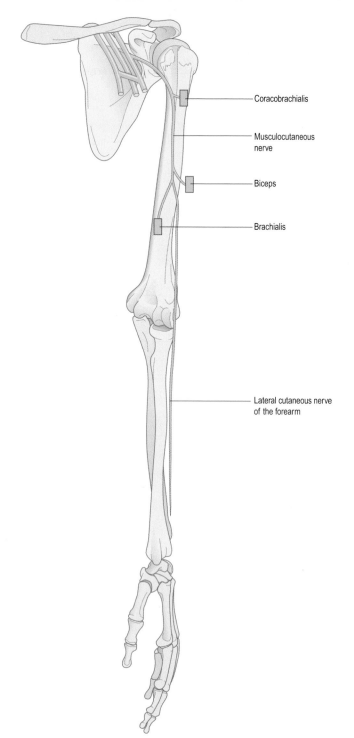

Fig. 18.5 *Motor and sensory branches of the musculocutaneous nerve. (From Aids to the Examination of the Peripheral Nervous System, 4th ed. 2000. Saunders, London. With permission of Guarantors of Brain.)*

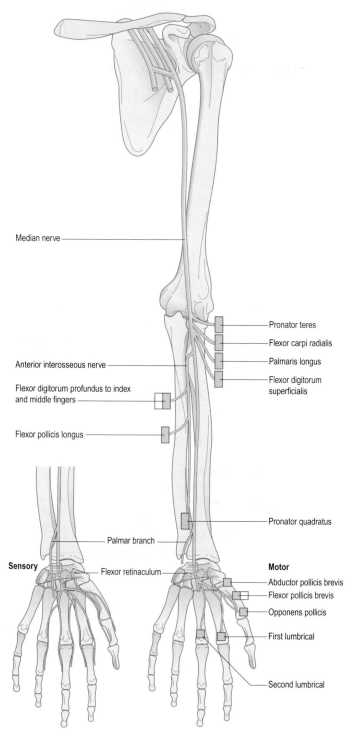

Fig. 18.6 *Motor and sensory branches of the median nerve. Flexor digitorum profundus to the ring and little fingers is supplied by the ulnar nerve. Flexor pollicis brevis may be supplied by both the median nerve and the ulnar nerve. (From Aids to the Examination of the Peripheral Nervous System, 4th ed. 2000. Saunders, London. With permission of Guarantors of Brain.)*

that normal can be differentiated from abnormal, so that slight weakness can be detected early with reliability. Some preference should be given to muscles with an easily elicited reflex.

Table 18.4 lists movements and muscles chosen according to these criteria. For example, with an upper motor neurone lesion, shoulder abduction, elbow extension, wrist and finger extension and finger abduction are weaker than their opposing movements. Because this weakness may be more distal than proximal, or vice versa, normal shoulder abduction and finger abduction excludes an upper motor neurone weakness of the arm. Some muscles are difficult to test but are included for special reasons. For example, brachioradialis strength is difficult to assess, but the muscle can be seen and felt, it is innervated mostly by the C6 root, and it has an easily elicited reflex.

To determine the root level of a lesion, it is necessary to know the appropriate muscle to test for each root, preferably with an easily elicited reflex.

Knowledge of the sequence in which motor branches leave a peripheral nerve to innervate specific muscles is very helpful in locating the level of the lesion. For example, with radial nerve lesions, if triceps is involved, the lesion must be high in the axilla. If, as is usual, triceps is spared but brachioradialis, wrist extensors, finger extensors and the superficial radial nerve are all involved, the lesion is in the arm, where the radial nerve is vulnerable to pressure against the humerus. If wrist extension is normal and the superficial radial nerve is not involved but finger extension is weak, the lesion involves the posterior interosseous branch of the radial nerve.

BRACHIAL PLEXUS AND NERVES OF THE SHOULDER

In the axilla, the lateral and posterior cords of the brachial plexus are lateral to the first part of the axillary artery, and the medial cord is behind it. The

CASE 1 ACUTE BRACHIAL PLEXUS NEUROPATHY

A 28-year-old man acutely develops severe pain in the region of his left shoulder blade, which radiates into his upper arm. Movement of his arm makes the pain worse. Ten days later, he notices weakness in his shoulder and upper arm muscles. The pain begins to improve at about the same time, but the weakness progresses, and muscle atrophy appears. He has no history of trauma or prior immunization, but he did have an upper respiratory infection 2 weeks before the onset of symptoms.

On examination, he has weakness and atrophy of the deltoid, serratus anterior, biceps and triceps muscles on the left, along with numbness of the outer arm in the distribution of the axillary nerve. The left biceps reflex is reduced. There is a mild Tinel's sign with pressure just over the left clavicle. His examination is otherwise normal.

Discussion: The acute onset of severe pain followed by weakness in the shoulder girdle and upper arm is a common presentation of acute brachial plexus neuropathy (neuralgic amyotrophy, Parsonage–Turner syndrome), generally involving part of the upper trunk of the plexus. The upper trunk supplies the suprascapular, lateral pectoral, musculocutaneous, lateral median, axillary and part of the radial nerves, but involvement can be patchy and may be sufficiently restricted to resemble a single neuropathy clinically. Involvement of other nerve distributions may be evident with needle electromyography.

The cause of acute brachial plexus neuropathy is unknown. It is often preceded by an infection or immunization, or it may appear following a non-specific and distant surgical procedure. It is thought to be an immune-mediated disorder, characterized primarily by axonal loss. Although usually unilateral, it may be bilateral and asymmetric. There are hereditary forms that occur as an autosomal dominant characteristic, and so-called hereditary neuropathy with liability for pressure palsies may mimic the disorder.

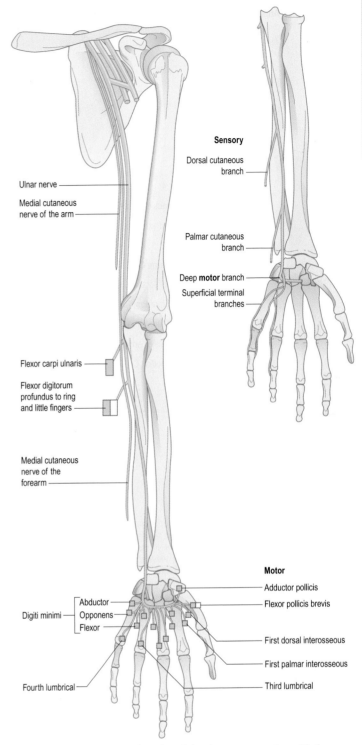

Sensory

Dorsal cutaneous branch

Ulnar nerve

Medial cutaneous nerve of the arm

Palmar cutaneous branch

Deep **motor** branch

Superficial terminal branches

Flexor carpi ulnaris

Flexor digitorum profundus to ring and little fingers

Medial cutaneous nerve of the forearm

Motor

Adductor pollicis

Flexor pollicis brevis

Abductor

Digiti minimi — Opponens

Flexor

First dorsal interosseous

First palmar interosseous

Third lumbrical

Fourth lumbrical

Fig. 18.7 *Motor and sensory branches of the ulnar nerve together with the medial cutaneous nerves of the arm and forearm. Flexor digitorum profundus to index and middle fingers is supplied by the median nerve. Flexor pollicis brevis may be supplied by both the median nerve and the ulnar nerve. (From Aids to the Examination of the Peripheral Nervous System, 4th ed. 2000. Saunders, London. With permission of Guarantors of Brain.)*

cords surround the second part of the artery; their names indicate their relationship. In the lower axillae the cords divide into nerves that supply the upper limb (see Fig. 18.2). Except for the medial root of the median nerve, these nerves are related to the third part of the artery, and their cords are related to the second part; that is, branches of the lateral cord are lateral, branches of the medial cord are medial, and branches of the posterior cord are posterior to the artery.

Branches of the brachial plexus may be described as supraclavicular or infraclavicular.

Supraclavicular Branches

Supraclavicular branches arise from roots or from trunks:

From roots	1. Nerves to scaleni and longus colli	C5, C6, C7, C8
	2. Branch to phrenic nerve	C5
	3. Dorsal scapular nerve	C5
	4. Long thoracic nerves	C5, C6 (C7)
From trunks	1. Nerve to subclavius	C5, C6
	2. Suprascapular nerve	C5, C6

Branches to the scaleni and longus colli arise from the lower cervical ventral rami near their exit from the intervertebral foramina. The phrenic nerve is joined by a branch from the fifth cervical ramus anterior to scalenus anterior.

Dorsal Scapular Nerve

The dorsal scapular nerve comes from the fifth cervical ventral ramus; pierces scalenus medius; passes behind levator scapulae, which it occasionally supplies; and runs with the deep branch of the dorsal scapular artery to the rhomboids, which it supplies.

Long Thoracic Nerve

The long thoracic nerve is usually formed by roots from the fifth to seventh cervical rami, although the last ramus may be absent (Fig. 18.9). The upper two roots pierce scalenus medius obliquely, uniting in or lateral to it. The nerve descends dorsal to the brachial plexus and the first part of the axillary artery and crosses the superior border of serratus anterior to reach its lateral surface.

A

Anterior   Posterior   **B**

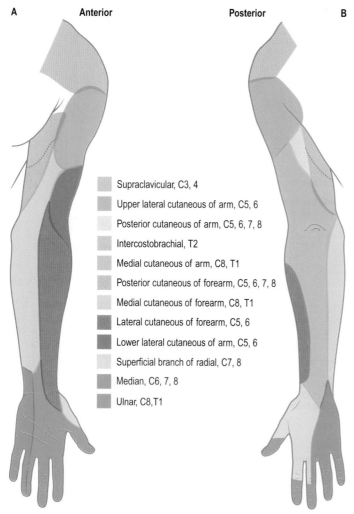

	Supraclavicular, C3, 4
	Upper lateral cutaneous of arm, C5, 6
	Posterior cutaneous of arm, C5, 6, 7, 8
	Intercostobrachial, T2
	Medial cutaneous of arm, C8, T1
	Posterior cutaneous of forearm, C5, 6, 7, 8
	Medial cutaneous of forearm, C8, T1
	Lateral cutaneous of forearm, C5, 6
	Lower lateral cutaneous of arm, C5, 6
	Superficial branch of radial, C7, 8
	Median, C6, 7, 8
	Ulnar, C8, T1

Fig. 18.8 *Arrangement of dermatomes and cutaneous nerves of the left upper limb.* **A,** *Viewed from the anterior aspect. The heavy black line represents the ventral axial line; overlap across it is minimal. In marked contrast, overlap is considerable across the interrupted lines.* **B,** *Viewed from the posterior aspect. The heavy black line represents the dorsal axial line; overlap across this line is minimal. Overlap is considerable across the interrupted lines.*

It may be joined by the root from C7, which emerges between scalenus anterior and scalenus medius, and descends on the lateral surface of medius. The nerve continues downward to the lower border of serratus anterior and supplies branches to each of its digitations.

The long thoracic nerve is the most common nerve to be affected by neuralgic amyotrophy. Winging of the scapula may be the only clinical manifestation; it is best demonstrated by asking the patient to push against resistance with the arm extended at the elbow and flexed to 90° at the shoulder (Fig. 18.10; see Case 1).

Nerve to Subclavius

The nerve to subclavius is small and arises near the junction of the fifth and sixth cervical ventral rami. It descends anterior to the plexus and the third part of the subclavian artery and is usually connected to the phrenic nerve. It passes above the subclavian vein to supply subclavius.

Suprascapular Nerve

The suprascapular nerve is a large branch of the superior trunk (Fig. 18.11). It runs laterally, deep to trapezius and omohyoid, and enters the supraspinous fossa through the suprascapular notch inferior to the superior transverse scapular ligament. It runs deep to supraspinatus and curves around the lateral border of the spine of the scapula with the suprascapular artery to reach the infraspinous fossa, where it gives two branches to supraspinatus and articular rami to the shoulder and acromioclavicular joints. The suprascapular nerve rarely has a cutaneous branch. When present, it pierces the deltoid close to the tip of the acromion and supplies the skin of the proximal third of the arm within the territory of the axillary nerve.

Lesions of the Suprascapular Nerve — The most common cause of lesions involving the suprascapular nerve is neuralgic amyotrophy, as described earlier. An entrapment neuropathy may occur in the scapular notch, or the

nerve may be damaged by trauma to the scapula and shoulder. There is pain in the shoulder and wasting and weakness of supraspinatus and infraspinatus.

Infraclavicular Branches

Infraclavicular branches come from the cords, but their axons may be traced back to the spinal nerves detailed below:

Lateral cord	Lateral pectoral	C5, C6, C7
	Musculocutaneous	C5, C6, C7
	Lateral root of median	(C5), C6, C7
Medial cord	Medial pectoral	C8, T1
	Medial cutaneous of forearm	C8, T1
	Medial cutaneous of arm	C8, T1
	Ulnar	(C7), C8, T1
	Medial root of median	C8, T1
Posterior cord	Upper subscapular	C5, C6
	Thoracodorsal	C6, C7, C8
	Lower subscapular	C5, C6
	Axillary	C5, C6
	Radial	C5, C6, C7, C8, (T1)

Lateral Pectoral Nerve

The lateral pectoral nerve (see Fig. 18.9) is larger than the medial and may arise from the anterior divisions of the upper and middle trunks or by a single root from the lateral cord. Its axons are from the fifth to seventh cervical rami. It crosses anterior to the axillary artery and vein, pierces the clavipectoral fascia and supplies the deep surface of pectoralis major. It sends a branch to the medial pectoral nerve, forming a loop in front of the first part of the axillary artery (see Fig. 18.9), to supply some fibres to pectoralis minor.

Medial Pectoral Nerve

The medial pectoral nerve is derived from the eighth cervical and first thoracic ventral rami and branches from the medial cord; the latter lies posterior to the axillary artery. It curves forward between the axillary artery and vein. Anterior to the artery it joins a ramus of the lateral pectoral nerve and enters the deep surface of pectoralis minor, which it supplies. Two or three branches pierce pectoralis minor, and others may pass around its inferior border to end in pectoralis major.

Upper (Superior) Subscapular Nerve

The superior subscapular nerve is smaller than the inferior. It arises from the posterior cord (C5 and C6), enters subscapularis at a high level and is frequently double.

Lower (Inferior) Subscapular Nerve

The inferior subscapular nerve arises from the posterior cord (C5 and C6). It supplies the lower part of subscapularis and ends in teres major, which is sometimes supplied by a separate branch.

Thoracodorsal Nerve

The thoracodorsal nerve arises from the posterior cord (C6–8) between the subscapular nerves. It accompanies the subscapular artery along the posterior axillary wall and supplies latissimus dorsi, reaching its distal border.

Axillary Nerve

The axillary nerve arises from the posterior cord (C5, C6). It is initially lateral to the radial nerve, posterior to the axillary artery and anterior to subscapularis (Fig. 18.12). At the lower border of subscapularis it curves back inferior to the humeroscapular articular capsule and, with the posterior circumflex humeral vessels, traverses a quadrangular space bounded above by subscapularis (anterior) and teres minor (posterior), below by teres major, medially by the long head of triceps and laterally by the surgical neck of the humerus. In the space it divides into anterior and posterior branches. The anterior branch curves around the neck of the humerus with the posterior circumflex humeral vessels, deep to deltoid. It reaches the anterior border of the muscle, supplies it and gives off a few small cutaneous branches that pierce deltoid and ramify in the skin over its lower part. The posterior branch courses medially and posteriorly along the attachment of the lateral head of triceps, inferior to the glenoid rim. It usually lies medial to the anterior branch in the quadrangular space. It gives off the nerve to teres minor and the upper lateral cutaneous nerve of the arm at the lateral edge of the origin of the long head of triceps. The nerve to teres minor enters the muscle on its inferior surface. The posterior branch frequently supplies the posterior aspect of deltoid, usually via a separate branch from the main stem, or occasionally from the superior

Table 18.1 Movements, muscles and segmental innervation in the upper limb

Joint	Movement	Muscle	Innervation	C3	C4	C5	C6	C7	C8	T1
SCAPULA	ELEVATION	Upper trapezius	Spinal accessory n.							
		Levator scapulae	Dorsal scapular n.							
	DEPRESSION	Lower trapezius	Spinal accessory n.							
	RETRACTION	Middle trapezius	Spinal accessory n.							
		Rhomboids	Dorsal scapular n.							
SHOULDER	PROTRACTION	Serratus anterior	Long thoracic n.							
	FLEXION	Anterior deltoid	Axillary n.							
		Pectoralis major (clavicular head)	Medial & lateral pectoral nn.							
		Pectoralis major (sternocostal head)	Medial & lateral pectoral nn.							
		Coracobrachialis	Musculocutaneous n.							
	EXTENSION	Posterior deltoid	Axillary n.							
		Infraspinatus	Suprascapular n.							
		Teres minor	Axillary n.							
		Teres major	Lower subscapular n.							
		Latissimus dorsi	Thoracodorsal n.							
	VERTICAL ABDUCTION	Middle deltoid	Axillary n.							
		Supraspinatus	Suprascapular n.							
	VERTICAL ADDUCTION	Pectoralis major (sternocostal head)	Medial & lateral pectoral nn.							
		Latissimus dorsi	Thoracodorsal n.							
		Coracobrachialis	Musculocutaneous n.							
	HORIZONTAL ABDUCTION	Posterior deltoid	Axillary n.							
	HORIZONTAL ADDUCTION	Pectoralis major (clavicular head)	Medial & lateral pectoral nn.							
		Pectoralis minor	Medial & lateral pectoral nn.							
		Anterior deltoid	Axillary n.							
	MEDIAL ROTATION	Subscapularis:								
		Teres major	Brachial plexus							
		Latissimus dorsi	Thoracodorsal n.							
		Anterior deltoid	Axillary n.							
	LATERAL ROTATION	Infraspinatus	Suprascapular n.							
		Teres minor	Axillary n.							
		Posterior deltoid	Axillary n.							
ELBOW	FLEXION	Biceps brachii	Musculocutaneous n.							
		Brachialis	Musculocutaneous & radial nn.							
		Brachioradialis	Radial n.							
	EXTENSION	Triceps	Radial n.							
	SUPINATION	Biceps brachii	Musculocutaneous n.							
		Supinator	Posterior interosseous n.							
	PRONATION	Pronator quadratus	Anterior interosseous n.							
		Pronator teres	Median n.							
WRIST	FLEXION	Flexor carpi radialis	Median n.							
		Palmaris longus	Median n.							
		Flexor carpi ulnaris	Ulnar n.							
	EXTENSION	Extensor carpi radialis longus	Radial n.							
		Extensor carpi radialis brevis	Posterior interosseous n.							
		Extensor carpi ulnaris	Posterior interosseous n.							
	ABDUCTION	Extensor carpi radialis longus	Radial n.							
		Extensor carpi radialis brevis	Posterior interosseous n.							
		Flexor carpi radialis	Median n.							
	ADDUCTION	Extensor carpi ulnaris	Posterior interosseous n.							
		Flexor carpi ulnaris	Ulnar n.							
FINGERS	FLEXION (MP/PIP Joints)	Flexor digitorum superficialis	Median n.							
	FLEXION (DIP Joints)	Flexor digitorum profundus (lateral)	Anterior interosseous n.							
		Flexor digitorum profundus (medial)	Ulnar n.							
		Dorsal interossei	Ulnar n.							
		Palmar interossei	Ulnar n.							
	FLEXION (MP Joint)	Flexor digiti minimi brevis	Ulnar n.							
	EXTENSION (MP/PIP/DIP Joints)	Extensor digitorum	Posterior interosseous n.							
		Extensor indicis	Posterior interosseous n.							
	EXTENSION (MP/PIP/DIP Joints)	Flexor digiti minimi	Posterior interosseous n.							
	EXTENSION (PIP/DIP Joints)	Lumbricals I & II	usu. Median n.							
		Lumbricals III & IV	usu. Ulnar n.							
	ABDUCTION	Dorsal interossei	Ulnar n.							
	ABDUCTION (thumb fixed)	Abductor pollicis brevis	Median n.							
	ABDUCTION	Abductor digiti minimi	Ulnar n.							
	ADDUCTION	Palmar interossei	Ulnar n.							
	OPPOSITION	Opponens digiti minimi	Ulnar n.							
THUMB	FLEXION (IP Joint)	Flexor pollicis longus	Anterior interosseous n.							
	FLEXION/ROTATION (MP Joint)	Flexor pollicis brevis	Median n. and/or ulnar n.							
	EXTENSION (MP Joint)	Extensor pollicis brevis	Posterior interosseous n.							
	EXTENSION (IP Joint)	Extensor pollicis longus	Posterior interosseous n.							
	ABDUCTION	Abductor pollicis longus	Posterior interosseous n.							
	ABDUCTION/ROTATION	Abductor pollicis brevis	Median n.							
	ADDUCTION/ROTATION	Adductor pollicis	Ulnar n.							
	ADDUCTION/FLEXION (MP Joint)	Palmar interosseous I	Ulnar n.							
	OPPOSITION	Opponens pollicis	Median n. and ulnar n.							

lateral cutaneous nerve of the arm. However, the posterior part of deltoid has a more consistent supply from the anterior branch of the axillary nerve, which should be remembered when performing a posterior deltoid-splitting approach to the shoulder. The upper lateral cutaneous nerve of the arm pierces the deep fascia at the medial border of the posterior aspect of deltoid and supplies the skin over the lower part of deltoid and upper part of the long head of triceps. The posterior branch is intimately related to the inferior aspects of the glenoid and shoulder joint capsule, which may place it at particular risk during capsular plication or thermal shrinkage procedures (Ball et al 2003). There is often an enlargement or pseudoganglion on the branch to teres minor. The axillary trunk supplies a branch to the shoulder joint below subscapularis.

Table 18.2 *Segmental innervation of muscles of the upper limb*

C3, C4	Trapezius, levator scapulae
C5	Rhomboids, deltoids, supraspinatus, infraspinatus, teres minor, biceps
C6	Serratus anterior, latissimus dorsi, subscapularis, teres major, pectoralis major (clavicular head), biceps, coracobrachialis, brachialis, brachioradialis, supinator, extensor carpi radialis longus
C7	Serratus anterior, latissimus dorsi, pectoralis major (sternal head), pectoralis minor, triceps, pronator teres, flexor carpi radialis, flexor digitorum superficialis, extensor carpi radialis longus, extensor carpi radialis brevis, extensor digitorum, extensor digiti minimi
C8	Pectoralis major (sternal head), pectoralis minor, triceps, flexor digitorum superficialis, flexor digitorum profundus, flexor pollicis longus, pronator quadratus, flexor carpi ulnaris, extensor carpi ulnaris, abductor pollicis longus, extensor pollicis longus, extensor pollicis brevis, extensor indicis, abductor pollicis brevis, flexor pollicis brevis, opponens pollicis
T1	Flexor digitorum profundus, intrinsic muscles of the hand (except abductor pollicis brevis, flexor pollicis brevis, opponens pollicis)

Table 18.3 / *Segmental innervation of joint movements of the upper limb*

Shoulder	Abductors and lateral rotators	C5
	Abductors and medial rotators	C6–8
Elbow	Flexors	C5, C6
	Extensors	C7, C8
Forearm	Supinators	C6
	Pronators	C7, C8
Wrist	Flexors and extensors	C6, C7
Digits	Long flexors and extensors	C7, C8
Hand	Intrinsic muscles	C8, T1

Lesions of the Axillary Nerve — The most common causes of axillary nerve lesions are trauma (dislocation of the shoulder, fracture of the surgical neck of the humerus) and neuralgic amyotrophy. There is deltoid wasting and weakness, which is usually clinically evident, and a patch of sensory loss on the outer aspect of the arm. This can be differentiated from a C5 root lesion by the finding of normal function in the distribution of the suprascapular nerve.

Musculocutaneous Nerve

The musculocutaneous nerve (see Fig. 18.9) arises from the lateral cord (C5–7), opposite the lower border of pectoralis minor. It pierces coracobrachialis and descends laterally between biceps and brachialis to the lateral side of the arm. Just below the elbow it pierces the deep fascia lateral to the biceps tendon and continues as the lateral cutaneous nerve of the forearm. A line drawn from the lateral side of the third part of the axillary artery across coracobrachialis and biceps to the lateral side of the biceps tendon is a surface projection for the nerve (but this varies according to its point of entry into coracobrachialis). It supplies coracobrachialis, both heads of the biceps and most of brachialis. The branch to coracobrachialis is given off before the musculocutaneous nerve enters the muscle; its fibres are from the seventh cervical ramus and may branch directly from the lateral cord. Branches to biceps and brachialis leave after the musculocutaneous has pierced coracobrachialis; the branch to brachialis also supplies the elbow joint. The musculocutaneous nerve supplies a small branch to the humerus, which enters the shaft with the nutrient artery.

Lesions of the Musculocutaneous Nerve — An isolated lesion of the musculocutaneous nerve is rare but may occur in injuries to the upper arm and shoulder (e.g. fracture of the humerus) and in patients with neuralgic amyotrophy. There is marked weakness of elbow flexion because biceps brachii and much of the brachialis are paralysed, as well as sensory impairment on the extensor aspect of the forearm in the distribution of the lateral cutaneous nerve of the forearm. Pain and paraesthesia may be aggravated by elbow extension.

Medial Cutaneous Nerve of the Arm

The medial cutaneous nerve of the arm is the smallest and most medial branch of the brachial plexus and arises from the medial cord (C8, T1). It crosses the axilla, either anterior or posterior to the axillary vein, then passes medial to the axillary vein, communicates with the intercostobrachial nerve and descends medial to the brachial artery and basilic vein. It pierces the deep fascia at the midpoint of the upper arm to supply the skin over the medial aspect of the distal third of the upper arm. It is described in further detail below.

Medial Cutaneous Nerve of the Forearm

The medial cutaneous nerve of the forearm arises from the medial cord (C8, T1). It is described in more detail below.

Median Nerve

The median nerve has two roots from the lateral (C5, C6, C7) and medial (C8, T1) cords, which embrace the third part of the axillary artery and unite anterior or lateral to it (see Fig. 18.9). Some fibres from C7 leave the lateral root in the lower part of the axilla and pass distomedially posterior to the medial root, and usually anterior to the axillary artery, to join the ulnar nerve. They may branch from the seventh cervical ventral ramus. Clinically, they are believed

Table 18.4 *Movements and muscles tested to determine the location of a lesion in the upper limb*

Arm Movement	Muscle	Upper Motor Neurone*	Root	Reflex	Nerve
Shoulder abduction	Deltoid	++	C5		Axillary
Elbow flexion	Biceps		C5–6	+	Musculocutaneous
	Brachioradialis		C6		Radial
Elbow extension	Triceps	+	C7	+	Radial
Radial wrist extensor	Extensor carpi radialis longus	+	C6		Radial
Finger extensors	Extensor digitorum	+	C7	(+)	Posterior interosseous
Finger flexors	Flexor pollicis longus + flexor digitorum profundus Index		C8	+	Anterior interosseous
	Flexor digitorum profundus Ring and little				Ulnar
Finger abduction	First dorsal interosseous	++	T1		Ulnar
	Abductor pollicis brevis		T1		Median

*The muscles indicated in this column are those preferentially affected in upper motor neurone lesions. The root level is the principal supply to a muscle.

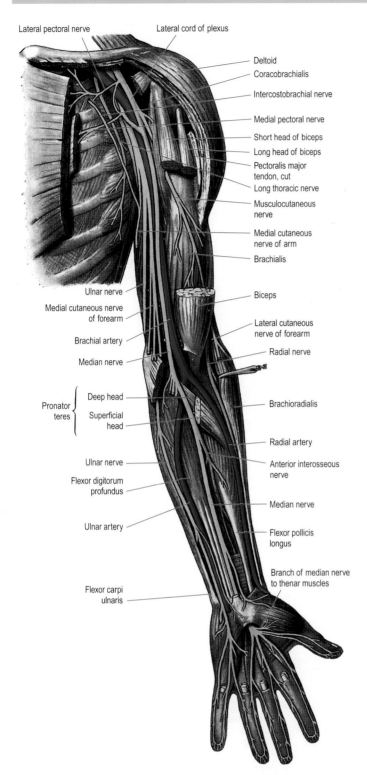

Lateral pectoral nerve

Lateral cord of plexus

Deltoid

Coracobrachialis

Intercostobrachial nerve

Medial pectoral nerve

Short head of biceps

Long head of biceps

Pectoralis major tendon, cut

Long thoracic nerve

Musculocutaneous nerve

Medial cutaneous nerve of arm

Brachialis

Ulnar nerve

Biceps

Medial cutaneous nerve of forearm

Lateral cutaneous nerve of forearm

Brachial artery

Radial nerve

Median nerve

Pronator teres {
Deep head
Superficial head
}

Brachioradialis

Radial artery

Ulnar nerve

Anterior interosseous nerve

Flexor digitorum profundus

Median nerve

Ulnar artery

Flexor pollicis longus

Flexor carpi ulnaris

Branch of median nerve to thenar muscles

Fig. 18.9 *Nerves of the left upper limb, dissected from the anterior aspect.*

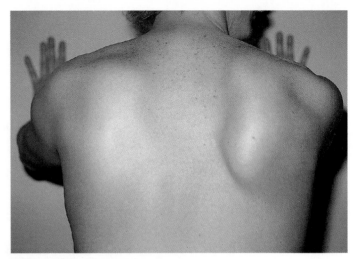

Fig. 18.10 *Winging of the right scapula. The patient is pushing against the wall at a 90° angle.*

triangular space below the lower border of teres major, between the long head of triceps and the humerus. It is described in more detail below.

Brachial Plexus Lesions

Lesions of the brachial plexus commonly affect either the upper part of the plexus (i.e. C5 and C6 roots and the upper trunk) or the lower part of the plexus (i.e. C8 and T1 roots and the lower trunk). Lesions affecting the upper part are usually traumatic, whereas those affecting the lower part may be caused by trauma, malignant infiltration or thoracic outlet syndrome. Severe trauma may affect the whole plexus.

Upper Plexus Palsies

Downward traction on an infant's arm during birth or, in adults, a severe fall on the side of the head and shoulder, forcing the two apart (as frequently occurs in a motorcycle crash), may tear the roots of C5 and C6. This results in paralysis of the deltoid, short muscles of the shoulder, brachialis and biceps. The last two are both elbow flexors, and biceps is also a powerful supinator of the superior radio-ulnar joint. The arm therefore hangs by the side, with the forearm pronated and the palm facing backward, like a waiter hinting for a tip (Erb–Duchenne paralysis). There is sensory loss over the lateral aspect of the upper arm.

Lower Plexus Palsies

Upward traction on the arm, such as in a forcible breech delivery, may tear the lowest root, T1, which provides the segmental supply to the intrinsic muscles of the hand. The hand assumes a clawed appearance, reflecting the unopposed action of the long flexors and extensors of the fingers (Klumpke's paralysis). There is sensory loss along the medial aspect of the forearm and often an associated Horner's syndrome (ptosis and constriction of the pupil), which occurs as a result of traction on the cervical sympathetic chain.

Malignant infiltration of the brachial plexus may result from extension of an apical lung carcinoma (Pancoast tumour) or from metastatic spread, often from carcinoma of the breast. There is slowly progressive weakness that usually starts in the small muscles of the hand (T1) and spreads to involve the finger flexors (C8). This is usually a painful condition, and the pain may be severe. There is sensory loss on the medial aspect of the forearm (T1), extending into the medial side of the hand and to the little finger (C8). Horner's syndrome may occur if there is involvement of the cervical sympathetic ganglia. A similar syndrome may occur following radiotherapy for breast carcinoma, but this is usually painless. Thoracic surgery involving a sternal split may cause traction on the brachial plexus and usually affects the lower part of the plexus.

The lower trunk of the brachial plexus (C8, T1), together with the subclavian artery, may be angulated over a cervical rib (thoracic outlet syndrome). Patients may present with vascular symptoms as a result of kinking of the subclavian artery (this is more likely to occur with large bony ribs), or they may present with neurological deficits (this is more likely in patients with small rudimentary ribs that extend into a fibrous band that joins the first rib anteriorly). Cervical ribs are quite common and are rarely associated with symptoms. There is a slow, insidious onset of wasting of the small muscles of the hand, which often starts on the lateral side with involvement of the thenar eminence and first dorsal interosseous. There is pain and paraesthesia in the

to be mainly motor and to supply flexor carpi ulnaris. If the lateral root is small, the musculocutaneous nerve (C5, C6, C7) connects with the median nerve in the arm. It is described in more detail below.

Ulnar Nerve

The ulnar nerve arises from the medial cord (C8, T1) but often receives fibres from the ventral ramus of C7 (see Fig. 18.9). It runs distally through the axilla medial to the axillary artery, between it and the vein. It is described in more detail below.

Radial Nerve

The radial nerve is the largest branch of the brachial plexus. It arises from the posterior cord (C5, C6, C7, C8, [T1]; see Fig. 18.12) and descends behind the third part of the axillary artery and the upper part of the brachial artery, anterior to subscapularis and the tendons of latissimus dorsi and teres major. With the arteria profunda brachii it inclines dorsally and passes through the

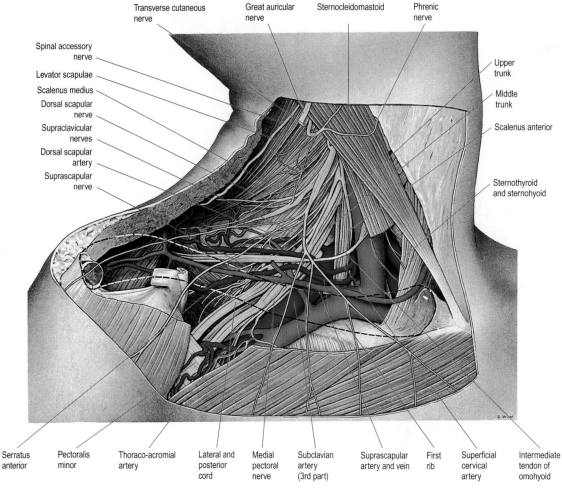

Transverse cutaneous nerve
Great auricular nerve
Sternocleidomastoid
Phrenic nerve
Spinal accessory nerve
Levator scapulae
Scalenus medius
Dorsal scapular nerve
Supraclavicular nerves
Dorsal scapular artery
Suprascapular nerve
Upper trunk
Middle trunk
Scalenus anterior
Sternothyroid and sternohyoid

Serratus anterior
Pectoralis minor
Thoraco-acromial artery
Lateral and posterior cord
Medial pectoral nerve
Subclavian artery (3rd part)
Suprascapular artery and vein
First rib
Superficial cervical artery
Intermediate tendon of omohyoid

Fig. 18.11 *Lower part of the posterior triangle showing the relations of the third part of the right subclavian artery. The clavicle has been removed, but its outline is indicated by a dashed line. In this dissection, the middle trunk of the brachial plexus gives an unusual contribution to the medial cord.*

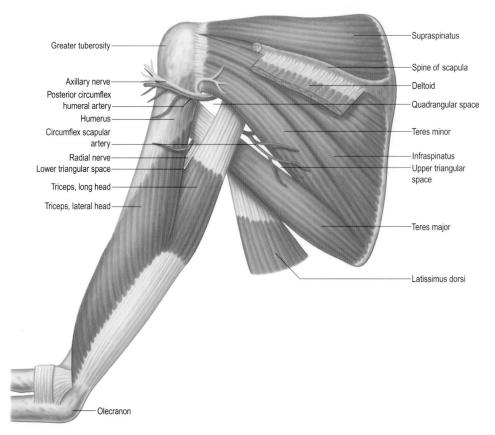

Greater tuberosity
Axillary nerve
Posterior circumflex humeral artery
Humerus
Circumflex scapular artery
Radial nerve
Lower triangular space
Triceps, long head
Triceps, lateral head
Olecranon

Supraspinatus
Spine of scapula
Deltoid
Quadrangular space
Teres minor
Infraspinatus
Upper triangular space
Teres major
Latissimus dorsi

Fig. 18.12 *Dorsal scapular muscles and triceps on the left side. The spine of the scapula has been divided near its lateral end, and the acromion has been removed along with a large part of deltoid. The humerus is laterally rotated, and the forearm is pronated.*

CASE 2   PANCOAST TUMOUR

A 59-year-old man, a heavy smoker for many years, develops posterior left shoulder pain radiating down the medial aspect of the left arm into the fourth and fifth digits of the hand, with weakness that ultimately involves the entire left hand. He has lost 35 pounds in the past 3 months. Examination demonstrates wasting and weakness of all intrinsic hand muscles on the left, as well as weakness of wrist flexion. There is decreased sensation in the left medial upper arm, forearm and hand, involving especially the fifth digit (Fig. 18.13). He has a mild left Horner's syndrome, with noticeable ptosis and miosis.

Discussion: Progressive lesions of the lower trunk of the brachial plexus associated with pain in the involved hand and accompanied by a history of weight loss and smoking are most suggestive of a Pancoast tumour, a tumour of the apex of the lung (Fig. 18.14). An enlarging tumour in the apex may erode bone locally and compress the lower trunk of the brachial plexus. Because the C8 and T1 nerve roots form the lower trunk of the brachial plexus, all median- and ulnar-innervated muscles are affected, as is the pectoralis muscle to some extent. Sensory loss appears in the distribution of C8 and T1 dermatomes. Extension of the mass superiorly into the stellate ganglion is responsible for an associated Horner's syndrome.

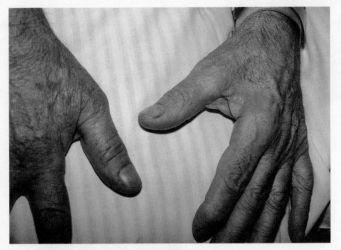

Fig. 18.13 *Brachial plexopathy (brachial neuritis). Atrophy of the intrinsic hand muscles due to denervation.*

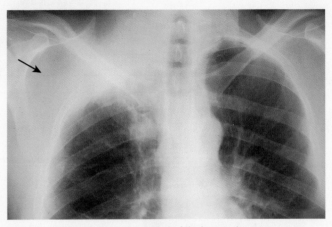

Fig. 18.14 *Pancoast tumour. Carcinoma of the lung at the superior apex (arrow) extending into the overlying brachial plexus.*

medial aspect of the forearm, extending to the little finger; this is often aggravated by carrying shopping bags or suitcases. A bruit may be heard over the subclavian artery, and the radial pulse may be easily obliterated by movements of the arm, particularly with the arm extended and abducted at the shoulder.

NERVES OF THE UPPER ARM AND ELBOW

Median Nerve

The median nerve enters the arm lateral to the brachial artery (see Fig. 18.9; Figs 18.15, 18.16). Near the insertion of coracobrachialis it crosses in front of (rarely behind) the artery, descending medial to it to the cubital fossa, where it is posterior to the bicipital aponeurosis and anterior to brachialis, separated by the latter from the elbow joint.

It gives off vascular branches to the brachial artery and usually a branch to pronator teres, a variable distance proximal to the elbow joint.

Pronator Syndrome

This is an uncommon entrapment neuropathy of the median nerve occurring in the elbow region. Entrapment typically occurs at one of four sites. One site is the ligament of Struthers, an anatomical variant that, when present, connects a small supracondyloid spur of bone to an accessory origin of pronator teres. The median nerve can be compressed as it passes under this ligament. The nerve can also be trapped as it passes deep to the bicipital aponeurosis, the aponeurotic edge of the deep head of pronator teres or the tendinous aponeurotic arch forming the proximal free edge of the radial attachment of flexor digitorum superficialis.

The syndrome presents with pain on the volar aspect of the distal arm and proximal forearm. The symptoms may be aggravated by flexing the elbow against resistance, pronating the forearm against resistance or flexion of superficialis to the middle finger against resistance, depending on the precise cause of the entrapment. If the anterior interosseous nerve is also compressed, there is weakness of all the muscles innervated by the median nerve, including abductor pollicis brevis and the long finger flexors, and sensory impairment in the palm of the hand.

Musculocutaneous Nerve

The musculocutaneous nerve is the nerve of the anterior compartment of the arm (see Fig. 18.9). It gives a branch to the shoulder joint and then passes through coracobrachialis, which it supplies, emerging to pass between biceps and brachialis. It sends branches to both these muscles. In the cubital fossa it lies at the lateral margin of the biceps tendon, where it continues as the lateral cutaneous nerve of the forearm.

The musculocutaneous nerve has frequent variations. It may run behind coracobrachialis or adhere for some distance to the median nerve and pass behind biceps. Some fibres of the median nerve may run in the musculocutaneous nerve, leaving it to join their proper trunk; less frequently, the reverse occurs, and the median nerve sends a branch to the musculocutaneous. Occasionally it supplies pronator teres and may replace radial branches to the dorsal surface of the thumb.

Ulnar Nerve

The ulnar nerve has no branches in the arm (see Figs 18.9, 18.15). It runs distally through the axilla medial to the axillary artery and between it and the vein, continuing distally medial to the brachial artery as far as the midarm. There it pierces the medial intermuscular septum, inclining medially as it descends anterior to the medial head of triceps to the interval between the medial epicondyle and the olecranon, along with the superior ulnar collateral artery. At the elbow, the ulnar nerve is in a groove on the dorsum of the epicondyle. It enters the forearm between the two heads of flexor carpi ulnaris superficial to the posterior and oblique parts of the ulnar collateral ligament (Figs 18.16, 18.17, 18.18).

Articular Branches

Articular branches to the elbow joint issue from the ulnar nerve between the medial epicondyle and olecranon.

Cubital Tunnel Syndrome

Typically, the ulnar nerve can be compressed in the tunnel formed by the tendinous arch connecting the two heads of flexor carpi ulnaris at their humeral and ulnar attachments. Other local causes of compression and

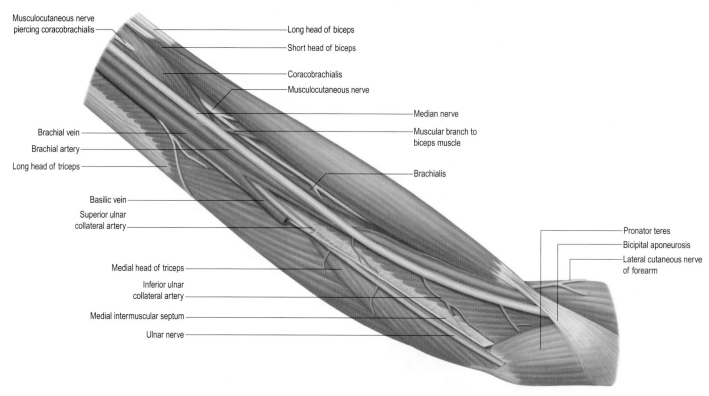

Fig. 18.15 *Muscles, vessels and nerves of the left upper arm viewed from the medial aspect.*

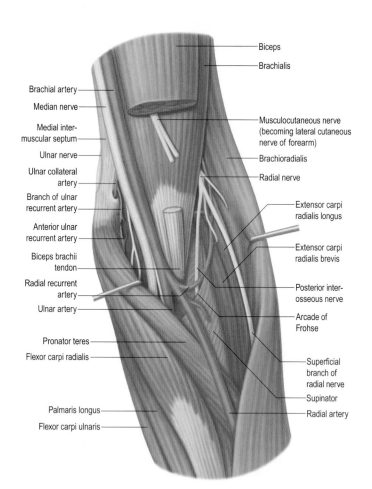

Fig. 18.16 / *Anterior aspect of the left elbow showing deep structures.*

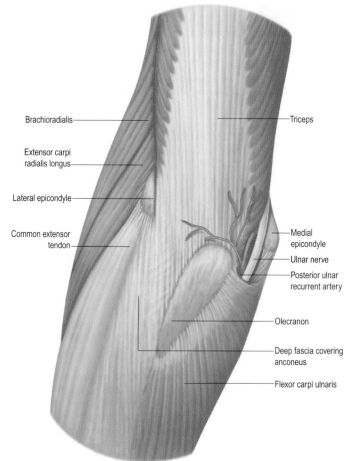

Fig. 18.17 *Posterior aspect of the left elbow showing superficial structures.*

neuritis at this site include trauma, compression by the medial head of the triceps, osteophytes, recurrent subluxation of the nerve across the medial epicondyle of the humerus and abnormal muscular variants such as the anconeus epitrochlearis.

The symptoms are pain at the medial aspect of the proximal forearm, together with paraesthesia and numbness of the little finger and ulnar half of the ring finger and the ulnar side of the dorsum of the hand. These symptoms are typically worse on forced elbow flexion. There may also be associated weakness of the muscles of the forearm and the intrinsic muscles of the hand innervated by the ulnar nerve. Interestingly, flexor carpi ulnaris and profundus to the ring and little fingers are frequently spared, presumably because the fascicles supplying these muscles are located on the deep aspect of the nerve. Clawing of the hand is therefore unusual in this syndrome.

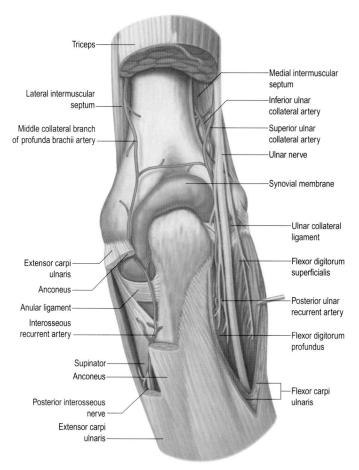

Fig. 18.18 *Posterior aspect of the left elbow region showing deep structures.*

Labels (clockwise from top):
Triceps
Medial intermuscular septum
Inferior ulnar collateral artery
Lateral intermuscular septum
Superior ulnar collateral artery
Middle collateral branch of profunda brachii artery
Ulnar nerve
Synovial membrane
Ulnar collateral ligament
Flexor digitorum superficialis
Extensor carpi ulnaris
Anconeus
Posterior ulnar recurrent artery
Anular ligament
Interosseous recurrent artery
Flexor digitorum profundus
Supinator
Anconeus
Posterior interosseous nerve
Flexor carpi ulnaris
Extensor carpi ulnaris

CASE 3   ULNAR NEUROPATHY AT
THE ELBOW

An 18-year-old fractured his distal right humerus while skiing. Following recovery, he was left with a mild bony deformity. He continued to play sports but then developed numbness and tingling in the fourth and fifth digits of the right hand, along with pain in the right elbow; he has also observed wasting of the muscles of his right hand. On examination, there is wasting and decreased strength of the interossei muscles. Flexion of the fourth and fifth digits is impaired, but wrist flexion is normal, as is strength elsewhere. Sensation is decreased in the medial half of the fourth digit and in the entire fifth digit on both the dorsal and palmar surfaces. Reflexes are normal. Percussion over the ulnar nerve proximal to the medial epicondyle elicits a shooting electric shock sensation radiating distally into the little finger (Tinel's sign).

Discussion: The term 'tardy ulnar palsy' usually refers to ulnar nerve compression at the elbow caused, in this case, by prior trauma at the level of the ulnar groove, bony deformity from an old fracture, or inflammation of bursae or subcutaneous tissues with compression of the nerve in the cubital tunnel (the nerve is injured at the level of the ulnar groove due to compression between two bony processes or compression within the cubital tunnel itself). The ulnar nerve does not branch throughout most of its course in the arm, proceeding through the axilla and along the medial upper arm and into the ulnar groove, between the medial epicondyle and the olecranon; it is here that trauma is such an important pathogenetic event. Distal to the medial epicondyle, the nerve travels in the cubital tunnel below the aponeurosis of the flexor carpi ulnaris muscle; its first branch is in fact to the flexor carpi ulnaris itself, which may be unaffected in typical cases of post-traumatic tardy ulnar palsy or cubital tunnel syndrome.

Surgical treatment involves decompression of the tunnel by division of the aponeurosis of flexor carpi ulnaris, with or without subsequent anterior transposition of the ulnar nerve.

Ulnar Nerve Division at the Elbow

The ulnar nerve is in a vulnerable position as it lies between the median epicondyle and the olecranon: it lies on bone covered only by a thin layer of skin. It is easily damaged if the ulnar groove is shallow, and the nerve may become more prominent than the medial epicondyle or the olecranon when the elbow is fully flexed.

Division of the nerve at the elbow paralyses flexor carpi ulnaris, flexor digitorum profundus to the ring and little fingers and all the intrinsic muscles of the hand (except for the radial two lumbricals). Clawing of the hand is less intense than that which occurs after division of the ulnar nerve at the wrist, reflecting the imbalance in action between the long flexors and extensors to the ring and little fingers when digit flexion is produced only by superficialis. In addition, there is sensory loss over the little finger and the ulnar half of the ring finger.

Radial Nerve

The branches of the radial nerve in the upper arm are as follows: muscular, cutaneous, articular and superficial terminal and posterior interosseous.

The radial nerve descends behind the third part of the axillary artery and the upper part of the brachial artery, anterior to subscapularis and the tendons of latissimus dorsi and teres major (see Fig. 18.9; Fig. 18.19). With the profunda brachii artery it inclines dorsally, passing through the triangular space below the lower border of teres major, between the long head of triceps and the humerus. There it supplies the long head of triceps and gives rise to the posterior cutaneous nerve of the arm, which supplies the skin along the posterior surface of the upper arm. It then spirals obliquely across the back of the humerus, lying posterior to the uppermost fibres of the medial head of triceps, which separate the nerve from the bone in the first part of the spiral groove. There it gives off a muscular branch to the lateral head of triceps and a branch that passes through the medial head of triceps to anconeus. On reaching the lateral side of the humerus it pierces the lateral intermuscular septum to enter the anterior compartment; it then descends deep in a furrow between brachialis and, proximally, brachioradialis, then, more distally, extensor carpi radialis longus. The radial nerve divides into the superficial terminal branch

and the posterior interosseous nerve just anterior to the lateral epicondyle (see Fig. 18.16).

Muscular Branches

Muscular branches supply triceps, anconeus, brachioradialis, extensor carpi radialis longus and brachialis in medial, posterior and lateral groups. Medial muscular branches arise from the radial nerve on the medial side of the arm. They supply the medial and long heads of triceps; the branch to the medial head is a long, slender filament that, lying close to the ulnar nerve as far as the distal third of the arm, is often termed the ulnar collateral nerve. A large posterior muscular branch arises from the nerve as it lies in the humeral groove. It divides to supply the medial and lateral heads of triceps and anconeus. The division for the latter is a long nerve that descends in the medial head of triceps and partially supplies it; it is accompanied by the middle collateral branch of the profunda brachii artery and passes behind the elbow joint to end in anconeus. Lateral muscular branches arise in front of the lateral intermuscular septum; they supply the lateral part of brachialis, brachioradialis and extensor carpi radialis longus.

Cutaneous Branches

Cutaneous branches are the posterior and lower lateral cutaneous nerves of the arm and the posterior cutaneous nerve of the forearm (see Fig. 18.8).

Lower Lateral Cutaneous Nerve of the Arm — The lower lateral cutaneous nerve of the arm perforates the lateral head of triceps distal to the deltoid tuberosity, passes to the front of the elbow close to the cephalic vein and supplies the skin of the lateral part of the lower half of the arm.

Posterior Cutaneous Nerve of the Arm — The small posterior cutaneous nerve of the arm arises in the axilla and passes medially to supply the skin on

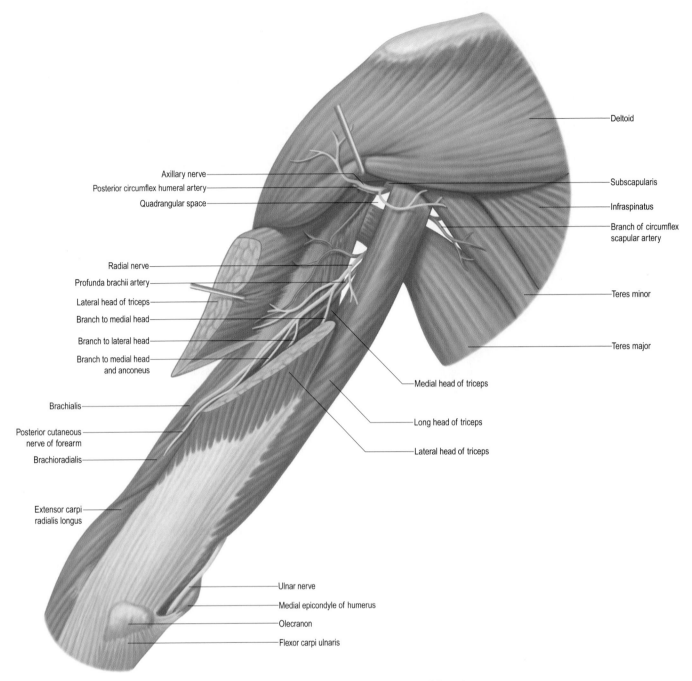

Fig. 18.19 *Muscles, vessels and nerves of the left upper arm viewed from the posterior aspect.*

the dorsal surface of the arm nearly as far as the olecranon. It crosses posterior to and communicates with the intercostobrachial nerve.

Posterior Cutaneous Nerve of the Forearm — The posterior cutaneous nerve of the forearm arises with the lower lateral cutaneous nerve of the arm. Perforating the lateral head of triceps, it descends first lateral in the arm, then along the dorsum of the forearm to the wrist, supplying the skin in its course and joining, near its end, with dorsal branches of the lateral cutaneous nerve of the forearm.

Articular Branches to the Elbow Joint

These articular nerves accompany blood vessels supplying the synovial membrane, fat pads and epiphyses; they presumably contain vasomotor fibres as well as afferent fibres serving pain and proprioception.

Lesions of the Radial Nerve in the Upper Arm

Lesions of the radial nerve at its origin from the posterior cord in the axilla may be caused by pressure from a long crutch (crutch palsy). Triceps is involved only when lesions occur at this level; it is usually spared in the more common lesions of the radial nerve in the arm because it lies alongside the spiral groove, where the nerve is commonly affected by fractures of the humerus. Compression of the nerve against the humerus occurs if the arm is rested on a sharp edge, such as the back of a chair (see Case 4, 'Saturday Night

Palsy'). Both these injuries cause weakness of brachioradialis, with wasting and loss of the reflex. There is both wristdrop and fingerdrop due to weakness of wrist and finger extensors, as well as weakness of extensor pollicis longus and abductor pollicis longus. There may be sensory impairment or paraesthesia in the distribution of the superficial radial nerve. However, nerve overlap means that usually only a small area of anaesthesia occurs on the dorsum of the hand between the first and second metacarpal bones.

Medial Cutaneous Nerve of the Arm

The medial cutaneous nerve of the arm supplies the skin of the medial aspect of the arm (see Figs 18.8, 18.9). It is the smallest branch of the brachial plexus, arises from the medial cord and contains fibres from the eighth cervical and first thoracic ventral rami. It traverses the axilla, crossing anterior or posterior to the axillary vein, to which it is then medial, and communicates with the intercostobrachial nerve; it descends medial to the brachial artery and basilic vein (see Fig. 18.9) to a point midway in the upper arm, where it pierces the deep fascia to supply a medial area in the distal third of the arm, extending to its anterior and posterior aspects. Rami reach the skin anterior to the medial epicondyle and over the olecranon. It connects with the posterior branch of the medial cutaneous nerve of the forearm. Sometimes the medial cutaneous nerve of the arm and the intercostobrachial nerve are connected in a plexiform manner in the axilla. The intercostobrachial nerve may be large

CASE 4 SATURDAY NIGHT PALSY

A 20-year-old man awakes after drinking heavily at a party. He had fallen asleep with his right arm resting on the top of a bench. The muscles in the right arm are stiff on awakening, but he then notices a marked right wristdrop. He also complains of numbness on the dorsal surface of the hand in the so-called radial snuff-box between the thumb and index fingers. Examination demonstrates weakness of the wrist and finger extensors and brachioradialis in the affected limb. Triceps strength is normal. There is loss of pinprick sensation in the pattern described earlier. The brachioradialis reflex is absent, although other reflexes are normal.

Discussion: 'Saturday night palsy' is a term used to describe an injury to the radial nerve at the level of the spiral groove of the humerus due to compression of the nerve against the bone as the nerve travels laterally. It often occurs during deep sleep following drug or alcohol abuse, most likely due to pressure as the arm is draped over a hard bench or a chair, as in this case. Sensory changes in the distribution of the radial nerve and wristdrop typically result from such nerve compression. Because triceps is innervated by a branch of the radial nerve that emerges above the spiral groove, it is usually spared. The nerve injury may be incomplete, with variable weakness of brachioradialis, as noted above. Reflex changes are also variable. Although the sensory branch of the radial nerve innervates a larger area than described in this patient, significant crossover in innervation restricts the sensory loss.

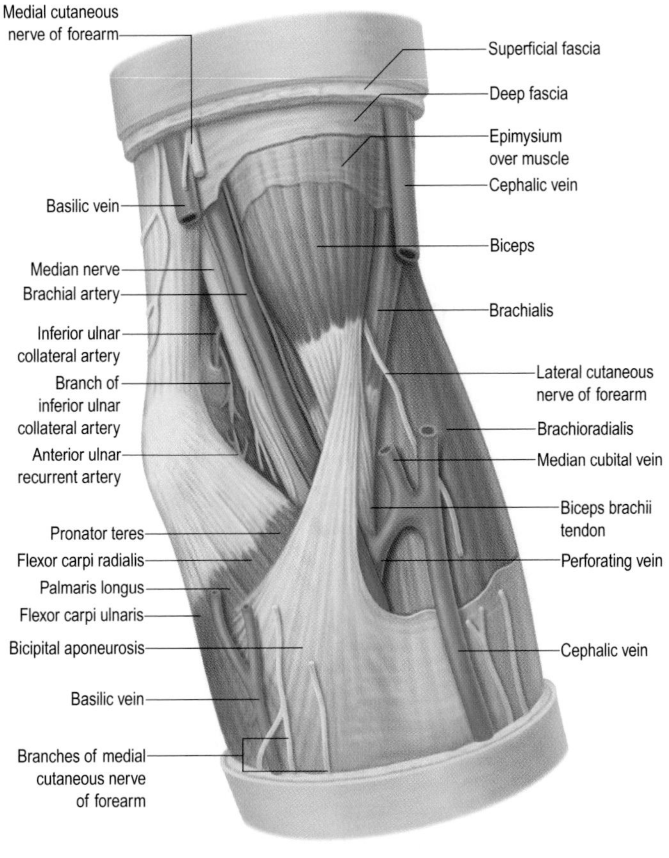

and reinforced by part of the lateral cutaneous branch of the third intercostal nerve. It then replaces the medial cutaneous nerve of the arm and receives a connection representing the latter from the brachial plexus (occasionally, this connection is absent).

Medial Cutaneous Nerve of the Forearm

The medial cutaneous nerve of forearm comes from the medial cord (see Fig. 18.9; Fig. 18.20). It is derived from the eighth cervical and first thoracic ventral rami. At first it is between the axillary artery and vein and gives off a ramus that pierces the deep fascia to supply the skin over biceps, almost to the elbow. The nerve descends medial to the brachial artery, pierces the deep fascia with the basilic vein midway in the arm and divides into anterior and posterior branches. The larger, anterior branch usually passes in front of, or occasionally behind, the median cubital vein, descending anteromedially in the forearm to supply the skin as far as the wrist and connecting with the palmar cutaneous branch of the ulnar nerve. The posterior branch descends obliquely medial to the basilic vein, anterior to the medial epicondyle, and curves around to the back of the forearm, descending on its medial border to the wrist, supplying the skin. It connects with the medial cutaneous nerve of the arm, posterior cutaneous nerve of the forearm and dorsal branch of the ulnar.

NERVES OF THE FOREARM

Median Nerve

The median nerve usually enters the forearm between the heads of pronator teres (Figs 18.21–18.25). (Occasionally, the nerve passes posterior to both heads of pronator teres, or it may pass through the humeral head.) It crosses to the

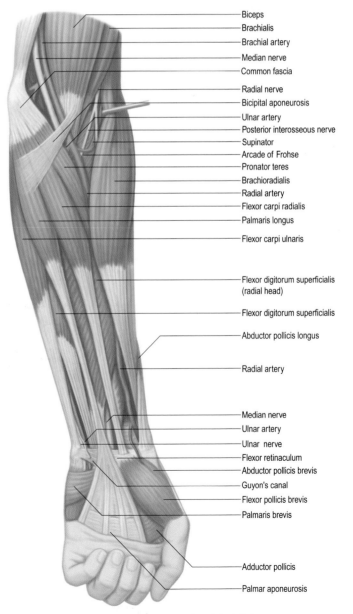

Fig. 18.20 *Anterior aspect of the left elbow, showing superficial structures.*

Medial cutaneous nerve of forearm
Superficial fascia
Deep fascia
Epimysium over muscle
Cephalic vein
Basilic vein
Biceps
Median nerve
Brachial artery
Inferior ulnar collateral artery
Brachialis
Branch of inferior ulnar collateral artery
Lateral cutaneous nerve of forearm
Anterior ulnar recurrent artery
Brachioradialis
Median cubital vein
Biceps brachii tendon
Pronator teres
Flexor carpi radialis
Palmaris longus
Flexor carpi ulnaris
Perforating vein
Bicipital aponeurosis
Basilic vein
Cephalic vein
Branches of medial cutaneous nerve of forearm

Fig. 18.21 *Superficial flexor muscles of the left forearm.*

Biceps
Brachialis
Brachial artery
Median nerve
Common fascia
Radial nerve
Bicipital aponeurosis
Ulnar artery
Posterior interosseous nerve
Supinator
Arcade of Frohse
Pronator teres
Brachioradialis
Radial artery
Flexor carpi radialis
Palmaris longus
Flexor carpi ulnaris
Flexor digitorum superficialis (radial head)
Flexor digitorum superficialis
Abductor pollicis longus
Radial artery
Median nerve
Ulnar artery
Ulnar nerve
Flexor retinaculum
Abductor pollicis brevis
Guyon's canal
Flexor pollicis brevis
Palmaris brevis
Adductor pollicis
Palmar aponeurosis

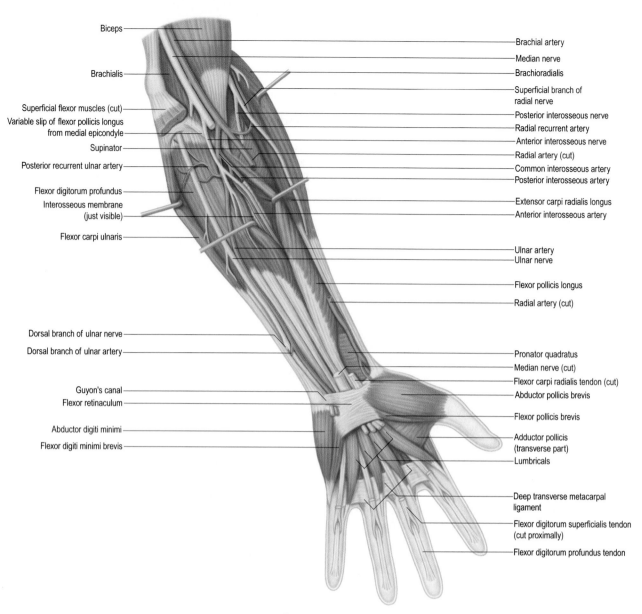

Biceps

Brachialis

Superficial flexor muscles (cut)

Variable slip of flexor pollicis longus
from medial epicondyle

Supinator

Posterior recurrent ulnar artery

Flexor digitorum profundus

Interosseous membrane
(just visible)

Flexor carpi ulnaris

Dorsal branch of ulnar nerve

Dorsal branch of ulnar artery

Guyon's canal

Flexor retinaculum

Abductor digiti minimi

Flexor digiti minimi brevis

Brachial artery

Median nerve

Brachioradialis

Superficial branch of
radial nerve

Posterior interosseous nerve

Radial recurrent artery

Anterior interosseous nerve

Radial artery (cut)

Common interosseous artery

Posterior interosseous artery

Extensor carpi radialis longus

Anterior interosseous artery

Ulnar artery

Ulnar nerve

Flexor pollicis longus

Radial artery (cut)

Pronator quadratus

Median nerve (cut)

Flexor carpi radialis tendon (cut)

Abductor pollicis brevis

Flexor pollicis brevis

Adductor pollicis
(transverse part)

Lumbricals

Deep transverse metacarpal
ligament

Flexor digitorum superficialis tendon
(cut proximally)

Flexor digitorum profundus tendon

Fig. 18.22 *Deep flexor muscles of the left forearm.*

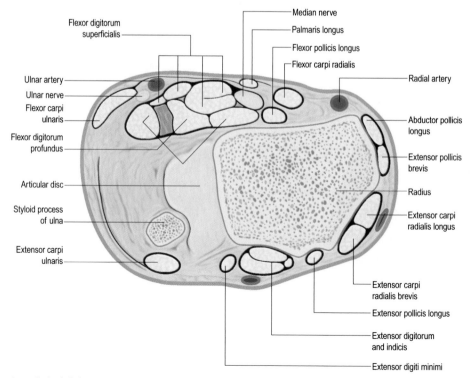

Flexor digitorum
superficialis

Ulnar artery

Ulnar nerve

Flexor carpi
ulnaris

Flexor digitorum
profundus

Articular disc

Styloid process
of ulna

Extensor carpi
ulnaris

Median nerve

Palmaris longus

Flexor pollicis longus

Flexor carpi radialis

Radial artery

Abductor pollicis
longus

Extensor pollicis
brevis

Radius

Extensor carpi
radialis longus

Extensor carpi
radialis brevis

Extensor pollicis longus

Extensor digitorum
and indicis

Extensor digiti minimi

Fig. 18.23 *Transverse section through the left forearm, passing through the distal end of the radius and the styloid process of the ulna, with the hand and forearm in full supination (distal [inferior] aspect).*

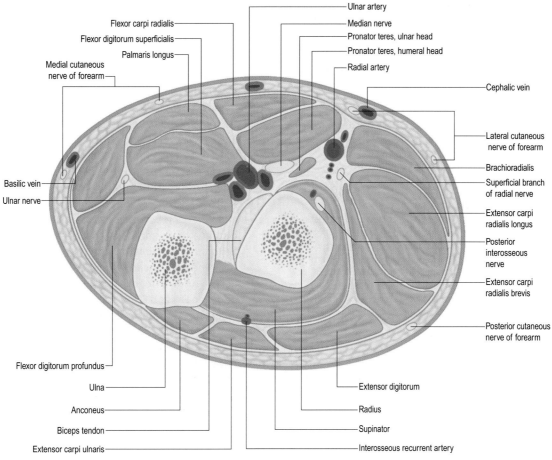

Flexor carpi radialis
Flexor digitorum superficialis
Palmaris longus
Medial cutaneous nerve of forearm
Basilic vein
Ulnar nerve
Flexor digitorum profundus
Ulna
Anconeus
Biceps tendon
Extensor carpi ulnaris

Ulnar artery
Median nerve
Pronator teres, ulnar head
Pronator teres, humeral head
Radial artery
Cephalic vein
Lateral cutaneous nerve of forearm
Brachioradialis
Superficial branch of radial nerve
Extensor carpi radialis longus
Posterior interosseous nerve
Extensor carpi radialis brevis
Posterior cutaneous nerve of forearm
Extensor digitorum
Radius
Supinator
Interosseous recurrent artery

Fig. 18.24 *Transverse section through the left forearm at the level of the radial tuberosity (proximal aspect).*

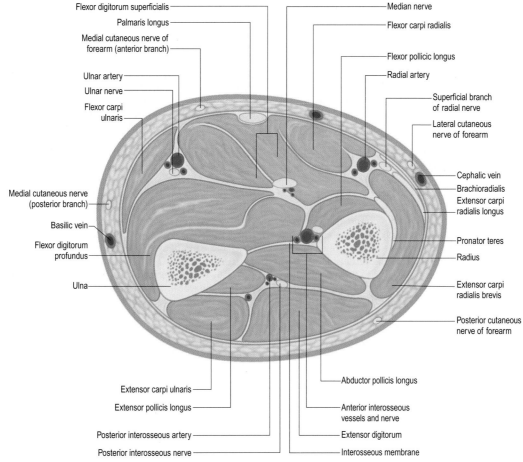

Flexor digitorum superficialis
Palmaris longus
Medial cutaneous nerve of forearm (anterior branch)
Ulnar artery
Ulnar nerve
Flexor carpi ulnaris
Medial cutaneous nerve (posterior branch)
Basilic vein
Flexor digitorum profundus
Ulna

Median nerve
Flexor carpi radialis
Flexor pollicic longus
Radial artery
Superficial branch of radial nerve
Lateral cutaneous nerve of forearm
Cephalic vein
Brachioradialis
Extensor carpi radialis longus
Pronator teres
Radius
Extensor carpi radialis brevis
Posterior cutaneous nerve of forearm

Extensor carpi ulnaris
Extensor pollicis longus
Posterior interosseous artery
Posterior interosseous nerve

Abductor pollicis longus
Anterior interosseous vessels and nerve
Extensor digitorum
Interosseous membrane

Fig. 18.25 *Transverse section through the middle of the left forearm (distal aspect).*

lateral side of the ulnar artery, from which it is separated by the deep head of pronator teres. It passes behind a tendinous bridge between the humero-ulnar and radial heads of flexor digitorum superficialis, and descends through the forearm posterior and adherent to flexor digitorum superficialis and anterior to flexor digitorum profundus. About 5 cm proximal to the flexor retinaculum it emerges from behind the lateral edge of flexor digitorum superficialis and becomes superficial just proximal to the wrist. There it lies between the tendons of flexor digitorum superficialis and flexor carpi radialis, projecting laterally from beneath the tendon of palmaris longus (see Fig. 18.23). It then passes deep to the flexor retinaculum into the palm. In the forearm the median nerve is accompanied by the median branch of the anterior interosseous artery.

The course and distribution of the median nerve in the wrist and hand are described below.

Martin–Gruber Connection

Multiple communicating branches between the median nerve (and sometimes the anterior interosseous nerve) arise proximally and pass medially between flexors digitorum superficialis and profundus, deep to the ulnar artery, and join the ulnar nerve. This motor fibre communication (commonly referred to as the Martin–Gruber connection) is estimated to be present in 17% of individuals. It results in median nerve innervation of a variable number of intrinsic muscles of the hand (Leibovic and Hastings 1992) and presumably explains why isolated ulnar and median nerve lesions can be unpredictable in terms of the pattern of intrinsic muscle paralysis.

Branches in the Forearm

Anterior Interosseous Nerve — The anterior interosseous nerve branches posteriorly from the median nerve between the two heads of pronator teres, just distal to the origin of its branches to the superficial forearm flexors and proximal to the point at which the median nerve passes under the tendinous arch of flexor digitorum superficialis. With the anterior interosseous artery it descends anterior to the interosseous membrane, between and deep to flexor pollicis longus and flexor digitorum profundus. It supplies flexor pollicis longus and the lateral part of flexor digitorum profundus (which sends tendons to the index and middle fingers). Terminally, the anterior interosseous nerve lies posterior to pronator quadratus, which it supplies via its deep surface. It also supplies articular branches to the distal radio-ulnar, radiocarpal and carpal joints.

Muscular Branches

Muscular branches are given off near the elbow to all the superficial flexor muscles except flexor carpi ulnaris—that is, to pronator teres, flexor carpi radialis, palmaris longus and flexor digitorum superficialis. The branch to the part of flexor digitorum superficialis that serves the index finger is given off near the mid-forearm and may be derived from the anterior interosseous nerve.

Other Branches

Articular branches, arising at or just distal to the elbow joint, supply the joint and the proximal radio-ulnar joint. The palmar cutaneous branch is described below.

Ulnar Nerve

The ulnar nerve descends on the medial side of the forearm, lying on flexor digitorum profundus (see Figs 18.22–18.25). Proximally, it is covered by flexor carpi ulnaris; its distal half lies lateral to the muscle and is covered only by skin and fasciae. In the upper third of the forearm, the nerve is distant from the ulnar artery, but more distally, it comes to lie close to the medial side of the artery. About 5 cm proximal to the wrist it gives off a dorsal branch that continues distally into the hand, anterior to the flexor retinaculum on the lateral side of the pisiform and posteromedial to the ulnar artery. It passes deep to the superficial part of the retinaculum (in Guyon's canal) with the artery and divides into superficial and deep terminal branches.

The course and distribution of the ulnar nerve in the hand are described below.

Muscular Branches

There are usually two muscular branches. They begin near the elbow and supply flexor carpi ulnaris and the medial half of flexor digitorum profundus.

Palmar Cutaneous Branch — The palmar cutaneous branch arises about mid-forearm. It descends on the ulnar artery, which it supplies, and then perforates the deep fascia to end in the palmar skin, after communicating with the palmar branch of the median nerve. It sometimes supplies palmaris brevis.

Dorsal Branch — The dorsal branch of the ulnar nerve is described below.

CASE 5 ANTERIOR INTEROSSEOUS SYNDROME

A 12-year-old boy fractures the midshaft of his right radius as a result of a skiing accident. Following removal of the cast, he has difficulty holding a pencil to write. Examination demonstrates weakness of his pinch grip between the thumb and index fingers, specifically involving flexor pollicis longus (FPL) and flexor digitorum profundus (FDP). Muscle testing is otherwise normal; pronation is spared. Reflexes and sensation are normal.

Discussion: The anterior interosseous nerve is a pure motor nerve, branching posteriorly from the median nerve and emerging between the heads of pronator teres, just distal to the branch that supplies the superficial forearm flexors but proximal to the median nerve passing under the tendinous arch of flexor digitorum superficialis. The nerve runs anterior to the interosseous membrane, between FPL and FDP, supplying FPL and lateral FDP. It also innervates the deep pronator quadratus muscle. Weakness of FPL and FDP, as occurs in anterior interosseous syndrome, causes a weak pinch between the thumb and index fingers. Pronator quadratus weakness may not be evident on testing owing to the normal strength of pronator teres. No sensory symptoms are present, distinguishing this syndrome from the so-called pronator syndrome, which reflects more proximal involvement of the median nerve, thus implicating a sensory branch as well. In the patient described here, a midshaft fracture of the radius resulted in injury to the anterior interosseous nerve distal to its branching from the median nerve.

Radial Nerve

There is some variation in the level at which branches of the radial nerve arise from the main trunk in different subjects (Fig. 18.26; see also Figs 18.23, 18.25). Branches to extensor carpi radialis brevis and supinator may arise from the main trunk of the radial nerve or from the proximal part of the posterior interosseous nerve, but almost invariably above the arcade of Frohse.

Radial Tunnel Syndrome

Radial tunnel syndrome is an entrapment neuropathy of the radial nerve near the elbow, where four structures can potentially cause compression of the nerve: (1) fibrous bands (which can tether the radial nerve to the radiohumeral joint), (2) the sharp tendinous medial border of extensor carpi radialis brevis, (3) a leash of vessels from the radial recurrent artery as it passes to supply brachioradialis and extensor carpi radialis longus and (4) the arcade of Frohse, which is the free aponeurotic proximal edge of the superficial part of supinator (see Fig. 18.16).

Usually the only presenting symptom is pain over the extensor mass just distal to the elbow. There is no sensory disturbance or motor loss, but there is frequently tenderness along the course of the radial nerve over the radial head. The pain is exacerbated when the elbow is extended and the wrist is passively flexed and pronated or extended and supinated against resistance. Extension of the middle finger against resistance when the elbow in fully extended may lead to increased pain. These manoeuvres tighten the anatomical structures, which cause compression.

Superficial Terminal Branch

The superficial terminal branch descends from the lateral epicondyle antero-laterally in the proximal two-thirds of the forearm, initially lying on supinator, lateral to the radial artery and behind brachioradialis. In the middle third of the forearm it lies behind brachioradialis, close to the lateral side of the artery, and is successively anterior to pronator teres, the radial head of flexor digitorum superficialis and flexor pollicis longus. It leaves the artery approximately 7 cm proximal to the wrist and passes deep to the brachioradialis tendon. It curves around the lateral side of the radius as it descends, pierces

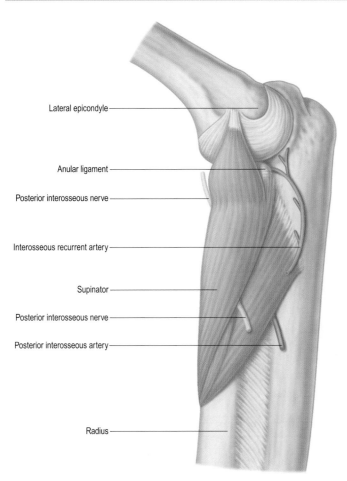

Fig. 18.26 *Left supinator muscle (posterolateral aspect).*

Labels on figure:
- Lateral epicondyle
- Anular ligament
- Posterior interosseous nerve
- Interosseous recurrent artery
- Supinator
- Posterior interosseous nerve
- Posterior interosseous artery
- Radius

the deep fascia and divides into five (sometimes four) dorsal digital nerves. On the dorsum of the hand it usually communicates with the posterior and lateral cutaneous nerves of the forearm.

As the nerve crosses the lateral aspect of the radius it is superficial and relatively unprotected; it is easily compressed here by tight bracelets, watch straps and handcuffs.

Radial Sensory Nerve Entrapment (Wartenberg's Disease) — Entrapment of the superficial radial nerve can occur as it emerges from beneath the edge of the brachioradialis tendon approximately 6 cm proximal to the radial styloid. The condition is frequently associated with previous trauma in this region. The symptoms are pain and paraesthesia over the radial aspect of the dorsum of the wrist and hand.

Posterior Interosseous Nerve

The posterior interosseous nerve is the deep terminal branch of the radial nerve (see Fig. 18.24). It reaches the back of the forearm by passing around the lateral aspect of the radius between the two heads of supinator. It supplies extensor carpi radialis brevis and supinator before entering supinator; as it passes through the muscle it supplies it with additional branches. The branch to extensor carpi radialis brevis may arise from the beginning of the superficial branch of the radial nerve. As it emerges from supinator posteriorly, the posterior interosseous nerve gives off three short branches to extensor digitorum, extensor digiti minimi and extensor carpi ulnaris; it also gives off two longer branches—a medial branch to extensor pollicis longus and extensor indicis, and a lateral branch that supplies abductor pollicis longus and extensor pollicis brevis. The nerve at first lies between the superficial and deep extensor muscles, but at the distal border of extensor pollicis brevis it passes deep to extensor pollicis longus and, diminished to a fine thread, descends on the interosseous membrane to the dorsum of the carpus. There it presents a flattened and somewhat expanded termination or 'pseudoganglion,' from which filaments supply the carpal ligaments and articulations. Articular branches from the posterior interosseous nerve supply carpal, distal radio-ulnar and some intercarpal and intermetacarpal joints. Digital branches supply the metacarpophalangeal and proximal interphalangeal joints.

The distal portion of the nerve lies in a separate fascial sheath in the radial, deep aspect of the fourth dorsal compartment of the extensor retinaculum of the wrist, where it is located deep to extensor digitorum and extensor indicis. This portion of the nerve can be used as a donor nerve for grafting

segmental digital nerve defects, as there is no clinically discernible donor site deficit.

Posterior Interosseous Nerve Palsy — There are many causes of posterior interosseous nerve palsy. These include trauma and inflammatory swelling, as well as entrapment at the same anatomical sites that can cause radial tunnel syndrome. Pain is similar in nature to that of radial tunnel syndrome and is later accompanied by weakness and paralysis. When fully developed, there is an inability to extend the fingers at the metacarpophalangeal joints and weakness of thumb extension and abduction. There is also weakness and radial deviation of wrist extension because extensor carpi ulnaris is usually affected, whereas the radial wrist extensors and brachioradialis are normal (because their nerve supply is given off proximal to the origin of the posterior interosseous nerve). There are no sensory disturbances, because the superficial radial nerve arises above this level.

Medial Cutaneous Nerve of the Forearm

The medial cutaneous nerve of the forearm has already divided into anterior and posterior branches before it enters the forearm (see Fig. 18.20). The larger anterior branch usually passes in front of, or occasionally behind, the median cubital vein and descends anteromedially in the forearm to supply the skin as far as the wrist. It curves around to the back of the forearm, descending on its medial border to the wrist, supplying the skin. It connects with the medial cutaneous nerve of the arm, posterior cutaneous nerve of the forearm and dorsal branch of the ulnar nerve.

Lateral Cutaneous Nerve of the Forearm

The lateral cutaneous nerve of the forearm is a direct continuation of the musculocutaneous nerve as it lies lateral to the biceps tendon in the antecubital fossa (see Figs 18.5, 18.8). It passes deep to the cephalic vein, descending along the radial border of the forearm to the wrist. It supplies the skin of the anterolateral surface of the forearm and connects with the posterior cutaneous nerve of the forearm and the terminal branch of the radial nerve by branches that pass around its radial border. Its trunk gives rise to a slender recurrent branch that extends along the cephalic vein as far as the middle third of the upper arm, distributing filaments to the skin over the distal third of the anterolateral surface of the upper arm close to the vein. At the wrist joint the lateral cutaneous nerve of the forearm is anterior to the radial artery. Some filaments pierce the deep fascia and accompany the artery to the dorsum of the carpus. The nerve then passes to the base of the thenar eminence, where it ends in cutaneous rami. It has branches that connect with the terminal branch of the radial nerve and the palmar cutaneous branch of the median nerve.

Posterior Cutaneous Nerve of the Forearm

The posterior cutaneous nerve of the forearm passes along the dorsum of the forearm to the wrist. It supplies the skin along its course and near its end joins the dorsal branches of the lateral cutaneous nerve of the forearm.

NERVES OF THE WRIST AND HAND
Median Nerve

The median nerve proximal to the flexor retinaculum is lateral to the tendons of flexor digitorum superficialis and lies between the tendons of flexor carpi radialis and palmaris longus. It passes under the retinaculum in the 'carpal tunnel' (see below), where its compression may lead to carpal tunnel syndrome. Distal to the retinaculum the nerve enlarges and flattens and usually divides into five or six branches; the mode and level of division are variable.

Palmar Cutaneous Branch

The palmar cutaneous branch starts just proximal to the flexor retinaculum. It pierces the retinaculum or the deep fascia and divides into lateral branches that supply the thenar skin and connect with the lateral cutaneous nerve of the forearm. Medial branches supply the central palmar skin and connect with the palmar cutaneous branch of the ulnar nerve.

Communicating branches, which may be multiple, often arise in the proximal forearm, sometimes from the anterior interosseous branch. They pass medially between flexors digitorum superficialis and profundus and behind the ulnar artery to join the ulnar nerve. This communication is a factor in explaining anomalous muscular innervation in the hand (see below).

Muscular Branch (Motor or Recurrent Branch)

The muscular branch is short and thick and arises from the lateral side of the nerve; it may be the first palmar branch or a terminal branch that arises level with the digital branches. It runs laterally, just distal to the flexor retinaculum, with a slight recurrent curve beneath the part of the palmar aponeurosis covering the thenar muscles. It turns around the distal border of the

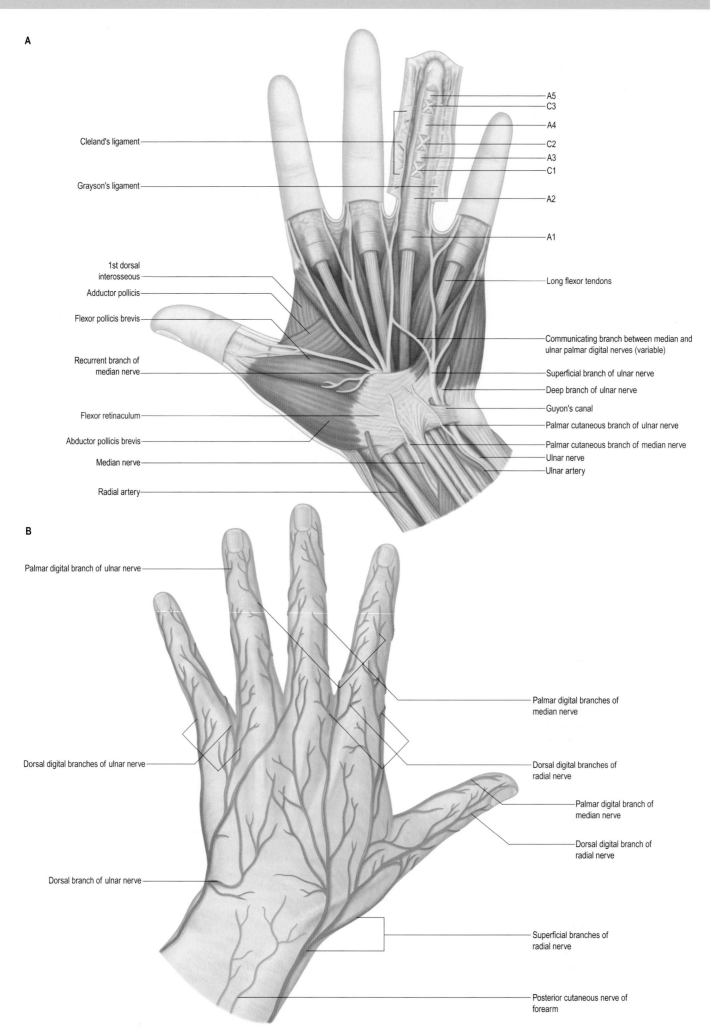

A

A5
C3
A4
C2
A3
C1

Cleland's ligament

Grayson's ligament

A2

A1

1st dorsal interosseous

Adductor pollicis

Flexor pollicis brevis

Long flexor tendons

Recurrent branch of median nerve

Communicating branch between median and ulnar palmar digital nerves (variable)

Superficial branch of ulnar nerve

Deep branch of ulnar nerve

Guyon's canal

Flexor retinaculum

Palmar cutaneous branch of ulnar nerve

Abductor pollicis brevis

Palmar cutaneous branch of median nerve

Median nerve

Ulnar nerve

Ulnar artery

Radial artery

B

Palmar digital branch of ulnar nerve

Palmar digital branches of median nerve

Dorsal digital branches of ulnar nerve

Dorsal digital branches of radial nerve

Palmar digital branch of median nerve

Dorsal digital branch of radial nerve

Dorsal branch of ulnar nerve

Superficial branches of radial nerve

Posterior cutaneous nerve of forearm

Fig. 18.27 *Cutaneous nerves of the hand.* **A**, *Palmar aspect.* **B**, *Dorsal aspect. The anular and cruciate pulleys are shown schematically in the ring finger.*

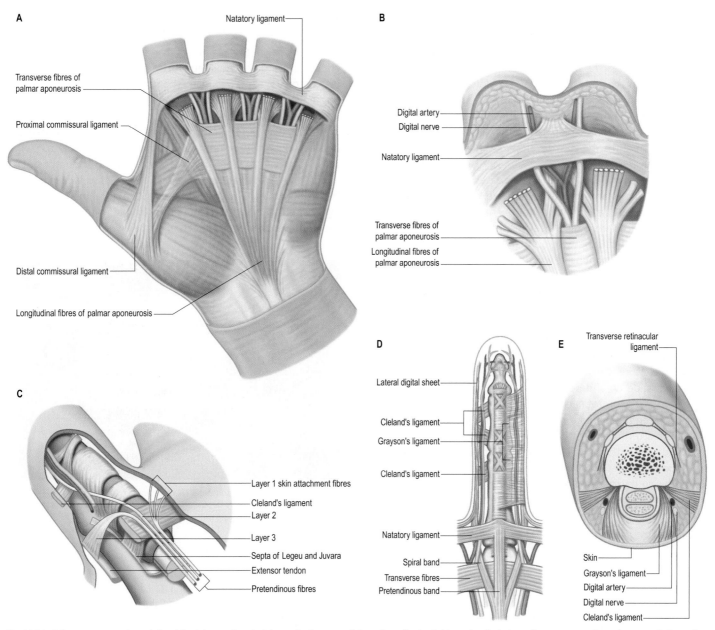

Fig. 18.28 *Palmar aponeurosis and distal fascial complex.* **A**, *Schematic diagram of the palmar fascia.* **B**, *More detailed view of structures at the web space.* **C**, *Fate of the distal longitudinal fibres.* **D** *and* **E**, *Normal digital fascia.*

retinaculum to lie superficial to flexor pollicis brevis, which it usually supplies, and continues either superficial to the muscle or traverses it. It gives a branch to abductor pollicis brevis, which enters the medial edge of the muscle and then passes deep to it to supply opponens pollicis, entering its medial edge. Its terminal part occasionally gives a branch to the first dorsal interosseous, which may be its sole or partial supply. The muscular branch may arise in the carpal tunnel and pierce the flexor retinaculum, which is a point of surgical importance.

Palmar Digital Branches (Figs 18.27, 18.28)

The median nerve usually divides into four or five digital branches. It often divides first into a lateral ramus, which provides digital branches to the thumb and radial side of the index finger, and a medial ramus, which supplies digital branches to adjacent sides of the index, middle and ring fingers. Other modes of termination can occur.

Digital branches are commonly arranged as follows. They pass distally, deep to the superficial palmar arch and its digital vessels, at first anterior to the long flexor tendons. Two proper palmar digital nerves, sometimes from a common stem, pass to the sides of the thumb; the nerve supplying its radial side crosses in front of the flexor pollicis longus tendon. The proper palmar digital nerve to the lateral side of the index also supplies the first lumbrical. Two common palmar digital nerves pass distally between the long flexor tendons. The lateral one divides in the distal palm into two proper palmar digital nerves that traverse adjacent sides of the index and middle fingers. The medial one divides into two proper palmar digital nerves that supply adjacent sides of the middle and ring fingers. The lateral common digital nerve supplies

the second lumbrical, and the medial receives a communicating twig from the common palmar digital branch of the ulnar nerve and may supply the third lumbrical. In the distal part of the palm the digital arteries pass deeply between the divisions of the digital nerves; the nerves lie anterior to the arteries on the sides of the digits. The median nerve usually supplies palmar cutaneous digital branches to the radial three and a half digits (thumb, index, middle and lateral sides of the ring finger); sometimes the radial side of the ring finger is supplied by the ulnar nerve. Occasionally, there is a communicating branch between the common digital nerve to the middle and ring fingers (derived from the median nerve) and the common digital nerve to the ring and little fingers (derived from the ulnar nerve). This can explain variations in sensory patterns that do not conform to the classic pattern.

The proper palmar digital nerves pass along the medial side of the index finger, both sides of the middle finger and the lateral side of the ring finger. They enter these digits in fat between slips of the palmar aponeurosis. Together with the lumbricals and palmar digital arteries, they pass dorsal to the superficial transverse metacarpal ligament and ventral to the deep transverse metacarpal ligament. In the digits, the nerves run distally beside the long flexor tendons (outside their fibrous sheaths), level with the anterior phalangeal surfaces and anterior to the digital arteries, between Grayson's and Cleland's ligaments . Each nerve gives off several branches to the skin on the front and sides of the digit, where many end in Pacinian corpuscles. It also sends branches to the metacarpophalangeal and interphalangeal joints.

The digital nerves supply the fibrous sheaths of the long flexor tendons, digital arteries (vasomotor) and sweat glands (secretomotor). Distal to the base of the distal phalanx, each digital nerve gives off a branch that passes

CASE 6   CARPAL TUNNEL SYNDROME

A 41-year-old right-handed man runs heavy machinery at work. In the last year he has developed progressive numbness and tingling in the thumb, index and middle fingers, plus half of the ring finger of the right hand. It is most prominent on arising in the morning and sometimes wakes him from sleep. He has mild difficulty twisting the tops off bottles. In the past 2 months, he has developed similar symptoms in the left hand.

On examination, there is decreased sensation over the thumb, index and middle fingers and half of the ring finger, with sparing of the remainder of the hand, including the thenar eminence. There is mild weakness of abductor pollicis brevis, but strength is otherwise normal (Fig. 18.29). Tapping distal to the proximal (dominant) wrist crease between the tendons of palmaris longus and flexor carpi radialis elicits an electric shock–like sensation in the hand (Tinel's sign). Reflexes are normal.

Discussion: Carpal tunnel syndrome, or median neuropathy at the wrist, reflects the close anatomical relationship between the flexor retinaculum and the deep branch of the median nerve. With wrist flexion and extension, the median nerve must slide up and down a fibro-osseous tunnel beneath the fibrous flexor retinaculum. The nerve can be compressed between these structures, especially if there are bony changes from arthritis or soft tissue thickening due to repetitive injury, with or without inflammation, at that site. The disorder appears in patients with diabetes, as a form of mononeuropathy, in myxoedema associated with acromegaly, in association with generalized oedema from obesity or pregnancy or in patients with arthritis of the wrist. Symptoms usually

predominate in the dominant hand, most likely owing to greater use and potential repeat compression. Numbness typically appears, as in this man. The sensory innervation of the ring finger is variable and is often spared by virtue of input from the ulnar nerve. Because the palmar cutaneous branch of the median nerve branches off before the median nerve dips below the flexor retinaculum and into the carpal tunnel, sensation over the thenar eminence is spared. Abductor pollicis brevis is innervated by the median nerve, so weakness of this muscle may be found. This indicates a distal median nerve injury; median-innervated muscles proximal to the flexor retinaculum are unaffected in carpal tunnel syndrome.

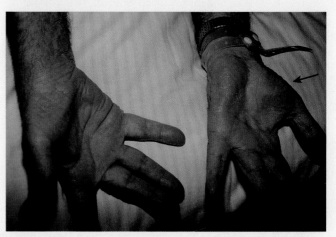

Fig. 18.29 *Carpal tunnel syndrome. There is marked wasting of the thenar eminence bilaterally* (arrow) *in an advanced case of carpal tunnel syndrome.*

---

dorsally to the nail bed. The main nerve frequently trifurcates to supply the pulp and skin of the terminal part of the digit. Distal to the base of the proximal phalanx, each proper digital nerve also gives off a dorsal branch to supply the skin over the back of the middle and distal phalanges. The proper palmar digital nerves to the thumb and lateral side of the index finger emerge with the long flexor tendons from under the lateral edge of the palmar aponeurosis. They are arranged in the digits as described earlier, but in the thumb, small distal branches supply the skin on the back of the distal phalanx only.

Other Branches

In addition to the branches of the median nerve already described, variable vasomotor branches supply the radial and ulnar arteries and their branches. Some of the intercarpal, carpometacarpal and intermetacarpal joints are thought to be supplied by the median nerve or its anterior interosseous branch; the precise details are uncertain.

Median Nerve Division at the Wrist

The median nerve is vulnerable to division from lacerations at the wrist. Division leads to paralysis of the lumbricals to the index and middle fingers and the thenar muscles (apart from adductor pollicis), as well as loss of sensation to the thumb, index, middle fingers and radial half of the ring finger. The radial half of the hand becomes flattened as a result of wasting of the thenar muscles and the adducted posture of the thumb.

Ulnar Nerve

At the wrist, the ulnar nerve passes under the superficial part of the retinaculum (in Guyon's canal) with the ulnar artery and divides into superficial and deep terminal branches.

Dorsal Branch

The dorsal branch arises approximately 5 cm proximal to the wrist. It passes distally and dorsally, deep to flexor carpi ulnaris; perforates the deep fascia; descends along the medial side of the back of the wrist and hand; and then

divides into two, or often three, dorsal digital nerves. The first supplies the medial side of the little finger; the second, the adjacent sides of the little and ring fingers; and the third, when present, supplies adjoining sides of the ring and middle fingers. The last may be replaced, wholly or partially, by a branch of the radial nerve, which always communicates with it on the dorsum of the hand (see Fig. 18.28). In the little finger, the dorsal digital nerves extend only to the base of the distal phalanx; in the ring finger, they extend only to the base of the middle phalanx. The most distal parts of the little finger and of the ulnar side of the ring finger are supplied by dorsal branches of the proper palmar digital branches of the ulnar nerve. The most distal part of the lateral side of the ring finger is supplied by dorsal branches of the proper palmar digital branch of the median nerve.

Superficial Terminal Branch

The superficial terminal branch supplies palmaris brevis and the medial palmar skin. It divides into two palmar digital nerves, which can be palpated against the hook of the hamate bone. One supplies the medial side of the little finger, and the other (a common palmar digital nerve) sends a twig to the median nerve and divides into two proper digital nerves to supply the adjoining sides of the little and ring fingers. The proper digital branches are distributed like those derived from the median nerve.

Deep Terminal Branch

The deep terminal branch accompanies the deep branch of the ulnar artery as it passes between abductor digiti minimi and flexor digiti minimi and then perforates the opponens digiti minimi to follow the deep palmar arch dorsal to the flexor tendons (Fig. 18.30). At its origin, it supplies the three short muscles of the little finger. As it crosses the hand, it supplies the interossei and the third and fourth lumbricals. It ends by supplying adductor pollicis, first palmar interosseous and usually flexor pollicis brevis. It sends articular filaments to the wrist joint.

The medial part of flexor digitorum profundus is supplied by the ulnar nerve, as are the third and fourth lumbricals, which are connected with the

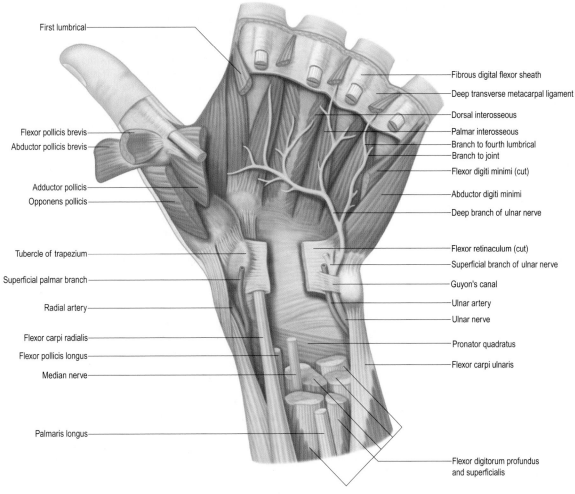

Fig. 18.30 *Deep structures in the left palm and wrist.*

Labels (clockwise from top left):
First lumbrical
Flexor pollicis brevis
Abductor pollicis brevis
Adductor pollicis
Opponens pollicis
Tubercle of trapezium
Superficial palmar branch
Radial artery
Flexor carpi radialis
Flexor pollicis longus
Median nerve
Palmaris longus
Fibrous digital flexor sheath
Deep transverse metacarpal ligament
Dorsal interosseous
Palmar interosseous
Branch to fourth lumbrical
Branch to joint
Flexor digiti minimi (cut)
Abductor digiti minimi
Deep branch of ulnar nerve
Flexor retinaculum (cut)
Superficial branch of ulnar nerve
Guyon's canal
Ulnar artery
Ulnar nerve
Pronator quadratus
Flexor carpi ulnaris
Flexor digitorum profundus and superficialis

tendons of this part of the muscle. Similarly, the lateral part of flexor digitorum profundus and the first and second lumbricals are supplied by the median nerve. The third lumbrical is often supplied by both nerves. The deep terminal branch is thought to give branches to some intercarpal, carpometacarpal and intermetacarpal joints; precise details are uncertain. Vasomotor branches, arising in the forearm and hand, supply the ulnar and palmar arteries.

Ulnar Tunnel Syndrome

Ulnar tunnel syndrome is an entrapment neuropathy of the ulnar nerve as it passes through Guyon's canal at the wrist (see Fig. 18.27). Causes of compression at this site include ganglion, trauma and proximity of aberrant or accessory muscles. Symptoms include pain in the hand or forearm and sensory changes in the palmar aspect of the little finger and ulnar half of the ring finger; however, sensation on the ulnar aspect of the dorsum of the hand is normal. In addition, there may be weakness and wasting of the intrinsic muscles of the hand supplied by the ulnar nerve, with clawing in extreme cases.

Surgical treatment involves decompression of the nerve by division of the roof of Guyon's canal.

Ulnar Nerve Division at the Wrist

Division of the ulnar nerve at the wrist paralyses all the intrinsic muscles of the hand (except for the radial two lumbricals). The intrinsic muscle action of flexing the metacarpophalangeal joints and extending the interphalangeal joints is therefore lost. The unopposed action of the long extensors and flexors of the fingers causes the hand to assume a clawed appearance with extension of the metacarpophalangeal joints and flexion of the interphalangeal joints. The clawing is less intense in the index and middle fingers because of their intact lumbricals, supplied by the median nerve. For a detailed account of the hand posture adopted in ulnar nerve lesions, see Smith 2002.

There is sensory loss over the little finger and the ulnar half of the ring finger. In comparison with an ulnar nerve division at the elbow, the skin over the ulnar aspect of the dorsum of the hand is spared because the dorsal branch of the ulnar nerve is given off approximately 5 cm proximal to the wrist joint.

A combined median and ulnar nerve palsy at the wrist results in a full claw hand, with thenar and hypothenar flattening and thumb adduction and flexion. This posture is known as 'simian hand' because of its similarity to the appearance of an ape's hand.

Radial Nerve

Branches of the superficial branch of the radial nerve reach the hand by curving around the wrist deep to the brachioradialis tendon. They divide into dorsal digital nerves. On the dorsum of the hand they usually communicate with the posterior and lateral cutaneous nerves of the forearm.

Dorsal Digital Nerves

There are usually four or five small dorsal digital nerves. The first supplies the skin of the radial side of the thumb and the adjoining thenar eminence and communicates with branches of the lateral cutaneous nerve of the forearm. The second supplies the medial side of the thumb; the third, the lateral side of the index finger; and the fourth, the adjoining sides of the index and middle fingers. The fifth communicates with a ramus of the dorsal branch of the ulnar nerve and supplies the adjoining sides of the middle and ring fingers, but it is frequently replaced by the dorsal branch of the ulnar nerve. The pollicial digital nerves reach only to the root of the nail; those in the index finger, midway along the middle phalanx; those to the middle and lateral parts of the ring finger may reach no farther than the proximal interphalangeal joints. The remaining distal dorsal areas of the skin in these digits are supplied by palmar digital branches of the median and ulnar nerves. The superficial terminal branch of the radial nerve may supply the whole dorsum of the hand.

AUTONOMIC INNERVATION

The autonomic supply to the limbs is exclusively sympathetic. The preganglionic sympathetic inflow to the upper limb is derived from neurones in the lateral horn of the upper thoracic spinal segments T2–6 (or 7). Fibres pass in white rami communicantes to the thoracic sympathetic chain and synapse in the stellate and second thoracic ganglia. Postganglionic fibres to the skin are distributed via cutaneous branches of the brachial plexus. The blood vessels to the upper limb receive their sympathetic supply via adjacent peripheral nerves; thus, the median nerve supplies postganglionic sympathetic fibres to the brachial artery and the palmar arches, and the ulnar nerve supplies the ulnar artery.

SPECIAL FUNCTIONS OF THE HAND

Closing the Hand

It is clear that the fingers and palm of the hand flex in gripping, grasping or making a fist, but there are subtle differences in hand posture in these various activities. The basic mechanisms of hand closure are described before special grips are considered.

As the digits flex, the wrist usually extends (dorsiflexes) at the same time. The involvement of the long digital flexors in this movement is considered first, followed by an analysis of the role of the wrist.

Role of the Long Digital Flexors

Flexor digitorum superficialis acts to flex principally the proximal interphalangeal joints, through its insertions into the middle phalanges. However, in each digit it also has an action on the metacarpophalangeal joint, because the tendon passes anterior to that joint. The muscle has the potential to produce flexion at the wrist for the same reason. The fact that each tendon arises from an individual muscle slip allows the clinician to test one finger at a time. The reader can verify this by attempting to flex each digit individually while using the other hand to keep the distal interphalangeal joints of the remaining fingers in extension. This test is frequently used in clinical practice and is useful for the middle and ring fingers, where flexion of one finger alone must be attributed to flexor digitorum superficialis. The index finger, however, has its own profundus musculotendinous unit and can therefore move independently under the action of this tendon. Many individuals cannot flex the proximal interphalangeal joint of the little finger alone, probably because the superficialis is deficient, although most can flex the metacarpophalangeal joint of the little finger using flexor digiti minimi.

Flexor digitorum profundus has similarities to superficialis; because it reaches farther (to the distal phalanx), it is the only muscle available for flexion of the distal interphalangeal joint. It also contributes, together with superficialis, to flexion at the proximal interphalangeal and metacarpophalangeal joints. These two long flexors (sometimes called extrinsic flexors, because the muscle bellies are outside the hand) can be considered to act together to flex the finger. However, their action alone would wind up the interphalangeal joints before the metacarpophalangeal joints, and the finger would not move in a normal arc of flexion. This is precisely what happens in ulnar nerve paralysis, in which the interossei and lumbricals are not functioning. These small (intrinsic) muscles have been described earlier in terms of their individual actions. For their role in coordinated activity, it is sufficient to appreciate that their contribution changes the arc produced by the long flexors, increasing flexion at the metacarpophalangeal joint and reducing flexion at the proximal interphalangeal joint. All three joints are then angulated to the same degree, and the fingers form a normal arc of flexion.

As the finger flexes, the long extensor tendons (extensor digitorum, extensor indicis and extensor digiti minimi) aid the process by relaxing and allowing the extensor apparatus to glide distally on the dorsa of the phalanges.

Role of the Wrist

As the fingers wind up to make a fist, the wrist tends to extend, particularly when force is applied. This extension has a marked effect on the excursion of the long flexor tendons. On its own, digital flexion would require the long tendons to move proximally in their sheaths, and the flexor muscles in the forearm would shorten. Dorsiflexion of the wrist tends to produce a lengthening of the same muscles, which in normal use is almost enough to balance the shortening due to finger flexion; the net effect is a very slight shortening (approximately 1 cm) of the long flexors in the forearm. The wrist can therefore be seen as a mechanism for maximizing force, because it allows the fingers to flex while maintaining the resting length of the extrinsic muscles near the peak of the force–length curve. It is, of course, possible to wind up the fingers with the wrist held in a neutral position, but the grip is somewhat weaker. With the wrist in full flexion, it is not possible to flex the fingers fully.

Flexion of the fingers on gripping tends to result in a distal excursion of the long extensors. However, this tendency is counteracted by dorsiflexion of the wrist. The net effect is a very small proximal excursion of the long extensor tendons on gripping, mirroring the effect on the flexor surface. If the movement of the wrist is exaggerated, so that the wrist is slightly flexed on opening the hand and fully dorsiflexed on closing it, the net excursion of the long flexors and extensors is zero; that is, this whole movement sequence can be completed with the forearm flexor and extensor muscles contracting isometrically.

The reader can observe the relationship between the digits and wrist by performing the following manoeuvre: Hold the wrist in a relaxed,

mid-supinated position, with the elbow flexed at 90°. If the forearm is rotated into pronation, the wrist falls into flexion, and the fingers automatically extend. If the forearm is rotated into supination, the wrist extends and the fingers flex. The finger movements compensate for the wrist movements and are entirely automatic; they are made without the need for any excursion of forearm flexor or extensor tendons. This test, the wrist tenodesis test, is a useful way to examine the limb for tendon injury. The pointing finger (which does not move with wrist motion) 'points to' a tendon injury.

Wrist motion is controlled principally by two wrist flexors (flexor carpi radialis and flexor carpi ulnaris) and three extensors (extensors carpi radialis longus and brevis, and extensor carpi ulnaris). Although the radiocarpal joint has some functional similarity to a ball and socket joint, it is possible to conceive of the wrist as a variable hinge joint, the axis of which may be set in a number of inclinations. For example, when using a hammer, it is useful to rotate the wrist backward and forward about an axis that permits not only wrist flexion but also ulnar deviation. It would be very restricting to have a pure hinge joint with collateral ligaments of fixed length. In this context, the wrist flexors and extensors may be regarded as variable collateral ligaments that allow the joint to be set about a number of different axes.

For movement about major axes, the wrist tendons can be considered to act in pairs:

> Wrist flexion: flexon carpi radialis and flexor carpi ulnaris
> Wrist extension: extensor carpi radialis longus and brevis, and extensor carpi ulnaris
> Ulnar deviation: extensor carpi ulnaris and flexor carpi ulnaris
> Radial deviation: flexor carpi radialis, extensor carpi radialis longus and brevis, extensor pollicis and abductor pollicis longus

Making a Tight Fist

It is possible to observe and palpate the muscle groups that are active in making a tight fist. The flexor compartment of the forearm is contracted tightly, and electromyographic evidence confirms that flexor digitorum profundus and flexor digitorum superficialis are active. Flexor carpi ulnaris may be seen and felt to contract strongly. The extensor compartment is tightly contracted, and the wrist extensors would certainly be expected to be active. Palpation of the long digital extensors on the back of the wrist shows that these are contracting as well. It seems that when the fingers are held tightly closed, the long digital extensors are unable to move the extensor apparatus; they have acquired a new fixed point on which to act—namely, the proximal limit of the extensor apparatus over the metacarpophalangeal joint. They therefore perform the only task available to them and act together as an additional wrist extensor.

In the thumb web, palpation confirms that the first dorsal interosseous is contracting, as are all the other interossei and the thenar and hypothenar muscles. As the firm fist is swung forward in anger, the brachioradialis stands out, and at the moment of impact, virtually every muscle in the limb is in a state of contraction, with the exception of the lumbricals.

Opening the Hand

The hand is opened from its relaxed balanced posture, such as when stretching out to reach an object. This motion is made up of extension of the distal interphalangeal, proximal interphalangeal and metacarpophalangeal joints. The hand is provided with an ingenious mechanism that allows this to happen. The laws of mechanics suggests that one motor would be required for every joint in a chain, together with some sort of controlling mechanism to ensure that the chain of joints moves together in a coordinated fashion. In the hand, this is achieved through an extensor apparatus that minimizes the number of motors required for movement by allowing the muscles to act on more than one joint and by linking different levels in the mechanism so that the arc of motion is controlled.

The tendons of extensor digitorum run distally over the metacarpal heads, forming the major component of the extensor apparatus. Extensor digitorum has no insertion into the proximal phalanx and therefore exerts its extensor action on the metacarpophalangeal joint indirectly through more distal insertions. The first point of insertion is at the base of the middle phalanx (in clinical practice, the term 'central slip' has been adopted). Acting at this insertion alone, extensor digitorum can extend both metacarpophalangeal and proximal interphalangeal joints together. The interossei are also active in hand opening because they tend to increase extension of the proximal interphalangeal joint. There is therefore a range of possibilities. At one extreme, with no interosseous contribution, the long extensor exerts all its action at the metacarpophalangeal joint; this leads to full extension or even hyperextension, while the proximal interphalangeal joint remains flexed (the typical claw hand of ulnar nerve paralysis, or 'intrinsic-minus' hand). At the other extreme, when the intrinsics act strongly together with extensor digitorum, the proximal interphalangeal joint extends completely while the metacarpophalangeal joint remains flexed ('intrinsic-plus' hand). Thus, in the proximal part of the extensor apparatus, the hand possesses a variable mechanism that allows different amounts of relative metacarpophalangeal or proximal interphalangeal joint motion.

In contrast, the more distal part of the extensor apparatus acts as an automatic or fixed mechanism, whereby the two interphalangeal joints, proximal and distal, move together. The lateral slips of the extensor apparatus arise from extensor digitorum and pass distally on either side of the central slip and thus over the proximal interphalangeal joint. Being farther lateral, they are nearer the joint axis, because the dorsal surface curves away on each side. A helpful analogy is to consider this arrangement as consisting of two pulleys of different sizes on one axle. The central slip can be regarded as a cord that passes over the larger wheel, and each lateral slip as a cord that passes over the smaller wheel. Because these latter pulleys are smaller, there is less longitudinal excursion for a given rotation of the wheel, and this allows some of the excursion to be used for another function—namely, extension at the distal joint. There is an additional mechanism by which the lateral slips move laterally during flexion of the proximal interphalangeal joint. The effect of this lateral movement is to further reduce the distance between the lateral slips and the joint axis, thereby reducing the amount of excursion at the proximal interphalangeal joint even more and allowing more excursion at the distal joint. When the hand flexes, this mechanical linkage system allows both interphalangeal joints to flex together in a coordinated way.

The extensor expansion also receives contributions from the interossei and lumbricals, which approach the digits from the webs and join the corresponding expansion in the proximal segment of the digit. These small muscles can therefore act on the extensor apparatus at two levels: they can extend the proximal interphalangeal joint through fibres that radiate toward the central slip, and they can act on the distal interphalangeal joint through fibres that join the lateral slip.

Apart from the components of the extensor expansion concerned with joint function, the whole structure requires additional anchorage. This must be arranged in such a way that it is not displaced from the underlying skeleton, yet it must not restrict longitudinal movement. These difficult requirements are met by transverse retinacular ligaments at the level of the joints, the transverse ligaments running to relatively fixed attachment points in the region of the joint axis. As the expansion glides backward and forward, the transverse fibres move like bucket handles. Smooth gliding layers are required under the expansion and retinacular ligaments to allow motion to occur without friction.

One final component of the extensor apparatus provides an additional automatic function. This is a fibrous anchorage system, Landsmeer's oblique retinacular ligament, which anchors the distal expansion to the middle phalanx. The role of the oblique retinacular ligament is controversial (reviewed by Bendz 1985). Some argue that it may act in a dynamic tenodesis effect to synchronize the movements of the interphalangeal joints; that is, it may initiate extension of the distal interphalangeal joint as the proximal interphalangeal joint is extended from a fully flexed position, and it may relax with proximal interphalangeal joint flexion to allow full distal interphalangeal joint flexion. Others argue that it becomes taut only when the proximal interphalangeal joint is fully extended and the distal interphalangeal joint is flexed, so that it functions as a restraining force to stabilize the fingertip when it is flexed against resistance (e.g. in the hook grip). Another possibility is that the ligament is merely a secondary lateral stabilizer of the proximal interphalangeal joint and that it acts to centralize the extensor components over the dorsum of the middle phalanx.

Movements of the Thumb

An opposable thumb requires a different system of control from the other digits. Because the metacarpal is much more mobile than in the digits, muscles are needed to control the extra freedom of movement.

The thumb does not easily assume the classic anatomical position. Therefore, the normal descriptive terms—anterior, posterior, medial and lateral—do not readily apply. The terms palmar, dorsal, ulnar and radial have been adopted in clinical practice.

The basic active movements are flexion–extension, abduction–adduction, rotation and circumduction. In the resting position of the first metacarpal, flexion and extension are parallel with the palmar plane, and abduction and adduction occur at right angles to this.

Flexion and extension should be confined to motion at the interphalangeal or metacarpophalangeal joints (Fig. 18.31A–C). Palmar abduction (Fig. 18.31D, E), in which the first metacarpal moves away from the second at right angles to

the plane of the palm, and radial abduction (Fig. 18.31D, F), in which the first metacarpal moves away from the second with the thumb in the plane of the palm, occur at the carpometacarpal joint. The opposite of radial abduction is ulnar adduction, or transpalmar adduction, in which the thumb crosses the palm toward its ulnar border. In clinical practice, the term adduction is generally used without qualification. Circumduction describes the angular motion of the first metacarpal, solely at the carpometacarpal joint, from a position of maximal radial abduction in the plane of the palm toward the ulnar border of the hand, maintaining the widest possible angle between the first and second metacarpals (Fig. 18.31G). Lateral inclinations of the first phalanx maximize the extent of excursion of the circumduction arc. Opposition is a composite position of the thumb achieved by circumduction of the first metacarpal, internal rotation of the thumb ray and maximal extension of the metacarpophalangeal and interphalangeal joints (Fig. 18.31H). Retroposition is the opposite of opposition (Fig. 18.31I). Flexion adduction is the position of maximal transpalmar adduction of the first metacarpal: the metacarpophalangeal and interphalangeal joints are flexed, and the thumb is in contact with the palm (Fig. 18.31J).

Rotary movements occur during circumduction. The simple angular movements described earlier combine with rotation about the long axis of the metacarpal shaft. In opposition, the shaft must rotate medially into pronation. In retroposition, the thumb must rotate laterally into supination. Axial rotation of the thumb metacarpal is produced by muscle activity (which moves the thumb through its arc of circumduction), the geometry of the articular surfaces of the trapeziometacarpal joint and tensile forces in the ligaments (which combine with forces exerted by the muscles of opposition and retroposition to produce axial rotation). The stability of the first metacarpal is greatest after complete pronation in the position of full opposition, when ligament tension, muscle contraction and joint congruence combine to maximal effect.

Position of Rest

The hand has a well-recognized position of rest, with the wrist in extension and the digits in some degree of flexion. The precise position of the thumb in the position of rest is variable. Typically, it is considered to be the midpoint between maximal palmar abduction and maximal retroposition. In this position, the carpometacarpal joint lies within 20° of radial abduction and 30° of palmar abduction. Based on clinical observations, it seems that the metacarpophalangeal joint lies within approximately 40° of flexion and the interphalangeal joint between extension and 10° of flexion.

From the position of rest, the tip of the thumb can approach the radial aspect of the fingers without incurring axial rotation because the palmar and dorsal trapeziometacarpal ligaments remain relaxed (see later).

Grips

From different positions of the arc of circumduction, numerous types of pinch grip are possible (Fig. 18.32). In clinical practice, these have been classified into two main types: tip pinch and lateral (or key) pinch. Many forces contribute to these configurations.

The thumb is a triarticular system, unlike the finger, which is a biarticular system. The thumb is activated by monoarticular muscles (abductor pollicis longus and opponens pollicis), biarticular muscles (extensor pollicis brevis, adductor pollicis, abductor pollicis brevis and flexor pollicis brevis), and triarticular muscles (extensor pollicis longus and flexor pollicis longus). It appears, however, that even a monoarticular muscle can change posture in all three joints by altering the overall balance of forces, making it very difficult to attribute function to the individual intrinsic muscles. However, the thumb muscles seem to provide two broad functions: they control metacarpal positioning (the guy-rope function), an activity that is automatically accompanied by rotation, and they control the axial stability of the skeleton of the thumb.

The thumb muscles can be classified into those used for retroposition, opposition and pinch grip.

Retroposition Muscles

The muscles that bring about retroposition are extensor pollicis longus, extensor pollicis brevis and abductor pollicis longus. As the thumb moves into retroposition, automatic axial rotation produces supination of the first metacarpal. This is produced by the off-axis action of two parallel but oppositely directed forces—one exerted by extensors pollicis longus and brevis, and the other by abductor pollicis longus and the anterior oblique carpometacarpal ligament.

Opposition Muscles

A succession of activity occurs in the thenar muscles during the movement of opposition. Three subgroups of radial (abductor pollicis longus and

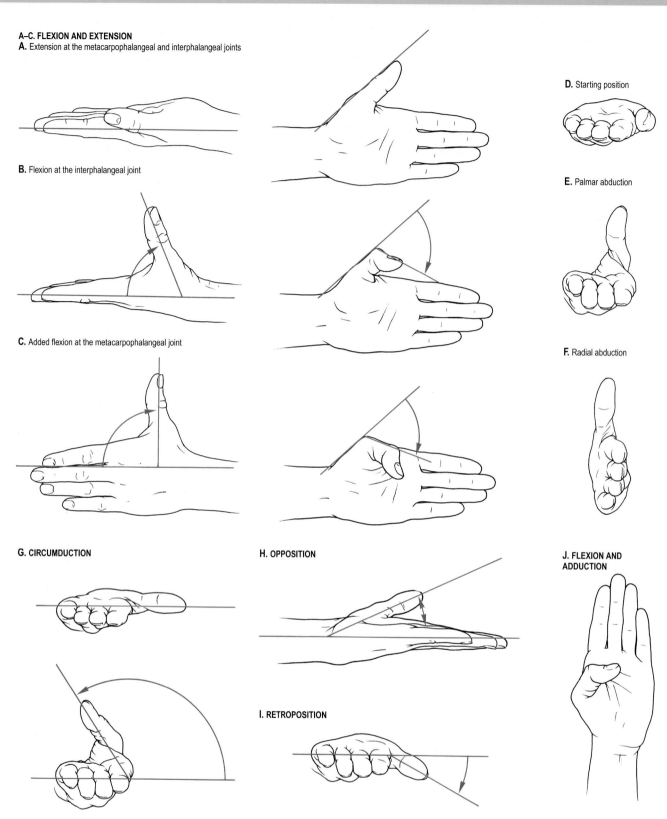

A–C. FLEXION AND EXTENSION
A. Extension at the metacarpophalangeal and interphalangeal joints

B. Flexion at the interphalangeal joint

C. Added flexion at the metacarpophalangeal joint

D. Starting position

E. Palmar abduction

F. Radial abduction

G. CIRCUMDUCTION

H. OPPOSITION

I. RETROPOSITION

J. FLEXION AND ADDUCTION

Fig. 18.31 *A–J, Movements of the thumb.*

extensor pollicis brevis), central (abductor pollicis brevis and opponens pollicis) and ulnar (flexor pollicis brevis) muscles are involved.

These forces act simultaneously but with different intensities, depending on the situation of the thumb. As the thumb moves into opposition, there is automatic axial rotation of the first metacarpal shaft to produce pronation. This is produced by the paired action of oppositely directed forces: the opposition muscles provide one force, and the posterior oblique carpometacarpal ligament provides the other.

Pinch Grip Muscles

The muscles of pinch grip can be divided into lateral, medial and intermediate subgroups. The lateral subgroup (opposition muscles) moves the first metacarpal into palmar abduction. The metacarpal shaft rotates medially into pronation. Radial angulation at the metacarpophalangeal joint increases the span of the hand. The metacarpophalangeal joint is stabilized principally by extensor pollicis brevis and flexor pollicis brevis. Flexion of the proximal and distal phalanges is controlled. Muscles of the medial subgroup (abductor pollicis brevis and first dorsal interosseous) produce an approach of the first metacarpal toward the palm. Because they act with the lateral group, they have a strong controlling effect on the position and rotation of the first metacarpal. The intermediate subgroup consists simply of flexor pollicis longus, which flexes the interphalangeal or metacarpophalangeal joint, as described earlier. Palpating the thenar eminence during tip and lateral pinch provides some appreciation of the action of the pinch grip muscles.

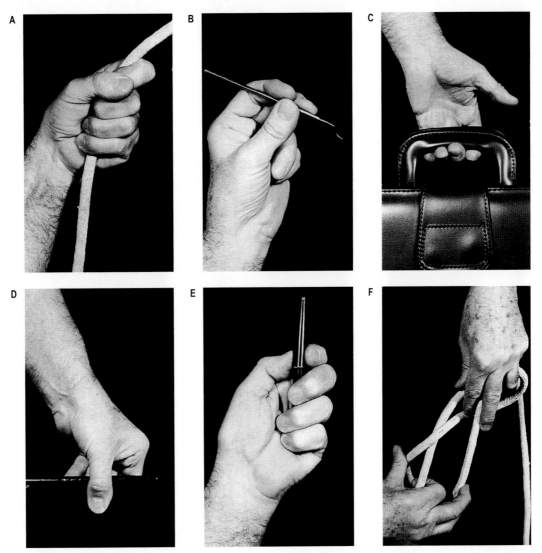

Fig. 18.32 *Some of the many functional postures that can be adopted by the human hand.* **A**, *In the power grip, the fingers are flexed around an object, with counterpressure from the thumb. Any skill in wielding the object derives from the limb, including the wrist; relative movements of the thumb and fingers are not involved.* **B**, *The precision grip, which varies considerably with the task, stabilizes the object between the tips of one or more fingers and the thumb. The gross position of the object can be adjusted by movements at the wrist, elbow or even shoulder, but the most skilled manipulations are carried out by the digits themselves, such as when advancing a thread through the eye of a needle.* **C**, *The hook grip is used to suspend or to pull open objects. The fingers are flexed around the object; the thumb may or may not be involved. It is a grip for the transmission of forces, not for skillful manipulation.* **D**, *Powerful opposition of the thumb to the radial side of the index finger produces a lateral pinch grip, such as to hold a door key; here the object is larger than a key, and all the fingers are involved.* **E**, *Many activities involve a combination of grips. Here a fountain pen is stabilized in a power grip by flexion of digits 4 and 5 against the palm, while the index finger and thumb, used in a precision grip, unscrew the cap.* **F**, *Complex manipulation.*

References

Ball, C.M., Steger, T., Galatz, L.M., Yamaguchi, K., 2003. The posterior branch of the axillary nerve: an anatomic study. J. Bone Joint Surg. 85, 1497–1501.

Bendz, P., 1985. The functional significance of the oblique retinacular ligament of Landsmeer: a review and new proposals. J. Hand Surg. 10, 25–29.

Leibovic, S.J., Hastings II H., 1992. Martin–Gruber revisited. J. Hand Surg. 17A, 47–53.

Smith, P.J., 2002. Lister's The Hand: Diagnosis and Indications, fourth ed. Churchill Livingstone, Edinburgh.

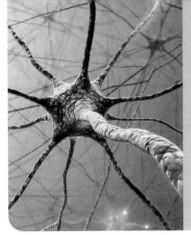

Chest and Abdominal Wall

Chapter 19

THORACIC VENTRAL SPINAL RAMI

There are 12 pairs of thoracic ventral rami. The upper 11 lie between the ribs (intercostal nerves), and the twelfth lies below the last rib (subcostal nerve) (Figs 19.1, 19.2). Each is connected with the adjoining ganglion of the sympathetic trunk by grey and white rami communicantes; the grey ramus joins the nerve proximal to the point at which the white ramus leaves it. Intercostal nerves are distributed primarily to the thoracic and abdominal walls. The first two nerves supply fibres to the upper limb in addition to their thoracic branches, the next four supply only the thoracic wall and the lower five supply both thoracic and abdominal walls. The subcostal nerve is distributed to the abdominal wall and the gluteal skin. Communicating branches link the intercostal nerves posteriorly in the intercostal spaces, and the lower five nerves communicate freely in the abdominal wall.

First to Sixth Thoracic Ventral Rami

The first thoracic ventral ramus divides unequally. A large branch ascends across the neck of the first rib, lateral to the superior intercostal artery, and enters the brachial plexus. The smaller branch is the first intercostal nerve; it runs in the first intercostal space and ends on the front of the chest as the first anterior cutaneous nerve of the thorax. It gives off a lateral cutaneous branch, which pierces the chest wall in front of the serratus anterior and supplies the axillary skin; it may communicate with the intercostobrachial nerve and sometimes joins the medial cutaneous nerve of the arm. The first thoracic ramus often receives a connecting ramus from the second, which ascends in front of the neck of the second rib.

The second to sixth thoracic ventral rami pass forward in their intercostal spaces below the intercostal vessels. At the back of the chest they lie between the pleura and external intercostal membranes, but in most of their course they run between the internal intercostals and the subcostals and innermost intercostals (see Fig. 19.2). Near the sternum, they cross anterior to the internal thoracic vessels and transversus thoracis; pierce the internal intercostals, external intercostal membranes and pectoralis major; and end as the anterior cutaneous nerves of the thorax, which supply the skin on the front of the thorax. The second anterior cutaneous nerve may be connected to the medial supraclavicular nerves of the cervical plexus; twigs from the sixth intercostal nerve supply abdominal skin in the upper part of the infrasternal angle.

Branches

Numerous slender muscular filaments supply the intercostals, serratus posterior superior and transversus thoracis. Anteriorly, some cross the costal cartilages from one intercostal space to another.

Each intercostal nerve gives off a collateral and a lateral cutaneous branch before it reaches the angle of the adjoining ribs. The collateral branch follows the inferior border of its space in the same intermuscular place as the main nerve, which it may rejoin before it is distributed as an additional anterior cutaneous nerve. The lateral cutaneous branch accompanies the main nerve a short way and then pierces the intercostal muscles obliquely. With the exception of the lateral cutaneous branches of the first and second intercostal nerves, each divides into anterior and posterior rami that subsequently pierce the serratus anterior. Anterior branches run forward over the border of the pectoralis major to supply the overlying skin; those of the fifth and sixth also supply twigs to a variable number of upper digitations of external oblique. Posterior branches run backward and supply the skin over the scapula and latissimus dorsi.

The lateral cutaneous branch of the second intercostal nerve is the intercostobrachial nerve (see Fig. 18.9). It crosses the axilla to gain the medial side of the arm and joins a branch of the medial cutaneous nerve of the arm. It then pierces the deep fascia of the arm and supplies the skin of the upper half of the posterior and medial parts of the arm, communicating with the posterior cutaneous branch of the radial nerve. Its size is in inverse proportion to the size of the medial cutaneous nerve. A second intercostobrachial nerve

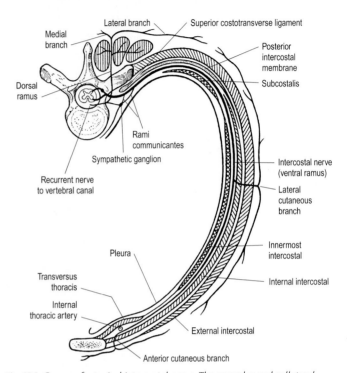

Fig. 19.1 *Course of a typical intercostal nerve. The muscular and collateral branches are not shown.*

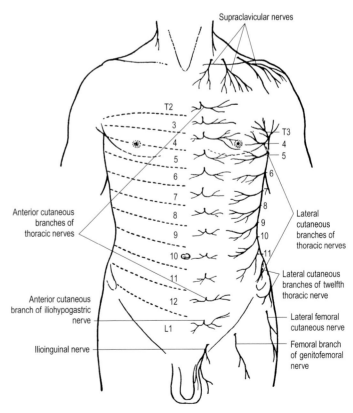

Fig. 19.2 *Approximate segmental distribution of the cutaneous nerves on the front of the trunk. The contribution from the first thoracic spinal nerve is not shown, and the considerable overlap between adjacent segments is not indicated.*

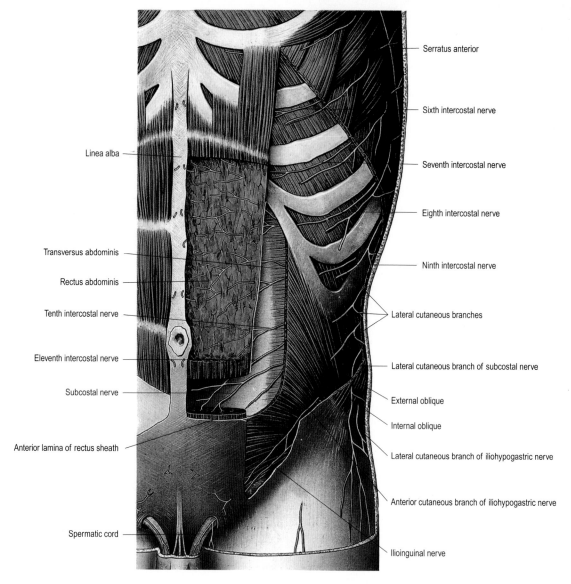

Fig. 19.3 *Course of the lower intercostal and cutaneous branches of some lumbar nerves. Portions of the muscles of the anterior abdominal wall have been removed, including most of the anterior layer of the rectus sheath and parts of rectus abdominis.*

often branches off from the anterior part of the third lateral cutaneous nerve and sends filaments to the axilla and the medial side of the arm.

Seventh to Twelfth Thoracic Ventral Rami

The seventh to twelfth lower thoracic ventral rami continue anteriorly from the intercostal spaces into the abdominal wall (Fig. 19.3). Approaching the anterior ends of their respective spaces, the seventh and eighth nerves curve superomedially across the deep surface of the costal cartilages between the digitations of the transverse abdominis. They reach the deep aspect of the posterior layer of the aponeurosis of internal oblique. Both the seventh and eighth nerves then run through this aponeurosis, pass posterior to the rectus abdominis and supply branches to the upper portion of the muscle. They pass through the muscle near its lateral edge and pierce the anterior rectus sheath to supply the skin of the epigastrium.

The ninth to eleventh intercostal nerves pass from their intercostal spaces between digitations of the diaphragm and transversus abdominis. They enter the layer between the transversus abdominis and internal oblique. Here, the ninth nerve runs forward almost horizontally, whereas the tenth and eleventh pass inferomedially. At the lateral edge of rectus abdominis, the nerves pierce the posterior layer of the aponeurosis of internal oblique and pass behind the muscle to end, like the seventh and eighth intercostal nerves, with cutaneous branches. The ninth nerve supplies skin above the umbilicus; the tenth supplies skin, which includes the umbilicus; and the eleventh supplies skin below the umbilicus (see Fig. 8.15). The twelfth thoracic nerve (subcostal nerve) connects with the first lumbar ventral ramus (dorsolumbar nerve). It accompanies the subcostal vessels along the inferior border of the twelfth rib, passing behind the lateral arcuate ligament and kidney and anterior to the upper part

of the quadratus lumborum. It perforates the transversus abdominis fascia, running deep to the internal oblique, to be distributed like the lower intercostal nerves. It supplies the anterior gluteal skin, reaching down to the greater trochanter.

The seventh to twelfth intercostal nerves supply the intercostal, subcostal and abdominal muscles. The tenth, eleventh and twelfth supply the serratus posterior inferior. All six nerves also provide sensory fibres to the costal parts of the diaphragm and related parietal pleura and peritoneum. Like the upper intercostal nerves, they give off collateral and lateral cutaneous branches before they reach the costal angles. The collateral branch may rejoin its parent nerve; if it does, it leaves again near the lateral border of rectus abdominis. It then runs forward, through the muscle and its anterior sheath near the linea alba to supply the overlying skin. The lateral cutaneous branches pierce the intercostal muscles and external oblique and divide into anterior and posterior branches. These branches supply the skin of the abdomen and back. The anterior branches supply external oblique. The posterior branches pass back to supply the skin over latissimus dorsi. Each lateral cutaneous nerve descends as it pierces external oblique and the superficial fascia and reaches the skin on a level with the anterior and posterior cutaneous nerves of the segment.

Twelfth Thoracic Ventral Ramus (Subcostal Nerve)

The ventral ramus of the twelfth thoracic nerve (subcostal nerve) is larger than the others. It gives a communicating branch to the first lumbar ventral ramus (sometimes termed the dorsolumbar nerve). Like the intercostal nerves, it soon gives off a collateral branch. It accompanies the subcostal vessels along the inferior border of the twelfth rib, passing behind the lateral arcuate ligament and kidney and in front of the upper part of quadratus lumborum. It perforates the aponeurosis of the origin of the transversus abdominis and passes forward between that muscle and internal oblique, to be distributed in the same manner as the lower intercostal nerves. It connects with the iliohypogastric nerve of the lumbar plexus and sends a branch to the pyramidalis. The lateral cutaneous branch of the subcostal nerve pierces the internal and external oblique muscles and supplies the lowest slip of the latter. It descends over the iliac crest approximately 5 cm behind the anterior superior iliac spine (see Fig. 19.3) and is distributed to the anterior gluteal skin; some filaments reach as low as the greater trochanter of the femur.

THORACIC DORSAL SPINAL RAMI

Thoracic dorsal rami pass backward close to the vertebral zygapophyseal joints and divide into medial and lateral branches. The medial branch emerges between the joint and the medial edge of the superior costotransverse ligament and intertransverse muscle. The lateral branch runs in the interval between the ligament and the muscle before inclining posteriorly on the medial side of levator costae.

Medial branches of the upper six thoracic dorsal rami pass between and supply the semispinalis thoracis and multifidus; they then pierce the rhomboids and trapezius and reach the skin near the vertebral spines (see Fig. 8.14). Medial branches of the lower six thoracic dorsal rami are distributed mainly to multifidus and longissimus thoracis; occasionally they give filaments to the skin in the median region. Lateral branches increase in size from above downward. They run through or deep to longissimus thoracis to the interval between it and iliocostalis cervicis, supplying these muscles and levatores costarum; the lower five or six also give off cutaneous branches that pierce serratus posterior inferior and latissimus dorsi in line with the costal angles (see Fig. 8.14). The lateral branches of a variable number of upper thoracic rami also supply the skin. The lateral branch of the twelfth sends a filament medially along the iliac crest, then passes down to the skin of the anterior part of the gluteal region.

Medial cutaneous branches of the thoracic dorsal rami descend for some distance close to the vertebral spines before reaching the skin. Lateral branches descend for a considerable distance—as much as the breadth of four ribs—before they become superficial; for example, the branch of the twelfth thoracic reaches the skin only slightly above the iliac crest.

LESIONS OF THE INTERCOSTAL NERVES

Subluxation of the interchondral joints between the lower costal cartilages may trap the intercostal nerves, causing referred abdominal pain. The dorsal cutaneous branch of an intercostal nerve can become entrapped as it penetrates the fascia of erector spinae. This produces an area of numbness, usually with painful paraesthesia, that extends from the midline laterally approximately 10 cm and for approximately 10 cm in length (notalgia paraesthetica). Commonly, the area between the medial edge of the scapula and the spine is affected. The anterior cutaneous branches of the intercostal nerves can become entrapped as they penetrate the fascia of rectus abdominis; this produces an area of numbness on the abdomen, usually with painful paraesthesia, that extends from the midline laterally 10 to 12 cm (rectus abdominis syndrome).

CASE 1 Herpes Zoster

An otherwise healthy 72-year-old woman acutely develops severe pain radiating from her back to below the left breast. In the emergency room, her electrocardiogram and cardiac enzymes are normal, but she is admitted for observation. She requires morphine sulphate for pain relief. Pain persists in the same distribution the next morning, but a few raised vesicular lesions are now noted in the left thoracic region in the distribution of the T6 dermatome, and the patient is exquisitely sensitive to mild cutaneous stimulation there. No other abnormalities are noted.

Discussion: This woman has typical herpes zoster infection ('shingles'), a remarkably painful but limited disorder of acute onset. Herpes zoster virus remains dormant in dorsal root ganglia following infection with chickenpox, generally for many years; it may be reactivated in immunocompromised individuals or in the non-immunocompromised elderly. Pain usually precedes the skin lesions and follows a dermatomal distribution in one or several adjacent dermatomes. The appearance of vesicular lesions in the same distribution clearly identifies the cause. The motor nerve and even the spinal cord may be involved, resulting in the appearance of an acute radiculopathy, sometimes leaving the patient with weakness and atrophy in that nerve root distribution. In some patients, severe and incapacitating pain lingers—so-called postherpetic neuralgia.

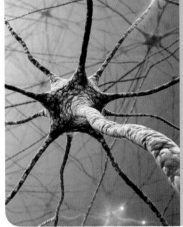

Lumbar Plexus and Sacral Plexus

OVERVIEW OF THE PLEXUSES

The lumbar and sacral plexuses innervate the lower limb. The lumbar plexus lies deep within psoas major, anterior to the transverse processes of the first three lumbar vertebrae. The sacral plexus lies in the pelvis on the anterior surface of piriformis, deep to the pelvic fascia, which separates it from the inferior gluteal and pudendal vessels. The lumbosacral trunk (L4 and L5) emerges medial to psoas major and lies on the ala of the sacrum before crossing the pelvic brim to join the anterior primary ramus of S1.

OVERVIEW OF THE PRINCIPAL NERVES OF THE LOWER LIMB (FIGS 20.1, 20.2)

Femoral Nerve (L2–4)

The femoral nerve is the nerve of the anterior compartment of the thigh. It arises from the posterior divisions of the second to fourth lumbar ventral rami, descends through psoas major and emerges on its lateral border to pass between psoas and iliacus and enter the thigh behind the inguinal ligament and lateral to the femoral sheath. Its terminal branches form in the femoral triangle approximately 2 cm distal to the inguinal ligament. In the abdomen the nerve supplies small branches to iliacus and a branch to the proximal part of the femoral artery. It subsequently supplies a large cutaneous area on the anterior and medial thigh and medial leg and foot and gives articular branches to the hip and knee. The femoral nerve is described in detail below.

Obturator Nerve (L2–4)

The obturator nerve is the nerve of the medial compartment of the thigh. It arises from the anterior divisions of the second to fourth lumbar ventral rami, descends through psoas major and emerges from its medial border at the pelvic brim. It crosses the sacroiliac joint behind the common iliac artery and lateral to the internal iliac vessels, runs along the lateral pelvic wall on obturator internus and enters the thigh through the upper part of the obturator foramen. Near the foramen it divides into anterior and posterior branches, separated at first by part of obturator externus and more distally by adductor brevis. It gives articular branches to the hip and knee and may supply skin on the medial thigh and leg. The obturator nerve is described in detail below.

Sciatic Nerve (L4, L5, S1–3)

The sciatic nerve is the nerve of the posterior compartment of the thigh and, via its major branches, of all the compartments of the lower leg and foot. Formed in the pelvis from the ventral rami of the fourth lumbar to third sacral spinal nerves, it is 2 cm wide at its origin and is the thickest nerve in the body. It enters the lower limb via the greater sciatic foramen below piriformis and descends between the greater trochanter and the ischial tuberosity. The nerve passes along the back of the thigh, where it is crossed by the long head of biceps femoris, and divides into the tibial and common peroneal (fibular) nerves proximal to the knee. The actual level of division is very variable because the tibial and common peroneal nerves are structurally separate and only loosely connected throughout their proximal course. The sciatic gives off articular branches that supply the hip joint through its posterior capsule (these are sometimes derived directly from the sacral plexus) and the knee joint. All the hamstring muscles, including the ischial part of adductor magnus but not the short head of biceps femoris, are supplied by the medial (tibial) component of the sciatic nerve. The short head of biceps is supplied by the lateral (common peroneal) component. The sciatic nerve is described in detail below.

Tibial Nerve (L4, L5, S1–3)

The tibial nerve arises from the anterior division of the sacral plexus. It descends along the back of the thigh and popliteal fossa to the distal border of popliteus, then passes anterior to the arch of soleus with the popliteal artery and continues into the leg. In the popliteal fossa it lies lateral to the popliteal vessels, becomes superficial to them at the knee and crosses to the medial side of the artery. In the leg it is the nerve of the posterior compartment and descends with the posterior tibial vessels to lie between the heel and the medial malleolus. It ends beneath the flexor retinaculum by dividing into the medial and lateral plantar nerves. The tibial nerve supplies articular branches to the knee and ankle. Its cutaneous area of supply, including its terminal branches, includes the back of the calf, the whole of the sole, the lateral border of the foot and the medial and lateral sides of the heel. The tibial nerve is described in detail below.

Common Peroneal Nerve (L4, L5, S1, S2)

The common peroneal nerve (common fibular nerve) is derived from the posterior division of the sacral plexus. In the leg it is the nerve of the anterior and lateral compartments. It descends obliquely along the lateral side of the popliteal fossa to the fibular head, lying between the tendon of biceps femoris and the lateral head of gastrocnemius. It curves lateral to the neck of the fibula deep to peroneus longus and divides into superficial and deep peroneal (fibular) nerves; the common peroneal nerve is easily injured at the fibular neck. Before it divides, it gives off articular branches to the knee and the superior tibiofibular joints and cutaneous branches. Its cutaneous area of supply, including its terminal branches, includes the anterolateral and lateral surfaces of the leg and most of the dorsum of the foot. The common peroneal nerve is described in detail below.

Gluteal Nerves

The gluteal nerves arise from the posterior division of the sacral plexus. The superior gluteal nerve (L4, L5, S1) leaves the pelvis through the greater sciatic notch above piriformis and supplies gluteus medius, gluteus minimus, tensor fasciae latae and the hip joint. The inferior gluteal nerve (L5, S1, S2) passes through the greater sciatic notch below piriformis and supplies gluteus maximus. The gluteal nerves are described in detail below.

Autonomic Innervation

The autonomic supply to the limbs is exclusively sympathetic. The preganglionic sympathetic inflow to the lower limb is derived from neurones in the lateral horn of the lower thoracic (T10, T11) and upper lumbar (L1, L2) spinal cord segments. Fibres pass in white rami communicantes to the sympathetic chain and synapse in the lumbar and sacral ganglia. Postganglionic fibres pass in grey rami communicantes to enter the lumbar and sacral plexuses, and many are distributed via the cutaneous branches of the nerves derived from these plexuses. The blood vessels to the lower limb receive their sympathetic supply via adjacent peripheral nerves. Postganglionic fibres accompanying the iliac arteries are destined mainly for the pelvis but may supply vessels in the upper thigh.

Dermatomes

Our knowledge of the extent of individual dermatomes, especially in the limbs, is based largely on clinical evidence. The dermatomes of the lower limb arise from spinal nerves T12 to S3 (Figs 20.3–20.5).

The preaxial border starts near the midpoint of the thigh and descends to the knee. It then curves medially, descending to the medial malleolus and the medial side of the foot and hallux. The postaxial border starts in the gluteal region and descends to the centre of the popliteal fossa, then deviates laterally to the lateral malleolus and the lateral side of the foot. The ventral and dorsal axial lines exhibit corresponding obliquity. The ventral axial line starts proximally at the medial end of the inguinal ligament and descends along the posteromedial aspect of the thigh and leg to end proximal to the heel. The dorsal axial line begins in the lateral gluteal region and descends posterolaterally in the thigh to the knee; it inclines medially and ends proximal to the ankle. Considerable overlap exists between adjacent dermatomes innervated by nerves derived from consecutive spinal cord segments.

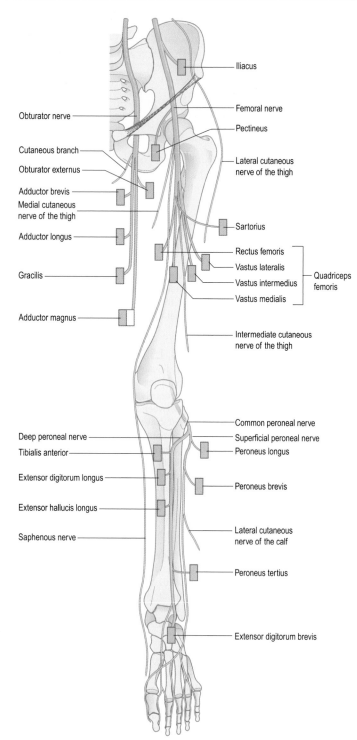

Fig. 20.1 *Nerves on the anterior aspect of the lower limb, their cutaneous branches and the muscles they supply. (From Aids to the Examination of the Peripheral Nervous System, 4th ed. 2000. Saunders, London. With permission of Guarantors of Brain.)*

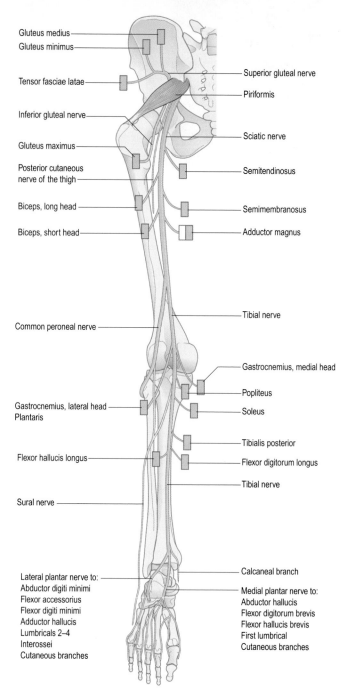

Fig. 20.2 *Nerves on the posterior aspect of the lower limb, their cutaneous branches and the muscles they supply. (From Aids to the Examination of the Peripheral Nervous System, 4th ed. 2000. Saunders, London. With permission of Guarantors of Brain.)*

Myotomes

Tables 20.1 to 20.4 summarize the predominant segmental origin of the nerve supply for each of the lower limb muscles and for movements that take place at the joints of the lower limb. Damage to these segments or to their motor roots results in maximal paralysis.

Reflexes

Knee Jerk (L2–4) — With the patient supine and the knee supported and partially flexed, the patellar tendon is struck at its midpoint; this should elicit quadriceps contraction, which extends the knee.

Ankle Jerk 'Achilles Reflex' (S1, S2) — With the patient supine and the lower limb externally rotated and partially flexed at the hip and knee, the foot is passively dorsiflexed to stretch the calcaneal tendon, which is then struck with a percussion hammer. Contraction of the calf muscles plantar-flexes the ankle. The reflex can also be examined with the patient kneeling on a chair.

Plantar Reflex — The plantar reflex is a superficial reflex, and its elicitation is an important part of the clinical examination of the central nervous system. With the foot relaxed and warm, the outer edge of the sole is stroked longitudinally with a hard object (traditionally, the examiner's fingernail or a key). This should elicit flexion of the toes, although the normal adult response varies with the strength of the stimulus. In adults with upper motor neurone lesions, the response includes extension of the great toe (Babinski's sign).

LUMBAR PLEXUS

The posterior abdominal wall contains the origin of the lumbar plexus (Fig. 20.6) and numerous autonomic plexuses and ganglia that lie close to the abdominal aorta and its branches.

Lumbar ventral rami increase in size from first to last and are joined, near their origins, by grey rami communicantes from the four lumbar sympathetic ganglia. These rami, long and slender, accompany the lumbar arteries around the sides of the vertebral bodies, behind psoas major. Their arrangement is irregular: one ganglion may give rami to two lumbar nerves, or one lumbar nerve may receive rami from two ganglia. Rami often leave the sympathetic trunk between ganglia. The first, second and sometimes third lumbar ventral which arise from different attachments. The lumbar plexus lies between these masses and hence is 'in line' with the intervertebral foramina. Although there may be minor variations, the most common arrangement of the plexus is described here.

The first lumbar ventral ramus, joined by a branch from the twelfth thoracic ventral ramus, bifurcates, and the upper and larger part divides again into the iliohypogastric and ilioinguinal nerves. The smaller lower part unites with a branch from the second lumbar ventral ramus to form the genitofemoral nerve. The remainder of the second, third and parts of the fourth lumbar ventral rami join the plexus and divide into ventral and dorsal branches. Ventral branches of the second to fourth rami join to form the obturator nerve. The main dorsal branches of the second to fourth rami join to form the femoral nerve. Small branches from the dorsal branches of the second and third rami join to form the lateral femoral cutaneous nerve. The accessory obturator nerve, when it exists, arises from the third and fourth ventral branches. The lumbar plexus is supplied by branches from the lumbar vessels, which supply the psoas major.

The branches of the lumbar plexus are as follows:

Muscular	T12, L1–4
Iliohypogastric	L1
Ilioinguinal	L1
Genitofemoral	L1, L2
Lateral femoral cutaneous	L2, L3
Femoral	L2–4 dorsal divisions
Obturator	L2–4 ventral divisions
Accessory obturator	L2, L3

Division of constituent ventral rami into ventral and dorsal branches is not as clear in the lumbar and lumbosacral plexuses as it is in the brachial plexus. Anatomically, the obturator and tibial nerves (via the sciatic) arise from ventral divisions, and the femoral and peroneal nerves (via the sciatic) arise from dorsal divisions. Lateral branches of the twelfth thoracic and first lumbar ventral rami are drawn into the gluteal skin, but otherwise, these nerves are typical. The second lumbar ramus is difficult to interpret. It not only contributes substantially to the femoral and obturator nerves but also has an anterior terminal branch (genital branch of the genitofemoral) and a lateral cutaneous branch (lateral femoral cutaneous nerve and femoral branch of the

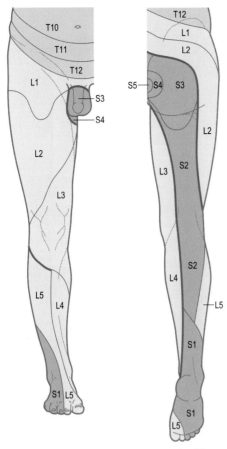

Fig. 20.3 *Dermatomes of the lower limb. There is considerable variation in and overlap between dermatomes, but the overlap across axial lines (heavy blue) is minimal.*

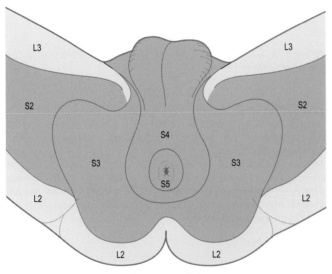

Fig. 20.4 *Dermatomes of the perineum.*

rami are each connected with the lumbar sympathetic trunk by a white ramus communicans. The lumbar ventral rami descend laterally into psoas major. The first three and most of the fourth form the lumbar plexus; the smaller moiety of the fourth joins the fifth as a lumbosacral trunk, which joins the sacral plexus. The fourth is often termed the nervus furcalis, being divided between the two plexuses; however, the third is occasionally the nervus furcalis. Alternatively, both the third and fourth may be furcal nerves, in which case the plexus is termed 'prefixed.' More frequently, the fifth nerve is furcal, and the plexus is then termed 'postfixed.' These variations modify the sacral plexus.

The lumbar plexus lies within the substance of the posterior part of psoas major, anterior to the transverse processes of the lumbar vertebrae. It is formed by the first three and most of the fourth lumbar ventral rami. The first lumbar ramus receives a branch from the last thoracic ventral ramus. The paravertebral part of psoas major consists of posterior and anterior masses,

CASE 1   RETROPERITONEAL HAEMATOMA

A 36-year-old man complains of increasing pain developing acutely in the right groin, thigh and leg. The pain, which is severe and increases with movement, is accompanied by modest weakness and tingling in the right leg. He is most comfortable in a sitting position with his right hip flexed. He was well until 1 month ago, when he developed paroxysmal atrial fibrillation and was placed on warfarin.

On examination, he is found lying on the bed with his right hip flexed. Iliopsoas and quadriceps muscle strength is 4/5, and hip adductors are 4+/5 on the right. The patellar reflex is absent on the right; reflexes are otherwise intact. Sensation is decreased over the right lateral, anterior and medial thigh, as well as the medial leg. Computed tomography scan of the pelvis demonstrates a right retroperitoneal haematoma.

Discussion: As noted above, the lumbar plexus is formed by L1–3 roots and part of L4, which traverse psoas major. Haemorrhage within the psoas muscle causes compression of the plexus between the muscle and the transverse processes of the vertebral bodies, which are themselves posterior to the plexus. In general, symptoms are in the distribution of the femoral, obturator and lateral femoral cutaneous nerves, but more extensive haemorrhage can result in more extensive weakness and numbness. Flexion of the hip reduces the pressure on the plexus by relaxing the psoas muscle.

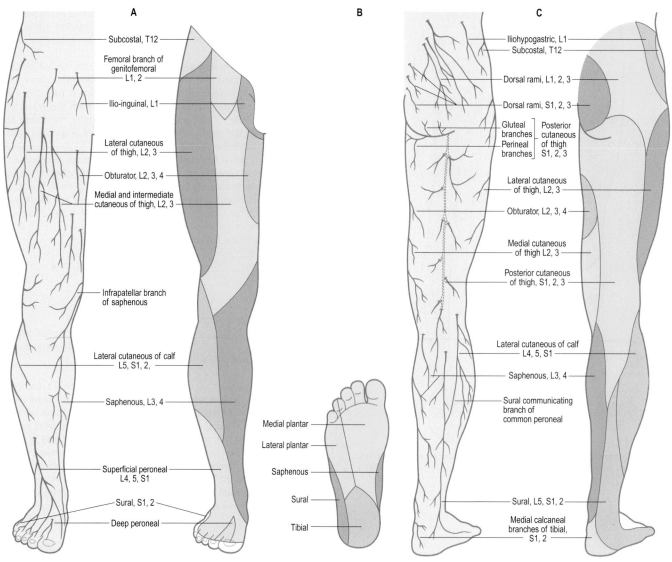

Fig. 20.5 *Cutaneous nerves of the right lower limb, their areas of distribution and segmental origins. **A,** Anterior aspect. **B,** Sole of the foot. **C,** Posterior aspect. In **C,** the interrupted line represents the trunk of the posterior cutaneous nerve of the thigh, most of which lies deep to the fascia lata.*

genitofemoral). Anterior terminal branches of the third to fifth lumbar and first sacral rami are suppressed, but the corresponding parts of the second and third sacral rami supply the skin of the perineum.

Inflammatory processes may occur in the posterior abdominal wall in the tissues anterior to psoas major, such as retrocaecal appendicitis on the right and diverticular abscess on the left. This may cause irritation of one or more of the branches of the lumbar plexus and lead to presenting symptoms of pain or dysaesthesia in the distribution of the affected nerves in the thigh, hip or buttock.

Muscular Branches
Small branches are derived from all five lumbar roots.

Iliohypogastric Nerve
Distribution — The iliohypogastric nerve originates from the L1 ventral ramus. It emerges from the upper lateral border of psoas major and crosses obliquely behind the lower renal pole and in front of quadratus lumborum. Above the iliac crest it enters the posterior part of transversus abdominis. Between transversus abdominis and internal oblique, it divides into lateral and anterior cutaneous branches and also supplies both muscles. The lateral cutaneous branch runs through the internal and external oblique above the iliac crest, a little behind the iliac branch of the twelfth thoracic nerve, and is distributed to the posterolateral gluteal skin. The anterior cutaneous branch runs between and supplies the internal oblique and transversus abdominis. It runs through the internal oblique approximately 2 cm medial to the anterior superior iliac spine and through the external oblique aponeurosis approximately 3 cm above the superficial inguinal ring; it is then distributed to the suprapubic skin. The iliohypogastric nerve connects with the subcostal and ilioinguinal nerves (see Fig. 19.3). It is occasionally injured during an oblique surgical approach to the appendix. However, because the suprapubic skin is

innervated from several sources, there is rarely any detectable sensory loss. Division of the iliohypogastric nerve above the anterior superior iliac spine may weaken the posterior wall of the inguinal canal and predispose to the formation of a direct hernia.

Motor — The iliohypogastric nerve supplies a small motor contribution to transversus abdominis and internal oblique, including the conjoint tendon.

Sensory — The iliohypogastric nerve supplies sensory fibres to transversus abdominis, internal oblique and external oblique and innervates the posterolateral gluteal and suprapubic skin.

Ilioinguinal Nerve
Distribution — The ilioinguinal nerve originates from the L1 ventral ramus. It is smaller than the iliohypogastric nerve and arises with it from the first lumbar ventral ramus, emerging from the lateral border of psoas major with or just inferior to the iliohypogastric nerve. It passes obliquely across quadratus lumborum and the upper part of iliacus and enters transversus abdominis near the anterior end of the iliac crest. It sometimes connects with the iliohypogastric nerve at this point. It pierces the internal oblique and supplies it and then traverses the inguinal canal below the spermatic cord. It emerges with the cord from the superficial inguinal ring to supply the proximal medial skin of the thigh and the skin over the root of the penis and upper part of the scrotum in males or the skin covering the mons pubis and adjoining labium majus in females. The ilioinguinal and iliohypogastric nerves are reciprocal in size. The ilioinguinal is occasionally very small and ends by joining the iliohypogastric, a branch of which then takes its place. Occasionally, the ilioinguinal nerve is completely absent when the iliohypogastric nerve supplies its territory. The nerve may be injured during inguinal surgery, particularly for hernia, which produces paraesthesia over the skin of the genitalia. Entrapment of the nerve during surgery may cause troublesome recurrent pain in this distribution.

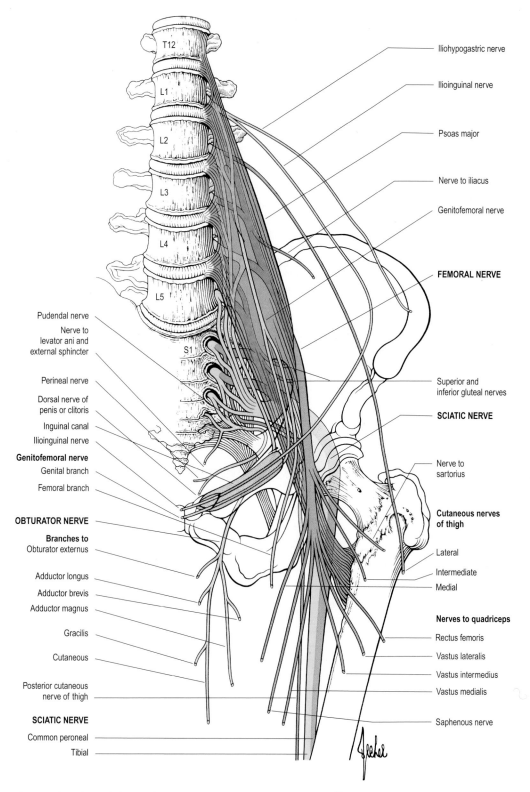

Fig. 20.6 *The lumbar plexus, its branches and the muscles they supply. The ventral branches of the ventral rami are coloured yellow, and the dorsal branches are coloured* orange.

Motor — The ilioinguinal nerve supplies motor nerves to transversus abdominis and internal oblique.

Sensory — The ilioinguinal nerve supplies sensory fibres to transversus abdominis and internal oblique. It innervates the medial skin of the thigh and the skin over the root of the penis and upper part of the scrotum in males or the skin covering the mons pubis and adjoining labium majus in females.

Genitofemoral Nerve

Distribution — The genitofemoral nerve originates from the L1 and L2 ventral rami. It is formed within the substance of psoas major and descends obliquely forward through the muscle to emerge on its abdominal surface near the medial border, opposite the third or fourth lumbar vertebra. It descends beneath the peritoneum on psoas major, crosses obliquely behind

the ureter and divides above the inguinal ligament into genital and femoral branches. It often divides close to its origin; its branches then emerge separately from psoas major. The genital branch crosses the lower part of the external iliac artery, enters the inguinal canal by the deep ring and supplies cremaster and the skin of the scrotum in males. In females, it accompanies the round ligament and ends in the skin of the mons pubis and labium majus. The femoral branch descends lateral to the external iliac artery and sends a few filaments around it. It then crosses the deep circumflex iliac artery, passes behind the inguinal ligament and enters the femoral sheath lateral to the femoral artery. It pierces the anterior layer of the femoral sheath and fascia lata and supplies the skin anterior to the upper part of the femoral triangle. It connects with the femoral intermediate cutaneous nerve and supplies the femoral artery. The genital branch may be injured during inguinal surgery, as may the ilioinguinal nerve.

Table 20.1 *Movements, muscles and segmental innervation in the lower limb*

Joint	Movement	Muscle	Innervation	L1	L2	L3	L4	L5	S1	S2	S3
HIP	FLEXION	Psoas major	Spinal nn. L1–3	■	■						
		Iliacus	Femoral n.		■						
		Pectineus	Femoral n.		■						
		Rectus femoris	Femoral n.			■	■				
		Adductor longus	Obturator n.		■	■					
		Sartorius	Femoral n.								
	EXTENSION	Gluteus maximus	Inferior gluteal n.					■	■		
		Adductor magnus	Obturator & tibial nn.								
		Hamstrings	Mainly tibial nn.						■		
	MEDIAL ROTATION	Iliacus	Femoral n.		■						
		Gluteus medius & minimus	Superior gluteal n.					■	■		
		Tensor fasciae latae	Superior gluteal n.					■	■		
	LATERAL ROTATION	Superior & inferior gemelli	Lumbosacral plexus								
		Quadratus femoris	Lumbosacral plexus								
		Piriformis	Lumbosacral plexus						■		
		Obturator internus	Lumbosacral plexus						■		
		Obturator externus	Obturator n.				■				
		Sartorius	Femoral n.								
	ADDUCTION	Gracilis	Obturator n.		■	■					
		Adductor longus	Obturator n.		■	■					
		Adductor magnus	Obturator & tibial nn.		■	■	■				
		Adductor brevis	Obturator n.								
		Pectineus	Femoral n.		■						
	ABDUCTION	Tensor fasciae latae	Superior gluteal n.					■	■		
		Gluteus medius & minimus	Superior gluteal n.					■	■		
		Piriformis	Lumbosacral plexus						■		
KNEE	FLEXION	Hamstrings:									
		Semimembranosus	Tibial n.						■		
		Semitendinosus	Tibial n.						■		
		Biceps femoris	Tibial & common peroneal nn.						■		
		Gastrocnemius	Tibial n.								
	EXTENSION	Quadriceps femoris:									
		Rectus femoris	Femoral n.			■	■				
		Vastus lateralis	Femoral n.			■	■				
		Vastus intermedius	Femoral n.			■	■				
		Vastus medialis	Femoral n.			■	■				
ANKLE	DORSIFLEXION	Tibialis anterior	Deep peroneal n.				■	■			
		Extensor digitorum longus	Deep peroneal n.					■	■		
		Extensor hallucis longus	Deep peroneal n.					■			
		Peroneus tertius	Deep peroneal n.					■	■		
	PLANTARFLEXION	Gastrocnemius	Tibial n.						■	■	
		Soleus	Tibial n.						■	■	
		Flexor digitorum longus	Tibial n.							■	■
		Flexor hallucis longus	Tibial n.							■	■
		Peroneus longus	Superficial peroneal n.						■		
		Tibialis posterior	Tibial n.								
	INVERSION	Tibialis anterior	Deep peroneal n.				■				
		Tibialis posterior	Tibial n.								
	EVERSION	Peroneus longus	Superficial peroneal n.								
		Peroneus tertius	Deep peroneal n.								
		Peroneus brevis	Superficial peroneal n.								
TOES	FLEXION	Flexor digitorum longus	Tibial n.						■	■	
		Flexor hallucis longus	Tibial n.						■	■	
		Flexor hallucis brevis	Medial plantar n.								
		Flexor digitorum brevis	Medial plantar n.								
		Flexor digitorum accessorius	Lateral plantar n.								
		Flexor digiti minimi brevis	Lateral plantar n.								
		Abductor hallucis	Medial plantar n.								
		Abductor digiti minimi	Lateral plantar n.								
		Lumbricals	Medial & lateral plantar nn.								
	EXTENSION	Extensor digitorum longus	Deep peroneal n.					■			
		Extensor hallucis longus	Deep peroneal n.								
		Extensor digitorum brevis	Deep peroneal n.								
	ABDUCTION	Abductor hallucis	Medial plantar n.								
		Abductor digiti minimi	Lateral plantar n.								
		Dorsal interossei	Lateral plantar n.								
	ADDUCTION	Plantar interossei	Lateral plantar n.								
		Adductor hallucis	Lateral plantar n.								

Motor — The genitofemoral nerve innervates cremaster via the genital branch.

Cutaneous — The genitofemoral nerve innervates the skin of the scrotum in males or mons pubis and labium majus in females via the genital branch, and the anteromedial skin of the thigh via the femoral branch.

Lateral Femoral Cutaneous Nerve of the Thigh

The lateral (femoral) cutaneous nerve of the thigh arises from the dorsal branches of the second and third lumbar ventral rami and emerges from the lateral border of psoas major, crossing the iliacus obliquely toward the anterior superior iliac spine. It supplies the parietal peritoneum in the iliac fossa. The right nerve passes posterolateral to the caecum, separated from it by the fascia iliaca and peritoneum; the left passes behind the lower part of the descending colon. Both pass behind or through the inguinal ligament, variably medial to the anterior superior iliac spine (commonly about 1 cm) and anterior to or through sartorius into the thigh, where they divide into anterior and posterior branches. The anterior branch becomes superficial approximately 10 cm distal to the anterior superior iliac spine and supplies the skin of the anterior and lateral thigh as far as the knee. It connects terminally with the cutaneous branches of the anterior division of the femoral nerve and the infrapatellar branch of the saphenous nerve, forming the peripatellar plexus. The posterior branch pierces the fascia lata higher than the anterior, and it divides to supply the skin on the lateral surface from the greater trochanter to about mid thigh. It may also supply the gluteal skin (see Case 2).

Femoral Nerve

The femoral nerve (Fig. 20.7), the largest branch of the lumbar plexus, arises from the dorsal branches (posterior divisions) of the second to fourth lumbar ventral rami. It descends through psoas major, emerging low on its lateral border, and then passes between psoas and iliacus, deep to the iliac fascia. Passing behind the inguinal ligament into the thigh, it splits into anterior and

CASE 2 MERALGIA PARAESTHETICA (LATERAL FEMORAL CUTANEOUS NEUROPATHY)

A 32-year-old woman, 30 weeks pregnant, develops pain and dysaesthesia in the left anterior and lateral thigh, which increase with standing or walking. She has no associated weakness and denies having any other symptoms. She has gained 45 pounds during her pregnancy to date. The neurological examination is entirely normal except for an area of hyperaesthesia in the left anterolateral thigh, involving the proximal two-thirds of the thigh but not extending past the midline anteriorly or posteriorly.

Discussion: The lateral cutaneous nerve of the thigh is formed by branches of the ventral primary rami of L2 and L3 spinal roots. The nerve passes through the lateral border of psoas, crosses iliacus, then usually runs under the inguinal ligament just medial to the anterior superior iliac spine. The nerve can be trapped under the inguinal ligament, resulting in paraesthesia or dysaesthesia or sensory loss in the cutaneous distribution of the nerve, generally referred to as meralgia paraesthetica. At this site, the nerve is susceptible to pressure due to increased weight, altered body mechanics, tight clothing or trauma. Entrapment of the nerve may also occur more distally, where the nerve pierces tensor fasciae latae.

Table 20.2 Segmental innervation of muscles of the lower limb

L1	Psoas major, psoas minor
L2	Psoas major, iliacus, sartorius, gracilis, pectineus, adductor longus, adductor brevis
L3	Quadriceps, adductors (magnus, longus, brevis)
L4	Quadriceps, tensor fasciae latae, adductor magnus, obturator externus, tibialis anterior, tibialis posterior
L5	Gluteus medius, gluteus minimus, obturator internus, semimembranosus, semitendinosus, extensor hallucis longus, extensor digitorum longus, peroneus tertius, popliteus
S1	Gluteus maximus, obturator internus, piriformis, biceps femoris, semitendinosus, popliteus, gastrocnemius, soleus, peronei (longus and brevis), extensor digitorum brevis
S2	Piriformis, biceps femoris, gastrocnemius, soleus, flexor digitorum longus, flexor hallucis longus, some intrinsic foot muscles
S3	Some intrinsic foot muscles (except abductor hallucis, flexor hallucis brevis, flexor digitorum brevis, extensor digitorum brevis)

Table 20.3 Segmental innervation of joint movements of the lower limb

Hip	Flexors, adductors, medial rotators	L1–3
	Extensors, abductors, lateral rotators	L5, S1
Knee	Extensors	L3, L4
	Flexors	L5, S1
Ankle	Dorsiflexors	L4, L5
	Plantar flexors	S1, S2
Foot	Inverters	L4, L5
	Everters	L5, S1
	Intrinsic muscles	S2, S3

Table 20.4 Movements and muscles tested to determine location of a lesion in the lower limb

Movement	Muscle	Upper Motor Neurone*	Root	Reflex	Nerve
Hip flexion	Iliopsoas	++	L1, L2		Femoral
Hip adduction	Adductors		L2, L3	(+)	Obturator
Hip extension	Gluteus maximus		L5, S1		Sciatic
Knee flexion	Hamstrings	+	S1		Sciatic
Knee extension	Quadriceps		L3, L4	++	Femoral
Ankle dorsiflexion	Tibialis anterior	++	L4		Deep peroneal
Ankle eversion	Peronei		L5, S1		Superficial peroneal
Ankle inversion	Tibialis posterior		L4, L5		Tibial
Ankle plantar flexion	Gastrocnemius/soleus		S1, S2	++	Tibial
Big toe extension	Extensor hallucis longus		L5	(Babinski's reflex)	Deep peroneal

*The muscles indicated in this column are those that are preferentially affected in upper motor neurone lesions. The root level is the principal supply to a muscle.

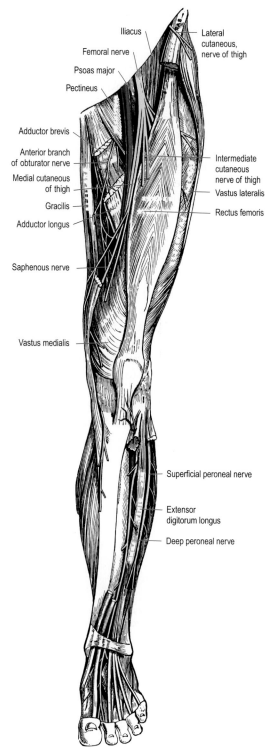

Iliacus

Femoral nerve

Psoas major

Pectineus

Lateral cutaneous, nerve of thigh

Adductor brevis

Anterior branch of obturator nerve

Medial cutaneous of thigh

Gracilis

Adductor longus

Intermediate cutaneous nerve of thigh

Vastus lateralis

Rectus femoris

Saphenous nerve

Vastus medialis

Superficial peroneal nerve

Extensor digitorum longus

Deep peroneal nerve

Fig. 20.7 *Nerves of the left lower limb (anterior aspect).*

The medial cutaneous nerve of the thigh is at first lateral to the femoral artery. It crosses anterior to the artery at the apex of the femoral triangle and divides into anterior and posterior branches. Before doing so, it sends a few rami through the fascia lata to supply the skin of the medial side of the thigh, near the long saphenous vein; one ramus emerges via the saphenous opening, and another becomes subcutaneous about mid thigh. The anterior branch descends on sartorius, perforates the fascia lata beyond mid thigh and divides into one branch that supplies the skin as low as the medial side of the knee and another branch that crosses to the lateral side of the patella and connects with the infrapatellar branch of the saphenous nerve. The posterior branch descends along the posterior border of sartorius to the knee, pierces the fascia lata, connects with the saphenous nerve and gives off several cutaneous rami, some as far as the medial side of the leg. The nerve contributes to the subsartorial plexus.

The main nerve to sartorius arises from the femoral nerve in common with the intermediate cutaneous nerve of the thigh.

Posterior Division of the Femoral Nerve — The branches of the posterior division of the femoral nerve are the saphenous nerve and branches to quadriceps femoris and the knee joint.

The saphenous nerve (see Fig. 20.7) is the largest cutaneous branch of the femoral nerve. It descends lateral to the femoral artery into the adductor canal, where it crosses anteriorly to become medial to the artery. At the distal end of the canal it leaves the artery and emerges through the aponeurotic covering with the saphenous branch of the descending genicular artery. As it leaves the adductor canal it gives off an infrapatellar branch that contributes to the peripatellar plexus and then pierces the fascia lata between the tendons of sartorius and gracilis, becoming subcutaneous to supply the prepatellar skin. It descends along the medial tibial border with the long saphenous vein and divides distally into one branch that continues along the tibia to the ankle and another branch that passes anterior to the ankle to supply the skin on the medial side of the foot, often as far as the first metatarsophalangeal joint. The saphenous nerve connects with the medial branch of the superficial peroneal nerve. Near mid thigh, it gives a branch to the subsartorial plexus (see below). The nerve may be subject to an entrapment neuropathy as it leaves the adductor canal.

The muscular branches of the posterior division of the femoral nerve supply quadriceps femoris. A branch to rectus femoris enters its proximal posterior surface and also supplies the hip joint. A larger branch to vastus lateralis forms a neurovascular bundle with the descending branch of the lateral circumflex femoral artery in its distal part and also supplies the knee joint. A branch to vastus medialis descends through the proximal part of the adductor canal, lateral to the saphenous nerve and femoral vessels. It enters the muscle at about its midpoint, sending a long articular filament distally along the muscle to the knee. Two or three branches to vastus intermedius enter its anterior surface about mid thigh; a small branch from one of these descends through the muscle to supply articularis genu and the knee joint.

Vascular branches of the femoral nerve supply the femoral artery and its branches.

Obturator Nerve

The obturator nerve arises from the ventral branches of the second to fourth lumbar ventral rami. The branch from the third is the largest, whereas that from the second is often very small. The nerve descends in psoas major, emerging from its medial border at the pelvic brim to pass behind the common iliac vessels and lateral to the internal iliac vessels. It then descends forward along the lateral wall of the lesser pelvis on obturator internus, anterosuperior to the obturator vessels and the obturator foramen, entering the thigh by its upper part. Near the foramen it divides into anterior and posterior branches, separated at first by part of obturator externus and lower by adductor brevis.

Anterior Branch — The anterior branch (see Fig. 20.7) leaves the pelvis anterior to obturator externus, descending in front of adductor brevis and behind pectineus and adductor longus. At the lower border of adductor longus it communicates with the medial cutaneous and saphenous branches of the femoral nerve, forming a subsartorial plexus that supplies the skin on the medial side of the thigh. It descends on the femoral artery, which its termination supplies. Near the obturator foramen, the anterior branch supplies the hip joint. Behind the pectineus, it supplies adductor longus, gracilis, usually adductor brevis and often pectineus, and it connects with the accessory obturator nerve when it is present. Occasionally the communicating branch to the femoral medial cutaneous and saphenous branches continues as a cutaneous branch to the thigh and leg, emerging from behind the distal border of adductor longus to descend along the posterior margin of sartorius to the knee, where it pierces the deep fascia, connects with the saphenous nerve and supplies the skin halfway down the medial side of the leg.

Posterior Branch — The posterior branch pierces obturator externus anteriorly, supplies it and passes behind adductor brevis to the front of adductor

posterior divisions. Behind the inguinal ligament it is separated from the femoral artery by part of psoas major. In the abdomen the nerve supplies small branches to iliacus and pectineus and a branch to the proximal part of the femoral artery; the latter branch sometimes arises in the thigh.

Nerve to Pectineus — The nerve to pectineus branches from the medial side of the femoral nerve near the inguinal ligament. It passes behind the femoral sheath and enters the anterior aspect of the muscle.

Anterior Division of the Femoral Nerve — The anterior division of the femoral nerve supplies intermediate and medial cutaneous nerves of the thigh and branches to sartorius.

The intermediate cutaneous nerve of the thigh pierces the fascia lata approximately 8 cm below the inguinal ligament, either as two branches or as one trunk that quickly divides into two. These descend on the front of the thigh, supplying the skin as far as the knee and ending in the peripatellar plexus (see later). The lateral branch of the intermediate cutaneous nerve communicates with the femoral branch of the genitofemoral nerve, frequently piercing sartorius and sometimes supplying it.

CASE 3   FEMORAL NEUROPATHY

Five days ago, a 55-year-old woman suddenly developed pain in the right anterior and medial thigh. She has a long-standing history of insulin-dependent diabetes mellitus. She now has difficulty walking due to both pain and perceived weakness of the right leg.

Examination documents right quadriceps muscle weakness with mild wasting, as well as sensory loss involving the anterior and medial thigh, extending distally down the medial aspect of the leg. Her patellar reflex cannot be elicited; reflex activity is otherwise normal.

Discussion: This woman has femoral neuropathy characterized by weakness and wasting of the quadriceps femoris muscle and loss of the patellar reflex. Medial and anterior thigh pain and tingling extending into the medial leg in the saphenous nerve distribution are due to the fact that the saphenous nerve, a sensory nerve, is a branch of the posterior division of the femoral nerve.

Originating in the upper lumbosacral plexus, the femoral nerve travels through psoas major, passing low and deep between psoas and iliacus, then behind the inguinal ligament, separated from the femoral artery by a part of the psoas major. Involvement of the femoral nerve may result from a retroperitoneal haemorrhage or, as in this case, may reflect a diabetic mononeuropathy (compare with Case 4, Proximal Diabetic Amyotrophy). Compression at the inguinal ligament by external or internal pressure can also result in femoral neuropathy.

CASE 4   PROXIMAL DIABETIC NEUROPATHY

A 60-year-old man with type 2 diabetes mellitus develops acute right anterior thigh pain so severe that he requires long-acting narcotics. Several weeks later he notes atrophy of the right thigh with weakness. He has no other sensory complaints. In the past, he has had difficulty controlling his glucose levels, with significant hyperglycemia, but he recently lost 15 pounds with better glucose control. On examination he has mild atrophy of all anterior thigh muscles on the right, with moderate weakness in the same muscles. Hamstring, hip flexors and extensors and all distal muscles exhibit normal strength. On sensory examination he has mild bilateral distal sensory loss, along with decreased Achilles reflexes.

Discussion: Diabetic amyotrophy (proximal diabetic neuropathy) often has an acute or subacute onset, affecting the anterior thigh muscles more than hip, posterior thigh or distal leg musculature. Ischaemic injury to the proximal lumbosacral plexus, probably due to a vasculitic process, is the most likely cause. Recent weight loss is common and suggests an additional metabolic component. Other portions of the lumbosacral plexus or spinal nerve may be involved.

magnus, dividing into branches to this and adductor brevis when the latter is not supplied by the anterior division. It usually sends an articular filament to the knee joint, which perforates adductor magnus distally or traverses its opening with the femoral artery to enter the popliteal fossa. There it descends on the popliteal artery to the back of the knee, pierces its oblique posterior ligament and supplies the articular capsule. It gives filaments to the popliteal artery.

Lesions of the Obturator Nerve — Isolated lesions of the obturator nerve are extremely rare but may occasionally occur as a result of direct trauma (sometimes during parturition) or in anterior dislocations of the hip. The nerve can also be damaged by a rare obturator hernia or may be involved, together with the femoral nerve, in retroperitoneal lesions close to their origins from the lumbar plexus. A nerve entrapment syndrome causing chronic medial thigh pain is described in athletes with large adductor muscles.

Accessory Obturator Nerve

Occasionally present (10% of cases), the accessory obturator nerve is small and arises from the ventral branches of the third and fourth lumbar ventral rami. It descends along the medial border of psoas major, crosses the superior pubic ramus behind pectineus and divides into branches; one branch enters the deep surface of pectineus, another supplies the hip joint and a third connects with the anterior branch of the obturator nerve. Sometimes the accessory obturator nerve is very small and supplies only pectineus. Any branch may be absent and others may occur; one sometimes supplies the adductor longus.

SACRAL PLEXUS

The sacral plexus provides the nerve supply to the pelvis and lower limb in addition to part of the autonomic supply to the pelvic viscera. It gives origin to the sciatic, inferior gluteal, superior gluteal and pudendal nerves, in addition to the nerves to quadratus femoris, obturator internus and the posterior cutaneous nerve of the thigh (Fig. 20.8).

The branches of the sacral plexus are as follows:

	Ventral Divisions	Dorsal Divisions
To quadratus femoris and gemellus inferior	L4, L5, S1	
To obturator internus and gemellus superior	L5, S1, S2	
To piriformis		(S1), S2
Superior gluteal		L4, L5, S1
Inferior gluteal		L5, S1, S2
Posterior femoral cutaneous	S2, S3	S1, S2
Tibial (sciatic)	L4, L5, S1, S2, S3	
Common peroneal (sciatic)		L4, L5, S1, S2
Perforating cutaneous		S2, S3
Pudendal	S2, S3, S4	
To levator ani, coccygeus and sphincter ani externus	S4	
Pelvic splanchnic	S2, S3, (S4)	

Sciatic Nerve

The sciatic nerve is 2 cm wide at its origin and is the thickest nerve in the body (Fig. 20.9). It leaves the pelvis via the greater sciatic foramen below piriformis and descends between the greater trochanter and the ischial tuberosity and along the back of the thigh, dividing into the tibial and common peroneal (fibular) nerves at a varying level proximal to the knee. Superiorly, it lies deep to gluteus maximus, resting first on the posterior ischial surface with the nerve to quadratus femoris between them. It then crosses posterior to obturator internus, the gemelli and quadratus femoris, separated by the last from obturator externus and the hip joint. It is accompanied medially by the posterior femoral cutaneous nerve and the inferior gluteal artery. More distally, it lies behind adductor magnus and is crossed posteriorly by the long head of biceps femoris. It corresponds to a line drawn from just medial to the midpoint between the ischial tuberosity and the greater trochanter to the apex of the popliteal fossa.

Articular branches arise proximally to supply the hip joint through its posterior capsule; these are sometimes derived directly from the sacral plexus. Muscular branches are distributed to biceps femoris, semitendinosus, semimembranosus and the ischial part of adductor magnus.

The point of division of the sciatic nerve into its major components (tibial and common peroneal) is very variable. A common site is at the junction of the middle and lower thirds of the thigh, near the apex of the popliteal fossa. The division may occur at any level above this, but rarely below it. It is not uncommon for the major components to leave the sacral plexus separately,

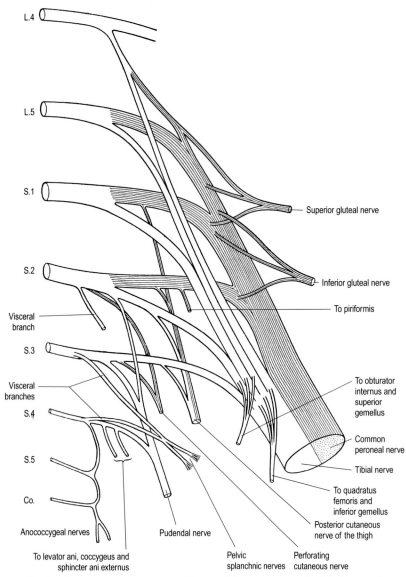

Fig. 20.8 *Sacral and coccygeal plexuses. The dorsal rami are not shown. Ventral (anterior) divisions are not shaded. The contribution from S2 to the pelvic splanchnic nerves has been cut before it joins those from S3 and S4.*

in which case the common peroneal component usually passes through piriformis at the greater sciatic notch, while the tibial component passes below the muscle.

Lesions of the Sciatic Nerve

The sciatic nerve supplies the knee flexors and all the muscles below the knee, so that a complete palsy of the sciatic nerve results in a flail foot and severe difficulty walking. This is rare and usually related to trauma. The nerve is vulnerable in posterior dislocation of the hip. As it leaves the pelvis it passes either behind piriformis or sometimes through the muscle, and at that point it may become entrapped (piriformis syndrome); this is a common anatomical variant, but an extremely rare entrapment neuropathy. External compression over the buttock (e.g. in patients who lie immobile on a hard surface for a considerable length of time) can injure the nerve. It may be damaged by misplaced therapeutic injections into gluteus maximus. The safe zone for deep intramuscular injections is the upper outer quadrant of the buttock. Perhaps safer still is to inject into quadriceps, although this can produce other problems such as haemorrhage, leading to contracture of the muscle, which limits knee motion. Sciatic nerve palsy occurs after total hip replacement or similar surgery in approximately 1% of cases. Haematoma is characterized by the development of severe pain in the immediate postoperative period. Early surgical exploration and evacuation of haematoma can reverse the nerve lesion. Unfortunately, the other causes may not be treatable; however, the majority are temporary. Complete sciatic nerve palsy is very rare. For some reason, possibly anatomical, the common peroneal part is usually affected alone. The patient so afflicted has a footdrop and a high-stepping gait.

Tibial Nerve

The tibial nerve, the larger sciatic component, is derived from the ventral branches (anterior division) of the fourth and fifth lumbar and first to third

sacral ventral rami. It descends along the back of the thigh and popliteal fossa to the distal border of popliteus. It then passes anterior to the arch of soleus with the popliteal artery and continues into the leg. In the thigh it is overlapped proximally by the hamstring muscles, but it becomes more superficial in the popliteal fossa, where it is lateral to the popliteal vessels. At the level of the knee the tibial nerve becomes superficial to the popliteal vessels and crosses to the medial side of the artery. In the distal popliteal fossa it is overlapped by the junction of the two heads of gastrocnemius.

In the leg the tibial nerve descends with the posterior tibial vessels to lie between the heel and the medial malleolus. Proximally, it is deep to soleus and gastrocnemius, but in its distal third it is covered only by skin and fasciae, overlapped sometimes by flexor hallucis longus. At first medial to the posterior tibial vessels, it crosses behind them and descends lateral to them until it bifurcates. It lies on tibialis posterior for most of its course except distally, where it adjoins the posterior surface of the tibia. The tibial nerve ends under the flexor retinaculum by dividing into the medial and lateral plantar nerves.

Branches

The branches of the tibial nerve are articular, muscular, sural, medial calcaneal and medial and lateral plantar. The sural and distal branches are described below.

Articular Branches — Articular branches accompany the superior, inferior medial and middle genicular arteries to the knee joint. They form a plexus with a branch from the obturator nerve and supply the oblique posterior ligament. The branches accompanying the superior and inferior genicular arteries also supply the medial part of the capsule. Just before the tibial nerve bifurcates it supplies the ankle joint.

Muscular Branches — Proximal muscular branches arise between the heads of gastrocnemius and supply gastrocnemius, plantaris, soleus and popliteus.

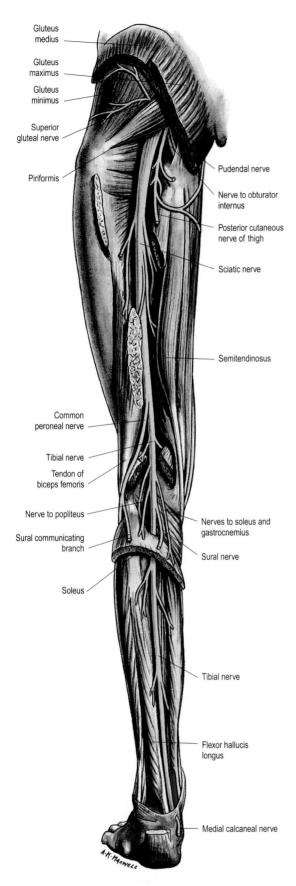

Fig. 20.9 *Nerves of the left lower limb (posterior aspect).*

The nerve to soleus enters its superficial aspect. The branch to popliteus descends obliquely across the popliteal vessels, curling around the distal border of the muscle to its anterior surface. It also supplies tibialis posterior, the proximal tibiofibular joint and the tibia and gives off an interosseous branch that descends near the fibula to reach the distal tibiofibular joint.

Muscular branches in the leg, either independently or by a common trunk, supply soleus (on its deep surface), tibialis posterior, flexor digitorum longus

CASE 5   SCIATICA

A 35-year-old man presents with the acute onset of low back pain radiating into his left hip and down the left leg. The pain began suddenly 2 days ago when he bent over to pick something up off the floor. He cannot stand erect due to increasing pain and is most comfortable leaning to the left. He also observes tingling discomfort in the left leg involving the sole, lateral foot and fifth toe. Pain and paraesthesia are worse with Valsalva's manoeuvres such as coughing, sneezing or straining.

Examination is hindered by the patient's pain, but weakness of plantar and toe flexion, of extension (dorsiflexion) of the great toe, and of hip extension and abduction is observed on the left. The left Achilles reflex is absent. There is decreased pinprick sensation over the left lateral foot and fifth toe. Straight leg testing on the left increases symptoms in the leg. He is very tender on percussion over the lumbar spine and exhibits moderate paravertebral muscle spasm.

Discussion: Sciatica is a term used to describe pain radiating down the leg, with or without back pain. It is most commonly associated with nerve root compression at L5 or S1. The most frequent cause of acute sciatica is disc herniation. L5 and S1 roots are most commonly compressed; both roots can be involved in dorsolateral or central disc herniation, with the disc compressing the roots in the lateral recess. A large and more lateral herniation may result in only a single root being compressed, usually within the intervertebral foramen. Owing to mixed root innervation to lower extremity muscles, motor and sensory symptoms and signs do not always precisely match the root injured. Sensory loss in the foot (lateral foot and fifth toe involvement) indicates S1 localization (Fig. 20.10), but in some instances, sensation is normal. Straight leg raising increases symptoms by stretching the roots already compromised. Loss of the Achilles reflex with a normal patellar reflex is typical of an S1 root lesion.

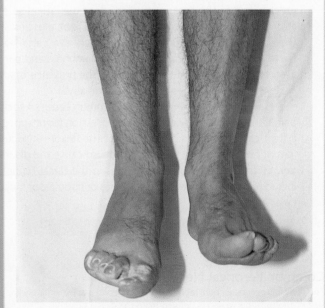

Fig. 20.10 Footdrop (right) in a case of sciatica. The foot cannot be dorsiflexed on command.

and flexor hallucis longus. The branch to flexor hallucis longus accompanies the peroneal vessels.

Lesions of the Tibial Nerve

The tibial nerve is vulnerable to direct injury in the popliteal fossa, where it lies superficial to the vessels at the level of the knee. It may be damaged in compartment syndrome affecting the deep flexor compartment of the calf. The nerve may be entrapped beneath the flexor retinaculum at the ankle, resulting in tarsal tunnel syndrome.

CASE 6 TARSAL TUNNEL SYNDROME

A 58-year-old woman with a 10-year history of rheumatoid arthritis complains of paraesthesia and pain in the right foot, present for 5 months. She has paraesthesia of the entire sole of the foot, along with medial ankle pain. On examination, she exhibits decreased sensation to pinprick on the sole, excluding the heel and the balls of all the toes. There is no definite weakness in any muscle of the foot or leg, but there is wasting of the intrinsic muscles of the right foot when compared with the left. There is mild tenderness to palpation just below the medial malleolus. Reflexes are normal.

Discussion: Symptoms consisting of ankle pain, foot pain or both, with or without paraesthesia of the sole of the foot, are the result of damage to the tibial nerve or its branches within the tarsal tunnel. The tibial nerve passes under the flexor retinaculum below the medial malleolus and divides into the calcaneal and plantar nerves. The distal branches of the nerve—the medial and lateral plantar nerves—travel beneath the flexor retinaculum at the ankle and may be entrapped there. The medial plantar nerve is the larger branch, supplying sensation to the anterior two-thirds of the medial sole of the foot and between the balls of all but the lateral fourth toe and the fifth toe, and including the skin around the toenails. It also gives branches to abductor hallucis, flexor digitorum brevis, flexor hallucis brevis and first lumbrical muscle. The lateral plantar nerve supplies sensory fibres to the remaining toes and to the anterior two-thirds of the lateral sole, and it is the motor to most of the deep foot muscles. If the entrapment or injury is high enough, the calcaneal nerve may also be entrapped, causing numbness and paraesthesia of the medial sole and heel. The presence of an ankle jerk places the lesion more proximally.

Tarsal tunnel syndrome is an uncommon cause of foot pain, usually caused by external compression (tight shoes, a tight cast) or trauma. Thickening of the flexor retinaculum or fibrosis around the nerve can also cause the disorder, as can a variety of mass lesions in the tarsal tunnel, including synovial cysts, schwannomas or lipomas, or muscular hypertrophy.

Common Peroneal Nerve

The common peroneal nerve (common fibular nerve) is approximately half the size of the tibial nerve and is derived from the dorsal branches of the fourth and fifth lumbar and first and second sacral ventral rami. It descends obliquely along the lateral side of the popliteal fossa to the fibular head, medial to biceps femoris. It lies between the bicipital tendon, to which it is bound by fascia, and the lateral head of gastrocnemius. The nerve then passes into the anterolateral muscle compartment through a tight opening in the thick fascia overlying tibialis anterior. It curves lateral to the fibular neck, deep to peroneus longus, and divides into superficial and deep peroneal nerves.

The course of the common peroneal nerve can be indicated by a line from the apex of the popliteal fossa, passing distally, medial to the biceps tendon, to the back of the head of the fibula, where the nerve can be rolled against the bone.

Branches

The common peroneal nerve has articular and cutaneous branches. It terminates as the superficial and deep peroneal nerves.

Articular Branches — There are three articular branches. Two accompany the superior and inferior lateral genicular arteries and may arise in common. The third, the recurrent articular nerve, arises near the termination of the common peroneal nerve. It ascends with the anterior recurrent tibial artery through tibialis anterior and supplies the anterolateral part of the knee joint capsule and the proximal tibiofibular joint.

Cutaneous Branches — The two cutaneous branches, often from a common trunk, are the lateral sural and sural communicating nerves. The lateral sural nerve (lateral cutaneous nerve of the calf) supplies the skin on the anterior, posterior and lateral surfaces of the proximal leg. The sural communicating nerve arises near the head of the fibula and crosses the lateral head of gastrocnemius to join the sural nerve. It may descend separately as far as the heel.

Lesions of the Common Peroneal Nerve

The common peroneal nerve is relatively unprotected as it traverses the lateral aspect of the neck of the fibula and is easily compressed at this site (e.g. by plaster casts or ganglia). The nerve may also become entrapped between the attachments of peroneus longus to the head and shaft of the fibula. Traction lesions can accompany dislocations of the lateral compartment of the knee and are most likely to occur if the distal attachments of biceps and the ligaments that insert into the fibular head are avulsed, possibly with a small part of the fibular head. Because it is tethered to the bicipital tendon by dense fascia, the nerve is pulled proximally. Patients with such injury present with footdrop, which is usually painless. Examination reveals weakness of ankle dorsiflexion and extensor hallucis longus and eversion of the foot; however, inversion and plantar flexion are normal, and the ankle reflex is preserved. Because the nerve divides at the fibular neck into the superficial and deep peroneal nerves, lesions damaging the nerve at this level may damage the main trunk of the nerve or either of its branches. A lesion of the superficial branch causes weakness of foot eversion with sensory loss on the lateral aspect of the leg, which extends onto the dorsum of the foot.

Superficial Peroneal Nerve

The superficial peroneal nerve (superficial fibular nerve) begins at the common peroneal bifurcation. It is at first deep to peroneus longus and passes anteroinferiorly between the peronei and extensor digitorum longus to pierce the deep fascia in the distal third of the leg, where it divides into medial and lateral branches. Between the muscles it supplies peroneus longus, peroneus brevis and the skin of the lower leg.

Branches

The medial branch passes anterior to the ankle and divides into two dorsal digital nerves: one supplies the medial side of the great toe, and the other supplies the adjacent sides of the second and third toes. The medial branch communicates with the saphenous and deep peroneal nerves. The smaller lateral branch traverses the dorsum of the foot laterally. It divides into dorsal digital branches that supply the contiguous sides of the third to fifth toes and the skin of the lateral aspect of the ankle, where it connects with the sural nerve. Both branches, especially the lateral, are at risk during the placement of portal incisions for arthroscopy. Branches of the superficial peroneal nerve supply the dorsal skin of all the toes except that of the lateral side of the fifth toe (supplied by the sural nerve) and the adjoining sides of the great and second toes (supplied by the medial terminal branch of the deep peroneal nerve). Some of the lateral branches of the superficial peroneal nerve are frequently absent and are replaced by sural branches.

Lesions of the Superficial Peroneal Nerve

The superficial peroneal nerve can be subject to entrapment as it penetrates the deep fascia of the leg. It may also be involved in compartment syndrome affecting the lateral compartment.

Deep Peroneal Nerve

The deep peroneal nerve (deep fibular nerve) begins at the common peroneal bifurcation, between the fibula and the proximal part of peroneus longus. It passes obliquely forward, deep to extensor digitorum longus, to the front of the interosseous membrane and reaches the anterior tibial artery in the proximal third of the leg. It descends with the artery to the ankle, dividing there into lateral and medial terminal branches. It is first lateral to the artery, then anterior and again lateral at the ankle.

Branches

The deep peroneal nerve supplies muscular branches to tibialis anterior, extensor hallucis longus, extensor digitorum longus and peroneus tertius, as well as an articular branch to the ankle joint. The lateral terminal branch crosses the ankle deep to extensor digitorum brevis, enlarges as a pseudoganglion and supplies extensor digitorum brevis. From the enlargement, three minute interosseous branches supply the tarsal and metatarsophalangeal joints of the middle three toes; the first branch also supplies the second dorsal interosseous. The medial terminal branch runs distally on the dorsum of the foot lateral to the dorsalis pedis artery and connects with the medial branch of the superficial peroneal nerve in the first interosseous space. It divides into two dorsal digital nerves, which supply adjacent sides of the great and second toes. Before dividing, it gives off an interosseous branch that supplies the first metatarsophalangeal joint and the first dorsal interosseous. The deep peroneal nerve may end as three terminal branches.

Lesions of the Deep Peroneal Nerve

The deep peroneal nerve supplies the muscles of the anterior tibial compartment. Consequently, damage to this nerve, as in compartment syndrome affecting the anterior compartment, results in weakness of ankle dorsiflexion and extension of all toes. Sensory impairment is confined to the first interdigital cleft.

CASE 7 PERONEAL PALSY

A 26-year-old woman presents with a painless left foot-drop of acute onset. She recently lost 50 pounds in a 3-month period through diet and exercise. She is otherwise healthy. Examination shows weakness of dorsiflexion of the ankle (tibialis anticus, extensor digitorum longus and peroneus tertius) and the great toe (extensor hallucis longus) and weakness of foot eversion (peronei tertius, longus and brevis); inversion of the foot and plantar flexion are normal. Reflexes are normal throughout.

Discussion: This woman has a peroneal palsy reflecting involvement of the common peroneal nerve, a nerve comprising branches of the fourth and fifth lumbar roots and first and second sacral roots. It travels laterally in the popliteal fossa along the medial border of the biceps femoris tendon, then emerges posterior to the tendon and around the fibular head. (The nerve can generally be palpated by rolling it manually against the head of the fibula.) It is there that the nerve can easily be compressed; mechanisms include significant weight loss, habitual leg crossing, or frequent squatting, with compression of the nerve in the popliteal fossa or by gastrocnemius. At the site of compression, the common peroneal nerve may be affected in its entirety, or the superficial or deep peroneal branches may be affected alone. Compression of the superficial peroneal nerve alone results in weakness of foot eversion and loss of sensation along the lateral leg and into the dorsal foot, whereas deep peroneal branch compression causes weakness of ankle dorsiflexion and toe extension, with sensory loss between the great toe and the second toe.

Sural Nerve

The sural nerve arises from the tibial nerve and descends between the heads of gastrocnemius, pierces the deep fascia proximally in the leg and is joined at a variable level by the sural communicating branch of the common peroneal nerve (Fig. 20.2). Some authors term this branch the lateral sural cutaneous nerve, and they call the main trunk (from the tibial nerve) the medial sural cutaneous nerve. The sural nerve descends lateral to the calcaneal

tendon, near the short saphenous vein, to the region between the lateral malleolus and the calcaneus and supplies the posterior and lateral skin of the distal third of the leg. It then passes distal to the lateral malleolus along the lateral side of the foot and little toe, supplying the overlying skin. It connects with the posterior femoral cutaneous nerve in the leg and with the superficial peroneal nerve on the dorsum of the foot. The surface marking at the ankle is a line parallel to the calcaneal tendon halfway between the tendon and the lateral malleolus. However, its position is variable, and it is at risk from any surgery in this region. Rather like the radial nerve at the wrist, the sural nerve has a tendency to form painful neuromas. The nerve is harvested for grafting on occasion because it is sensory only, superficial, and easily identified.

Inferior Gluteal Nerve

The inferior gluteal nerve arises from the dorsal branches of the fifth lumbar and first and second sacral ventral rami. It leaves the pelvis via the greater sciatic foramen below piriformis and divides into branches that enter the deep surface of gluteus maximus.

Superior Gluteal Nerve

The superior gluteal nerve arises from the dorsal branches of the fourth and fifth lumbar and first sacral ventral rami. It leaves the pelvis via the greater sciatic foramen above piriformis, with the superior gluteal vessels, and divides into superior and inferior branches. The superior branch accompanies the upper branch of the deep division of the superior gluteal artery to supply gluteus medius and occasionally gluteus minimus. The inferior branch runs with the lower ramus of the deep division of the superior gluteal artery across gluteus minimus, supplying glutei medius and minimus and ending in tensor fasciae latae.

Perforating Cutaneous Nerve

The perforating cutaneous nerve usually arises from the posterior aspects of the second and third sacral ventral spinal rami. It pierces the sacrotuberous ligament, curves around the inferior border of gluteus maximus and supplies the skin over the inferomedial aspect of this muscle. The nerve may arise from the pudendal nerve or, if absent, may be replaced by a branch from either the posterior femoral cutaneous nerve or the third and fourth, or fourth and fifth, sacral ventral rami.

Nerve to Quadratus Femoris and Gemellus Inferior

The nerve to quadratus femoris and gemellus inferior arises from the ventral branches of the fourth lumbar to first sacral ventral rami. It leaves the pelvis via the greater sciatic foramen below piriformis; descends on the ischium deep to the sciatic nerve, gemelli and the tendon of obturator internus; and supplies gemellus inferior, quadratus femoris and the hip joint.

Nerve to Obturator Internus and Gemellus Superior

The nerve to obturator internus and gemellus superior arises from the ventral branches of the fifth lumbar and first and second sacral ventral rami. It leaves the pelvis like the nerve to quadratus femoris and gemellus inferior, supplies a branch to the upper posterior surface of gemellus superior, crosses the ischial spine lateral to the internal pudendal vessels, reenters the pelvis via the lesser sciatic foramen and enters the pelvic surface of obturator internus.

Posterior Cutaneous Nerve of the Thigh

The posterior cutaneous nerve of the thigh arises from the dorsal branches of the first and second sacral rami and the ventral branches of the second and third sacral rami. It leaves the pelvis via the greater sciatic foramen below piriformis and descends under gluteus maximus with the inferior gluteal vessels, lying posterior or medial to the sciatic nerve. It descends in the back of the thigh superficial to the long head of biceps femoris, deep to the fascia lata. Behind the knee it pierces the deep fascia and accompanies the short saphenous vein to midcalf, its terminal twigs connecting with the sural nerve. Its branches are all cutaneous and are distributed to the gluteal region, perineum and flexor aspect of the thigh and leg. Three or four gluteal branches curl around the lower border of gluteus maximus to supply the skin over its inferolateral area. The perineal branch supplies the superomedial skin in the thigh, curves forward across the hamstrings below the ischial tuberosity, pierces the fascia lata and runs in the superficial perineal fascia to the scrotal or labial skin, communicating with the inferior rectal and posterior scrotal branches of the perineal nerve. It gives numerous branches to the skin of the back and medial side of the thigh, the popliteal fossa and the proximal part of the back of the leg.

Nerve to Piriformis

The nerve to piriformis usually arises from the dorsal branches of the first and second sacral ventral rami (sometimes only the second) and enters the anterior surface of piriformis.

INNERVATION OF THE FOOT

Superficial Peroneal Nerve

The superficial peroneal nerve was described earlier.

Deep Peroneal Nerve

The deep peroneal nerve was described earlier.

Tibial Nerve

The branches of the tibial nerve are the articular, muscular, sural, medial calcaneal and medial and lateral plantar nerves. The articular, muscular and sural nerves were described earlier.

Medial Calcaneal Nerve

The medial calcaneal nerve arises from the tibial nerve and perforates the flexor retinaculum to supply the skin of the heel and medial side of the sole.

Medial Plantar Nerve

The medial plantar nerve (Fig 20.11) is the larger terminal division of the tibial nerve, and it lies lateral to the medial plantar artery. From its origin under the flexor retinaculum, it passes deep to abductor hallucis, then appears between it and flexor digitorum brevis, gives off a medial proper digital nerve to the hallux and divides near the metatarsal bases into three common plantar digital nerves.

Cutaneous branches pierce the plantar aponeurosis between abductor hallucis and flexor digitorum brevis to supply the skin of the sole of the foot. Muscular branches supply abductor hallucis, flexor digitorum brevis, flexor hallucis brevis and first lumbrical. The first two arise near the origin of the nerve and enter the deep surfaces of the muscles. The branch to flexor hallucis brevis is from the hallucal medial digital nerve, and that to the first lumbrical is from the first common plantar digital nerve. Articular branches supply the joints of the tarsus and metatarsus.

Three common plantar digital nerves pass between the slips of the plantar aponeurosis, each dividing into two proper digital branches. The first supplies adjacent sides of the hallux and second toe, and the second supplies adjacent

sides of the second and third toes; the third supplies adjacent sides of the third and fourth toes and also connects with the lateral plantar nerve. The first gives a branch to the first lumbrical. Each proper digital nerve has cutaneous and articular branches; near the distal phalanges, a dorsal branch supplies structures around the nail, and the termination of each nerve supplies the ball of the toe. The common digital branches of the medial plantar nerve are distributed in a manner similar to those of the median nerve, as are the motor branches of the two nerves. In the hand, the median nerve supplies abductor and flexor pollicis brevis, opponens pollicis and first and second lumbricals. An opponens is absent in the foot, but abductor hallucis, flexor hallucis brevis and first lumbrical are all supplied by the medial plantar nerve. Because flexor digitorum brevis and flexor digitorum superficialis (median nerve) correspond, only the innervation of the second lumbrical differs.

Lateral Plantar Nerve

The lateral plantar nerve (see Fig. 20.11) supplies the skin of the fifth toe, the lateral half of the fourth toe and most of the deep muscles of the foot. Its distribution therefore closely resembles that of the ulnar nerve in the hand. It passes laterally forward, medial to the lateral plantar artery, toward the tubercle of the fifth metatarsal. It next passes between flexor digitorum brevis and accessorius and ends between brevis and abductor digiti minimi by dividing into superficial and deep branches. Before division, it supplies flexor digitorum accessorius and abductor digiti minimi and gives rise to small branches that pierce the plantar fascia to supply the skin of the lateral part of the sole (Fig. 20.12). The superficial branch splits into two common plantar digital nerves: the lateral supplies the lateral side of the fifth toe, flexor digiti minimi brevis and the two interossei in the fourth intermetatarsal space; the medial connects with the third common plantar digital branch of the medial plantar nerve and divides into two to supply the adjoining sides of the fourth and fifth toes. The deep branch accompanies the lateral plantar artery deep to the flexor tendons and adductor hallucis and supplies the second to fourth lumbricals, adductor hallucis and all interossei (except those of the fourth intermetatarsal space). Branches to the second and third lumbricals pass distally, deep to the transverse head of adductor hallucis, and curl around its distal border to reach them (Fig. 20.13).

Nerve Entrapment Syndromes in the Foot

Any nerve of the foot can be affected by entrapment, classically leading to a burning sensation in the distribution of that nerve. Tarsal tunnel syndrome (see Case 6) is much less common than carpal tunnel syndrome. The flexor retinaculum can compress the tibial nerve or either of its branches (medial and lateral plantar nerves), but it is most commonly compressed by a space-occupying lesion (e.g. ganglion), a leash of vessels or the deep fascia associated with abductor hallucis. Compression of the first branch of the lateral plantar nerve by the deep fascia of abductor hallucis can lead to heel pain. The medial plantar nerve can be irritated at the master knot of Henry; this is usually related to jogging. The superficial peroneal nerve can be damaged in severe inversion injuries of the ankle, and the deep peroneal nerve is sometimes compressed by osteophytes in the region of the second tarsometatarsal

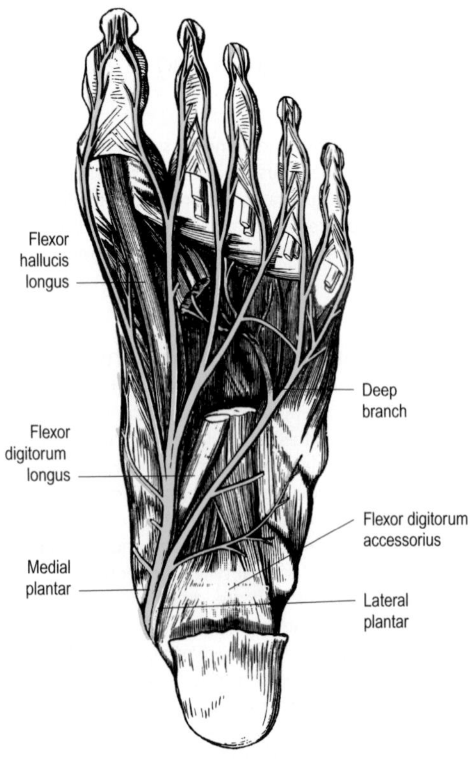

Flexor hallucis longus

Flexor digitorum longus

Medial plantar

Deep branch

Flexor digitorum accessorius

Lateral plantar

Fig. 20.11 *Plantar nerves of the left foot.*

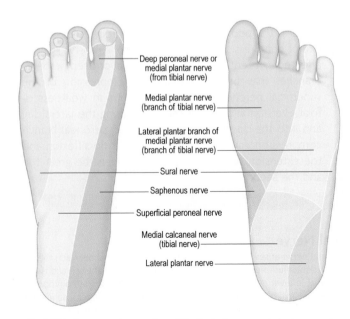

Deep peroneal nerve or medial plantar nerve (from tibial nerve)

Medial plantar nerve (branch of tibial nerve)

Lateral plantar branch of medial plantar nerve (branch of tibial nerve)

Sural nerve

Saphenous nerve

Superficial peroneal nerve

Medial calcaneal nerve (tibial nerve)

Lateral plantar nerve

Fig. 20.12 *Cutaneous innervation of the foot: dorsum and plantar aspect.*

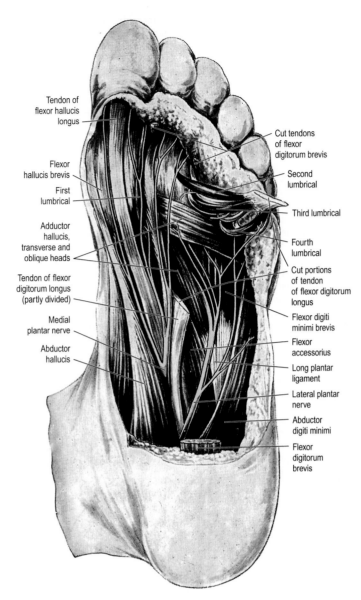

Fig. 20.13 *Dissection of the lateral and medial plantar nerves of the left foot. Most of flexor digitorum brevis has been removed. Flexor digitorum longus has been partially divided, and its distal end has been displaced, together with the second, third, and fourth lumbricals.*

joint. Sural nerve entrapment does not occur from compression by fascial elements; rather, it follows trauma and subsequent scar formation around the nerve. Entrapment of the common digital nerve as it passes under the intermetatarsal ligament of the third (or, less commonly, second) web space can result in Morton's neuroma, which is probably the most common form of nerve entrapment in the foot.

INNERVATION OF THE PELVIS

Pudendal Nerve
The pudendal nerve arises from the ventral divisions of the second, third and fourth sacral ventral rami and is formed just above the superior border of the sacrotuberous ligament and the upper fibres of ischiococcygeus. It leaves the pelvis via the greater sciatic foramen between piriformis and ischiococcygeus, enters the gluteal region and crosses the sacrospinous ligament close to its attachment to the ischial spine. The nerve lies medial to the internal pudendal vessels on the spine. It accompanies the internal pudendal artery through the lesser sciatic foramen into the pudendal (Alcock's) canal on the lateral wall of the ischioanal fossa. In the posterior part of the canal it gives rise to the inferior rectal nerve, the perineal nerve and the dorsal nerve of the penis or clitoris.

Sacral Visceral Branches
These arise from the second to fourth sacral ventral rami to innervate the pelvic viscera; they are termed pelvic splanchnic nerves.

Sacral Muscular Branches
Several muscular branches arise from the fourth sacral ventral ramus to supply the superior surface of levator ani and the upper part of the external anal sphincter. The branches to levator ani enter the superior (pelvic) surface of the muscle, while the branch to the external anal sphincter (also referred to as the perineal branch of the fourth sacral nerve) reaches the ischioanal fossa by running through ischiococcygeus or between ischiococcygeus and iliococcygeus. It supplies the skin between the anus and coccyx via its cutaneous branches.

Coccygeal Plexus
The coccygeal plexus is formed by a small descending branch from the fourth sacral ramus and by the fifth sacral and coccygeal ventral rami. The fifth sacral ventral ramus emerges from the sacral hiatus, curves around the lateral margin of the sacrum below its cornu and pierces ischiococcygeus from below to reach its upper, pelvic surface. There it is joined by a descending branch of the fourth sacral ventral ramus, and the small trunk so formed descends on the pelvic surface of ischiococcygeus. They join the minute coccygeal ventral ramus, which emerges from the sacral hiatus and curves around the lateral coccygeal margin to pierce coccygeus to reach the pelvis. This small trunk is the coccygeal plexus. Anococcygeal nerves arise from it and form a few fine filaments that pierce the sacrotuberous ligament to supply the adjacent skin.

Pelvic Part of the Sympathetic System
The pelvic sympathetic trunk lies in the extraperitoneal tissue anterior to the sacrum beneath the presacral fascia. It lies medial or anterior to the anterior sacral foramina and has four or five interconnected ganglia. Above, it is continuous with the lumbar sympathetic trunk. Below the lowest ganglia, the two trunks converge to unite in the small ganglion impar anterior to the coccyx. Grey rami communicantes pass from the ganglia to sacral and coccygeal spinal nerves, but there are no white rami communicantes. Medial branches connect across the midline, and twigs from the first two ganglia join the inferior hypogastric plexus or the hypogastric 'nerve.' Other branches form a plexus on the median sacral artery.

Vascular Branches
Postganglionic fibres pass through the grey rami communicantes to the roots of the sacral plexus. Those forming the tibial nerve are conveyed to the popliteal artery and its branches in the leg and foot, while those in the pudendal and superior and inferior gluteal nerves accompany the same named arteries to the gluteal and perineal tissues. Branches may also supply the pelvic lymph nodes.

Preganglionic fibres for the rest of the lower limb are derived from the lower three thoracic and upper two or three lumbar spinal segments. They reach the lower thoracic and upper lumbar ganglia through white rami communicantes and descend through the sympathetic trunk to synapse in the lumbar ganglia. Postganglionic fibres pass from these ganglia via grey rami communicantes to the femoral nerve, which carries them to the distribution of the femoral artery and its branches. Some fibres descend through the lumbar ganglia to synapse in the upper two or three sacral ganglia, from which postganglionic axons join the tibial nerve to supply the popliteal artery and its branches in the leg and foot.

Sympathetic denervation of vessels in the lower limb can be effected by removing or ablating the upper three lumbar ganglia and the intervening parts of the sympathetic trunk, which is rarely useful in treating vascular insufficiency of the lower limb.

INNERVATION OF THE PERINEUM
The pudendal nerve gives rise to the inferior rectal, perineal and dorsal nerves of the penis or clitoris. The pudendal nerve is readily found in its constant position over the ischial spine. It can be 'blocked' by infiltration with a local anaesthetic applied via a needle passed through the lateral wall of the vagina to cause anaesthesia of the perineal and anal skin. It can also be palpated there through the lateral wall of the rectum, and motor terminal latencies can be measured.

Inferior Rectal Nerve
The inferior rectal nerve runs through the medial wall of the pudendal canal with the inferior rectal vessels. It crosses the ischioanal fossa to supply the external anal sphincter, the lining of the lower part of the anal canal and the circumanal skin. It frequently breaks into terminal branches just before reaching the lateral border of the sphincter. Its cutaneous branches distributed around the anus overlap the perineal branch of the posterior femoral cutaneous nerve and the scrotal or labial nerves. The inferior rectal nerve occasionally arises directly from the sacral plexus and crosses the

sacrospinous ligament or reconnects with the pudendal nerve. In females the inferior rectal nerve may supply sensory branches to the lower part of the vagina.

Perineal Nerve

The perineal nerve is the inferior and larger terminal branch of the pudendal nerve in the pudendal canal. It runs forward, below the internal pudendal artery, and accompanies the perineal artery, dividing into posterior scrotal or labial and muscular branches. The posterior scrotal or labial nerves are usually double and have medial and lateral branches that run over the perineal membrane and pass forward in the lateral part of the urogenital triangle with the scrotal (or labial) branches of the perineal artery. They supply the skin of the scrotum or labia majora, overlapping the distribution of the perineal branch of the posterior femoral cutaneous and inferior rectal nerves. In females, the posterior labial branches also supply sensory fibres to the skin of the lower vagina.

Muscular branches arise directly from the pudendal nerve to supply the superficial transverse perinei, bulbospongiosus, ischiocavernosus, deep transverse perinei, sphincter urethrae and anterior parts of the external anal sphincter and levator ani. In males, a nerve to the bulb of the urethra leaves the nerve to the bulbospongiosus, piercing it to supply the corpus spongiosum penis, and ends in the urethral mucosa.

Dorsal Nerve of the Penis or Clitoris

The dorsal nerve of the penis or clitoris runs anteriorly above the internal pudendal artery along the ischiopubic ramus deep to the inferior fascia of the urogenital diaphragm. It supplies the corpus cavernosum and accompanies the dorsal artery of the penis or clitoris between the layers of the suspensory ligament. In males, it runs on the dorsum of the penis to end in the glans. In females, the dorsal nerve of the clitoris is very small.

LUMBAR SYMPATHETIC SYSTEM

The lumbar part of each sympathetic trunk usually contains four interconnected ganglia. It runs in the extraperitoneal connective tissue anterior to the vertebral column and along the medial margin of psoas major. Superiorly, it is continuous with the thoracic trunk posterior to the medial arcuate ligament. Inferiorly, it passes posterior to the common iliac artery and is continuous with the pelvic sympathetic trunk. On the right side, it lies posterior to the inferior vena cava, and on the left, it is posterior to the lateral aortic lymph nodes. It is anterior to most of the lumbar vessels but may pass behind some lumbar veins.

The first, second and sometimes third lumbar ventral spinal rami send white rami communicantes to the corresponding ganglia. Grey rami communicantes pass from all four lumbar ganglia to the lumbar spinal nerves. They are long and accompany the lumbar arteries around the sides of the vertebral bodies, medial to the fibrous arches to which psoas major is attached. Four lumbar splanchnic nerves pass from the ganglia to join the coeliac, inferior mesenteric (or occasionally abdominal aortic) and superior hypogastric plexuses. The first lumbar splanchnic nerve, from the first ganglion, gives branches to the coeliac, renal and inferior mesenteric plexuses. The second nerve joins the inferior part of the intermesenteric or inferior mesenteric plexus. The third nerve arises from the third or fourth ganglion and passes anterior to the common iliac vessels to join the superior hypogastric plexus. The fourth lumbar splanchnic nerve from the lowest ganglion passes above the common iliac vessels to join the lower part of the superior hypogastric plexus or the inferior hypogastric 'nerve.'

Vascular branches from all lumbar ganglia join the abdominal aortic plexus. Fibres of the lower lumbar splanchnic nerves pass to the common iliac arteries and form a plexus, which continues along the internal and external iliac arteries as far as the proximal part of the femoral artery. Many postganglionic fibres travel in the muscular, cutaneous and saphenous branches of the femoral nerve, supplying vasoconstrictor nerves to the femoral artery and its branches in the thigh. Other postganglionic fibres travel via the obturator nerve to the obturator artery.

LUMBAR PARASYMPATHETIC SYSTEM

The parasympathetic supply to the abdominal viscera is provided by the vagus nerve to the coeliac and superior mesenteric plexuses, and from the pelvic splanchnic nerves to the inferior mesenteric, superior hypogastric and inferior hypogastric plexuses.

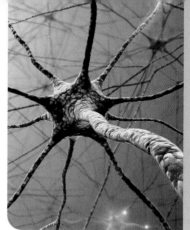

Autonomic Nervous System

The autonomic nervous system represents the visceral component of the nervous system. It consists of neurones located within both the central nervous system (CNS) and the peripheral nervous system (PNS) and is concerned with control of the internal environment through innervation of secretory glands and with cardiac and smooth muscle. The term 'autonomic' is a convenient rather than appropriate title, because the functional autonomy of this part of the nervous system is illusory. Rather, its functions are normally closely integrated with changes in somatic activities, although the anatomical bases for such interactions are not always clear.

Visceral afferent pathways resemble somatic afferent pathways. The cell bodies of origin are unipolar neurones located in cranial and dorsal root ganglia. Their peripheral processes are distributed through autonomic ganglia or plexuses, or possibly through somatic nerves, without interruption. Their central processes (axons) accompany somatic afferent fibres through cranial nerves or dorsal spinal roots into the CNS, where they establish connections that mediate autonomic reflexes and visceral sensation.

Visceral efferent pathways differ from their somatic equivalents, in that the former are interrupted by peripheral synapses; there is a sequence of at least two neurones between the CNS and the target structure (Fig. 21.1). These are referred to as preganglionic and postganglionic neurones. The somata of preganglionic neurones are located in the visceral efferent nuclei of the brain stem and in the lateral grey columns of the spinal cord. Their axons, which are usually finely myelinated, exit from the CNS in certain cranial and spinal nerves and then pass to peripheral ganglia, where they synapse with the postganglionic neurones. The axons of postganglionic neurones are usually non-myelinated. Postganglionic neurones are more numerous than preganglionic ones; one preganglionic neurone may synapse with 15 to 20 postganglionic neurones, which permits the wide diffusion of many autonomic effects.

The autonomic nervous system can be divided into three major parts: sympathetic, parasympathetic and enteric. These differ in organization and structure but are closely integrated functionally. Most but not all structures innervated by the autonomic nervous system receive both sympathetic and parasympathetic fibres, whereas the enteric nervous system is a network of neurones intrinsic to the wall of the gastrointestinal tract.

Two long-held assumptions about the sympathetic and parasympathetic nervous systems are that they are functionally antagonistic (because activation of their respective efferents has opposing actions on target structures) and that sympathetic reactions are mass responses, whereas parasympathetic reactions are usually localized. A more realistic notion is that these sets of neurones represent an integrated system for the coordinated neural regulation of visceral and homeostatic functions. Moreover, even though widespread activation of the sympathetic nervous system may occur (e.g. in association with fear or rage), it is now recognized that the sympathetic nervous system is also capable of discrete activation, and many different patterns of activation of sympathetic nerves throughout the body occur in response to a wide variety of stimuli. Thus, sympathetic activity may result in the general constriction of cutaneous arteries (increasing blood supply to the heart, muscles and brain), cardiac acceleration, increased blood pressure, contraction of sphincters and depression of peristalsis, all of which mobilize body energy stores to deal with increased activity. Parasympathetic activity results in cardiac slowing and an increase in intestinal glandular and peristaltic activities, which may be considered to conserve body energy stores.

Autonomic activity is not initiated or controlled solely by the reflex connections of general visceral afferent pathways, nor do impulses in these pathways necessarily activate general visceral efferents. For example, in many situations demanding general sympathetic activity, the initiator is somatic and typically arises from either the special senses or the skin. Rises in blood pressure and pupillary dilatation may result from the stimulation of somatic receptors in the skin and other tissues. Peripheral autonomic activity is integrated at higher levels in the brain stem and cerebrum, including various nuclei of the brain stem reticular formation, thalamus and hypothalamus; the limbic lobe and prefrontal neocortex; and the ascending and descending pathways that connect these regions.

The traditional concept of autonomic neurotransmission is that preganglionic neurones of both sympathetic and parasympathetic systems are cholinergic, as are postganglionic parasympathetic neurones, whereas those of the sympathetic nervous system are noradrenergic. The discovery of neurones that do not use either acetylcholine or noradrenaline (norepinephrine) as their primary transmitter, and the recognition of a multitude of substances in autonomic nerves that fulfill the criteria for a neurotransmitter or neuromodulator, have greatly complicated the neuropharmacological concepts of the autonomic nervous system. Thus, adenosine 5′-triphosphate (ATP), numerous peptides and nitric oxide have all been implicated in the mechanisms of cell signalling in the autonomic nervous system. The principal cotransmitters in sympathetic nerves are ATP and neuropeptide Y, vasoactive intestinal polypeptide (VIP) in parasympathetic nerves and ATP, VIP and substance P in enteric nerves.

SYMPATHETIC NERVOUS SYSTEM

The sympathetic trunks are two ganglionated nerve cords that extend from the cranial base to the coccyx. The ganglia are joined to spinal nerves by short connecting nerves called white and grey rami communicantes. Preganglionic axons join the trunk through the white rami communicantes, whereas postganglionic axons leave the trunk in the grey rami. In the neck, each sympathetic trunk lies posterior to the carotid sheath and anterior to the transverse processes of the cervical vertebrae. In the thorax, the trunks are anterior to the heads of the ribs; in the abdomen, they lie anterolateral to the bodies of the lumbar vertebrae; and in the pelvis, they are anterior to the sacrum and medial to the anterior sacral foramina. Anterior to the coccyx the two trunks meet in a single median, terminal ganglion. Cervical sympathetic ganglia are usually reduced to three by fusion. The internal carotid nerve, a continuation of the sympathetic trunk, issues from the cranial pole of the superior ganglion and accompanies the internal carotid artery through its canal into the cranial cavity. There are from 10 to 12 (usually 11) thoracic ganglia, 4 lumbar ganglia and 4 or 5 ganglia in the sacral region.

The cell bodies of preganglionic sympathetic neurones are located in the lateral horn of the spinal grey matter of all thoracic segments and the upper two or three lumbar segments (Fig. 21.2). Their axons are myelinated, with diameters of 1.5 to 4 μm. These leave the cord in corresponding ventral nerve roots and pass into the spinal nerves, but they soon leave in white rami communicantes to join the sympathetic trunk (Fig. 21.3). Neurones like those in the lateral grey column exist at other levels of the cord above and below the thoracolumbar outflow, and small numbers of their fibres leave in other ventral roots. Preganglionic sympathetic neurones release acetylcholine as their principal neurotransmitter.

On reaching the sympathetic trunk, preganglionic fibres may behave in one of several ways (see Fig. 21.3). They may synapse with neurones in the nearest ganglion or traverse the nearest ganglion and ascend or descend in the sympathetic chain to end in another ganglion. A preganglionic fibre may terminate in a single ganglion or, through collateral branches, synapse with neurones in several ganglia. Preganglionic fibres may traverse the nearest ganglion, ascend or descend and, without synapsing, emerge in one of the medially directed branches of the sympathetic trunk to synapse in the ganglia of autonomic plexuses (situated mainly in the midline, such as around the coeliac and mesenteric arteries). More than one preganglionic fibre may synapse with a single postganglionic neurone. Uniquely, the suprarenal gland is innervated directly by preganglionic sympathetic neurones that traverse the sympathetic trunk and coeliac ganglion without synapse.

The somata of sympathetic postganglionic neurones are located mostly in ganglia of the sympathetic trunk or ganglia in more peripheral plexuses. Therefore, the axons of postganglionic neurones are generally longer than those of preganglionic neurones; an exception is some of those that innervate

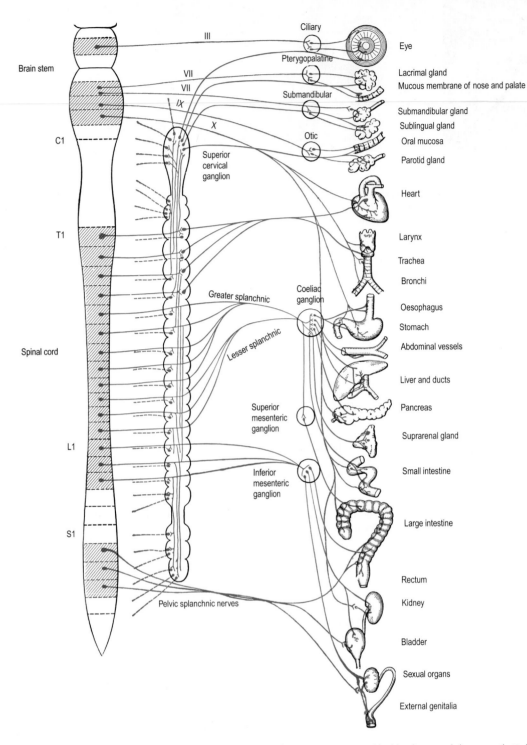

Fig. 21.1 *Efferent pathways of the autonomic nervous system. The parasympathetic pathways are represented by* blue lines, *and the sympathetic by* red lines. *The* interrupted red lines *indicate postganglionic rami to the cranial and spinal nerves. (After Meyer, Gottlieb. 1914. Die Exper. Pharmacol. (Wien) 36, 260.)*

pelvic viscera. The axons of ganglionic cells are non-myelinated. They are distributed to target organs in various ways. Those from a ganglion of the sympathetic trunk may return to the spinal nerve of preganglionic origin through a grey ramus communicans, which usually joins the nerve just proximal to the white ramus; they are then distributed through ventral and dorsal spinal rami to blood vessels, sweat glands, hairs and so forth in their zone of supply. Segmental areas vary in extent and overlap considerably. The extent of innervation of different effector systems (e.g. vasomotor, sudomotor) by a particular nerve may not be the same. Alternatively, postganglionic fibres may pass in a medial branch of a ganglion directly to particular viscera, or they may innervate adjacent blood vessels or pass along them externally to their peripheral distribution. They may ascend or descend before leaving the sympathetic trunk. Many fibres are distributed along arteries and ducts as plexuses to distant effectors.

The principal neurotransmitter released by postganglionic sympathetic neurones is noradrenaline. The sympathetic system has a much wider distribution than the parasympathetic one. It innervates all sweat glands, the arrector pili muscles, the muscular walls of many blood vessels, the heart, the lungs and respiratory tree, the abdominopelvic viscera, the oesophagus, the muscles of the iris and the non-striated muscle of the urogenital tract, eyelids and elsewhere.

Postganglionic sympathetic fibres that return to the spinal nerves are vasoconstrictor to blood vessels, secretomotor to sweat glands and motor to the arrector pili muscles within their dermatomes. Those that accompany the motor nerves to voluntary muscles are probably only dilatatory. Most if not all peripheral nerves contain postganglionic sympathetic fibres. Those reaching the viscera are concerned with general vasoconstriction, bronchial and bronchiolar dilatation, modification of glandular secretion, pupillary dilatation, inhibition of alimentary muscle contraction and the like. A single preganglionic fibre probably synapses with the postganglionic neurones in only one effector system, which means that effects such as sudomotor and vasomotor actions can be separate.

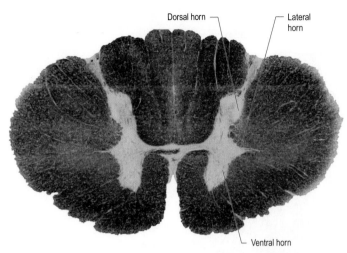

Fig. 21.2 *Transverse section through the thoracic spinal cord showing the lateral horn, where preganglionic sympathetic neurones are located. (Enhanced by B. Crossman.)*

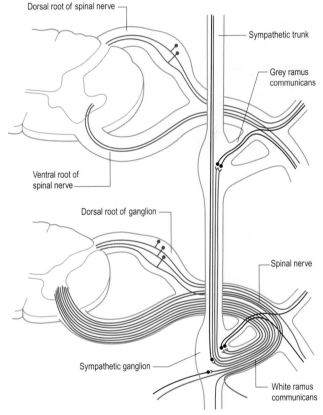

Fig. 21.3 *Relationship between spinal nerves and the sympathetic trunk. The somatic components of spinal nerve roots are illustrated in the* upper part *of the diagram, and the visceral components are shown in the* lower part. *Somatic and preganglionic sympathetic fibres are coloured* red, *somatic and visceral afferent fibres are coloured* blue *and postganglionic sympathetic fibres are coloured* black.

Cervical Sympathetic Trunk

The cervical sympathetic trunk (Figs 21.4, 21.5) lies on the prevertebral fascia behind the carotid sheath and contains three interconnected ganglia: the superior, middle and inferior (stellate or cervicothoracic). However, there may occasionally be two or four ganglia. The cervical sympathetic ganglia send grey rami communicantes to all the cervical spinal nerves but receive no white rami communicantes from them. Their spinal preganglionic fibres emerge in the white rami communicantes of the upper five thoracic spinal nerves (mainly the upper three) and ascend in the sympathetic trunk to synapse in the cervical ganglia. In their course, the grey rami communicantes may pierce longus capitis or scalenus anterior.

Superior Cervical Ganglion

The superior cervical ganglion is the largest of the three ganglia. It lies on the transverse processes of the second and third cervical vertebrae and is probably formed from four fused ganglia, judging by its grey rami to C1–4. The internal carotid artery within the carotid sheath is anterior, and longus capitis is posterior (see Fig. 21.4). The lower end of the ganglion is united by a connecting trunk to the middle cervical ganglion. Postganglionic branches are distributed in the internal carotid nerve, which ascends with the internal carotid artery into the carotid canal to enter the cranial cavity, and in lateral, medial and anterior branches. They supply vasoconstrictor and sudomotor nerves to the face and neck, dilator pupillae and smooth muscle in the eyelids and orbitalis.

Lateral Branches — The lateral branches are grey rami communicantes to the upper four cervical spinal nerves and to some of the cranial nerves. Branches pass to the inferior vagal ganglion, hypoglossal nerve, superior jugular bulb and associated jugular glomus and meninges in the posterior cranial fossa. Another branch, the jugular nerve, ascends to the cranial base and divides into two; one part joins the inferior glossopharyngeal ganglion, and the other joins the superior vagal ganglion.

Medial Branches — The medial branches of the superior cervical ganglion are the laryngopharyngeal and cardiac. The laryngopharyngeal branches supply the carotid body and pass to the side of the pharynx, joining glossopharyngeal and vagal rami to form the pharyngeal plexus. A cardiac branch arises by two or more filaments from the lower part of the superior cervical ganglion and occasionally receives a twig from the trunk between the superior and middle cervical ganglia. It is thought to contain only efferent fibres (the preganglionic outflow being from the upper thoracic segments of the spinal cord) and to be devoid of pain fibres from the heart. It descends behind the common carotid artery and in front of longus colli and crosses anterior to the inferior thyroid artery and recurrent laryngeal nerve. The courses on the two sides then differ. The right cardiac branch usually passes behind, but sometimes in front of, the subclavian artery and runs posterolateral to the brachiocephalic trunk to join the deep (dorsal) part of the cardiac plexus behind the aortic arch. It has other sympathetic connections. About mid neck, it receives filaments from the external laryngeal nerve. Inferiorly, one or two vagal cardiac branches join it. As it enters the thorax, it is joined by a filament from the recurrent laryngeal nerve. Filaments from the nerve also communicate with the thyroid branches of the middle cervical ganglion. The left cardiac branch, in the thorax, is anterior to the left common carotid artery and crosses in front of the left side of the aortic arch to reach the superficial (ventral) part of the cardiac plexus. Sometimes it descends on the right of the aorta to end in the deep (dorsal) part of the cardiac plexus. It communicates with the cardiac branches of the middle and inferior cervical sympathetic ganglia and sometimes with the inferior cervical cardiac branches of the left vagus; branches from these mixed nerves form a plexus on the ascending aorta.

Anterior Branches — The anterior branches of the superior cervical ganglion ramify on the common and external carotid arteries and the branches of the external carotid, and they form a delicate plexus around each one, in which small ganglia are occasionally found. The plexus around the facial artery supplies a filament to the submandibular ganglion; the plexus on the middle meningeal artery sends one ramus to the otic ganglion and another, the external petrosal nerve, to the facial ganglion. Many of the fibres coursing along the external carotid and its branches ultimately leave them to travel to facial sweat glands via branches of the trigeminal nerve.

Middle Cervical Ganglion

The middle cervical ganglion (Figs 21.6, 21.7) is the smallest of the three; it is occasionally absent, in which case it may be replaced by minute ganglia in the sympathetic trunk or fused with the superior ganglion. It is usually found at the level of the sixth cervical vertebra, anterior or just superior to the inferior thyroid artery, or it may adjoin the inferior cervical ganglion. It probably represents a coalescence of the ganglia of the fifth and sixth cervical segments, judging by its postganglionic rami, which join the fifth and sixth cervical spinal nerves (but sometimes also the fourth and seventh). It is connected to the inferior cervical ganglion by two or more very variable cords. The posterior cord usually splits to enclose the vertebral artery, whereas the anterior cord loops down anterior to, and then below, the first part of the subclavian artery, medial to the origin of its internal thoracic branch, and supplies rami to it. This loop, the ansa subclavia, is frequently multiple, lies in close contact with the cervical pleura and typically connects with the phrenic nerve and sometimes with the vagus.

The middle cervical ganglion gives off thyroid and cardiac branches. The thyroid branches accompany the inferior thyroid artery to the thyroid gland. They communicate with the superior cardiac, external laryngeal and recurrent laryngeal nerves and send branches to the parathyroid glands. Fibres to both glands are largely vasomotor, but some reach the secretory cells. The cardiac branch, the largest sympathetic cardiac nerve, arises either from the ganglion itself or, more often, from the sympathetic trunk cranial or caudal to it. On

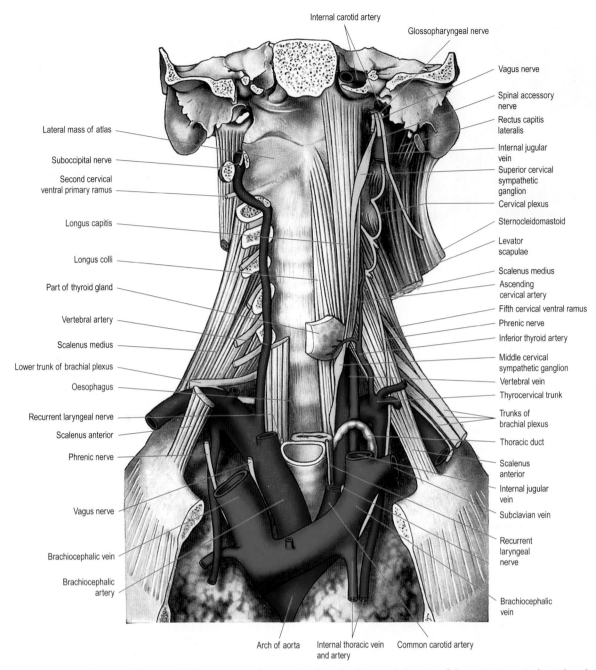

Internal carotid artery

Glossopharyngeal nerve

Vagus nerve

Spinal accessory nerve

Rectus capitis lateralis

Internal jugular vein

Superior cervical sympathetic ganglion

Cervical plexus

Sternocleidomastoid

Levator scapulae

Scalenus medius

Ascending cervical artery

Fifth cervical ventral ramus

Phrenic nerve

Inferior thyroid artery

Middle cervical sympathetic ganglion

Vertebral vein

Thyrocervical trunk

Trunks of brachial plexus

Thoracic duct

Scalenus anterior

Internal jugular vein

Subclavian vein

Recurrent laryngeal nerve

Brachiocephalic vein

Lateral mass of atlas

Suboccipital nerve

Second cervical ventral primary ramus

Longus capitis

Longus colli

Part of thyroid gland

Vertebral artery

Scalenus medius

Lower trunk of brachial plexus

Oesophagus

Recurrent laryngeal nerve

Scalenus anterior

Phrenic nerve

Vagus nerve

Brachiocephalic vein

Brachiocephalic artery

Arch of aorta

Internal thoracic vein and artery

Common carotid artery

Fig. 21.4 *Dissection showing the prevertebral region and the superior mediastinum. On the right,* the costal elements of the upper six cervical vertebrae have been removed to expose the cervical part of the vertebral artery. On the left, *most of the deep relations of the common carotid artery and the internal jugular vein are exposed.*

the right side it descends behind the common carotid artery, in front of or behind the subclavian artery, to the trachea, where it receives a few filaments from the recurrent laryngeal nerve before joining the right half of the deep (dorsal) part of the cardiac plexus. In the neck, it connects with the superior cardiac and recurrent laryngeal nerves. On the left side, the cardiac nerve enters the thorax between the left common carotid and subclavian arteries to join the left half of the deep (dorsal) part of the cardiac plexus. Fine branches from the middle cervical ganglion also pass to the trachea and oesophagus.

Inferior (Cervicothoracic Stellate) Ganglion

The inferior cervical (cervicothoracic stellate) ganglion is irregular in shape and much larger than the middle cervical ganglion (see Figs 21.6, 21.7). It is probably formed by a fusion of the lower two cervical and first thoracic segmental ganglia, sometimes including the second and even the third and fourth thoracic ganglia. The first thoracic ganglion may be separate, leaving an inferior cervical ganglion above it. The sympathetic trunk turns backward at the junction of the neck and thorax, so the long axis of the cervicothoracic ganglion becomes almost anteroposterior. The ganglion lies on or just lateral to the lateral border of longus colli between the base of the seventh cervical transverse process and the neck of the first rib (which are both posterior to it). The vertebral vessels are anterior, and the ganglion is separated from the

posterior aspect of the cervical pleura inferiorly by the suprapleural membrane. The costocervical trunk of the subclavian artery branches near the lower pole of the ganglion, and the superior intercostal artery is lateral.

A small vertebral ganglion may be present on the sympathetic trunk anterior or anteromedial to the origin of the vertebral artery and directly above the subclavian artery. When present, it may provide the ansa subclavia and is also joined to the inferior cervical ganglion by fibres enclosing the vertebral artery. It is usually regarded as a detached part of the middle cervical or inferior cervical ganglion. Like the middle cervical ganglion, it may supply grey rami communicantes to the fourth and fifth cervical spinal nerves. The inferior cervical ganglion sends grey rami communicantes to the seventh and eighth cervical and first thoracic spinal nerves, and it gives off a cardiac branch, branches to nearby vessels and sometimes a branch to the vagus nerve.

The grey rami communicantes to the seventh cervical spinal nerve vary from one to five (two being the usual number). A third often ascends medial to the vertebral artery in front of the seventh cervical transverse process. It connects with the seventh cervical nerve and sends a filament upward through the sixth cervical transverse foramen, accompanied by the vertebral vessels, to join the sixth cervical spinal nerve as it emerges from the intervertebral foramen. An inconstant ramus may traverse the seventh cervical transverse foramen. The number of grey rami to the eighth cervical spinal nerve ranges from three to six.

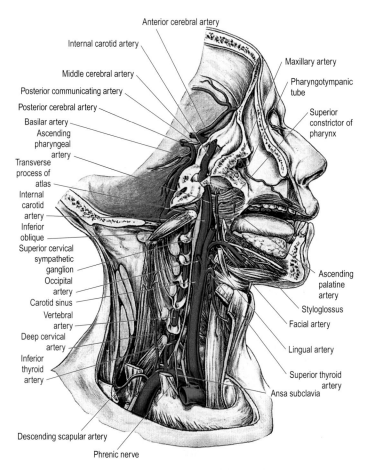

Fig. 21.5 *Dissection showing the course of the right vertebral and internal carotid arteries and some of their branches.*

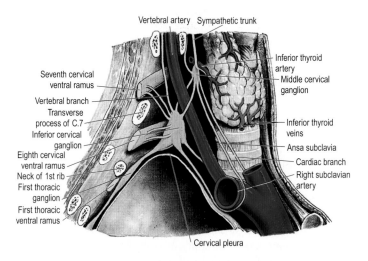

Fig. 21.6 *Middle and inferior cervical ganglia of the right side, viewed from the right. Note the proximity of the inferior cervical and first thoracic ganglia, which often fuse to form a cervicothoracic (stellate) ganglion.*

The cardiac branch descends behind the subclavian artery and along the front of the trachea to the deep cardiac plexus. Behind the artery it connects with the recurrent laryngeal nerve and the cardiac branch of the middle cervical ganglion (the latter is often replaced by fine branches of the inferior cervical ganglion and ansa subclavia).

The branches to blood vessels form plexuses on the subclavian artery and its branches. The subclavian supply is derived from the inferior cervical ganglion and ansa subclavia and typically extends to the first part of the axillary artery, although a few fibres may extend farther. An extension of the subclavian plexus to the internal thoracic artery may be joined by a branch of the phrenic nerve. The vertebral plexus is derived mainly from a large branch of the inferior cervical ganglion that ascends behind the vertebral artery to the sixth transverse foramen. There it is reinforced by branches of the vertebral ganglion or the cervical sympathetic trunk that pass cranially on the ventral aspect of the artery. Deep rami communicantes from this plexus join the

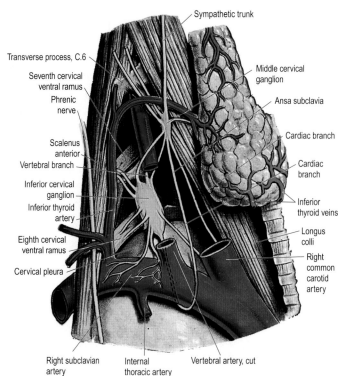

Fig. 21.7 *Middle and inferior cervical ganglia of the right side, anterior view. Part of the vertebral artery has been excised to show the inferior cervical ganglion.*

ventral rami of the upper five or six cervical spinal nerves. The plexus, which contains some neuronal cell bodies, continues into the skull along the vertebral and basilar arteries and their branches as far as the posterior cerebral artery, where it meets a plexus from the internal carotid artery. The plexus on the inferior thyroid artery reaches the thyroid gland and connects with the recurrent and external laryngeal nerves, the cardiac branch of the superior cervical ganglion and the common carotid plexus.

Horner's Syndrome — Any condition or injury that destroys the sympathetic trunk ascending from the thorax through the neck into the face results in Horner's syndrome (Fig. 21.8), characterized by a drooping eyelid (ptosis), sunken globe (enophthalmos), narrow palpebral fissure, contracted pupil (miosis), vasodilatation and lack of thermal sweating (anhidrosis) on the affected side. Classically, this occurs when a bronchial carcinoma invades the sympathetic trunk (see Ch. 18, Case 2). It also occurs as a complication of cervical sympathectomy or radical neck dissection.

PARASYMPATHETIC NERVOUS SYSTEM

Preganglionic parasympathetic neurone cell bodies are located in certain cranial nerve nuclei of the brain stem (see Fig. 5.6) and in the grey matter of the second to fourth sacral segments of the spinal cord. Efferent fibres, which are myelinated, emerge from the CNS only in certain cranial nerves (oculomotor, facial, glossopharyngeal, vagus) and the second to fourth sacral spinal nerves. The preganglionic parasympathetic neurones are cholinergic.

The cell bodies of postganglionic parasympathetic neurones are mostly sited distant from the CNS, either in discrete ganglia located near the structures innervated or dispersed in the walls of viscera. In the cranial part of the parasympathetic system there are four small peripheral ganglia—ciliary, pterygopalatine, submandibular and otic—which are all described on a regional basis. These are solely efferent parasympathetic ganglia, unlike the trigeminal, facial, glossopharyngeal and vagal ganglia, all of which are concerned exclusively with afferent impulses and contain the cell bodies of sensory neurones. However, the cranial parasympathetic ganglia are traversed by afferent fibres, postganglionic sympathetic fibres and, in the case of the otic ganglion, branchial efferent fibres, but none of these are interrupted in the ganglia. Postganglionic parasympathetic fibres are usually non-myelinated and shorter than those in the sympathetic system, because the ganglia in which the former synapse are in or near the viscera they supply. In contrast to the sympathetic system, postganglionic parasympathetic neurones are cholinergic.

Oculomotor preganglionic parasympathetic fibres originate in the Edinger–Westphal nucleus of the midbrain and travel in the nerve along its branch to the inferior oblique, reaching the ciliary ganglion, where they synapse. Postganglionic fibres, which are thinly myelinated, travel in the short ciliary nerves that pierce the sclera to run forward in the perichoroidal space to the

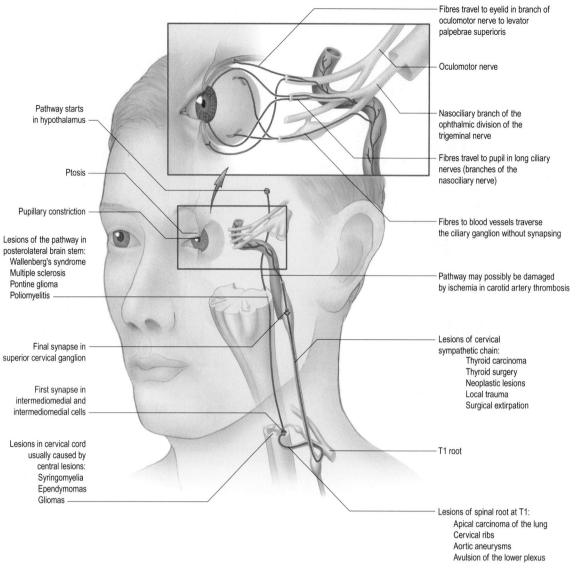

Fibres travel to eyelid in branch of
oculomotor nerve to levator
palpebrae superioris

Oculomotor nerve

Nasociliary branch of the
ophthalmic division of the
trigeminal nerve

Fibres travel to pupil in long ciliary
nerves (branches of the
nasociliary nerve)

Fibres to blood vessels traverse
the ciliary ganglion without synapsing

Pathway may possibly be damaged
by ischemia in carotid artery thrombosis

Lesions of cervical
sympathetic chain:
   Thyroid carcinoma
   Thyroid surgery
   Neoplastic lesions
   Local trauma
   Surgical extirpation

T1 root

Lesions of spinal root at T1:
   Apical carcinoma of the lung
   Cervical ribs
   Aortic aneurysms
   Avulsion of the lower plexus

Pathway starts
in hypothalamus

Ptosis

Pupillary constriction

Lesions of the pathway in
posterolateral brain stem:
   Wallenberg's syndrome
   Multiple sclerosis
   Pontine glioma
   Poliomyelitis

Final synapse in
superior cervical ganglion

First synapse in
intermediomedial and
intermediomedial cells

Lesions in cervical cord
usually caused by
central lesions:
   Syringomyelia
   Ependymomas
   Gliomas

Fig. 21.8 *Horner's syndrome.*

CASE 1   HARLEQUIN SYNDROME

A 55-year-old woman presents with a 3-month history of exercise-induced anhidrosis and lack of flushing on the left side of the face, with normal autonomic responses on the right. Examination demonstrates a left Horner's syndrome with miosis and ptosis. Provocative manoeuvres such as controlled exercise confirm loss of flushing on the left side of the face, as described historically, along with hemifacial anhidrosis. No other neurological abnormalities are found.

Discussion: Asymmetric facial flushing and sweating suggest a diagnosis of harlequin syndrome, with asymmetric involvement of vasomotor and sudomotor fibres. Because one entire side of the face is involved, the autonomic lesion must be below the bifurcation of the carotid artery, presumably a preganglionic sympathetic lesion below the superior cervical ganglion but distal to the stellate ganglion. It has been suggested that the lesion involves preganglionic fibres originating at T2 and T3. Occasionally, segmental autonomic dysfunction is observed in an upper extremity as well. The presence of the ocular features of Horner's syndrome suggests involvement of the ciliary ganglia in at least some cases. A relationship to Ross syndrome (segmental anhidrosis, tonic pupils and hyporeflexia) has also been suggested.

ciliary muscle and sphincter pupillae. Their activation mediates accommodation of the eye to near objects and pupillary constriction.

The facial nerve contains preganglionic parasympathetic axons of neurones with their somata in the superior salivatory nucleus (see Ch. 10). The fibres emerge from the brain stem in the nervus intermedius, leave the main facial nerve trunk above the stylomastoid foramen and travel in the chorda tympani, which subsequently joins the lingual nerve (see Ch. 11). In this way, preganglionic fibres are conveyed to the submandibular ganglion, where they synapse on ganglionic neurones. Postganglionic fibres innervate the submandibular and sublingual salivary glands and are said to travel in the lingual nerve. Some preganglionic fibres may synapse around cells in the hilum of the submandibular gland. Stimulation of the chorda tympani dilates the arterioles in both glands, in addition to having a direct secretomotor effect. The facial nerve also contains efferent parasympathetic lacrimal secretomotor axons, which travel in its greater petrosal branch and then via the nerve of the pterygoid canal, to relay in the pterygopalatine ganglion. Postganglionic axons are thought to travel by the zygomatic nerve to the lacrimal gland and by ganglionic branches to the nasal and palatal glands.

The glossopharyngeal nerve contains preganglionic parasympathetic secretomotor fibres for the parotid gland. These originate in the inferior salivatory nucleus and travel in the glossopharyngeal nerve and its tympanic branch. They traverse the tympanic plexus and lesser petrosal nerve to reach the otic

CASE 2   PARINAUD'S SYNDROME

A 13-year-old boy has complained of headaches for several months. On examination, he is found to have bilateral disc oedema (papilloedema), with paresis of up-gaze. His pupils fail to constrict in bright light but constrict normally with accommodation. He also has convergence retraction nystagmus. Magnetic resonance imaging reveals a tumour involving the dorsal midbrain (collicular plate) that is also responsible for obstructive hydrocephalus.

Discussion: This boy has classic Parinaud's (dorsal midbrain) syndrome, with prominent light-near dissociation along with paresis of up-gaze convergence, retraction nystagmus and eyelid retraction. It is caused by lesions affecting the dorsal midbrain (tectum) in the region of the superior colliculi and involving the pretectal nuclei. Supranuclear fibres destined for the oculomotor nerve complex are spared. Pupils are midsize or enlarged. Light-near dissociation (characterized by a poor pupillary response (reflex) to light, but with preservation of pupillary constriction to a near target) usually results from bilateral midbrain lesions, but not necessarily. Responsible lesions include tumour (e.g. pinealoma), hydrocephalus or infarction. It is of interest that Argyll Robertson pupils, which are seen, for example, in cases of neurosyphilis, may also exhibit pupillary-near dissociation, but the Argyll Robertson pupil is typically very small and irregular, with reduced dilatation in the dark. Again, the supranuclear connection between the pretectum and the midbrain Edinger–Westphal nucleus is spared, so that the pupillary-near reflex is preserved. The so-called tonic pupil of Adie's syndrome, with a lesion involving primarily the ciliary ganglia, similarly exhibits light-near dissociation.

ENTERIC NERVOUS SYSTEM

The traditional view of the autonomic nervous system was that intrinsic neurones in peripheral organs such as the heart, airways and bladder were postganglionic parasympathetic neurones, which acted as simple cholinergic relay stations. However, many peripheral ganglia contain circuits that are capable of sustaining and modulating visceral activities by local reflex mechanisms. Large populations of intrinsic neurones exist that are derived from the neural crest and are independent of sympathetic and parasympathetic nerves. The enteric nervous system consists of ganglionated plexuses localized in the wall of the gastrointestinal tract. It contains reflex pathways through which contractions of the muscular coats of the alimentary tract, secretion of gastric acid, intestinal transport of water and electrolytes, mucosal bloodflow and other functions are controlled. Although complex interactions occur between the enteric and sympathetic and parasympathetic nervous systems, the enteric nervous system is capable of sustaining local reflex activity independent of the CNS. Thus, because intrinsic neurones survive following section of the extrinsic sympathetic and parasympathetic nerves, organs that are transplanted are not truly denervated. It is worth noting that separation from their autonomic input often has no obvious impact on the non-striated muscle or glands innervated by autonomic fibres; contraction may be unaffected, and no structural changes ensue. This has been variously attributed to the continued activity of local plexuses or the intrinsic activity of visceral muscle. In some important instances, however, denervation does result in cessation of activity, such as in sweat glands, pilomotor muscle, orbital non-striated muscle and the suprarenal medulla.

VISCERAL AFFERENT PATHWAYS

General visceral afferent fibres from the viscera and blood vessels accompany their efferent counterparts and are the peripheral processes of unipolar cell bodies located in some cranial nerve and dorsal root ganglia. They are contained in the vagus, glossopharyngeal and possibly other cranial nerves; the second to fourth sacral spinal nerves, distributed with the pelvic splanchnic nerves; and in thoracic and upper lumbar spinal nerves, distributed through rami communicantes and alongside the efferent sympathetic innervation of viscera and blood vessels.

The cell bodies of vagal general visceral afferent fibres are in the superior and inferior vagal ganglia. Their peripheral processes are distributed to terminals in the pharyngeal and oesophageal walls, where, acting synergistically with glossopharyngeal visceral afferents in the pharynx, they are concerned with swallowing reflexes. Vagal afferents are also believed to innervate the thyroid and parathyroid glands. In the heart, vagal afferents innervate the walls of the great vessels, the aortic bodies and pressor receptors, where they are stimulated by raised intravascular pressure. In the lungs, they are distributed via the pulmonary plexuses. They supply bronchial mucosa, where they are probably involved in cough reflexes; bronchial muscle, where they encircle myocytes and end in tendrils, which are sometimes regarded as 'muscle spindles' and are believed to be stimulated by changes in the length of myocytes; interalveolar connective tissue, where their knob-like endings, together with terminals on myocytes, may evoke Hering–Breuer reflexes; the adventitia of pulmonary arteries, where they may be pressor receptors; and the intima of pulmonary veins, where they may be chemoreceptors. Vagal visceral afferent fibres also end in the gastric and intestinal walls, digestive glands and kidneys. Fibres ending in the gut and its ducts respond to stretch or contraction. Gastric impulses may evoke sensations of hunger and nausea.

The cell bodies of glossopharyngeal general visceral afferents are in the glossopharyngeal ganglia. Their peripheral processes innervate the posterior lingual region, tonsils and pharynx, but they do not innervate taste buds. They also innervate the carotid sinus and the carotid body, which contain receptors sensitive to tension and changes in the chemical composition of the blood. Impulses from these receptors are essential to circulatory and respiratory reflexes.

Visceral afferents that enter the spinal cord through spinal nerve roots terminate in the spinal grey matter. The central processes of vagal and glossopharyngeal afferent fibres end in the vagal nucleus or the nucleus solitarius of the medulla. Visceral afferents establish connections within the CNS that mediate autonomic reflexes. In addition, afferent impulses probably mediate visceral sensations such as hunger, nausea, sexual excitement, vesical distension and so forth. Visceral pain fibres may follow these routes. Although viscera are insensitive to cutting, crushing or burning, excessive tension in smooth muscle and some pathological conditions produce visceral pain. In visceral disease, vague pain may be felt near the viscus itself (visceral pain) or in a cutaneous area or other tissue whose somatic afferents enter spinal segments receiving afferents from the viscus—a phenomenon known as referred pain. If inflammation spreads from a diseased viscus to the adjacent parietal serosa (e.g. the peritoneum), somatic afferents will be stimulated, causing local

ganglion, where they synapse. Postganglionic fibres pass by communicating branches to the auriculotemporal nerve, which conveys them to the parotid gland. Stimulation of the lesser petrosal nerve produces vasodilator and secretomotor effects.

The vagal nucleus (dorsal motor nucleus of the vagus) in the medulla is a major source of preganglionic parasympathetic fibres. Efferent fibres travel in the vagus nerve and its pulmonary, cardiac, oesophageal, gastric, intestinal and other branches. They synapse in minute ganglia in the visceral walls. Cardiac branches, which act to slow the cardiac cycle, join the cardiac plexuses, and fibres relay in ganglia distributed over both atria. Pulmonary branches contain fibres that relay in ganglia of the pulmonary plexuses. They are motor in function to the circular non-striated muscle fibres of the bronchi and bronchioles and are bronchoconstrictor in function. With the exception of the pyloric sphincter, gastric branches are secretomotor and motor to the non-striated muscle of the stomach, which they inhibit. Intestinal branches have a corresponding action in the small intestine, caecum, vermiform appendix, ascending colon, right colic flexure and most of the transverse colon. They are secretomotor to the glands and motor to the intestinal muscular coats, but inhibitory to the ileocaecal sphincter. Their synaptic relays with postganglionic neurones are situated in the myenteric (Auerbach's) and submucosal (Meissner's) plexuses.

Pelvic splanchnic nerves to the pelvic viscera travel in anterior rami of the second, third and fourth sacral spinal nerves. These nerves unite with branches of the sympathetic pelvic plexuses. Minute ganglia occur at the points of union and in the visceral walls, and sacral preganglionic parasympathetic fibres relay synaptically in these ganglia. The pelvic splanchnic nerves are motor to the muscle of the rectum and bladder wall but inhibitory to the vesical sphincter. They supply vasodilator fibres to the erectile tissue of the penis and clitoris and are probably also vasodilator to the testes, ovaries, uterine tubes and uterus. Filaments from the pelvic splanchnic nerves ascend in the hypogastric plexus and are visceromotor to the sigmoid and descending colon, left colic flexure and terminal transverse colon.

somatic pain, which is commonly spasmodic. Referred pain is often associated with local cutaneous tenderness.

Afferent fibres in pelvic splanchnic nerves innervate pelvic viscera and the distal part of the colon. Vesical receptors are widespread; those in muscle strata are associated with thickly myelinated fibres and are believed to be stretch receptors, possibly activated by contraction. Pain fibres from the bladder and proximal urethra traverse both pelvic splanchnic nerves and the inferior hypogastric plexus, hypogastric nerves, superior hypogastric plexus and lumbar splanchnic nerves to reach their cell bodies in ganglia on the lower thoracic and upper lumbar dorsal spinal roots. The significance of this dual sensory pathway is uncertain. Lesions of the cauda equina abolish pain from vesical overdistension, but hypogastric section is ineffective. Pain fibres from the uterus traverse the hypogastric plexus and lumbar splanchnic nerves to reach somata in the lowest thoracic and upper lumbar spinal ganglia; hypogastric division may relieve dysmenorrhoea. However, afferents from the uterine cervix traverse the pelvic splanchnic nerves to somata in the upper sacral spinal ganglia. Stretch of the cervix uteri causes pain, but cauterization and biopsy excisions do not.

In general, afferent fibres that accompany pre- and postganglionic sympathetic fibres have a segmental arrangement. They end in spinal cord segments from which preganglionic fibres innervate the region or viscus concerned. General visceral afferents entering thoracic and upper lumbar spinal segments are largely concerned with pain. Nociceptive impulses from the pharynx, oesophagus, stomach, intestines, kidneys, ureter, gallbladder and bile ducts seem to be carried in sympathetic pathways. Cardiac nociceptive impulses enter the spinal cord via the first to fifth thoracic spinal nerves, mainly in the middle and inferior cardiac nerves, but a few pass directly to the spinal nerves. It is thought that there are no general visceral afferents in the superior cardiac nerves. Peripherally, the fibres pass through the cardiac plexuses and along the coronary arteries. Myocardial anoxia may evoke symptoms of angina pectoris, in which pain is typically presternal and is also referred to much of the left chest and radiates to the left shoulder, medial aspect of the left arm, along the left side of the neck to the jaw and occiput and down to the epigastrium. Cardiac afferents carried in vagal cardiac branches are concerned with the reflex depression of cardiac activity. Ureteric pain fibres, also running with sympathetic fibres, are presumably involved in the agonizing renal colic that follows obstruction by calculi. Afferent fibres from the testis and ovary run through the corresponding plexuses to somata in the tenth and eleventh thoracic dorsal root ganglia.

Certain primary afferent nerve fibres, which have their cell bodies in cranial and dorsal root ganglia, also have an efferent function (so-called sensory–motor nerves). The importance of sensory–motor nerve regulation in many organs, such as the gut, lungs, heart and blood vessels, is now recognized. Although most such nerves are, presumably, purely sensory, some of them have been termed sensory–motor because they release transmitter from their peripheral endings during the axon reflex and have a motor rather than a sensory role. The primary substances so released are substance P, calcitonin gene-related peptide and ATP. These substances act on target cells to produce several biological actions, including vasodilatation, increased venular permeability, changes in smooth muscle contractility, degranulation of mast cells and a variety of effects on leukocytes and fibroblasts—a process collectively known as 'neurogenic inflammation.' The local release of such substances may play a trophic role in the maintenance of tissue integrity and repair in response to injury.

References

Benarroch, E.E., 2007. The autonomic nervous system: basic anatomy and physiology. CONTINUUM Lifelong learning in neurology 1 (6), 13–32.

CASE 3   AUTONOMIC NEUROPATHY

A 60-year-old man has suffered from non-insulin-dependent diabetes mellitus for many years. He now complains of the insidious onset of bowel difficulties, with chronic constipation alternating with diarrhea, as well as epigastric discomfort. For several years he has been impotent.

Discussion: Autonomic dysfunction with gastroenteropathy is common among diabetic patients, often accompanied by features of a mixed sensory–motor neuropathy. Colonic distension (atony) is often found radiographically. Gastric atrophy (gastroparesis) is also common and may produce symptoms of gastric distress. Sexual and bladder dysfunction caused by diabetic autonomic neuropathy is well recognized.

Autonomic neuropathies may be hereditary or acquired. The hereditary sensory autonomic neuropathies (HSANs) are rare disorders, usually presenting at birth or in early childhood. HSAN III (Riley–Day syndrome) is characterized by the loss of unmyelinated nerve fibres; afflicted children suffer from instability of blood pressure and temperature regulation. Acquired autonomic neuropathies have diverse causes, including paraneoplastic or autoimmune disorders, toxic (thallium) or metabolic (uremia) insults, vitamin deficiency syndromes, infection (leprosy) or amyloid deposition.

Benarroch, E.E., 2007. Enteric nervous system: functional organization and neurologic implications. Neurology 69, 1953–1958.

Björklund, A., Hökfelt, T., Owman, C. (Eds.), 1988. The Peripheral Nervous Systems: Handbook of Chemical Neuroanatomy. Vol. 6. Elsevier, Amsterdam. *Description of sensory–motor nerves.*

Burnstock, G., 1990. Co-transmission: The fifth Heymans lecture. Arch. Int. Pharmacodyn. Ther. 304, 7–33. *Review of neurotransmission in the autonomic nervous system.*

Burnstock, G. (Ed.), 1992–1995. The Autonomic Nervous System. Vols 1–14. Harwood Academic Publishers, Switzerland. *Extensive material on the neurotransmitters of the autonomic nervous system.*

Freeman, R., Kaufmann, H., 2007. Disorders of orthostatic tolerance—orthostatic hypotension, postural tachycardia syndrome, and syncope. CONTINUUM Lifelong learning in neurology 1 (6), 50–88.

Kaufmann, H., Goldstein, D.S., 2007. Autonomic failure in neurodegenerative disorders. CONTINUUM Lifelong learning in neurology 1 (6), 111–142.

Maggi, C.A., 1991. The pharmacology of the efferent function of sensory nerves. J. Auton. Pharmacol. 11, 173–208.

Vernino, S., Freeman, R., 2007. Peripheral autonomic neuropathies. CONTINUUM Lifelong learning in neurology 1 (6), 89–110.

Vinken, P.J., Bruyn, G.W. (Eds.), 1999. The Autonomic Nervous System. Part 1. Normal Functions. Appenzeller O (volume ed) Elsevier Science Publishers, Amsterdam and London.

Vinken, P.J., Bruyn, G.W. (Eds.), 2000. The Autonomic Nervous System. Part 2. Dysfunctions. Appenzeller O (volume ed) Elsevier Science Publishers, Amsterdam and London.

Wasner, G., Maag, R., Ludwig, J., Binder, A., Schattschneider, J., Stingele, R., Baron, R., 2005. Harlequin syndrome: one face of many etiologies. Neurology 1, 54–59.

Section VII

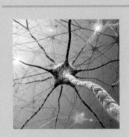

The Neuromuscular Junction and Muscle

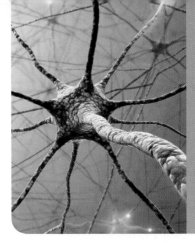

Neuromuscular Junction

Chapter 22

SKELETAL MUSCLE

The most intensively studied effector endings are those that innervate muscle, particularly skeletal muscle. All neuromuscular (myoneural) junctions are axon terminals of somatic motor neurones. They are specialized for the release of neurotransmitter onto the sarcolemma of skeletal muscle fibres, causing a change in their electrical state that leads to contraction. Each axon branches near its terminal and subsequently innervates from several to hundreds of muscle fibres, depending on the precision of motor control required. The detailed structure of a motor terminal varies with the type of muscle innervated. Two major endings are recognized: those typical of extrafusal muscle fibres, and endings on the intrafusal fibres of neuromuscular spindles. In the former, each axon terminal usually ends midway along a muscle fibre in a discoidal motor end-plate (Figs 22.1–22.3). This type usually initiates action potentials, which are rapidly conducted to all parts of the muscle fibre. In the latter, the axon has numerous subsidiary branches that form a cluster of small expansions extending along the muscle fibre. In the absence of propagated muscle excitation, these excite the fibre at several points. Both types are associated with a specialized receptive region of the muscle fibre, the sole plate, where a number of muscle cell nuclei are grouped within the granular sarcoplasm.

The sole plate contains numerous mitochondria, endoplasmic reticulum and Golgi complexes (see Figs 22.2, 22.3). The neuronal terminal branches are plugged into shallow grooves in the surface of the sole plate (primary clefts), from which numerous pleats extend for a short distance into the underlying sarcoplasm (secondary clefts). The axon terminal contains mitochondria and many clear 60-nm spherical vesicles, similar to those in presynaptic boutons, clustered over the zone of membrane apposition. The motor terminal is ensheathed by Schwann cells whose cytoplasmic projections extend into the synaptic cleft. The plasma membranes of the nerve terminal and the muscle cell are separated by a 30- to 50-nm gap, with a basal lamina interposed. The basal lamina follows the surface folding of the sole plate membrane into the secondary clefts. It contains specialized components, including specific isoforms of type IV collagen and laminin and agrin, a heparan sulphate proteoglycan. Endings of fast and slow twitch muscle fibres differ in detail: the sarcolemmal grooves are deeper, and the presynaptic vesicles more numerous, in the fast fibres.

Junctions with skeletal muscle are cholinergic, and the release of acetylcholine (ACh) changes the ionic permeability of the muscle fibre. Clustering of ACh receptors at the neuromuscular junction depends in part on the presence of agrin, synthesized by the motor neurone. Agrin affects muscle cytoskeletal attachments to the ACh receptor cytoplasmic domain and prevents their lateral diffusion out of the junction. When the depolarization of the sarcolemma reaches a particular threshold, it initiates an all-or-none action potential in the sarcolemma, which is then propagated rapidly over the whole cell surface and also deep within the fibre via the invaginations (T-tubules) of the sarcolemma, causing contraction. The amount of ACh released by the arrival of a single nerve impulse is sufficient to trigger an action potential. However, because ACh is very rapidly hydrolysed by the enzyme acetylcholinesterase (AChE), present at the sarcolemmal surface of the sole plate, a single nerve impulse gives rise to only one muscle action potential—that is, there is a one-to-one relationship between neural and muscle action potentials. Thus, the contraction of a muscle fibre is controlled by the firing frequency of its motor neurone. Neuromuscular junctions are partially blocked by high concentrations of lactic acid, as in some types of muscle fatigue.

CONDUCTION OF THE NERVOUS IMPULSE

All cells generate a steady electrochemical potential across their plasma membranes (a membrane potential) because of the different ionic concentrations inside and outside the cell (Fig. 22.4). Neurones use minute fluctuations in this potential to receive, conduct and transmit information across their surfaces.

The membrane potential of a neurone, known as the resting potential, is similar to that of non-excitable cells. In most neurones it is approximately 80 mV, being negative inside. The entry into neurones of sodium or, in some sites, calcium ions causes depolarization of the cell, whereas an increased chloride influx or an increased potassium efflux results in hyperpolarization. Plasma membrane permeability to these ions is altered by the opening or closing of ion-specific transmembrane channels, triggered by chemical or electrical stimuli. Chemically triggered ionic fluxes occur at synapses and may be either direct, whereby the chemical agent (neurotransmitter) binds to the channel itself to cause it to open, or indirect, whereby the neurotransmitter is bound by a transmembrane receptor molecule that is not itself a channel but that activates a complex second messenger system within the cell to open separate transmembrane channels. Electrically induced changes in membrane potential depend on the presence of voltage-sensitive ion channels that, when the transmembrane potential reaches a critical level, open to allow the influx or efflux of specific ions. In all cases, the channels remain open only transiently, and the numbers that open and close determine the total flux of ions across the membrane.

The types and concentrations of transmembrane channels and related proteins, and therefore the electrical activity of the membranes, vary in different parts of the cell. Dendrites and neuronal somata depend mainly on neurotransmitter action and show graded potentials, whereas axons have voltage-gated channels that give rise to action potentials.

In graded potentials, a flow of current from or into adjacent areas of the cell occurs when a synapse is activated, and this contributes to the total degree of polarization of the membrane covering the cell body. However, the influence of an individual synapse on neighbouring regions decreases with distance, so that, for instance, synapses on the distal tips of dendrites may, on their own, have relatively little effect. The electrical state of a neurone therefore depends on many factors, including the number and position of thousands of excitatory and inhibitory synapses, their degree of activation, the branching pattern of the dendritic tree and the geometry of the cell body. The target of these integrated factors is a small part of the neurone surface, the axon hillock, where voltage-sensitive channels are concentrated (unlike the dendrites or somata). The axon hillock is the site where action potentials are generated before being conducted along the axon.

Autonomic Motor Terminations

Autonomic neuromuscular junctions differ in several important ways from the skeletal neuromuscular junction and from synapses in the central nervous system (CNS) and peripheral nervous system (PNS). There is no fixed junction with well-defined pre- and postjunctional specializations. Unmyelinated, highly branched postganglionic autonomic axons become beaded or varicose as they reach the effector smooth muscle. These varicosities are not static but are able to move along axons. They are packed with mitochondria and vesicles containing neurotransmitters, which are released from the varicosities during conduction of an impulse along the axon. The distance (cleft) between the varicosity and smooth muscle membrane varies considerably, depending on the tissue—from 20 nm in densely innervated structures, such as the vas deferens, to 1 to 2 μm in large elastic arteries. Unlike skeletal muscle, the effector tissue is a muscle bundle rather than a single cell. Gap junctions between individual smooth muscle cells are low-resistance pathways, allowing electronic coupling and the spread of activity within the effector bundle. They vary in size from punctate junctions to junctional areas of more than 1 μm in diameter.

Adrenergic sympathetic postganglionic terminals contain dense-core vesicles. Cholinergic terminals, which are typical of all parasympathetic and some sympathetic endings, contain clear spherical vesicles like those in motor end-plates of skeletal muscle. A third category of autonomic neurones has non-adrenergic, non-cholinergic endings that contain a wide variety of chemicals with transmitter properties. Conjugated purine (ATP, a nucleoside), is probably the neurotransmitter at these terminals, which are thus classed as purinergic.

CASE 1 BOTULISM

A 22-year-old woman presents in the early morning with double vision, slurred speech and swallowing difficulties, preceded the night before by dry mouth, blurred vision, abdominal cramping and constipation. During the next several hours, she develops limb weakness and finally shortness of breath requiring intubation. She has otherwise been well. However, she participated in a covered-dish dinner at a family reunion on the day the symptoms began. Several other family members who attended also complained of abdominal cramps and diarrhea or constipation, and later the same day her mother experienced double vision and slurred speech.

On examination, she exhibits eyelid ptosis and complete bilateral ophthalmoplegia. Her pupils fail to react to light. She has marked facial and tongue weakness. Strength is reduced throughout, with absent reflexes.

Discussion: Botulinum toxin ingestion in adults initially causes gastrointestinal symptoms, followed by weakness, especially of ocular and bulbar muscles. Because the toxin's site of action is presynaptic, decreased or lack of ACh release occurs at all peripheral cholinergic nerve endings, both nicotinic (neuromuscular junction) and muscarinic (autonomic) receptors. The toxin is taken up into the nerve terminal by endocytosis, then cleaves proteins required for the docking and fusing of vesicles to the presynaptic member, thereby blocking exocytosis and release of ACh. The binding of the toxin is permanent and results in destruction of the axon terminal. Regrowth of the nerve terminal must occur for function to return. Those affected early after ingestion usually have a more devastating course than those affected later. Clustering of cases frequently occurs.

CASE 2 LAMBERT–EATON SYNDROME

A 68-year-old man presents with generalized weakness of 3 months' duration. He finds it most difficult to climb stairs or rise from a chair. He has a dry mouth most of the time but denies other symptoms, except for a recent 20-pound weight loss. He has a 50–pack-year smoking history. Examination shows a dry mouth; proximal muscle weakness, especially in the lower extremities; and decreased reflexes throughout. Following a brief full contraction of biceps, the biceps reflex is briefly normal but diminishes again within 1 minute. When asked to grip the examiner's hand, his grip gets stronger as it is maintained.

Discussion: This man has Lambert–Eaton ("myasthenic") syndrome. In this disorder, the presynaptic release of ACh at the neuromuscular junction and in autonomic nerves is abnormal. Antibodies to presynaptic calcium channels block calcium flow into the presynaptic nerve following its depolarization; with a decreased influx of calcium, synaptic vesicles containing ACh cannot bind to the presynaptic membrane, and ACh cannot be released. The result is weakness, often generalized, along with autonomic complaints such as dry mouth and impotence. Because this is a presynaptic issue, both nicotinic and muscarinic receptors are affected. Increasing strength and reflexes following muscle contraction occur by virtue of the fact that exercise forces more calcium into the presynaptic nerve terminal, resulting in increased release of ACh and a temporary increase in strength or reflex, as in this man. These pathophysiological events are also reflected in electrophysiological studies; the initial amplitude of a compound muscle action potential is very low, but following a brief period of exercise of the tested muscle or repetitive stimulation of a motor nerve, the compound muscle action potential amplitude increases in an incremental manner (opposite the response seen in true myasthenia gravis).

Lambert–Eaton syndrome is a paraneoplastic syndrome in more than 50% of affected individuals, most commonly associated with small cell carcinoma of the lung. In this man, his weight loss and smoking history underscore this possibility and should prompt appropriate laboratory and radiographic investigations.

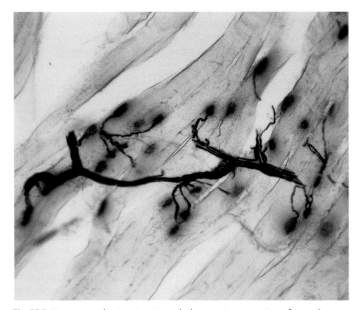

Fig. 22.1 *Neuromuscular junction in a whole-mount preparation of teased skeletal muscle fibres (pale, faintly striated, diagonally oriented structures). The terminal part of the axon (silver-stained, brown) branches to form motor end-plates on adjacent muscle fibres. The sole plate recesses in the sarcolemma, into which the motor end-plates fit, are demonstrated by the presence of AChE (shown by enzyme histochemistry, blue). (Courtesy of Dr. Norman Gregson, Division of Neurology, GKT School of Medicine, London. Photograph by Sarah-Jane Smith.)*

Typically, their axons contain large (80- to 200-nm), dense, opaque vesicles congregated in varicosities at intervals along axons. They are formed in many sites, including the external muscle layers and sphincters of the alimentary tract, lungs, vascular walls, urogenital tract and CNS. In the intestinal wall, neuronal somata lie in the myenteric plexus, and their axons spread caudally for a few millimetres, mainly to innervate circular muscle. Purinergic neurones are under cholinergic control from preganglionic sympathetic neurones. Their endings mainly hyperpolarize smooth muscle cells, causing relaxation (e.g. preceding peristaltic waves), opening sphincters and probably causing reflex distension in gastric filling.

Autonomic efferents also innervate glands, myoepithelial cells and adipose and lymphoid tissue.

Action Potential

The action potential is a brief complete reversal of polarity that propagates itself along membranes. It depends on an initial influx of sodium ions, which causes a reversal of polarity to about 40 mV (positive inside), followed by a rapid return to the resting potential as potassium ions flow out (the detailed mechanism differs somewhat between CNS and PNS). The whole process is

CASE 3   MYASTHENIA GRAVIS

A 24-year-old woman complains of difficulty holding her arms over her head to wash her hair. For the last 6 months she has also noted bilateral eyelid ptosis, worse at the end of the day, and intermittent diplopia, especially when driving at night. She has occasional difficulty swallowing, and if she drinks water quickly, she may cough, resulting in nasal regurgitation of the liquid. She has no pain and otherwise feels well. On examination, she has mild bilateral ptosis, increasing after 60 seconds of up-gaze. There is no diplopia in primary gaze, but she develops diplopia after 20 seconds of sustained up-gaze. She has palatal weakness, especially after repeated phonation, and has a nasal voice. Routine testing of strength demonstrates only mild neck flexor weakness, but she cannot keep her arms extended for more than 30 seconds. She is able to rise from a chair six times before exhibiting difficulty. The remainder of the neurological examination is normal. A bedside edrophonium test results in a transient improvement in strength.

Discussion: Myasthenia gravis (MG) is a postsynaptic disorder of the neuromuscular junction, with antibodies to ACh receptors being demonstrated there. Ocular, bulbar and systemic muscles may all be affected to varying degrees. As noted, ACh is released from synaptic vesicles in the terminal twigs of motor axons, then diffuses across the discontinuous neuromuscular junction to find receptors in the synaptic cleft in the postsynaptic sarcolemma. Binding of ACh to the receptors causes end-plate depolarization by opening sodium channels, and an all-or-none action potential ensues, spreading rapidly over the cell surface and inducing muscle contraction. ACh is then rapidly hydrolysed by AChE at the sarcolemmal surface. In MG, muscle weakness worsens with repetition, as available stores of ACh released from the presynaptic nerve terminal are depleted. Administration of edrophonium, an AChE inhibitor, produces improvement by slowing the breakdown of ACh, allowing more effective binding of the neurotransmitter with more postsynaptic receptors, and transiently improving strength.

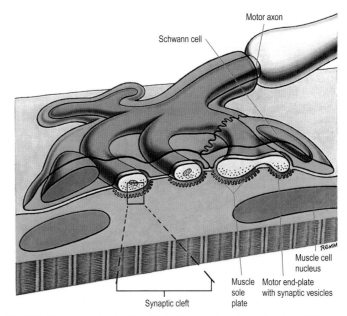

Fig. 22.2 *Neuromuscular junction. Note the axonal motor end-plate and the deeply infolded sarcolemma.*

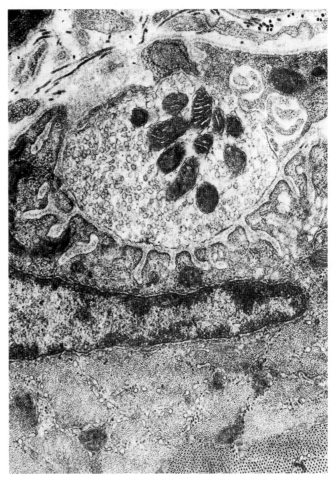

Fig. 22.3 *Neuromuscular junction in skeletal muscle. The expanded motor end-plate of the axon is filled with vesicles containing synaptic transmitter (ACh; above), and the deep infoldings of the sarcolemmal sole plate (below) form subsynaptic gutters. (Courtesy of D. N. Landon, Institute of Neurology, University College London.)*

completed in approximately 5 msec. For a particular neurone, the size and duration of action potentials are always the same (described as all or none), no matter how much a stimulus exceeds the threshold value.

Once initiated, an action potential spreads rapidly and at a constant velocity because it triggers the opening of neighbouring voltage-gated channels of the same sort. The velocity of conduction, ranging from 4 to 120 m/sec, depends on a number of factors related to the way the current spreads, including axonal cross-sectional area, membrane capacitance (influenced by the presence of myelin) and the number and position of ion channels. At the end of an action potential, there is an irreducible delay—the refractory period—during which another action potential cannot be triggered. This determines the maximum frequency at which action potentials can be conducted along a nerve fibre; its value differs in different neurones and affects the amount of information that can be carried by an individual fibre.

Myelinated fibres are electrically insulated along most of their lengths, except at nodes of Ranvier. Voltage-gated sodium channels are clustered at nodes, and the nodal membrane is the only place where an action potential can be propagated down the axon. The action potential thus jumps from node to node across internodal distances of 0.2 to 2.0 mm, depending on the axon diameter—a process known as saltatory conduction. This greatly speeds the rate of conduction. In demyelinating disease, the speed and security of conduction are severely compromised.

Axonal conduction is naturally unidirectional, from dendrites and somata to axon terminals. When an action potential reaches the axon terminals, it causes depolarization of the presynaptic membrane, and as a result, quanta of neurotransmitter (corresponding to the content of individual vesicles) are released to change the degree of excitation of the next neurone, muscle fibre or glandular cell (Kandel and Schwartz 2000).

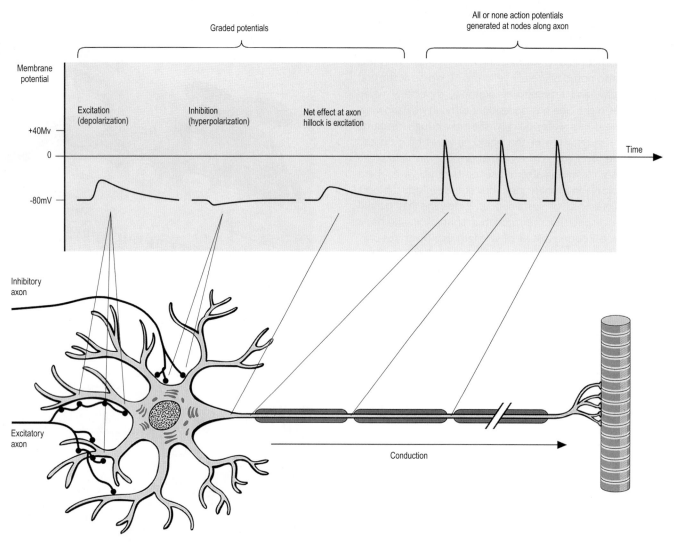

Fig. 22.4 *Types of changes in electrical potential that can be recorded across the cell membrane of a motor neurone at the points indicated by the arrows. Excitatory and inhibitory synapses on the surfaces of the dendrites and somata cause local graded changes of potential that summate at the axon hillock and may initiate a series of all-or-none action potentials, which in turn are conducted along the axon to the effector terminals.*

References

Kandel, E.R., Schwartz, J.H., 2000. Principles of Neural Science, fourth ed. McGraw-Hill, New York.

Lehmann-Horn, F., Jurkat-Rott, K., Rudel, R., 2006. Periodic paralysis: understanding channelopathies. Neurology 66 (Suppl. 1), 62–69.

Miller, A.E. (Ed.), 2009. Myasthenic disorders and ALS: CONTINUUM Lifelong learning in neurology. Lippincott Williams & Wilkins, Philadelphia.

Ohno, K., Engel, A.G., 2006. Congenital myasthenic syndromes: genetic defects of the neuromuscular junction. Neurology 66 (Suppl. 1), 77–88.

Muscle

Chapter 23

CLASSIFICATION OF MUSCLE

Muscle cells (fibres) are also known as myocytes (the prefixes myo- and sarco-are frequently used when naming structures associated with muscle). They differentiate along one of three main pathways to form skeletal, cardiac or smooth muscle. Both skeletal muscle and cardiac muscle are called striated muscle, because their myosin and actin filaments are organized into regular, repeating elements that give the cells a finely cross-striated appearance when they are viewed microscopically. Smooth muscle, in contrast, lacks such repeating elements and thus has no striations.

Other contractile cells, including myofibroblasts and myoepithelial cells, are different in character and origin. They contain smooth muscle–like contractile proteins and are found singly or in small groups.

Striated Muscle
Skeletal Muscle

Skeletal muscle is innervated by somatic motor nerves and forms the bulk of the muscular tissue of the body. It consists of parallel bundles of long, multinucleate fibres. This type of muscle is capable of powerful contractions (approximately 100 watts/kg) by virtue of the regular organization of its contractile proteins. The price paid for this organization is a limited contractile range. Wherever a larger range of movement is required, it is achieved through the amplification provided by the lever systems of the skeleton to which the muscle is attached (hence the name skeletal muscle).

Skeletal muscle is sometimes referred to as voluntary muscle because the movements in which it participates are often initiated under conscious control. However, this term is misleading; skeletal muscle is also involved in many movements (e.g. breathing, blinking, swallowing and actions of muscles in the perineum and middle ear) that are usually or exclusively driven at an unconscious level.

Cardiac Muscle

Cardiac muscle is found only in the heart and in the walls of large veins where they enter the heart. It consists of a branching network of individual cells that are linked electrically and mechanically to function as a unit. Compared with skeletal muscle, cardiac muscle is much less powerful (approximately 3 to 5 watts/kg) but far more resistant to fatigue. It is provided with a continuous supply of energy by numerous blood vessels around the fibres and abundant mitochondria within them. Cardiac muscle differs structurally and functionally from skeletal muscle in some important respects. It is, for example, intrinsically capable of rhythmic contraction with a rate and strength that are nevertheless responsive to hormonal and autonomic nervous control.

Smooth Muscle

Smooth muscle contains actin and myosin, but they are not organized into repeating units, so its microscopic appearance is unstriated (smooth). The elongated cells are smaller than those of striated muscle, and they taper at the ends. They are capable of slow but sustained contractions, and although this type of muscle is less powerful than striated muscle, the amount of shortening can be much greater. These functional attributes are well illustrated by smooth muscle's role in the walls of tubes and sacs, where its action regulates the size of the enclosed lumen and, in some cases, the movement of luminal contents.

A smooth muscle cell may be excited in several ways, most commonly by an autonomic nerve fibre, a blood-borne neurohormone, or conduction from a neighbouring smooth muscle cell. Because none of these routes is under conscious control, smooth muscle is sometimes referred to as involuntary muscle. It is found in all systems of the body; in the walls of the viscera, including most of the gastrointestinal, respiratory, urinary and reproductive tracts; in the tunica media of blood vessels; in the dermis (as the arrector pili muscles); in the intrinsic muscles of the eye; and in the dartos muscular layer of the scrotum. In some places, smooth muscle fasciculi are associated with those of skeletal muscle, including the sphincters of the anus and the urinary bladder, the tarsal muscles of the upper and lower eyelids, the suspensory muscle of the duodenum, a transitional zone in the oesophagus and fasciae and ligaments on the pelvic aspect of the pelvic diaphragm.

SKELETAL MUSCLE
Shape and Fibre Architecture

It is possible to classify muscles based on their general shape and the predominant orientation of their fibres relative to the direction of pull (Fig. 23.1). Muscles with fibres that are largely parallel to the line of pull vary in form from flat, short and quadrilateral (e.g. thyrohyoid) to long and strap-like (e.g. sternohyoid, sartorius). In such muscles, individual fibres may run for the entire length of the muscle or over shorter segments when there are transverse, tendinous intersections at intervals (e.g. rectus abdominis). In a fusiform muscle, the fibres may be close to parallel in the belly but converge to a tendon at one or both ends. Where fibres are oblique to the line of pull, muscles may be triangular (e.g. temporalis, adductor longus) or pennate (feather-like) in construction. The latter vary in complexity (see Fig. 23.1) from unipennate (e.g. flexor pollicis longus) and bipennate (e.g. rectus femoris, dorsal interossei) to multipennate (e.g. deltoid). In some muscles, the fibres pass obliquely between deep and superficial aponeuroses, in a type of unipennate form (e.g. soleus). In other sites, muscle fibres start from the walls of osteofascial compartments and converge obliquely on a central tendon in circumpennate fashion (e.g. tibialis anterior). Some muscles have a spiral or twisted arrangement (e.g. sternocostal fibres of pectoralis major and latissimus dorsi, which undergo a 180° twist between their median and lateral attachments). Others spiral around a bone (e.g. supinator, which winds obliquely around the proximal radial shaft) or contain two or more planes of fibres arranged in different directions, a type of spiral sometimes referred to as cruciate; sternocleidomastoid, masseter and adductor magnus are all partially spiral and cruciate. Many muscles display more than one of these major types of arrangement and show regional variations that correspond to contrasting and, in some cases, independent actions.

Muscle Nomenclature

The names given to individual muscles are usually descriptive, based on their shape, size, number of heads or bellies, position, depth, attachments or actions. The meanings of some of these terms are given in Table 23.1.

These terms are often used in combination—for example, flexor digitorum longus (long flexor of the digits) and latissimus dorsi (broadest muscle of the back). The names given to individual muscles or muscle groups are often oversimplified, and terms denoting action emphasize only one of a number of usual actions. A given muscle may play different roles in different movements, and these roles may change if the movements are assisted or opposed by gravity. The functional roles implied by names should therefore be interpreted with caution.

Microstructure

The cellular units of skeletal muscle are the muscle fibres (Fig. 23.2). These long, cylindrical structures tend to be consistent in size within a given muscle, but in different muscles they may range from 10 to 100 μm in diameter and from millimetres to many centimetres in length. Some typical skeletal muscle fibres are seen in longitudinal section in Figure 23.3. Their staining characteristics are dominated by the contractile apparatus, which constitutes much of the cytoplasm or sarcoplasm. The contractile proteins are organized into cylindrical myofibrils that are too tightly packed to be visible by routine light microscopy. Of greater significance are transverse striations, which are the result of alignment across the fibre of repeating elements, the sarcomeres, within neighbouring myofibrils. These cross-striations are usually evident in sections stained conventionally, but they may be demonstrated more effectively using special stains (Fig. 23.4).

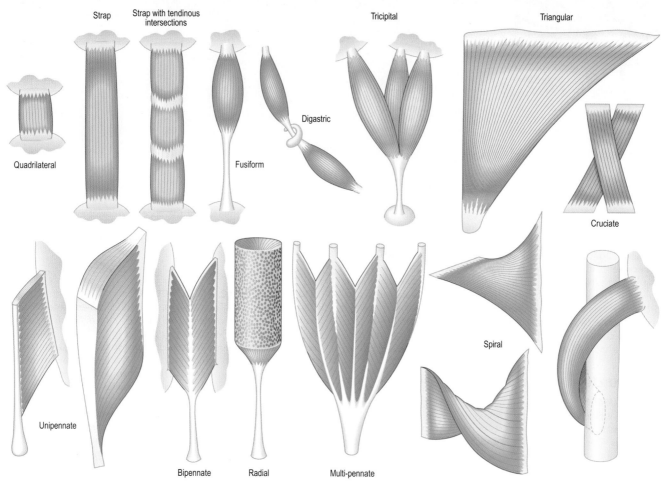

Fig. 23.1 *Morphological types of muscle based on their general form and fascicular architecture.*

Table 23.1 *Terms used in naming muscles*

Shape	Position
Deltoid (triangular)	Anterior, posterior, medial, lateral, superior, inferior, supra-, infra-
Quadratus (square)	Interosseous (between bones)
Rhomboid (diamond shaped)	Dorsi (of the back)
Teres (round)	Abdominis (of the abdomen)
Gracilis (slender)	Pectoralis (of the chest)
Rectus (straight)	Brachii (of the arm)
Lumbrical (worm-like)	Femoris (of the thigh)
	Oris (of the mouth)
Size	Oculi (of the eye)
Major, minor, longus (long)	**Attachment**
Brevis (short)	
Latissimus (broadest)	Sternocleidomastoid (from sternum and clavicle to mastoid process)
Longissimus (longest)	Coracobrachialis (from the coracoid process to the arm)
Number of Heads or Bellies	**Action**
Biceps (two heads)	Extensor, flexor
Triceps (three heads)	Abductor, adductor
Quadriceps (four heads)	Levator, depressor
Digastric (two bellies)	Supinator, pronator
	Constrictor, dilator
Depth	
Superficialis (superficial)	
Profundus (deep)	
Externus/externi (external)	
Internus/interni (internal)	

Under polarized light, the striations are even more striking and are seen as a pattern of alternating dark and light bands. The darker bands are birefringent, rotating the plane of polarized light strongly, and are known as anisotropic or A-bands; the lighter bands rotate the plane of polarized light to a negligible degree and are known as isotropic or I-bands. The structures responsible for this appearance are described more readily at the ultrastructural level.

The multiple nuclei are oval and are located at the periphery of the fibres, under the plasma membrane or sarcolemma. They are especially numerous in the region of the neuromuscular junction. The nuclei are moderately euchromatic and usually have one or more nucleoli. They occupy a thin, transparent rim of sarcoplasm between the myofibrils and the sarcolemma and are seen most clearly in transverse sections (Fig. 23.5). Other nuclei belonging to vascular endothelial cells, Schwann cells, fibroblasts, and so forth may be present in the spaces between the fibres, where blood vessels and nerve fibres travel through layers of fine connective tissue, the endomysium. Nuclei of satellite cells lie between the sarcolemma and the surrounding basal lamina.

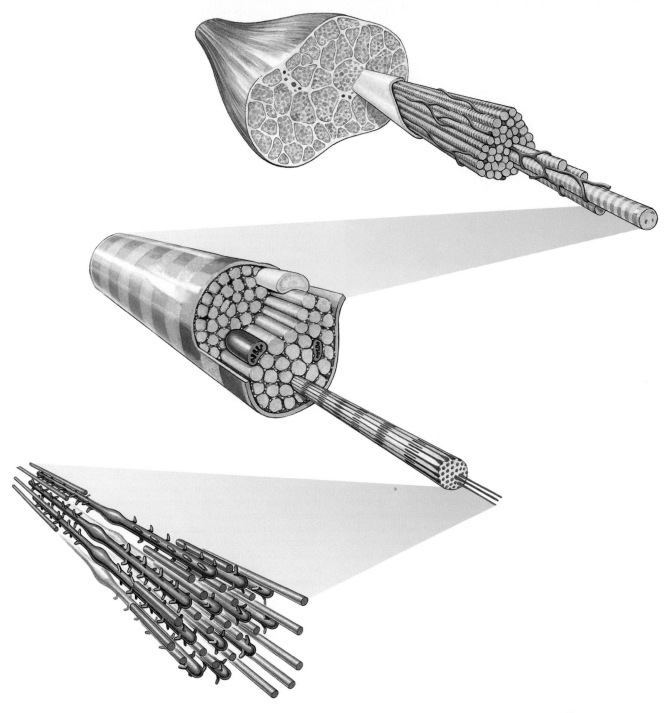

Fig. 23.2 *Levels of organization within a skeletal muscle, from whole muscle to fasciculi, single fibres, myofibrils and myofilaments.*

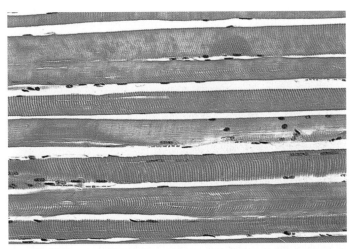

Fig. 23.3 *Skeletal muscle fibres in longitudinal section. Note the numerous peripherally placed nuclei in these extremely elongated, unbranched syncytial cells and the faint transverse striations in their cytoplasm. The central fibre is sectioned in part through its periphery, close to the sarcolemma, so several nuclei appear to be lying centrally. (By permission from Young, B., Heath, J.W., 2000. Wheater's Functional Histology. Churchill Livingstone, Edinburgh.)*

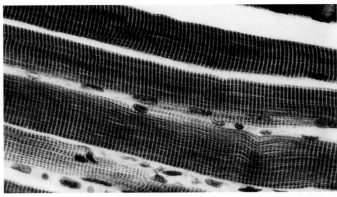

Fig. 23.4 *Skeletal muscle fibres in longitudinal section. Cross-striations reflect the sarcomeric organization of actin and myosin within the myofibrils and the alignment of myofibrils in register within the cytoplasm. The nuclei between fibres are those of endomysial connective tissue and capillaries, and some may be of satellite cells (phosphotungstic acid–stained preparation). (Photograph by Sarah-Jane Smith.)*

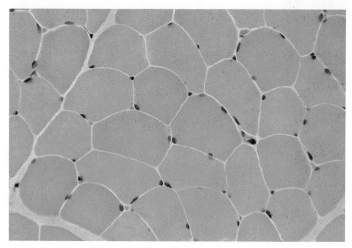

Fig. 23.5 *Transverse cryostat section of adult human skeletal muscle. Note the tight packing of the fibres and the peripheral location of the dark-stained nuclei. (Photograph by Stanley Salmons, from a specimen provided by Tim Helliwell, Department of Pathology, University of Liverpool.)*

In transverse section, the profiles of the fibres are usually polygonal (see Fig. 23.5). Some muscles, such as the extrinsic muscles of the larynx, tend to be less tightly packed. In such situations, as well as in conditions of generalized wasting or muscle damage, the fibres may adopt a more rounded profile; however, in some normal muscles, such as those that close the jaw, the fibres are closely packed but have rounded profiles. The sarcoplasm often has a stippled appearance because the transversely sectioned myofibrils are resolved as dots.

Skeletal muscle fibres are large (with a few exceptions, such as the laryngeal muscles), and unless electron micrographs are taken at very low magnification, they seldom show more than part of the interior of a fibre (Fig. 23.6A). Myofibrils are the dominant ultrastructural feature of such micrographs. They are cylindrical structures approximately 1 μm in diameter, which appear as ribbons in longitudinal section. Thin, very densely stained transverse lines, which correspond to discs in the parent cylindrical structure, appear at regular intervals along these ribbons. They are called Z-lines or, more properly, Z-discs (*Zwischenscheiben*, or 'between discs'). They divide the myofibril into a linear series of identical contractile units called sarcomeres, each of which is approximately 2.2 μm long in resting muscle.

At higher power, sarcomeres are seen to consist of two types of filament—thick and thin—organized into regular arrays (Fig. 23.6B). The thick filaments, which are approximately 15 nm in diameter, are composed mainly of myosin. The thin filaments, which are 8 nm in diameter, are composed mainly of actin. The arrays of thick and thin filaments form a partially overlapping structure in which the electron density varies according to the amount of protein present. The A-band consists of the thick filaments, together with lengths of thin filaments that interdigitate with, and thus overlap, the thick filaments at either end (see Fig. 23.6B; Fig. 23.7). The central, paler region of the A-band, into which the thin filaments have not penetrated, is called the H zone (*helle*, or 'light'). At their centres, the thick filaments are linked together transversely by material that constitutes the M line (*Mittelscheibe*, or 'middle (of) disc'), which is visible in most muscles.

The I-band consists of the adjacent portions of two neighbouring sarcomeres in which the thin filaments are not overlapped by thick filaments. It is bisected by the Z-disc, into which the thin filaments of adjacent sarcomeres are anchored. In addition to the thick and thin filaments, there is a third type of filament composed of the elastic protein titin. The high degree of organization of the filament arrays is equally evident in electron micrographs of transverse sections (see Fig. 23.7; Fig. 23.8). The thick myosin filaments form a hexagonal lattice; in the regions where they overlap with the thin filaments, each myosin filament is surrounded by six actin filaments at the trigonal points of the lattice. In the I-band, the thin filament pattern changes from hexagonal to square as the filaments approach the Z-disc, where they are incorporated into a square lattice structure.

The banded appearance of individual myofibrils is thus attributable to the regular alternation of the thick and thin filament arrays. However, myofibrils are at the limit of resolution of light microscopy; the fact that cross-striations are also visible at that level is the result of alignment in register of the bands in adjacent myofibrils across the breadth of the whole muscle fibre. In suitably stained, relaxed material, the A-bands, I-bands and H zones are quite distinct, but the Z-discs, which are such a prominent feature of electron micrographs, are thin and much less conspicuous under the light microscope, and M lines cannot be seen at all.

Muscle Proteins

Myosin, the protein of the thick filament, is the most abundant contractile protein (60% of the total myofibrillar protein). The thick filaments of skeletal (and cardiac) muscle are 1.5 μm long. Actin is the next most abundant contractile protein (20% of the total myofibrillar protein). In its filamentous form (F-actin), it is the principal protein of the thin filaments; the other components, the regulatory proteins tropomyosin and troponin, play a major part in the control of contraction.

The third type of long sarcomeric filament, which connects the thick filaments to the Z-disc, is formed by the giant protein titin, with a molecular mass in the millions. Single titin molecules span the half-sarcomere between the M lines and the Z-discs, into which they are inserted, with a bound portion in the A-band and an elastic portion in the I-band. In the A-band, titin is attached to thick filaments as far as the M line. Its physical properties endow the myosin filaments with elastic recoil after stretching.

A number of proteins that are neither contractile nor regulatory are responsible for the structural integrity of the myofibrils, particularly their regular internal arrangement. A component of the Z-disc, α-actinin, is a rod-shaped molecule that anchors the plus-ends of actin filaments from adjacent sarcomeres to the Z-disc. Nebulin inserts into the Z-disc, associated with the thin filaments, and regulates the length of actin filaments. An intermediate filament protein characteristic of muscle, desmin, encircles the myofibrils at the Z-disc and, with the linking molecule plectin, forms a meshwork that connects myofibrils together within the muscle fibre. Myomesin holds myosin filaments in their regular lattice arrangement in the region of the M line. Dystrophin is confined to the periphery of the muscle fibre, close to the cytoplasmic face of the sarcolemma. It binds to actin intracellularly and is also associated with a large oligomeric complex of glycoproteins that spans the membrane and links specifically with merosin, the laminin isoform of the muscle basal lamina. This stabilizes the muscle fibre and transmits forces generated internally on contraction to the extracellular matrix.

Dystrophin is the product of the gene affected in Duchenne's muscular dystrophy, a fatal disorder that develops when mutation of the gene leads to the absence of this protein. A milder form of the disease, Becker's muscular dystrophy, is associated with reduced size or abundance of dystrophin. Female carriers (heterozygous for the mutant gene) of Duchenne's muscular dystrophy may also have mild symptoms of muscle weakness. At approximately 2500 kb, the gene is one of the largest yet discovered, which may account for the high mutation rate of Duchenne's muscular dystrophy (approximately 35% of cases are new mutations).

Other Sarcoplasmic Structures

Although myofibrils are the dominant ultrastructural feature of skeletal muscle, the fibres contain other organelles essential for cellular function, such as ribosomes, Golgi apparatus and mitochondria. Most of them are located around the nuclei, between the myofibrils and the sarcolemma and, to a lesser extent, between the myofibrils. Mitochondria, lipid droplets and glycogen provide the metabolic support needed by active muscle. The mitochondria are elongated, and their cristae are closely packed. Their profiles are usually seen in longitudinal orientation between the myofibrils (see Fig. 23.6A). The number of mitochondria in an adult muscle fibre is not fixed, but it can increase or decrease quite readily in response to sustained changes in activity. Spherical lipid droplets, approximately 0.25 μm in diameter, are distributed uniformly throughout the sarcoplasm between myofibrils. They represent a rich source of energy that can be tapped only by oxidative metabolic pathways; they are therefore more common in fibres that have a high mitochondrial content and good capillary blood supply. Glycogen is distributed in small clusters of granules between myofibrils and among the thin filaments. With brief bursts of activity, it provides an important source of anaerobic energy that is not dependent on nutrient blood flow to the muscle fibre.

At the ends of the muscle fibre, where force is transmitted to adjacent connective tissue structures, the sarcolemma is folded into numerous finger-like projections that strengthen the junctional region by increasing the area of attachment. Tubular invaginations of the sarcolemma penetrate between the myofibrils in a transverse plane at the limit of each A-band (Fig. 23.10). The lumina of these transverse tubules (T-tubules) are thus in continuity with the extracellular space. T-tubules play an important role in excitation–contraction coupling.

The sarcoplasmic reticulum is a specialized form of smooth endoplasmic reticulum. It consists of a plexus of anastomosing membrane cisternae that fill much of the space between myofibrils and expand into larger sacs, the junctional sarcoplasmic reticulum or terminal cisternae, where they come into close contact with T-tubules. At this point, they form part of a structure called a triad, consisting of a central T-tubule flanked on either side by two terminal cisternae, the latter filled with dense, granular material (see Fig. 23.6B). The membranes of the sarcoplasmic reticulum contain calcium–ATPase pumps

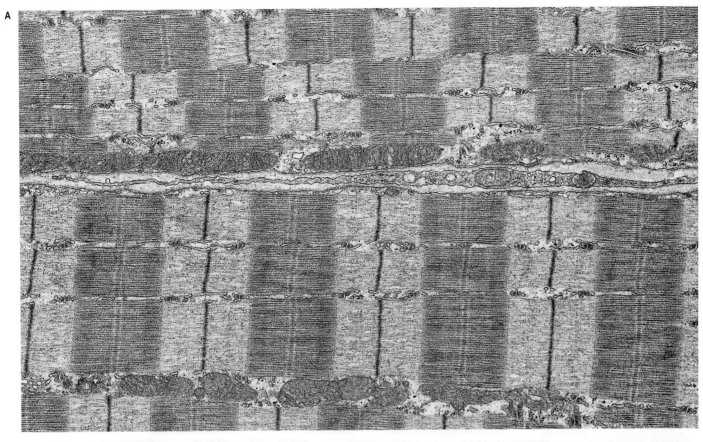

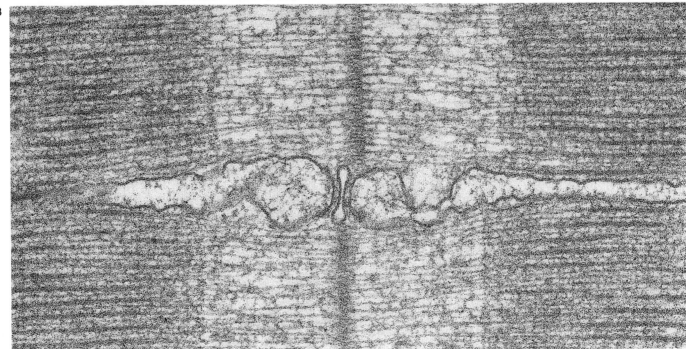

Fig. 23.6 *A, Low-power electron micrograph of parts of two skeletal muscle fibres in longitudinal section. B, High-power electron micrograph of frog skeletal muscle in longitudinal section, showing a triad, thick and thin filaments and cross-bridges in the spaces between them. Note the overlap of thin filaments within the Z-disc at the top of the micrograph. (The human triad lies at the junction between the A-bands and I-bands, not at the Z-disc as shown here.) (Photographs by Brenda Russell, Department of Physiology and Biophysics, University of Illinois at Chicago.)*

that transport calcium ions into the terminal cisternae, where the ions are bound to calsequestrin, a protein with a high affinity for calcium, in dense storage granules. In this way, calcium can be accumulated and retained in the terminal cisternae at a much higher concentration than anywhere else in the sarcoplasm. Ca^{2+} release channels (made of ryanodine receptor molecules) are concentrated mainly in the terminal cisternae. They form half of the junctional 'feet' or 'pillars' that bridge the sarcoplasmic reticulum and T-tubules at the triads, forming a critical communication point between them. The other half of the junctional feet is the T-tubule receptor, which constitutes the voltage sensor.

Connective Tissues

The endomysium is a delicate network of connective tissue that surrounds muscle fibres and forms their immediate external environment. It is the site of metabolic exchange between muscle and blood and contains capillaries and bundles of small nerve fibres. Ion fluxes associated with the electrical excitation of muscle fibres take place through its proteoglycan matrix. The endomysium is continuous with more substantial septa of connective tissue that constitute the perimysium. The latter ensheathes groups of muscle fibres to form parallel bundles or fasciculi, carries larger blood vessels and nerves and accommodates neuromuscular spindles. Perimysial septa are themselves

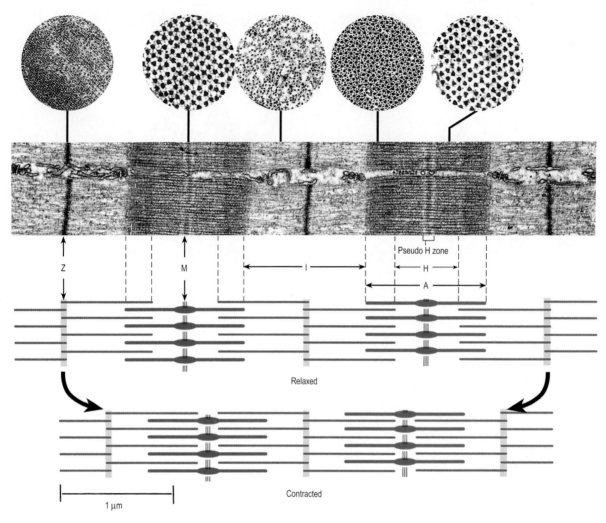

Z

M

Pseudo H zone

H

A

I

Relaxed

1 μm

Contracted

Fig. 23.7 *Sarcomeric structures. The drawings below the electron micrograph (of two myofibrils sectioned longitudinally) indicate the corresponding arrangements of thick and thin filaments. Relaxed and contracted states are shown to illustrate the changes that occur during shortening. Insets at the top show the electron micrographic appearance of transverse sections through the sarcomere at the levels shown. Note that the packing geometry of the thin filaments changes from a square array at the Z-disc to a hexagonal array where they interdigitate with thick filaments in the A-band. (Photographs by Brenda Russell, Department of Physiology and Biophysics, University of Illinois at Chicago; artwork by Lesley Skeates.)*

the inward extensions of a collagenous sheath, the epimysium, which forms part of the fascia that invests whole muscle groups.

Epimysium consists mainly of type I collagen, perimysium contains type I and type III collagen and endomysium contains type III and type IV collagen. Type IV collagen is particularly associated with the basal lamina that invests each muscle fibre.

The epimysial, perimysial and endomysial sheaths coalesce where the muscles connect to adjacent structures at tendons, aponeuroses and fasciae; this gives the attachments great strength, because the tensile forces are distributed in the forms of shear stresses, which are more easily resisted. This principle is also seen at the ends of the muscle fibres, which divide into finger-like processes separated by collagen fibres. Although there are no desmosomal attachments at these myotendinous junctions, there are other specializations that assist in the transmission of force from the interior of the fibre to the extracellular matrix. Actin filaments from the adjacent sarcomeres, which would normally insert into a Z-disc at this point, penetrate instead into a dense, subsarcolemmal filamentous matrix that provides attachment to the plasma membrane. This matrix is similar in character to the cytoplasmic face of an adherens junction. The structure as a whole is homologous to the intercalated discs of cardiac muscle. Beyond the surface of the sarcolemma, fine junctional microfibrils, 5 to 10 nm thick and of unknown composition, bridge across the lamina lucida to the prominent lamina densa of the junctional basal lamina. This, in turn, adheres closely to collagen and reticular fibres (type III collagen) of the adjacent tendon or other connective tissue structure.

Attachments

The forces developed by skeletal muscles are transferred to bones by connective tissue structures: tendons, aponeuroses and fasciae. The microstructure of tendons is considered here.

Tendons — Tendons take the forms of cords or straps that are round or oval in cross-section and consist of dense, regular connective tissue (Fig. 23.11). They contain fascicles of type I collagen that are oriented mainly parallel to the long axis but are, to some extent, interwoven. The fasciculi may be conspicuous enough to give tendons a longitudinally striated appearance to the unaided eye. Tendons generally have smooth surfaces, although large tendons may be ridged longitudinally by coarse fasciculi (e.g. the osseous aspect of the angulated tendon of obturator internus). Loose connective tissue between fascicles provides a pathway for small vessels and nerves and condenses on the surface as a sheath or epitendineum, which may contain elastic and irregularly arranged collagen fibres. The loose attachments between this sheath and the surrounding tissue present little resistance to movement of the tendon, but where greater freedom of movement is required, a tendon is separated from adjacent structures by a synovial sheath.

Tendons are strongly attached to bones, both at the periosteum and through fasciculi (extrinsic collagen fibres), which continue deep into the bone cortex. Sections of fresh bone show that at sites of tendinous attachment there is often a smooth plate of white fibrocartilage, which may cushion and reinforce the attachment zone. Tendons are slightly elastic and may be stretched by up to 6% of their length without damage. Recovery of the elastic energy stored in tendons can make movement more economical. Although they resist extension, tendons are flexible. They can therefore be diverted around osseous surfaces or deflected under retinacula to redirect the angle of pull.

Because tendons are composed of collagen and their vascular supply is sparse, they appear white. However, the blood supply to tendons is not unimportant; small arterioles from adjacent muscle tissue pass longitudinally between the fascicles, branching and anastomosing freely, and are accompanied by venae commitantes and lymphatic vessels. This longitudinal plexus is

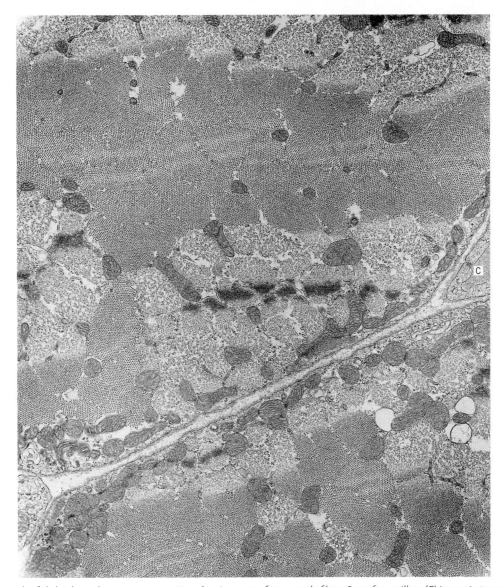

Fig. 23.8 *Electron micrograph of skeletal muscle in transverse section, showing parts of two muscle fibres. Part of a capillary (C) is seen in transverse section in the endomysial space* (right). *The variation in the appearance of myofibrils in cross-section is explained in Figure 23-7. (Photograph by Brenda Russell, Department of Physiology and Biophysics, University of Illinois at Chicago.)*

augmented by small vessels from adjacent loose connective tissue or synovial sheaths. Vessels rarely pass between bone and tendon at osseous attachments, and the junctional surfaces are usually devoid of foramina. A notable exception is the calcaneal (Achilles) tendon, which receives a blood supply across the osseotendinous junction. During postnatal development, tendons enlarge by interstitial growth, particularly at myotendinous junctions, where there are high concentrations of fibroblasts. Growth decreases along the tendon from the muscle to the osseous attachments. The thickness finally attained by a tendon depends on the size and strength of the associated muscle, but it also appears to be influenced by other factors, such as the degree of pennation of the muscle. The metabolic rate of tendons is very low but increases during infection or injury. Repair involves the initial proliferation of fibroblasts, followed by interstitial deposition of new fibres.

The nerve supply to tendons is largely sensory, and there is no evidence of any capacity for vasomotor control. Specialized endings that are sensitive to force (Golgi tendon organs) are found near myotendinous junctions; their large myelinated afferent axons run centrally within branches of muscular nerves or in small rami of adjacent peripheral nerves.

Innervation

Every skeletal muscle is supplied by one or more nerves. In the limbs, face and neck there is usually a single nerve, although its axons may be derived from neurones in several spinal cord segments. Muscles such as those of the abdominal wall, which originate from several embryonic segments, are supplied by more than one nerve. In most cases, the nerve travels with the principal blood vessels within a neurovascular bundle, approaches the muscle near its least mobile attachment and enters the deep surface at a position that is more or less constant for each muscle.

Nerves supplying muscle are frequently referred to as 'motor nerves,' but they contain both motor and sensory components. The motor component is composed mainly of large, myelinated α-efferent axons that supply the muscle fibres, supplemented by small, thinly myelinated γ-efferents, or fusimotor fibres, that innervate the intrafusal muscle fibres of neuromuscular spindles and fine, non-myelinated autonomic efferents (C fibres) that innervate vascular smooth muscle. The sensory component consists of large, myelinated IA and smaller group II afferents from the neuromuscular spindles, large myelinated IB afferents from the Golgi tendon organs and fine myelinated and non-myelinated axons that convey pain and other sensations from free terminals in the connective tissue sheaths of the muscle.

Within muscles, nerves follow the connective tissue sheaths, coursing in the epimysial and perimysial septa before entering the fine endomysial tissue around the muscle fibres. The α motor axons branch repeatedly before they lose their myelinated sheaths and terminate near the middle of muscle fibres. These terminals tend to cluster in a narrow zone toward the centre of the muscle belly known as the motor point. Clinically, this is the place on the muscle where it is easiest to elicit a contraction with stimulating electrodes. Long muscles generally have two or more terminals, or end-plate bands, because many muscle fibres do not run the full length of the anatomical muscle.

A specialized synapse, the neuromuscular junction (Ch. 22), is formed where the terminal branch of an α motor axon contacts the muscle fibre. The axon terminal gives off several short, tortuous branches, each ending in an elliptical area, the motor end-plate. Within the underlying discoidal patch of sarcolemma—the sole plate or subneural apparatus—the sarcolemma is thrown into deep synaptic folds. This discrete type of neuromuscular junction is an example of an *en plaque* ending and is found on muscle

CASE 1   DUCHENNE'S MUSCULAR DYSTROPHY

A 4-year-old boy presents with difficulty rising from the floor. His parents report that he has always walked on his toes and has had trouble climbing stairs and running, but now he must get on all fours, push himself into a squat and then push off his legs with his hands to stand (Gowers' sign).

On examination, he has large, firm calves (Fig. 23.9). His gait is waddling, with a broad base and marked lumbar lordosis. He has proximal lower extremity weakness, significant neck flexor weakness and Gowers' sign when rising from the floor. The remainder of the examination is normal.

Discussion: Duchenne's muscular dystrophy is an X-linked recessive disorder caused by a mutation in the gene located on the short arm of the X chromosome (Xp21) that produces dystrophin. Mutation results in the absence of this protein in skeletal muscle fibres (as well as in heart, brain and smooth muscle). The dystrophin gene is very large, and multiple gene mutations can result in the defect. Some mutations result in incomplete loss of dystrophin and milder clinical disease (i.e. Becker's muscular dystrophy). Within muscle, dystrophin is found in the periphery of the fibres, close to the cytoplasmic face of the sarcolemma. It is part of a large complex of gly-coproteins that spans the muscle membrane, binding intracellular actin with merosin in the muscle basal lamina, thus stabilizing the sarcolemmal membrane and allowing the transmission of forces of contraction and relaxation from internally to the extracellular matrix. The exact function of dystrophin is not fully understood, but it most likely acts as a stabilizer in skeletal muscle. Without dystrophin, the muscle membrane may be more susceptible to disruption, with destruction of muscle fibres and increasing fibrosis.

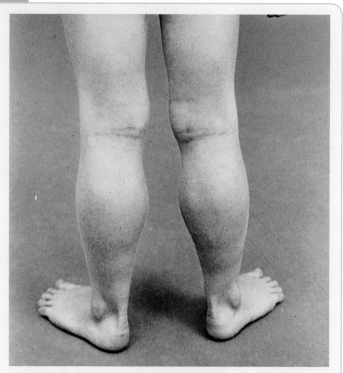

Fig. 23.9 *Duchenne's muscular dystrophy. Although the muscles of both calves are enlarged, they are weak (pseudohypertrophy rather than true muscular hypertrophy with enhanced strength).*

CASE 2   MYOTONIC DYSTROPHY

A 34-year-old man is referred for shortness of breath with exercise. Past medical history is significant for bilateral cataract removal at age 31, diabetes mellitus of 2 years' duration, recurrent pneumonia and testicular atrophy. His father and paternal uncle both experienced sudden cardiac death in their 50s; although neither had significant muscle weakness, his father had cataracts removed in his 30s. The patient's younger sister has had recurrent respiratory problems.

Examination demonstrates facial weakness (diplegia), with mild bilateral eyelid ptosis and marked frontal balding. He has bilateral distal upper extremity weakness and both proximal and distal lower extremity weakness. Delayed relaxation of grip is striking (myotonia), and percussion of the thenar eminence documents delayed relaxation. Testicles are reduced in size. Creatine kinase is mildly elevated.

Discussion: This man has typical myotonic dystrophy, an autosomal dominant disorder with variable expression. There are two types of myotonic dystrophy: DM1 and DM2. DM1 usually appears earlier, with more severe weakness. Many patients do not present until early adulthood, but when the mother has the disease, infants may exhibit hypotonia and poor feeding at birth. Anticipation is seen in DM1 from one generation to the next. Pathophysiologically, the disease is due to expansion of a trinucleotide (CTG trinucleotide repeat). The myotonic phenomenon exhibited on both physical examination and electrophysiological testing is due to repetitive spontaneous and contraction-induced muscle fibre activation. The diseased muscle fibre has increased expression of calcium-activated potassium channels, but it is not clear how this results in the repetitive muscle fibre activation to which the rubric 'myotonia' is applied. Chloride conductance may also be affected. Muscle biopsy shows a mixture of findings, including muscle fibre atrophy and hypertrophy, some necrotic fibres, fibrosis and adipose deposition, with rare eosinophilic cytoplasmic inclusions. Ring and split fibres can also be seen. Ringbinden (aberrant muscle fibres encircling normally oriented fibres) may be found.

It is noteworthy that whereas muscular involvement is proximal in the great majority of muscular dystrophies, in myotonic dystrophy a distal distribution is characteristic.

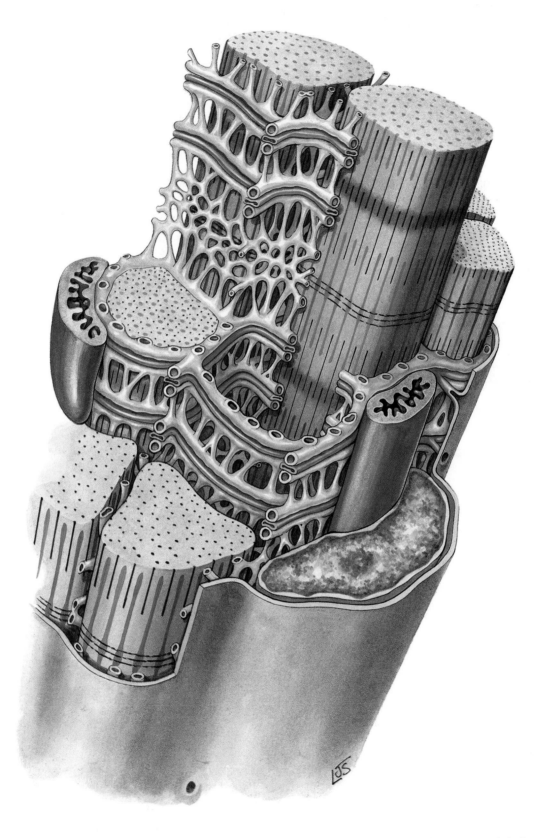

Fig. 23.10 *Three-dimensional reconstruction of a mammalian skeletal muscle fibre, showing in particular the organization of the transverse tubules (orange) and sarcoplasmic reticulum (buff). Mitochondria (blue) lie between the myofibrils and a muscle nucleus (green) at the periphery. Note that T-tubules are found at the level of the A–I junctions, where they form triads with the terminal cisternae of the sarcoplasmic reticulum. (Artwork by Lesley Skeates.)*

fibres that are capable of propagating action potentials. A different type of ending is found on slow tonic muscle fibres that do not have this capability (e.g. the extrinsic ocular muscles), where these fibres form a minor component of the muscle. In this case, the propagation of excitation is taken over by the nerve terminals, which branch over an extended distance to form a number of small neuromuscular junctions (*en grappe* endings). Some muscle fibres of this type receive the terminal branches of more than one motor neurone. The terminals of the γ-efferents that innervate

the intrafusal muscle fibres of the neuromuscular spindle also take a variety of forms.

The terminal branches of α motor axons are normally in a 'one-to-one' relationship with their muscle fibres: a muscle fibre receives only one branch, and any one branch innervates only one muscle fibre. When a motor neurone is excited, an action potential is propagated along the axon and all its branches to all the muscle fibres it supplies. The motor neurone and the muscle fibres it innervates can therefore be regarded as a functional unit, the motor unit, which accounts for the more or less simultaneous contraction of a number of fibres within the muscle.

The size of a motor unit varies considerably. In muscles employed for precision tasks (e.g. extraocular muscles, interossei and intrinsic laryngeal muscles), each motor neurone innervates only about 10 muscle fibres, whereas in a large limb muscle, a motor neurone may innervate several hundred muscle fibres. Within a muscle, the fibres belonging to one motor unit are distributed over a wide territory, without regard to fascicular boundaries, and they intermingle with the fibres of other motor units. The motor units become larger in cases of nerve damage, because denervated fibres induce collateral or terminal sprouting of the remaining axons. Each new branch can reinnervate a fibre, thus increasing the territory of its parent motor neurone.

Muscle Contraction: Basic Physiology

The arrival of an action potential at the motor end-plate causes acetylcholine (ACh) to be released from storage vesicles into the 30- to 50-nm synaptic

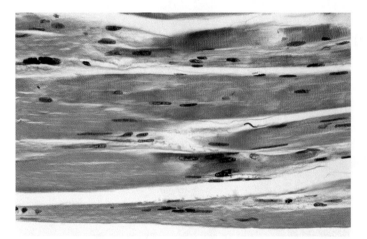

Fig. 23.11 *Attachment of a tendon (orange) to skeletal muscle (pink). The regular dense connective tissue of the tendon consists of parallel bundles of type I collagen fibres that are oriented in the long axis of the tendon and the muscle to which it is attached. A few elongated fibroblast nuclei are visible. (Photograph by Sarah-Jane Smith.)*

cleft that separates the nerve ending from the sarcolemma. ACh is rapidly bound by receptor molecules located in the junctional folds, triggering an almost instantaneous increase in the permeability, and hence conductance, of the postsynaptic membrane. This generates a local depolarization (the end-plate potential), which initiates an action potential in the surrounding area of sarcolemma. The activity of the neurotransmitter is rapidly terminated by the enzyme acetylcholinesterase (AChE), which is bound to the basal lamina in the sarcolemmal junctional folds. The sarcolemma is an excitable membrane, and action potentials generated at the neuromuscular junction propagate rapidly over the entire surface of the muscle fibre.

The action potentials are conducted radially into the interior of the fibre via the T-tubules, which are extensions of the sarcolemma; this ensures that all parts of the muscle fibre are activated rapidly and almost synchronously. Excitation–contraction coupling is the process whereby an action potential triggers the release of calcium from the terminal cisternae of the sarcoplasmic reticulum into the cytosol. This activates a calcium-sensitive switch in the thin filaments and thus initiates contraction. At the end of excitation, the T-tubular membrane repolarizes, calcium release ceases, calcium ions are actively transported back to the calsequestrin stores by the calcium–ATPase pumps and the muscle relaxes.

Electron microscopy shows that the length of the thick and thin filaments does not change during muscle contraction. The sarcomere shortens by means of the thick and thin filaments sliding past each other, which draws the Z-discs toward the middle of each sarcomere (see Fig. 23.7). As the overlap increases, the I-bands and H zones narrow to extinction, while the width of the A-bands remains constant. Filament sliding depends on the making and breaking of bonds (cross-bridge cycling) between myosin head regions and actin filaments. Myosin heads 'walk' along actin filaments (sliding the filaments past each other) using a series of short power strokes, each resulting in a relative movement of 5 to 10 nm. Actin filament binding sites for myosin are revealed only in the presence of calcium, which is released into the sarcoplasm from the sarcoplasmic reticulum, with the consequent repositioning of the troponin–tropomyosin complex on actin (the calcium-sensitive switch). Both myosin head binding and release are energy dependent (adenosine triphosphate (ATP) binding is required for detachment of bound myosin heads as part of the normal cycle). In the absence of ATP (as occurs postmortem), the bound state is maintained and is responsible for the muscle stiffness known as rigor mortis.

The summation of myosin power strokes leads to an average sarcomere shortening of up to 1 μm. Because each muscle has thousands of sarcomeres in series along its length, the anatomical muscle shortens by a centimetre or more, depending on the muscle.

	Fibres Types		
Characteristics	**TYPE I**	**TYPE IIA**	**TYPE IIB**
Physiological			
Function	Sustained forces, as in posture	Powerful, fast movements	
Motor neurone firing threshold	Low	Intermediate	High
Motor unit size	Small	Large	Large
Firing pattern	Tonic, low-frequency	Phasic, high-frequency	
Maximum shortening velocity	Slow	Fast	Fast
Rate of relaxation	Slow	Fast	Fast
Resistance to fatigue	Fatigue resistant	Fatigue resistant	Fatigue susceptible
Power output	Low	Intermediate	High
Structural			
Capillary density	High		Low
Mitochondrial volume	High	Intermediate*	Low
Z-band	Broad	Narrow	Narrow
T and SR systems	Sparse		Extensive
Biochemical			
Myosin ATPase activity	Low		High
Oxidative metabolism	High	Intermediate*	Low
Anaerobic glycolysis	Low	Intermediate*	High
Calcium transport ATPase	Low		High

Table 23-2 *Physiological, structural and biochemical characteristics of the major histochemical fibre types*

*Metabolic characteristics vary among species and may show considerable overlap between fibre types. (See text for further details.)

Slow Twitch versus Fast Twitch

The passage of a single action potential through a motor unit elicits a twitch contraction whereby peak force is reached within 25 to 100 msec, depending on the motor unit type involved. However, the motor neurone can deliver a second nervous impulse in less time than it takes for the muscle fibres to relax. When this happens, the muscle fibres contract again, building the tension to a higher level. Because of this mechanical summation, a sequence of impulses can evoke a larger force than a single impulse; within certain limits, the higher the impulse frequency, the more force is produced ('rate recruitment'). The other strategy is to recruit more motor units. In practice, the two mechanisms appear to operate in parallel, but their relative importance may depend on the size or function of the muscle; in large muscles with many motor units, motor unit recruitment is probably the more important mechanism.

With the exception of rare tonic fibres, skeletal muscles are composed entirely of fibres of the twitch type. These fibres can all conduct action potentials, but they are not the same in other respects. Some fibres obtain their energy very efficiently by aerobic oxidation of substrates, particularly fats and fatty acids. They have large numbers of mitochondria and contain myoglobin, an oxygen-transport pigment related to haemoglobin. They are supported by a well-developed network of capillaries, which maintains a steady nutrient supply of oxygen and substrates. Such fibres are well suited to functions such as postural maintenance, in which moderate forces must be sustained for prolonged periods. At the other extreme are fibres that have few mitochondria, little myoglobin and a sparse capillary network. Their immediate energy requirements are met largely through anaerobic glycolysis, a route that provides prompt access to energy stores but is less sustainable than oxidative metabolism. Such fibres are capable of brief bursts of intense activity, but these must be separated by extended quiescent periods during which intracellular pH and phosphate concentrations, perturbed in fatigue, are restored to normal values, and glycogen and other reserves are replenished.

These types of fibres tend to be segregated into different muscles in some animals; thus, some muscles have a conspicuously red appearance, derived from the rich blood supply and high myoglobin content associated with a predominantly aerobic metabolism, whereas others have a much paler appearance, reflecting a more anaerobic character. These variations in colour led to the early classification of red and white muscles.

In humans, all muscles are, in fact, mixed, with fibres specialized for aerobic working conditions intermingled with fibres of a more anaerobic or intermediate metabolic character. The different types of fibres are not readily distinguished in routine histological preparations but are clear when specialized enzyme histochemical techniques are used. On the basis of metabolic differences, the individual fibres can be classified as predominantly oxidative, slow twitch (red) fibres or glycolytic, fast twitch (white) fibres. Muscles composed mainly of oxidative, slow twitch fibres thus correspond to the red muscles of classic descriptions. This classification has now been largely superseded by myosin-based typing and the presence of specific disease-related enzymes (see later).

Muscles that are predominantly oxidative in their metabolism contract and relax more slowly than muscles that rely on glycolytic metabolism. This difference in contractile speed is due in part to the activation mechanism (volume density of sarcotubular system and proteins of the calcium 'switch' mechanism) and in part to molecular differences between the myosin heavy chains of these types of muscle, which affect the ATPase activity of the myosin head; this in turn alters the kinetics of its interaction with actin and hence the rate of cross-bridge cycling. Differences between myosin isoforms may be detected histochemically; ATPase histochemistry continues to play a significant role in diagnostic typing (Table 23.2). Two main categories have been described: type I fibres, which are slow contracting, and type II fibres, which are fast contracting. Molecular analyses have revealed that type II fibres can be subdivided according to their content of myosin heavy-chain isoforms into types IIA, IIB and IIX (Schiaffino and Reggiani 1996). There is a correlation between categories and metabolism and therefore with fatigue resistance: type I fibres are generally oxidative (slow oxidative) and resistant to fatigue; type IIA are moderately oxidative, glycolytic (fast oxidative glycolytic) and fatigue resistant; and type IIB largely rely on glycolytic metabolism (fast glycolytic) and so are easily fatigued. Fibre type grouping (Fig. 23.12) occurs when there are repeated cycles of denervation and reinnervation and is seen in a variety of conditions, including disuse atrophy, ageing, demyelination neuropathies and some forms of muscular dystrophy.

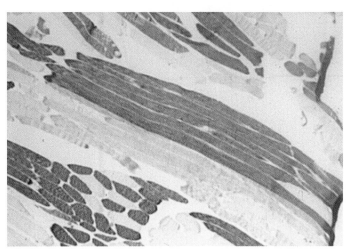

Fig. 23.12 *ATPase stain of skeletal muscle demonstrating fibre type grouping. Muscle fibers are clustered into large groups by type: type I (dark) and type II (light). (Courtesy of Mark Curtis, MD, Jefferson Medical College, Philadelphia, PA.)*

CASE 3 INCLUSION BODY MYOSITIS

A 62-year-old man has a 2-year history of progressive weakness of his hands and fingers, hindering his ability to perform some activities of daily living. In the last 8 months, he has experienced frequent falls due to leg weakness. Increased difficulty swallowing has led to a 10-pound weight loss.

On examination, there is decreased strength in the finger and wrist flexors, worse on the right, and bilateral quadriceps weakness. Neck flexors are weak. Creatine kinase is slightly elevated.

Discussion: Inclusion body myositis is the most common acquired inflammatory myopathy. The predominantly distal pattern of weakness helps distinguish this disease from other inflammatory myopathies that involve primarily proximal muscles. Muscle biopsy in such cases shows endomysial mononuclear cell inflammation; scattered muscle fibre degeneration and regeneration, with characteristic rimmed vacuoles (Fig. 23.13); clustering of small fibres; and both intranuclear and intracytoplasmic inclusions that stain for amyloid.

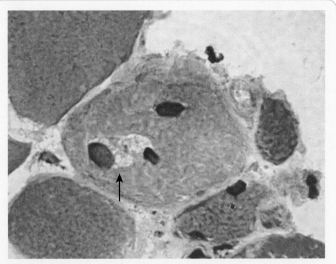

Fig. 23.13 *Photomicrograph of rimmed vacuoles (arrow). Rimmed vacuoles are a typical finding in inclusion body myositis but may be seen in other pathological conditions, including polymyositis, congenital myopathies and some limb girdle muscular dystrophies. (Courtesy of Mark Curtis, MD, Jefferson Medical College, Philadelphia, PA.)*

References

Bishopric, N.H., Gahlmann, R., Wade, R., Kedes, L., 1991. Gene expression during skeletal and cardiac muscle development. In: Fozzard, H.A., Haber, E., Jennings, R.B., Katz, A.M., Morgan, H.E. (Eds.), The Heart and Cardiovascular System, second ed. Raven Press, New York, pp. 1587–1598.

Brand-Saberi, B., Christ, B., 2000. Evolution and development of distinct cell lineages derived from somites: Current Topics in Developmental Biology, Vol. 48. Academic Press, New York.

Buckingham, M., Bajard, L., Chang, T., et al., 2003. The formation of skeletal muscle: from somite to limb. J. Anat. 202, 59–68.

Buller, A.J., Eccles, J.C., Eccles, R.M., 1960. Interactions between motoneurones and muscles in respect of the characteristic speeds of their responses. J. Physiol. 150, 417–439.

Edgerton, V.R., Roy, R.R., Allen, D.L., Monti, R.J., 2002. Adaptations in skeletal muscle disuse or decreased-use atrophy. Am. J. Phys. Med. Rehabil. 81 (11 Suppl.), S127–S147.

Goldring, K., Partridge, T., Watt, D., 2002. Muscle stem cells. J. Pathol. 197, 457–467. *Reviews the role of the satellite cell in growth and repair of muscle fibres.*

King Engel, W., Askanas, V., 2006. Inclusion-body myositis: clinical, diagnostic and pathologic aspects. Neurology Suppl. 1 (66),S20–S29.

Ko, C.P., Thompson, W.J. (Guest Eds.), 2003. The Neuromuscular Junction. J. Neurocytol. 32, 421–1037.

Lieber, R.L., Friden, J., 2000. Functional and clinical significance of skeletal muscle architecture. Muscle Nerve. 23, 1647–1666.

Maltin, C.A., Delday, M.I., Sinclair, K.D., Steven, J., Sneddon, A.A., 2001. Impact of manipulations of myogenesis in utero on the performance of adult skeletal muscle. Reproduction 122, 359–374.

Mathes, S.J., Nahai, F., 1981. Classification of the vascular anatomy of muscles: experimental and clinical correlation. Plast. Reconstr. Surg. 67, 177–187.

Mizuno, H., Zuk, P.A., Zhu, M., Lorenz, H.P., Benhaim, P., Hedrick, M.H., 2002. Myogenic differentiation by human processed lipoaspirate cells. Plast. Reconstr. Surg. 109, 199–209.

Muntoni, F., Brown, S., Sewry, C., Patel, K., 2002. Muscle development genes: their relevance in neuromuscular disorders. Neuromuscul. Disord. 12, 438–446.

Salmons, S., 1967. An implantable muscle stimulator. J. Physiol. 188, 13P–14P.

Schiaffino, S., Reggiani, C., 1996. Molecular diversity of myofibrillar proteins: gene regulation and functional significance. Physiol. Rev. 76, 371–423.

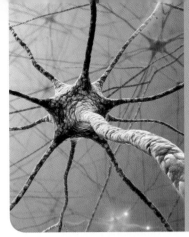

Index